Proceedings in Life Sciences

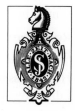

IUBS Section of Comparative Physiology and Biochemistry
1st International Congress, Liège, Belgium, August 27–31, 1984

Conference Organization

Organizing Board
R. Gilles, Chairman, Liège, Belgium
M. Gilles-Baillien and L. Bolis, Liège, Belgium/Messina, Italy

Host Society
European Society for Comparative Physiology
and Biochemistry.

Under the Patronage of
The European Economic Community
The Fonds National de la Recherche Scientifique
The Ministère de l'Education Nationale
et de la Culture Française
The Fondation Léon Fredericq
The University of Liège

The European Society for Comparative Physiology
and Biochemistry
The American Society of Zoologists
The Canadian Society of Zoologists
The Japanese Society for General and Comparative Physiology.

The Congress has been organized in relation with the 100th
Anniversary of the School of Comparative Physiology and
Biochemistry of the University of Liege.

The proceedings of the invited lectures to the different symposia
of the congress have been gathered in five different volumes
published by Springer-Verlag under the following titles:

Circulation, Respiration, and Metabolism
Current Comparative Approaches. Edited by R. Gilles

Transport Processes, Iono- and Osmoregulation
Current Comparative Approaches
Edited by R. Gilles and M. Gilles-Baillien

Neurobiology, Current Comparative Approaches
Edited by R. Gilles and J. Balthazart

Respiratory Pigments in Animals: Relation Structure-Function
Edited by J. Lamy, J.P. Truchot and R. Gilles

High Pressure Effects on Selected Biological Systems
Edited by A. Pequeux and R. Gilles

Neurobiology
Current Comparative Approaches

Edited by
R. Gilles and J. Balthazart

With 162 Figures

Springer-Verlag
Berlin Heidelberg New York Tokyo

Professor Dr. RAYMOND GILLES (Coordinating Editor)
Laboratory of Animal Physiology
University of Liège, 22, Quai Van Beneden
B-4020 Liège, Belgium

Dr. JACQUES BALTHAZART, (Scientific Editor)
Laboratory of Biochemistry
University of Liège, 17, Place Delcour
B-4020 Liège, Belgium

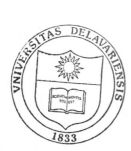

ISBN 3-540-15480-9 Springer-Verlag Berlin Heidelberg New York Tokyo
ISBN 0-387-15480-9 Springer-Verlag New York Heidelberg Berlin Tokyo

Library of Congress Cataloging in Publication Data. International Congress of Comparative Physiology and Biochemistry (1st: 1984: Liège, Belgium) Neurobiology: current comparative approaches. (Proceedings in life sciences) "Proceedings of the invited lectures to the First International Congress of Comparative Physiology and Biochemistry organized at Liège, Belgium, in August 1984 under the auspices of the Section of Comparative Physiology and Biochemistry of the International Union of Biological Sciences" – Foreword. Bibliography: p. Includes index. 1. Psychoneuroendocrinology – Congresses. 2. Neurobiology – Congresses. 3. Physiology, Comparative – Congresses. I. Gilles, R. II. Balthazart, J. (Jacques), 1949–. III. Title. IV. Series. QP356.45.I57 1984   591.1'88   85-12654

Typesetting, offsetprinting and bookbinding: Brühlsche Universitätsdruckerei, Giessen
2131/3130-543210

Foreword

This volume is one of those published from the proceedings of the invited lectures to the First International Congress of Comparative Physiology and Biochemistry I organized at Liège (Belgium) in August 1984 under the auspices of the Section of Comparative Physiology and Biochemistry of the International Union of Biological Sciences. In a general foreword to these different volumes, it seems to me appropriate to consider briefly what may be the comparative approach.

Living organisms, beyond the diversity of their morphological forms, have evolved a widespread range of basic solutions to cope with the different problems, both organismal and environmental with which they are faced. Soon after the turn of the century, some biologists realized that these solutions can be best comprehended in the framework of a comparative approach integrating results of physiological and biochemical studies done at the organismic, cellular and molecular levels. The development of this approach amongst both physiologists and biochemists remained, however, extremely slow until recently. Physiology and biochemistry have indeed long been mainly devoted to the service of medicine, finding scope enough for their activities in the study of a few species, particularly mammals. This has tended to keep many physiologists and biochemists from the comparative approach, which demands either the widest possible survey of animals forms or an integrated knowledge of the specific adaptive features of the species considered. These particular characteristics of the comparative approach have, on the other hand, been very attractive for biologists interested in the mechanisms of evolution and environmental adaptations. This diversity of requirements of the comparative approach, at the conceptual as well as at the technological level, can easily account for the fact that it emerged only slowly amongst the other new, more rapidly growing, disciplines of the biological sciences. Although a few pioneers have been working in the field since the beginning of the century, it only started effectively in the early 1960's. 1960 was the date of the organization of the periodical *Comparative Physiology and Biochemistry* by Kerkut and Scheer and of the publication of the first volumes of the comprehensive treatise *Comparative Biochemistry* edited by Florkin and Mason. These publications can be considered as milestones in the evolution of the comparative approach. They have been followed by many others which have greatly contributed to giving the field the international status it deserved. Since the 1960's, the comparative approach has been maturing and developing more and more rapidly into the independent discipline it now is, widely recognized by the international communities of physiologists, biochemists, and biologists. It is currently used as an effective tool of great help in the understanding of many research problems: biological as well as clinical, applied as well as fundamental.

The actual development of the field and the interest it arouses in a growing portion of the biological scientific community led some of us to consider the organization of an international structure, bringing together the major representative societies and groups around the world, which would aim at the general advancement and promotion of the comparative approach. This was done in 1979 with the incorporation, within the international Union of Biological Sciences, of a Section of Comparative Physiology and Biochemistry. The first International Congress of CPB I organized in Liège with the help of a few friends and colleagues, is the first activity of this newly founded Section. In 22 symposia it gathered some 146 invited lectures given by internationally renowned scientists on all major current topics and trends in the field. The proceedings of these lectures have been collected in 5 volumes produced by Springer-Verlag, a publisher long associated with the development of CPB. The organization of the CPB Section of IUBS, its first Congress and these proceedings volumes can well be considered as milestones reflecting the international status and the maturity that the comparative approach has gained, as a recognized independent discipline, in the beginning of the 1980's, some 20 years after it was effectively launched.

Finally, I would like to consider that the selection of Liège for this first International Congress has not been simply coincidental. I thus feel that this brief foreword would not be complete without noting the privileged role Liège has played in some events associated with the development of the comparative approach. Liège had a pioneer in comparative physiology already at the end of the last century with Léon Fredericq. With Marcel Florkin, Liège had its first Professor of biochemistry and one of the founding fathers of comparative biochemistry. These two major figureheads of the comparative approach founded and developed what is actually called the Liège School of Comparative Physiology and Biochemistry, which was, at the time of the Congress, celebrating its 100th anniversary. This school provided early support to the European Society for Comparative Physiology and Biochemistry organized by Marcel Florkin and myself some years ago. The society, still headquartered in Liège, was, with the CPB division of the American Society of Zoologists, at the origin of the formation of the CPB Section of IUBS under the auspices of which this first International Congress, specifically devoted to the comparative approach has been organized. An essential particularly of the Liège school of CPB is that its two founding fathers, scientists interested in general, basic aspects of the organization of living organisms, were also professors at the faculty of medicine. This largely contributed in Liège to avoiding the undesirable structuration of a so-called "zoophysiology" or "zoobiochemistry" independent of the rest of the field. The conditions were thus realized very early in Liège for CPB to play its key role in canalizing the necessary interactions between the general, pre-clinical or clinical and the environmental, ecological or evolutionary tendences of physiology and biochemistry. The possibility of stimulating such interactions has served as a major guide line in the selection of the symposia and invited lectures from which these proceedings have issued.

Liège, Belgium, June 1985   R. GILLES

Preface

Comparative neurobiology is a rapidly growing field in the biological sciences. The discipline has taken advantage of major advances and refinements in a number of techniques including biochemistry, endocrinology, electrophysiology, neuroanatomy, and immunocytochemistry, and is now able to ask and answer questions which would have been considered science-fiction only a few years ago. This has certainly justified the inclusion of five symposia on comparative neurobiology within the first International Congress of Comparative Physiology and Biochemistry which was held in Liège in August 1984. This volume presents the proceedings of these symposia.

Five themes were developed, three of which are directly related to the control of behavior by the central nervous system and more specifically by steroid hormones. The first one presents recent views on the control of male and female sexual behaviour in mammals. This topic is considered at all levels of integration from population dynamics to interaction of steroids with their intracellular brain receptors.

Current trends in behavioural endocrinology of birds are presented in a second series of chapters. Birds have frequently been used as experimental tools in behavioural endocrinology and neurobiology in general, and have been instrumental in stimulating the emergence of new concepts and directions of research. Let us only mention in this context the fact that the first demonstration of the behavioural effects of testicular secretions was obtained in a bird, the domestic cock, by Berthold in 1849 about 50 years before this subject was studied in mammals. We can also quote the discovery by Nottebohm and collaborators of the neuronal multiplication in the brain of adult song birds in relationship with season and song control. This has undoubtedly renewed interest in studies on neuronal plasticity in adult vertebrates. Behavioral endocrinology of birds is still a very active field, and new trends such as the endocrine study of free-living animals in the field or the analysis of steroid metabolism in the brain and its behavioural implications are presented here.

The third "behavioural" section is devoted to the problem of sexual differentiation and its hormonal control. Important conceptual and technical advances have been made in this area during the last few years and they are presented here by renowned scientists from Europe and the United States.

The fourth section of the book presents current views on the aminergic neurons in the brain. Special efforts have been made here to present broad reviews of this complex and rapidly growing field and much emphasis is laid on the comparative aspects. Detailed information can be found on assay methods, distribution across the phylogenetic scale from protozoa to mammals, interaction with peptidergic systems and involvement in behaviour control.

The last series of chapters concerns photo-transduction in invertebrates. The visual system has always been a subject of intensive research and as a consequence it is now possible to analyze vision in refined electrophysiological and biochemical terms. These different approaches are exemplified here, together with genetical studies relating mutations affecting the visual system in *Drosophila* to specific biochemical alterations.

This book thus offers specific information, as well as broad reviews on selected topics of neurobiology. It will be of interest for all neurobiologists and neuroendocrinologists, as well as for biologists in general, by showing how modern techniques in neurobiology can turn the wildest dreams into reality.

Liège, Belgium, June 1985   J. BALTHAZART

Contents

Symposium V   **Photo-Transduction in Invertebrate Visual Cells**
Organizers: T. Yoshizawa and H. Langer

List of Contributors

You will find the addresses of the beginning of the respective contribution

Symposium I
Behavioural Endocrinology of Mammals

Organizer J. BALTHAZART

Neuroendocrine Control of Population Size in Rodents with Special Emphasis on the Mongolian Gerbil

H. H. SWANSON[1]

1 Introduction

Only rodents will be considered in this paper, although most premises will also apply to other mammals. In order for a species to survive, two major drives must exist in its members: (1) a drive for survival of the individual and (2) a drive for propagation of the species. Personal survival requires maintenance activities such as eating and drinking, as well as taking precautions against being destroyed by predators or unfavourable environmental conditions. At first glance these activities seem to operate within an individual which presumably takes appropriate action to alleviate unpleasant internal stimuli of hunger or thirst, or external stimuli such as heat or cold. Indeed most studies of the physiological mechanisms which regulate these homeostatic behaviours have concentrated on the stimulus-response sequence within an individual. On second thought it becomes obvious that social factors are also involved. Young animals must learn which foods are edible, where and how they can be obtained, and how predators may be recognized and avoided. As adults, individuals may cooperate in hunting, foraging, and warning of danger, or alternately, compete for food either directly or indirectly through competition for territory or a position in the social hierarchy.

Neuroendocrine interactions are involved in most of these processes. The interaction between the nervous and endocrine systems may be in either direction, i.e. neural stimuli may trigger hormone production or changes in hormone levels may affect neural input (such as changes in sensitivity to environmental cues) or output (behaviour). The action of hormones on behaviour is usually permissive. A particular endocrine state allows or facilitates the expression of certain behaviours if the conditions are appropriate. Hormones do not cause behaviour.

The second major drive, propagation of the species, requires the interaction of at least two individuals. Copulation, however, is only one link in the chain which begins at conception with sexual differentiation, progresses through maturation of the reproductive system, attraction of a mate, copulation, preparation of a nest, and culminates in birth and subsequent care of the young. At each stage neuroendocrine factors come into play.

The genetic sex of an individual is determined at conception, but the development of the reproductive tract and other sexually dimorphic structures is influenced by the

---

1 Netherlands Institute for Brain Research, Meibergdreef 33, 1105 AZ Amsterdam ZO,
  The Netherlands

Neurobiology
(ed. by R. Gilles and J. Balthazart)
© Springer-Verlag Berlin Heidelberg 1985

presence or absence of androgens and other hormones secreted by the foetal testis. Structural and functional sex differences in the brain may also be programmed through androgen action during early development (De Vries et al. 1984; Swanson 1985). In the male, foetal testosterone is taken up by specific receptors in the brain, where it is aromatized to oestrogen and exerts permanent effects on the developing nervous system. Certain brain centres become "masculinized" whereas others become "feminized". The result is that the individual, when adult, will not only secrete gonadotrophins in the typical male acyclic manner, but will also make the appropriate behavioural responses to cues from receptive female (copulation) or male (perhaps territorial aggression) conspecifics.

The next important phase in reproductive development is sexual maturation. The mechanisms which trigger the sequence of events leading to first ovulation in females is still uncertain. One view is that an oestrogen-sensitive "negative feedback" system controlled by the hypothalamus becomes less sensitive to oestrogen as puberty progresses and ultimately, as oestrogen levels rise, a "positive feedback" threshold of oestrogen on luteinizing hormone (LH) is reached and phasic gonadotrophin release initiated (Ramirez and McCann 1963; Smith and Davidson 1968). An alternate suggestion is that the "positive feedback" threshold is reached well before sexual maturation, but that prior to this event LH release is inhibited by a "negative feedback" effect of prolactin or progesterone on the central nervous system (Wuttke et al. 1976; Döhler and Wuttke 1975). The rhythm of the oestrus cycle is regulated by neural stimuli produced daily at a precise time related to the onset of the light period.

Similar mechanisms may initiate sperm production and maturation of accessory sex organs in the male. It is clear, however, that in both sexes the timing of sexual maturity is influenced both by internal factors such as body size (Kennedy and Mitra 1963) and external seasonal factors such as light and temperature (reviewed by Sadleir 1969; Kappers and Pevet 1979). Social factors may also be involved. These have been extensively studied in the mouse, in which generally olfactory stimuli from females have been found to delay and those from males to accelerate the rate of sexual maturation in young females (Bronson 1971; Vandenbergh 1973; Drickamer 1977; Cowley 1978).

The attainment of sexual maturity is usually synchronized with the seasons, so that young will be born at the most advantageous time of year (Hutchinson 1978). Indeed, the gonads of many rodents living in the lower latitudes regress during the winter and undergo changes similar to puberty every spring. The endocrine changes may produce alterations in character usually manifested in the male by increased aggressiveness towards other males. Success in defeating rivals will allow an individual to either gain access to a desirable territory or to attain a sufficiently high place in the social hierarchy to allow him to participate in breeding. The same hormones then cause him to become receptive to stimuli from females and to seek a mate. At the same time females will show proceptive (soliciting) and receptive behaviour towards the advances of a male. Most female rodents are only sexually motivated during the oestrous phase of their cycle, which coincides with ovulation and thereby maximizes the chance that fertilization will follow mating.

If the female becomes pregnant, she will engage in maternal activities, which include building a nest and feeding and caring for the young after birth (Gubernick and Klopfer 1981; Elwood 1983a). Maternal behaviour seems to be initiated and maintained by a combination of the appropriate endocrine balance and stimulation by pups (Rosenblatt 1967). Depending on the species, the father may or may not engage in parental care (Kleinman and Malcolm 1981; Elwood 1983b). Stimuli from the pups are able to induce parental care in males or virgin females if exposure is prolonged over several days (Rosenblatt 1967). In parturient females, hormones serve to increase sensitivity to pup stimulation, thus reducing the latency to a few minutes after birth (Pedersen and Prange 1979; Bolwerk and Swanson 1984). Weaning of the young completes the reproductive process, which may of course be reinitiated at an appropriate interval.

Most studies on the neuroendocrine control of reproduction have focussed on a specific phase, i.e. sexual differentiation, puberty, the oestrous cycle, intermale aggression, sexual, or maternal behaviour, rather than examining how the system is integrated as a whole to ensure that the species will survive in a particular ecological niche.

2 Studies on the Mongolian Gerbil

In the present paper I will try to present a picture of how neural and endocrine factors interact in regulating population size in one particular species, the Mongolian gerbil *(Meriones unguiculatus)*. This work was done over several years in the Department of Anatomy at the University of Birmingham and formed the basis of a Ph.D. thesis by B. Payman (1980). Although the studies were carried out in the artificial conditions of laboratory enclosures, what is known about the ecology of the gerbil suggests that the mechanisms observed may also operate under natural conditions. Field observations indicate that in this rodent, which inhabits desert and semi-desert regions of Mongolia and northern China, young of the season spend the winter in a burrow with their parents, but do not hibernate (Bannikov 1954). Hence, exposure of young to their parents beyond weaning is a situation which could be encountered in the wild.

Rodents and other small mammals with a high reproductive capacity use various strategies to limit population size so as not overexploit their habitat (Wynne-Edwards 1962; Ebling and Stoddart 1978; Lidicker 1975, 1978; Swanson 1983). In most mammals the family is the basic social unit. The size, complexity, and cohesion of the family group is characteristic of the species. One or more families form a social group or colony within which stable relationships between individuals become established (Lidicker 1965). In the case of the gerbil, each colony occupies a complex burrow system which is defended against intruders. The spacing between colonies depends on the local availability of food and shelter.

In the present study family groups of gerbils were established in enclosures in which all extrinsic factors for population control were absent (climate, predators, food shortage). As there was no opportunity for emigration or immigration, stabilization of such a freely breeding population must be accomplished by social controls. Behavioural interactions between individuals were systematically observed and related to their position in the social hierarchy and their breeding performance. Each family group showed a distinct pattern. This variability suggests that rodents show individual differences which are worthy of study in their own right. This is an alternative to the usual approach of observing the behaviour of a sufficient number of animals so that individual differences are obscured in order for statistically significant results to be obtained. Once an overall picture had emerged, specific experiments were designed to elucidate the nature of the sensory cues and the role of sex hormones in establishing and maintaining the social structure.

In the first study we examined the formation of family groups of gerbils under two different housing conditions (Swanson and Lockley 1978). Adult pairs with a litter of juveniles were placed in six indoor enclosures ($1 \ m^2$) containing several wire-mesh nest boxes, as well as food, water and nesting material. Control pairs were housed in standard

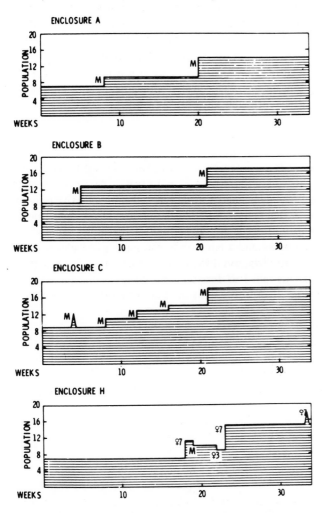

Fig. 1. Population dynamics in colonies of gerbils founded by an adult pair plus one or two litters in four selected enclosures. The founding mothers (*M*) in enclosures *A*, *B*, and *C* gave birth to 2,2 and 5 litters, respectively, during a 34-week period, whereas none of the daughters was fertile. In contrast, in enclosure *H*, the mother failed to breed for 18 weeks; several daughters became reproductively active and one (♀ 7) gave birth to a litter. Following a period of conflict, the mother (*M*) and another daughter (♀ 3) died, whereupon ♀ 7 became the sole breeding female. (Swanson and Lockley 1978)

cages. All couples produced a litter within a few weeks and most females immediately became pregnant again. The founding females stopped breeding after three or four litters, when the population was between 17 and 24 animals. Although occasional pregnancies occurred thereafter, litters failed to survive. The reproductive pattern in four enclosures is shown in Fig. 1. The asymptotic population size was the same in both cages and enclosures, and was of the same magnitude as the largest number found in any one burrow system in Leontjev's (1964) survey of 120 burrows in Mongolia. Agren (1976) released four families of gerbils in a 100 m² outdoor enclosure. The families established separate territories but the total population remained stable at 18 animals, i.e. the same range as in cages, indoor enclosures, and natural burrows.

Lidicker (1965) observed that the asymptotic population reached by several species of rodents (mouse, rice rat, deer mouse, and pinyon mouse) did not depend on the size of their enclosures. He concluded that in a confined space it was not possible for the population to divide itself into more than one social grouping, and hence limitations on the size of a single social unit was probably the critical factor.

3 The Female Gerbil

In the female gerbil, the oestrogen-dependent ventral scent gland appears at puberty and may be used as an index of sexual maturation. Females removed from their parents at 4 weeks of age and housed in litter-mate groups attain such glands around 12 to 16 weeks. However in both the initial and a later study (Swanson and Payman 1978; Payman and Swanson 1978, 1980; Swanson 1983), it was found that females living in family groups with their parents failed to develop scent glands at this age although they had reached adult size (Fig. 2). Autopsy confirmed that ovaries and uterus were

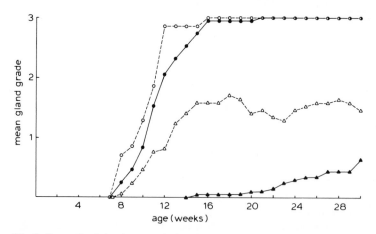

Fig. 2. Scent gland development in female gerbils growing up under various social and housing conditions. Mean gland grade is expressed in arbitrary units (max = 3) and the points represent the mean per group at each age. ○−−−−−−○ brother-sister pairs (cage); ●————● whole litters without parents (cage); △−−−−−−△ whole litters *with* parents (cage); ▲————▲ whole litters *with* parents (enclosure). (Swanson in Elwood 1983a)

immature. Sexual maturation thus seemed to be retarded in females staying with their parents beyond weaning age.

The delay in sexual development in daughters living with parents was greater in enclosures than in cages. This finding was interesting in view of the frequency with which delayed sexual maturation has been attributed to crowding (Brain 1971; Lidicker 1975). Clearly, in our studies where retardation was less severe in the more crowded environment, such an explanation does not apply. Following a long term quantitative study of the behaviour of individuals within family groups in enclosures, Payman (1980) reported an association between dominance, as judged by the exchange of submissive and aggressive acts, and breeding performance in females (Fig. 3). It seems likely that animals in cages would have less opportunity to avoid or seek selective interactions with specific individuals, thus reducing their chance of establishing a structured social organization. Earlier observations in the colonies suggested that the retardation of sexual development in young females is directly associated with the presence of the mother. Thus experimental removal or natural death of the mother (but not that of the father) resulted in a sudden increase in the proportion of daughters reaching sexual maturity and breeding. During this period there was much fighting between daughters and some animals were killed. Finally one female emerged as the only successful breeder (Fig. 1, Enclosure H). The scent glands of the others regressed and sample autopsies confirmed that their reproductive tracts had reverted to a juvenile condition. Eventually, peaceful conditions were reestablished within the colony, with the successful breeder showing all the behavioural signs of dominance and the rest directing submissive acts towards her (Swanson and Lockley 1978).

A series of experiments was then designed to investigate the source and nature of cues responsible for the retardation of reproductive development of young females. Breeding pairs were established in cages and the litter subsequently born was left with

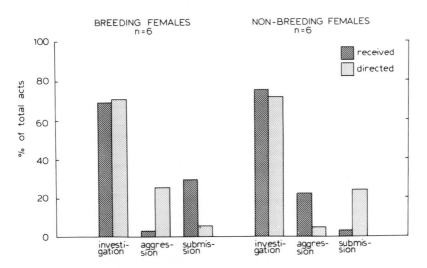

Fig. 3. Social behaviour of breeding and non-breeding females living in colonies in enclosures. Although the total amount of social contact was the same, breeding females *directed* more aggression and *received* more submission than non-breeding females. (Courtesy of Payman 1980)

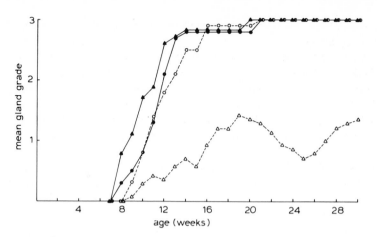

Fig. 4. Influence of mother (with or without litter) on scent gland development of young female gerbils. ▲————————▲ three daughters without mother; ○——————○ two daughters with non-pregnant mother; ●————————● two daughters with mother, who had a litter which was removed at birth; △——————△ two daughters with mother plus litter. (Swanson in Elwood 1983a)

both parents up to the age of 4 weeks, at which time the composition of the group was manipulated. A surprising initial observation was that in the absence of other social cues from 4 weeks of age, sexual maturation of daughters was not retarded in the presence of their mother alone. An examination of the possibility that the mother's reproductive condition was relevant to her effect on her daughters revealed that sexual development was retarded in females reared with their mother in the continuing presence of her second litter, but not in those housed with a mother who had either failed to conceive again or whose second litter was removed at birth (Payman and Swanson 1980; Swanson 1983) (Fig. 4).

Further experiments failed to determine the precise nature of cues involved in delayed sexual development. However, it was ascertained that any female with young pups was as effective as the natural mother with litter in causing retardation. In some other rodents, it has been shown that females can become imprinted to odours experienced in the preweaning period (Porter and Etscorn 1974). Obviously, in gerbils olfactory or other cues derived from the natural mother during the suckling period are not important. Also, by segregating the juvenile daughters by a wire partition, it was found that tactile cues dependent on direct physical contact between the young females and their mother and/or her newborn litter were not critical for this effect (Payman 1980). Pheromonal influences on sexual maturation of rodents have been reported in several studies (Cowley 1978; Bronson 1971; Vandenbergh 1973). The possibility that maternal scent gland odours in the gerbil are involved was investigated because female marking activity rises during lactation (Wallace et al. 1973) and gerbils are able to recognize individual scent gland odours (Halpin 1976). In our experiments, excision of the mother's scent gland, however, did not prevent inhibition of her daughters' maturation. Other possible sources of maternal odour whose influences were not examined are the faeces (which in rats contain a specific maternal pheromone; Leon 1974), urine, and milk (Porter 1983). Alternately, relevant olfactory cues may have come from the body odour or excretory products of the infants (Smotherman et al. 1978; Elwood and McCauley 1983). Indeed, we did not determine whether the cues responsible for delayed development of juvenile females originated from the mother and/or her second litter, since it was not possible to separate the sucklings from their mother for a prolonged period. Finally, in many rodents, including gerbils, both mothers and pups emit ultrasounds (Noirot 1972; Bell 1974; Sales and Smith 1978; Elwood 1979). The possibility that such cues are relevant to the retardation of sexual maturation cannot be dismissed, since audible and ultrasonic signals associated with mating may activate neuroendocrine responses.

Inhibition of sexual maturation in young females has been reported in experimental colonies of deer mice when emigration was prevented (Terman 1965) as well as in overwintering natural populations of deer mice (Sadleir 1969) and wood mice (Flowerdew 1978). There is good evidence that an olfactory component is involved although stress associated with agonistic interaction may also play a role. Both factors may induce changes in gonadotrophin secretion through neural input to the pituitary which results in reproductive inhibition (Christian et al. 1965; Bronson 1979). In our experimental situation, there was no impairment of body weight and the animals all seemed in good condition. Furthermore the adrenals were not enlarged. It therefore seems unlikely that stress was a causal factor. In a number of the sexually inhibited females the scent gland was not completely absent (see Fig. 2), which suggests that a low level of oestrogen was circulating. Psychic stimuli may exert their effect on sexual maturation at the level of the hypothalamic "negative feedback controller", so that in the retarded females the sensitivity of the negative feedback system to oestrogen decreases at a slower rate than normal and that consequently oestrogen fails to rise sufficiently to trigger ovulation.

It is interesting to consider the significance of retardation of female sexual development to the species in its natural habitat. The breeding season extends from February to September. Young born in the autumn overwinter with their parents. The situation could therefore arise whereby daughters of potential reproductive age are living with their parents in a burrow whose resources cannot support more than one breeding female. Under these circumstances temporary inhibition of sexual maturation of females living with an actively breeding mother may be in the long term interests of all the females concerned (Payman 1980). Indeed if mating only occurs between the original parents, and there is evidence to support this (see below), siblings would be genetically as closely related to daughters as their own offspring. By sociobiological principles there would be no advantage for the young females to start breeding as long as their mother was reproducing and there was no opportunity for dispersal (Trivers 1974; Wilson 1975; Dawkins 1976; Bekoff 1981). All our experimental data supports the general conclusion that female gerbils only attain sexual maturity (and breed) in the absence of a breeding mother.

4 The Male Gerbil

Parallel to the mother's influence on her daughters, there is evidence of a paternal influence on reproductive activity of sons. Ågren (personal communication) compared

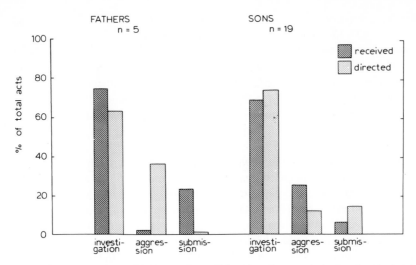

Fig. 5. Social behaviour of fathers and sons living in enclosures. As in females, the total amount of social contact was the same, but fathers *directed* more aggression and *received* more submission than sons. (Courtesy of Payman 1980)

the number of litters born before and after vasectomy of the father in cages containing a father, mother, and one adult offspring of each sex. Whereas litters were born in all cages in the 12-month period before the father's operation (which impaired his fertility without altering his hormonal state) no litters were born during a similar period thereafter. Reproduction continued in control cages in which the father was not vasectomized. Sons were thus inhibited from mating by the mere presence of the father.

Payman (1980), in her quantitative study of family relationships in gerbil enclosures, found that the founding male (father) was indeed dominant to his sons with respect to aggressive acts directed and submissive acts received (Fig. 5). Of further significance to Ågren's findings was the observation that the father influenced scent marking by sons, a behaviour which, like sexual activity, is testosterone-dependent in the male (Thiessen et al. 1968; Swanson and Norman 1978). Very few sons living with their father marked when placed individually in a novel arena. In contrast, almost all young males removed from their father at weaning marked as actively as the father (Fig. 6). Removal of the father from the enclosure had a similar effect on sons as removal of the mother had on daughters. There was a period of social disruption with much fighting, during which several males were killed. The final result was the emergence of a new dominant male, towards whom the remaining males showed submissive behaviour. Moreover the new dominant was the only who engaged in a significant amount of marking behaviour (Swanson and Lockley 1978; Payman 1980).

Neither scent gland excision nor castration of the father attenuated his inhibitory influence on scent marking by his sons (Fig. 7) (Swanson 1983). Suppression of marking was therefore not mediated by olfactory cues emanating from the father's very active scent gland, nor by other testosterone dependent sensory or behavioural cues. The fact that the castrated father did not mark did not reactivate this behaviour in the young males. That the sons were sufficiently mature to engage in marking was confirmed

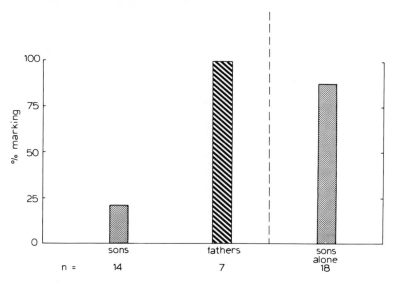

Fig. 6. Marking behaviour of fathers and sons living in cages. *Left* two sons with father in cage from weaning. *Right* three sons alone in cage. (Courtesy of Payman 1980)

by the marking activity of sons of the same age living in a cage without their father. In this context it is interesting that a castrated father provided effective inhibitory cues whereas another large adult, i.e. the mother had no such effect. A foster father was just as effective as the natural father (Payman 1980).

In rodent encounters a variety of acts and postures may be used in communication between conspecifics. A wire-mesh partition was placed in a cage between father and sons in order to determine whether scent marking is depressed in sons which are prevented from direct physical interactions with their father but maintain olfactory, visual, auditory, and very restricted tactile contact with him. The proportion of sons which marked in a neutral arena was about half-way between sons living in intimate contact with their father and sons alone (Fig. 8). Direct physical interaction between father and sons is involved in depression of sons' marking, but such cues are not solely responsible for the effect. Observations in the enclosure suggest that aggressive postures may be effective visual signals (Payman 1980).

Since marking is testosterone-dependent (Thiessen et al. 1968; Thiessen and Yahr 1977; Swanson and Norman 1978), the question arises whether testosterone secretion is depressed in sons living with their father. Although sexual development (as estimated by the rate of development of the scent glands) is somewhat delayed in young males growing up in enclosures with their parents, the inhibition is much less severe than in females (Swanson and Lockley 1978). At autopsy, the weights of testes, seminal vesicles, and scent glands were in the normal range. Subcutaneous testosterone implants (25 mg), which restored marking in castrated males had no such effect on adult sons living with their father (Swanson 1980). This dose of testosterone had previously been shown to increase the blood level above normal and to cause hypertrophy of both scent glands and seminal vesicles. These results suggest that the suppression of marking in

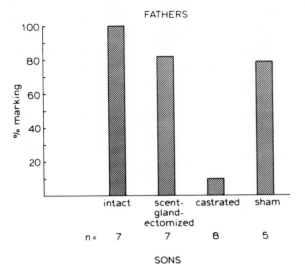

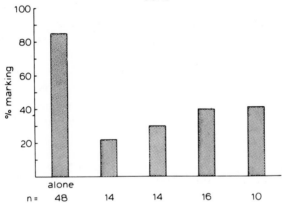

Fig. 7. Effects of scent gland excision or castration of father on marking behaviour of fathers and sons. *Column 1* three sons alone in cage from weaning. *All other columns* two sons with father from weaning. Marking behaviour was tested when sons were 20-weeks-old. (Swanson in Elwood 1983a)

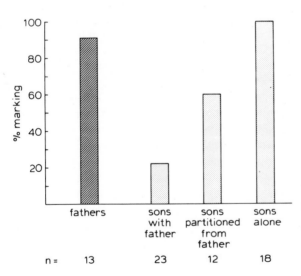

Fig. 8. Paternal influence of scent marking on sons. Effects of separating fathers and sons by a wire-mesh partition from the time of weaning until testing when sons were 20-weeks-old. (Courtesy of Payman 1980)

sons is not mediated through inhibition of testosterone secretion. Social factors are thus of primary importance in the control of marking behaviour in the Mongolian gerbil. The action of testosterone on scent marking is permissive. Marking does not occur under any circumstances following castration. But although castrated fathers living with their sons ceased to mark, they were still able to suppress marking in their sons (Swanson 1983).

The behavioural act of marking is mediated through the action of testosterone on the brain, as shown by Thiessen and Yahr (1970), who found that doses of testosterone propionate ($1.25-2.5$ μg), too small to have a systemic effect on either scent glands or marking, induced marking when injected into the lateral ventricles of the brain. In an attempt to localize the site of action, they implanted crystals of testosterone in the brain. They found that such implants were most effective in the preoptic area of the hypothalamus, whereas testosterone implants in the hippocampus or cortex were ineffective, as were cholesterol implants in the hypothalamus. The authors suggested that, since actinomycin-D blocked the effects of testosterone by preventing transcription of DNA, the hormone acts by stimulating genetic transcription. Testosterone was the only naturally occurring steroid which induced marking when implanted in the brain; Dihydrotestosterone (DHT) was ineffective (Yahr and Thiessen 1972; Thiessen et al. 1973). It is interesting that the neural site controlling marking behaviour (preoptic area) is believed to be the same as that controlling sexual behaviour (De Vries et al. 1984). It seems possible that in the gerbil, a paternal influence on male behaviour is mediated via modifications at this site.

5 Discussion

The control of scent marking in the Mongolian gerbil is an excellent illustration of neuroendocrine integration as an evolutionary adaptation. Thus sex hormones, in addition to their obvious effects on the reproductive tract and sexual behaviour, lead to aggression and scent marking in the male, both of which are probably important in territorial defence and in maintaining the integrity of the social unit. At the same time they provide the physical substrate for marking by peripheral stimulation of specialized sebaceous glands which have become modified for the production of pheromones.

Females, who usually mark at very low levels, are stimulated to mark almost as much as males by the administration of testosterone (Swanson and Norman 1978). It would be interesting to see whether testosterone-implanted females would be inhibited from marking in the presence of their father (or mother?) in the same way as sons.

The normal size of testes, seminal vesicles, and scent glands in sons living with fathers compared to sons living alone, suggests that their lack of marking was not due to depressed testosterone secretion. A massive increase in testosterone through implantation of pellets did not increase marking (Swanson 1980). These results are similar to those reported by Bronson in mice (Bronson 1976). Using fluorescence under ultraviolet light to trace urine trails in enclosures, Bronson found that dominant males deposited small amounts of urine all over their territory, saturating the area with their scent. In contrast, subordinate males deposited their urine in large pools in just a few spots, thus fulfilling only an excretory function. Implanting testosterone in subordinate males did not alter the pattern of urine deposition. Thus a similar mechanism seems to control the deliberate act of marking with a specialized sebaceous gland in gerbils, and the deliberate use of natural excretory product for the same purpose in the mouse.

The fact that rodents can be readily maintained in the laboratory and occupy an extremely wide range of natural habitats renders them particularly suitable mammalian subjects for integrated ecological, ethological, and physiological studies. The results of our study highlight the dramatic impact which an individual's social environment can have on aspects of physiology and behaviour and thus, ultimately, reproductive fitness. More specifically, they illustrate social mechanisms which would apparently enable individuals of a species to exploit a harsh, and therefore problematical, habitat.

In a recent round-table on signals in reproductive neuroendocrinology, it became apparent that although a great deal is known about which environmental factors influence reproduction, and that various signals interact with the hypothalamus to modulate secretion of pituitary hormones and thereby control reproduction, the brain mechanisms mediating the endocrine responses to these signals are still mostly concealed within the "black box" (Dyer 1984a,b). Much work has been done on how daily and seasonal rhythms of light and darkness entrain physiological changes (Kappers and Pevet 1979; Oksche and Pevet 1981). In rodents, the circadian photoperiod determines the time of ovulation, implantation, and parturition. It seems that retinohypothalamic fibres project to the suprachiasmatic nuclei, and changes in illumination are associated with electrophysiological and metabolic changes in these nuclei. These signals entrain the suprachiasmatic nuclei and govern the timing of all reproductive events dependent thereon. In many species, day length is transcribed into a seasonal time cue so as to ensure that mating and birth are timed to maximize reproductive potential. Substantial evidence now indicates that the seasonal control, mediated via the pineal, involves changes in the "negative feedback" sensitivity of the brain to gonadal steroids and the development of refractoriness with time. It is not known whether the pineal may be involved in the retardation of sexual maturation in gerbils through social factors, or whether later common pathways are involved.

Among environmental factors which interfere with ovulation, fasting may prevent hypothalamic neurones from initiating an LH surge in response to rising titres of plasma oestrogen. Recent experiments have shown that whereas hypothalamic neurones are normally excited by stimulation of the ventral noradrenergic tract, after a 72-h fast the response changes to one of inhibition (Dyer 1984a,b). Prolactin, on the other hand, is also involved in the control of ovulation and it is known that social factors can block ovulation by increasing prolactin. Keverne et al. (1982) have shown that in colonies of talapoin monkeys, only the dominant female ovulates. The subordinate females are prevented, presumably through social stimuli, from initiating a preovulatory LH surge. This is due to a high prolactin titre, which can be reversed by bromocriptine, a drug which depresses prolactin. Such a mechanism may also operate in gerbil colonies.

Lactation, which constitutes the final stage of reproduction is controlled by the hypothalamus through two major processes: one, hypothalamic control of prolactin secretion and two, hypothalamic secretion of oxytocin in response to the milk ejection reflex induced by suckling (Drewett 1983). The latter is one of the few examples where a direct link between an environmental stimulus and a specific neuronal response has been established.

6 Conclusions

In this review the impact of social factors on reproduction in the Mongolian gerbil has been examined. The family is the basic social unit. The number of individuals in the group is dependent on the social relationships within the colony rather than the size of the living space. In circumstances in which dispersal is restricted, neuroendocrine mechanisms come into play which curtail population growth. These factors act selectively on certain individuals through the establishment of a dominant breeding pair. Displays of dominance which elicit submissive postures from subordinates result in the suppression of sexual development in young females and of marking behaviour in young males. This strategy ensures the stability of the social group and its survival under conditions where dispersal is impossible, e.g. in laboratory enclosures or in overwintering burrows.

References

Ågren G (1976) Social and territorial behaviour in the Mongolian gerbil (Meriones unguiculatus) under semi-natural conditions. Biol Behav 1:267–285

Bannikov AG (1954) The places inhabited and natural history of Meriones unguiculatus. In: Mammals of the Mongolian Peoples' Republic. USSR Academy of Sciences, p 410

Bekoff M (1981) Mammalian sibling interactions: genes, facilitative environments, and the coefficient of familiarity. In: Gubernick DJ, Klopfer P (eds) Parental care in mammals. Plenum, New York, p 307

Bell RW (1974) Ultrasound in small rodents: arousal produced and arousal producing. Dev Psychobiol 7:39–42

Bolwerk ELM, Swanson HH (1984) Does oxytocin play a role in the onset of maternal behaviour in the rat? J Endocrinol 101:353–357

Brain PF (1971) The physiology of population limitation in rodents – a review. Commun Behav Biol 6:115–123

Bronson FH (1971) Rodent pheromones. Biol Reprod 4:344–357

Bronson FH (1976) Urine marking in mice: causes and effects. In: Doty RL (ed) Mammalian olfaction, reproductive processes and behaviour. Academic, New York, p 119

Bronson FH (1979) The reproductive ecology of the house mouse. Q Rev Biol 54:265–299

Christian JJ, Lloyd JA, Davis DE (1965) The role of endocrines in the self-regulation of mammalian populations. Recent Prog Horm Res 21:501–578

Cowley JJ (1978) Olfaction and the development of sexual behaviour. In: Hutchison JB (ed) Biological determinants of sexual behaviour. Wiley, Chichester, p 87

Dawkins R (1976) The selfish gene. Oxford Univ Press, London

De Vries GJ, De Bruin JPC, Uylings HBM, Corner MA (eds) (1984) Sex differences in the brain. Prog Brain Res, vol 61. Elsevier, Amsterdam

Döhler DW, Wuttke W (1975) Changes with age in levels of serum gonadotrophins, prolactin and gonadal steroids in prepubertal male and female rats. Endocrinology 97:898–907

Drewett RF (1983) Sucking, milk synthesis, and milk ejection in the Norway rat. In: Elwood RW (ed) Parental behaviour in rodents. Wiley, Chichester, p 181

Drickamer LC (1977) Delay in sexual maturation in female house mice by exposure to grouped females or urine from grouped females. J Reprod Fertil 51:77–81

Dyer RG (1984a) Signals in reproductive neuroendocrinology. Abstracts: Europ Winter Conf Brain Res (unpublished)

Dyer RG (1984b) Sexual differentiation of the forebrain – relationship to gonadotrophin secretion. In: De Vries GJ, De Bruin JPC, Uylings HMB, Corner MA (eds) Sex differences in the brain. Prog Brain Res, vol 61. Elsevier, Amsterdam, p 223

Ebling FJ, Stoddart DM (eds) (1978) Population control by social behaviour. Symp Inst Biol, vol 23. Inst Biol, London

Elwood RW (1979) Ultrasounds and maternal behaviour in the Mongolian gerbil. Dev Psychobiol 12:281−284

Elwood RW (ed) (1983a) Parental behaviour in rodents. Wiley, Chichester

Elwood RW (ed) (1983b) Paternal care in rodents. In: Parental behaviour in rodents. Wiley, Chichester, p 235

Elwood RW, McCauley (1983) Communication in rodents: infants to adults. In: Elwood RW (ed) Parental behaviour in rodents. Wiley, Chichester, p 127

Flowerdew JR (1978) Residents and transients in wood mouse populations. In: Ebling FJ, Stoddart DM (eds) Population control by social behaviour. Symp Inst Biol, vol 23. London, p 49

Gubernick DJ, Klopfer PH (eds) (1981) Parental care in mammals. Plenum, New York

Halpin ZT (1976) The role of individual recognition by odors in the Mongolian gerbil. Behaviour 58:117−130

Hutchison JB (ed) (1978) Biological determinants of sexual behaviour. Wiley, Chichester

Kappers JA, Pevet P (eds) (1979) The pineal gland of vertebrates including man. Prog Brain Res, vol 52. Elsevier, Amsterdam

Kennedy GC, Mitra J (1963) Body weight and food intake as initiating factors for puberty in the rat. J Physiol (Lond) 166:408−418

Keverne EB, Eberhart JA, Meller RE (1982) Social influences on behaviour and neuroendocrine responsiveness of talapoin monkeys. Scand J Psychol Supp 1:37−47

Kleinman DG, Malcolm JR (1981) The evolution of male parental investment in mammals. In: Gubernick DJ, Klopfer PH (eds) Parental care in mammals. Plenum, New York, p 347

Leon M (1974) Maternal pheromone. Physiol Behav 13:441−453

Leontjev AN (1964) Studying Meriones unguiculatus by the method of marking. Biol Abstr 1964, Abstract No 103056

Lidicker WZ (1965) Comparative studies of density regulation in confined colonies of four species of rodents. Res Popul Ecol (Kyoto) 7:57−72

Lidicker WZ (1975) The role of dispersal in the demography of small mammals. In: Golley FP, Petrusewicz K, Ryszkowki L (eds) Small mammals: their productivity and population dynamics. Cambridge Univ Press, p 103

Lidicker WZ (1978) Regulations of numbers in small mammal populations − historical reflections and a synthesis. In: Snyder DP (ed) Populations of small mammals under natural conditions. Univ Pittsburgh Press, p 122

Noirot E (1972) Ultrasounds and maternal behaviour in small rodents. Dev Psychobiol 5:371−387

Oksche A, Pevet P (eds) (1981) The pineal organ. Dev Endocrinol, vol 14. Elsevier, Amsterdam

Payman B (1980) Social factors influencing scent marking and reproduction in the Mongolian gerbil (Meriones unguiculatus). PhD Thesis, Univ Birmingham

Payman B, Swanson HH (1978) Maternal influence on sexual development of female offspring in the Mongolian gerbil (Meriones unguiculatus). J Endocrinol 79:30P−31P

Payman B, Swanson HH (1980) Social influence on sexual maturation and breeding in the female Mongolian gerbil (Meriones unguiculatus). Anim Behav 28:528−535

Pedersen CA, Prange Jr AJ (1979) Induction of maternal behaviour in virgin rats after intracerebroventricular administration of oxytocin. Proc Natl Acad Sci USA 76:6661−6665

Porter RH (1983) Communication in rodents: adults to infants. In: Elwood RW (ed) Parental behaviour in rodents. Wiley, Chichester, p 95

Porter RH, Etscorn F (1974) Olfactory imprinting resulting from brief exposures in Acomys cahirinus. Nature (Lond) 250:732−733

Ramirez DV, McCann SM (1963) Comparison of the regulation of luteinizing hormone (LH) secretion in immature and adult rats. Endocrinology 72:452−474

Rosenblatt JS (1967) Nonhormonal basis of maternal behavior in the rat. Science (Wash DC) 156:1512−1514

Sadleir RMFS (1969) The ecology of reproduction in wild and domestic mammals. Methuen, London

Sales GD, Smith JC (1978) Comparative studies of the ultrasonic calls of infant murid rodents. Dev Psychobiol 11:595−619

Smith ER, Davidson JM (1968) Role of estrogen in the cerebral control of puberty in female rats. Endocrinology 82:100−108

Smotherman WP, Bell RW, Hershberger WA, Coover GD (1978) Orientation to rat pup cues: effects of maternal experiential history. Anim Behav 26:265−273

Swanson HH (1980) Social and hormonal influences on scent marking in the Mongolian gerbil. Physiol Behav 24:839−842

Swanson HH (1983) Parental behaviour and population control. In: Elwood RW (ed) Parental behaviour in rodents. Wiley, Chichester, p 259

Swanson HH (1985) Sex differences in the brain. In: Gupta D, Borelli B, Hanasio A (eds) Paediatric neuroendocrinology. Croom-Helm, London, p 1

Swanson HH, Lockley MR (1978) Population growth and social structure of confined colonies of Mongolian gerbils: scent gland size and marking behaviour as indices of social status. Aggressive Behav 4:57−89. Liss, New York

Swanson HH, Norman ME (1978) Central and peripheral action of testosterone propionate on scent gland morphology and marking behaviour in the Mongolian gerbil. Behav Processes 3:9−19

Swanson HH, Payman B (1978) Social and spatial influences on puberty in the female Mongolian gerbil. In: Dörner G, Kawakami M (eds) Hormones and brain development. Elsevier, Amsterdam, p 375

Terman CR (1965) A study of population growth and control exhibited in the laboratory by prairie deermice. Ecology 46:890−895

Thiessen DD, Yahr P (1970) Central control of territorial marking in the Mongolian gerbil. Physiol Behav 5:275−278

Thiessen DD, Yahr P (1977) The gerbil in behavioural investigations: mechanisms of territoriality and olfactory communication. Univ Texas Press, Austin London

Thiessen DD, Lindzey G, Friend H (1968) Androgen control of territorial marking in the Mongolian gerbil (Meriones unguiculatus). Science (Wash DC) 160:432−434

Thiessen DD, Yahr P, Owen K (1973) Regulatory mechanisms of territorial marking in the Mongolian gerbil. J Comp Physiol Psychol 82:382−393

Trivers RL (1974) Parent-offspring conflict. Am Zool 14:249−264

Vandenbergh JG (1973) Acceleration and inhibition of puberty in female mice by pheromones. J Reprod Fertil Suppl 19:411−419

Wallace P, Owen K, Thiessen DD (1973) The control and function of maternal scent marking in the Mongolian gerbil. Physiol Behav 10:463−466

Wilson EO (1975) Sociobiology: the new synthesis. Belknap, Harvard

Wuttke W, Döhler KD, Gelato M (1976) Oestrogens and prolactin as possible regulators of puberty. J Endocrinol 68:391−396

Wynne-Edwards WC (1962) Animal dispersion in relation to social behaviour. Oliver Boyd, Edinburgh

Yahr P, Thiessen DD (1972) Steroid regulation of territorial scent marking in the Mongolian gerbil (Meriones unguiculatus). Horm Behav 3:359−368

Social and Hormonal Determinants of Reproductive Patterns in the Prairie Vole

C.S. CARTER [1,2] and L.L. GETZ [1]

1 Introduction

The prairie vole, *Microtus ochrogaster*, is a small North American rodent which has been studied intensively by ecologists. Like many other microtine rodents, the prairie vole shows dramatic population fluctuations. The factors regulating population levels in this species in nature are not fully known, but may relate to the social organization and reproductive physiology of the species (Getz 1978; Getz and Carter 1980).

The prairie vole also provides a laboratory-compatible and potentially powerful model system for the analysis of social factors in reproduction. The species is readily bred and studied in the laboratory. In addition, field data, obtained from free-living animals through the use of live trapping (Getz et al. 1981), and radiotelemetry (Hofmann et al. 1984), provide uniquely detailed information on population structure, social organization, and mating systems in the prairie vole.

An overview of some of the major features of reproduction in this species is shown in Table 1. The prairie vole can be monogamous and a number of aspects of reproduction in this species apparently reflect adaptations to monogamy. At low population densities male and female prairie voles live together and defend a territory. Even under laboratory conditions there is incest avoidance, and offspring are reproductively suppressed as long as they remain in the natal nest. Oestrus induction and maintenance in the virgin female prairie vole depends on stimuli from the male. Like other microtine rodents, females of this species generally require copulatory stimulation to trigger ovu-

Table 1. Features of reproduction in the prairie vole (*Microtus ochrogaster*)

Dramatic population fluctuations
Monogamy
Incest avoidance
Reproductive suppression of offspring
Induced oestrus (in non-reproductive females)
Postpartum oestrus
Induced ovulation

1 Departments of Ecology, Ethology and Evolution, and Psychology, University of Illinois at Urbana-Champaign, Champaign, IL 61820, USA
2 Mailing address: Department of Zoology, University of Maryland, College Park, MD 20742, USA

Neurobiology
(ed. by R. Gilles and J. Balthazart)
© Springer-Verlag Berlin Heidelberg 1985

lation and are considered to be reflex ovulators (Richmond and Conaway 1969). Established pairs of adult males and females may remain together over prolonged periods of time and, after the first mating, reproduction relies on a postpartum oestrus.

In this paper we will summarize the current laboratory and field evidence for monogamy and pair-bonding and behavioural and physiological events that lead to oestrus induction in the prairie vole. The social interactions and mating patterns among male and female prairie voles will be described as a function of the social and sexual history of the animals being observed. In particular, time-lapse videotaping has been used to examine the copulatory (or in some cases, lack of copulatory) interactions among unfamiliar pairs and also among animals from known family groups. These observations also allow an analysis of the nature of incest avoidance and offspring suppression in this species.

2 Monogamy in the Prairie Vole

It has been estimated that only about 3% of mammals have a monogamous mating system (Kleiman 1977). Of the known monogamous species the prairie vole is probably the most accessible for detailed physiological and behavioural study. The following are some of the characteristics of prairie vole behaviour and reproduction which appear to conform to the criteria suggested by Kleiman (1977) and others as indicative of a monogamous mating system.

Laboratory evidence for monogamy in the prairie vole is abundant (Thomas and Birney 1979; Getz et al. 1981). In the laboratory, females in postpartum oestrus show a clear preference for mating with the male with which they have been cohabiting (i.e. their mate) and will often rebuff the mating advance of unfamiliar males (Getz and Carter 1980; Getz et al. 1981; Figs. 1 and 2). Observations in laboratory cages (Gavish et al. 1983) and in a semi-natural, undisturbed setting (Gruder-Adams and Getz 1985) suggest that female breeders living in establishing pairs attempt to maintain mating exclusivity. In contrast, when females are in their first (induced) oestrus (Fig. 3) they are equally likely to mate with familiar or unfamiliar males. (In this case the familiar males were previously unfamiliar animals with which the female was housed for 18 h and which were then maintained across a perforated metal barrier for 24 h before

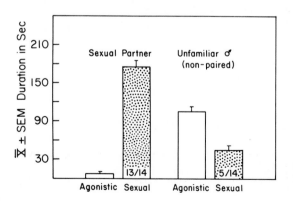

Fig. 1. Mating preference and aggression in females in postpartum oestrus in a 10-min test

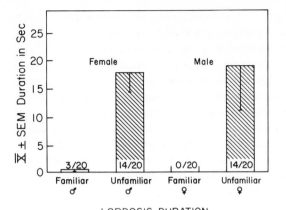

Fig. 2. Aggression toward strangers in paired male and female prairie voles in a 5-min test

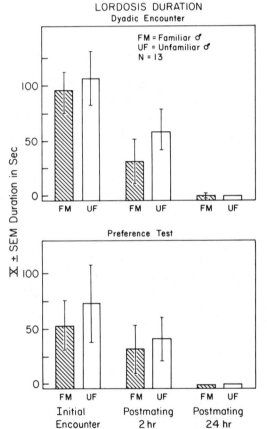

Fig. 3. Mating preferences in females in induced (first) oestrus. In dyadic encounters oestrous females were placed with a familiar or unfamiliar male. In preference tests a familiar and unfamiliar male were tethered at opposite ends of a test arena and the female could choose to spend time with either male or in a neutral center area in a 10-min test

they were reintroduced for testing. Thus, these were the males that had activated the female's behavioural oestrus.)

The mating exclusivity of the previously mated female prairie vole is not absolute or permanent. When the postpartum oestrous female is forced into continued association with a strange male, mating occurs in about 80% of the cases. The mating pattern of females that do mate when tested with unfamiliar males is similar to that seen between established pairs. Males from established pairs ("breeder" males in our terminology) show a pattern of initial response to strange non-oestrous females that is characterized by somewhat more chasing and attacking than that seen in sexually experienced "non-breeder" males. Aggression is rare between inexperienced males and young females (Gavish et al. 1983). Breeder males also do not *initially* engage in the olfactory investigation patterns that may play an important role in normal courtship. Males from established family groups in nature have also been live-trapped and immediately placed in a neutral test cage with females in hormone-induced oestrous or with naive non-oestrous females. In 10-min field trials the oestrous female elicited less aggression than non-oestrous females, but in neither case did these males immediately attempt to copulate with the female. Sexually mature males that were known to be living in the absence of an established mate were also live-trapped. Such (non-breeder) males spent significantly more time in physical (side-by-side) contact with a non-oestrous female (Getz, unpublished observations).

The postcopulatory changes in behaviour in this species may be part of the mechanism responsible for pair-bonding and thus help to establish the monogamy. Aggression toward strangers is pronounced in pregnant females and their mates. It is our hypothesis that physiological changes during and following mating play an important role in the pair-bonding process, and that protracted mating bouts (often lasting more than 24 h) in naive pairs (to be described, Fig. 4) may provide stimuli relevant to pregnancy induction and pair-bonding. Studies examining this hypothesis are in progress.

Males participate actively in parental care (Hartung and Dewsbury 1979). Within a day or two following delivery the male tends to spend nearly as much time on the nest as does the female (Gruder-Adams and Getz 1985). Older siblings may also assist in care of younger offspring. In nature older siblings, and especially females, are found in the natal nest well beyond weaning and probably provide thermal and physical support for the younger siblings.

Male-female pairs are more reproductively successful than trios or females living alone. In one study in our laboratory we found that pregnancies in male-female pairs living alone produced an average of five live births, while in trios (see Table 2 for group composition) composed of either related (sibling) or unrelated individuals the average litter sizes of those females that delivered were fewer than four pups ($p < 0.05$; Gavish et al. 1981). For the latter study, a variety of types of trios were constituted and left relatively undisturbed for 2 months. When two females were placed with a single unfamiliar (non-sib) male, survival and reproductive success were highest if the females were sisters (sibs; Table 2). When trios were composed of two unrelated females and an unfamiliar male, usually only one female bore young, and it was not uncommon to find the second female dead within a few days after the animals were placed together. When an established breeder female with a history of prior reproduction was placed with an unrelated young male and female, the breeder female was the only female to reproduce, and in 3 of 10 groupings the other younger female died. When trios were composed of one female and two males survival was high, except in the trios composed of a breeder male and an unrelated younger male; 70% of the younger males died in the latter groups. Unisex trios cohabited relatively peacefully, with the exception of one grouping of 3 non-sibling females, in which 2 of the females died.

Table 2. Survival and reproduction in groups of prairie voles

Group	Female	Males	Male survival (%)[a]	Females reproducing
A	1 non-sib	1 non-sib	100	11/14 (79%)
B	1 non-sib	1 non-sib and 1 non-sib	100	9/10 (90%)
C	1 non-sib	1 sib and 1 sib	100	10/10 (100%)
D	1 non-sib	1 breeder 1 non-sib	100 30	10/10 (100%)
E	0	3 non-sib	100 (30/30)	–
F	0	3 sib	100 (30/30)	–

Group	Females	Male	Female survival (%)	Females reproducing of survivors	% of total females
G	1 non-sib and 1 non-sib	1 non-sib	64 (14/22)	9/14	(41%)
H	1 sib and 1 sib	1 non-sib	100 (22/22)	16/22	(73%)
I	1 breeder and 1 non-sib	1 non-sib	100 (10/10) 70 (7/10)	7/10 0/ 7	(70%) (0%)
J	3 non-sib	0	93 (28/30)	–	
K	3 sib	0	100 (30/30)	–	

[a] All females survived in groups A–D. (After Gavish et al. 1981)

Fuentes and Dewsbury (1984) have also studied the mating preferences of male prairie voles given the opportunity to mate with more than one female. They have observed that males of this species show a tendency to select one female, rather than distributing copulatory behaviour (and thus sperm) equally among several females. We have obtained similar findings from videotaping trios of two oestrous females and one male (see later Section on female-female suppression and Fig. 5). These findings also support the assumption that this species is in someway adapted to monogamy.

In field studies that have continued over a period of many years, Getz and his associates have discovered that prairie voles, under conditions of low population densities, tend to live in stable male-female pairs, as long as both members of the pair remain alive. For example, in one recent study, at low densities, 17 family groups were followed by live-trapping continually for a period of several months. Fifteen (88%) of the family groups were monogamous and virtually no adult strangers were allowed in the family nest area for a period of time that spanned the production of several litters. When population densities increased, the percentage of females living with a single male dropped to between 30% and 50% (n = 48 family groups). At higher densities females were occasionally found living in multi-female groups. These unpublished studies and earlier live-trapping data (Getz et al. 1981) support the conclusion that during periods of low population density males and females remain together in the same territory and share a home nest. Other adult males and females are unlikely to enter the pair's territory or nest as long as both members of the original pair are alive. These live-trapping observations have been confirmed by radiotelemetry over periods of 3–10 days (Hofmann et al. 1984).

Comparable observations are available for the sympatric species, *Microtus pennsylvanicus*, the meadow vole. Meadow voles are apparently not monogamous and males are believed to mate with more than one female. Males and females do not engage in nest cohabitation and rarely spend time together outside of the actual mating period (Getz et al. 1981; Madison 1980; Gruder-Adams and Getz 1985). Laboratory studies of the meadow vole reveal lower levels of paternal care (Hartung and Dewsbury 1979) and no indications of monogamy.

3 Oestrus Induction: Behavioural Events

Oestrus induction in the intact female prairie vole depends on the presence of a male (Richmond and Conaway 1969), and primarily on pheromonal cues from an unfamiliar male. Using uterine weight as an index of reproductive activation, we have observed (Carter et al. 1980) that either brief (1 h or less) direct physical contact or applications of male urine will induce essentially equivalent increases in uterine weight. (Uterine weights in these animals approx. double.) Visual, auditory, or airborne-olfactory cues from the male are not effective in inducing uterine weight changes.

The uterine changes that follow either the application of male urine or brief male exposure are highly reliable, occurring in most females. However, females treated in this manner do not usually show behavioural receptivity. In order to reliably induce and maintain behavioural oestrus females must receive not only an initial exposure to an unfamiliar male or male urine, but must also be in the continued presence of stimuli from a male. Thus, about 60%–70% of females that are briefly exposed to a male and then placed in a freshly soiled male cage will show behavioural oestrus and increases in uterine weight that are often 3–4 times, or more, greater than those of unstimulated naive females (Carter et al., submitted for publication).

To assess the characteristics of mating interactions in the prairie vole we have found it useful to monitor behaviour using time-lapse videotape. Voles (usually in pairs or small families) are placed together in a plexiglas-fronted semicircular arena (1,645 cm^2 in area), and maintained under a 14-h light, 10-h dark cycle (using red-light which permits taping during the dark phase). Videotape data collected over 12 or 18 h is typically replayed in a 1-h-period for data analysis. Thus, the frequency of behaviours such as male mounting and female lordosis can be efficiently and accurately quantified over a period of several days.

Using time-lapse videotaping we have found that when unfamiliar young male and female prairie voles of approximately 50 days of age are placed together the latency to the onset of mating ranges from about 20–70 h (Fig. 4). Mating bouts, which usually include many mounts and lordosis, often last for periods of over 24 h. Lordosis frequencies average around 124 per 100 h of videotaping. The latency to the onset of copulation and the mount/lordosis frequencies are not dependent on the sexual history of the male, since similar patterns are seen in experienced and inexperienced males. When females are already in oestrus at the time of introduction to the male the patterns

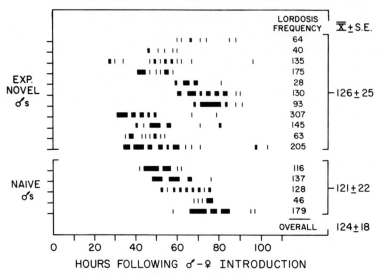

Fig. 4. Time-lapse videotaping data for mating patterns in females in induced oestrus. Unfamiliar males (either sexually experienced or naive) and reproductively inactive (naive) females were paired at the beginning of a 100-h undisturbed taping session. Each *horizontal line* contains data for one pair with *darkened areas* used to indicate periods of relatively uninterrupted mating

of behaviour are similar to those described above, although most pairs will begin to mate within minutes of introduction.

These findings differ somewhat from the description of prairie vole copulatory behaviour by Gray and Dewsbury (1973). Using a "satiety" criterion of 30 min without intromission, the latter authors typically observed only two ejaculations prior to satiety. It seems likely that had Gray and Dewsbury observed their animals over a longer period of time that they would have seen the protracted mating bouts observed in prairie voles in our laboratory (Fig. 4). It is, however, also possible that differences in the reproductive condition or history of the males and/or females they used contributed to the much abbreviated duration of mating reported by Gray and Dewsbury.

4 Incest Avoidance

Suppression of breeding in sibling prairie voles has been reported by Hasler and Nalbandov (1974), Richmond and Stehn (1976), and Batzli et al. (1977). Females living in established families do not typically sniff their father, brothers or other familiar males, and therefore, presumably do not encounter high levels of the activational pheromone.

We have observed that when novel females and males are introduced to each other there is mutual anogenital investigation and contact (Getz and Carter 1980; Gavish et al. 1983). In contrast, even when males and female siblings are disrupted by placing them in a novel area they engage in little or no olfactory investigation.

When male and female siblings are placed together, even in the absence of their parents, they rarely produce litters (6% in comparison to 78% producing litters in non-sibling pairs, McGuire and Getz 1981). Separations of 1 or 2 weeks will overcome the incest avoidance and cross-fostered pups that are maintained together from an early age do not breed (Gavish et al. 1984). When urine from a brother is placed directly on his sister's nose, the incest avoidance may be disrupted and sibling pairs will then breed (Carter et al. 1980). Thus, the major factor regulating the suppression of reproduction in sibling prairie voles is not genetic relatedness. Rather, it appears that siblings, due to familiarity, fail to interact in a manner that would lead to the transfer of pheromones in quantities that are sufficient to *initiate* the physiological changes necessary for oestrus induction.

5 Female-Female Suppression

There appear to be additional factors capable of suppressing reproduction in young prairie voles that remain in their family groups. Getz et al. (1983) found that the presence of another female or female urine prevented or reversed the activational effects of brief male exposure. Uterine weights averaged about 37 mg in females exposed to an unfamiliar male for 1 h, while those of unstimulated females, maintained either alone or with a sibling female, averaged about 17 mg. Male-exposed females that were housed with either another female or that simply received one drop of female urine on their upper lip, immediately following the 1 h male exposure, showed only slight (not statistically significant) increases in uterine weight (averaging between about 21 and 24 mg).

We have also obtained evidence that the reproductive condition of female prairie voles can be inhibited, even after the female is already in behavioural oestrus (Carter et al., unpublished data). In this experiment (Table 3) females were brought into behavioural oestrus and then paired with either another unfamiliar oestrous female, an unfamiliar female that was not in oestrous (naive female) or housed alone. To maintain their oestrous condition each female or pair was maintained in a male-soiled cage which

Table 3. Uterine weights in activated, oestrous females 24 h after exposure to other females or living alone. Dirty cages (male-soiled) were those used to activate the female herself (Own) or the one used to activate another female (Strange). Naive females were not male exposed

♀ Measured	Paired with	Dirty cage	n	X ± S.E. uterine weight
Oestrous	Alone	Own	14	39 ± 3
Oestrous	Alone	Strange	18	32 ± 1.5
Oestrous	Oestrous ♀	Own	15	33 ± 3
Oestrous	Oestrous ♀	Strange	14	32 ± 3
Oestrous	Naive ♀	Own	14	31 ± 3
Naive	Oestrous ♀	Strange	9	15 ± 2

was either the one that had been used to help bring them into oestrus (own dirty cage) or one that had been used to bring another female into oestrus (strange dirty cage). There was a significant decrease in uterine weight measured 24 h after the onset of the pairing with another female. Uterine weight was essentially the same in females housed with other oestrous females or with naive, non-oestrous females and did not vary as a function of the caging condition of the female. (Naive non-oestrous females showed the low uterine weights typical of females that have not been directly exposed to a male). The behavioural oestrus of females in this study was also monitored by periodically testing (4- to 8-h intervals) each female briefly with a freshly screened, highly motivated strange male. Although, there was considerable variability in the duration of behavioural receptivity, the females that lived alone tended to show lordosis for several hours longer than did the paired females.

We are currently using time-lapse videotaping to study the mating patterns of trios composed of one male and two females. In three trios (Fig. 5) in which both females were known to be in oestrus at the onset of testing, neither female mated in one case, only one female mated in a second case and the male mated briefly with one female, then more extensively with the second in the third case. In all cases the cumulative frequency of mating bouts was less than that typical of comparable male-female pairs (Figs. 4, 6). We have also tested six trios in which two reproductively *inactive* females

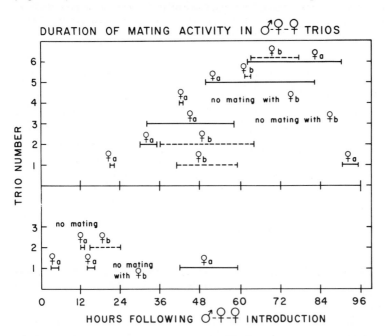

Fig. 5. Time-lapse videotape observations of mating activity duration in trios of one male and two females. In the upper sex trios all females were reproductively inactive when placed with an unfamiliar male. In the lower three trios two oestrous females and one male were placed together at hour 0. Duration of sexual behaviour is represented as a line connecting the first and last mount/lordosis observed. However, in those cases in which mating with a given female stopped for several hours, the line was discontinued until the onset of later mating activity. The female that was mounted first was designated *a*

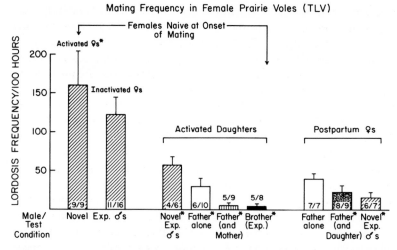

Fig. 6. Time-lapse videotaping (TLV) data summarized as lordosis frequencies in 100 h of taping. Males used for testing females were either novel experienced males (not pair-bonded), or fathers (i.e. paired "breeder" males) or brothers (immediately removed from family groups, screened for mounting behaviour with another oestrous female and thus defined as experienced. *These females were activated and in behavioural oestrus prior to male introduction. Lordosis frequencies are shown as mean ± S.E. for only those females that mated. The ratio enclosed at the base of each *vertical bar* is the number of females that responded over the number tested

were placed with an unfamiliar male (Fig. 5). In 4 of 6 trios both females mated with the male within 4 days, but again the mating directed toward at least one of the females was less extensive than that expected in pairs. The mean frequency of lordosis/mount bouts in the preferred female in these trios was 88 ± 18, and in the non-preferred female, the average bout frequency was 16 ± 9. (Only results from responding females were used to determine these averages and standard errors.) In general, the presence of more than one female seems to disrupt reproductive behaviour in this species.

6 Activated Daughters

We have also looked at the possibility that the mother or other family members may have direct suppressive effects on the young females even after the female is in behavioural oestrus. To examine this possibility, females were allowed to remain with their family groups until about 45 days of age, when they were briefly removed and exposed to an unfamiliar male. Those females that came into behavioural oestrus ("activated" daughters in Fig. 6) were then observed on time-lapse videotape for a 4-day period under one of four different test conditions: Females were tested either with a novel experienced male, alone with their father, alone with an experienced brother (recently screened with another female), or with both their father and mother. A number of these females (Fig. 6) did not continue to mate in spite of having shown at least one clear lordosis posture in a pretest with an experienced male. In those activated daughters that did mate, lordosis frequencies were highest with novel experienced males. However, lordosis frequencies in these females were well below those seen in females that have previously been isolated from their family before attempted activation. Females mated more extensively with their fathers if the mother was not present, but again the frequencies of mount/lordosis bouts was relatively low. Activated females mated infrequently with their father if the mother was present and also only rarely mated with their brothers.

7 Postpartum Oestrus

Postpartum oestrous females (Figs. 6, 7) show markedly less mating behaviour than that seen in young females in induced oestrus (Figs. 4, 6). Videotaping indicates that mating may begin before, during or after the birth of the litter. The average lordosis frequency was 38 and the duration of the mating ranged from a few minutes to, in rare cases, 16 or more h. When females in postpartum oestrus were tested with novel males (in those cases in which they did mate), the lordosis frequency was even lower (Fig. 7) than with an established partner, suggesting that the duration of the mating episode is primarily a function of the female rather than the male. Postpartum oestrous mating may be slightly inhibited by the presence of an oestrous daughter as well.

We have also examined the interactions of postpartum oestrous females and their sons. In general, sons do not attempt to mate with their mothers. We have observed mating in only one of 15 encounters. In 7 of those tests the males were defined as experienced before testing by virtue of their willingness to mount unfamiliar oestrous females just prior to being placed with the mother for videotaping.

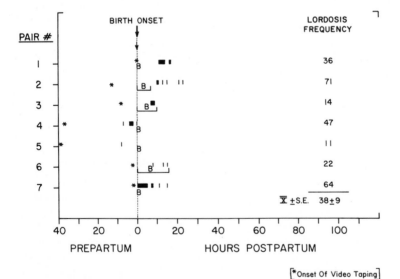

Fig. 7. Time-lapse videotaping data for mating patterns in pre- and postpartum oestrous females. Birth is indicated by *B* and *brackets* ([]) in those cases when birth extended over several hours. Each small *vertical line* or *darkened area* represents lordosis/mount bouts

8 Reproductive Suppression of Young Males

Batzli et al. (1977) have previously observed that body weight and reproduction are suppressed in both males and females when they are held together in sibling groups. Pairing these animals with opposite-sexed strangers caused a rapid acceleration of growth curves and in most cases eventual fertility. Suppression could be prevented or broken by placing animals in an independent air-space or by the physical introduction of a (non-suppressed) stranger of the opposite sex.

In more direct analysis of reproductive suppression in young male prairie voles, we have found evidence for suppression in males maintained in their natal family groups (mother, father, male, and female siblings). For males of approx. 42–45 days of age, on the first day of testing with an oestrous female only 1 male of 27 (less than 4%) showed any mounting behaviour. (Animals were returned to their natal groups between tests.) By the fourth day of testing about 60% of these males were showing mounting behaviour. We have also tested other groups of males that have been reared from weaning in male-sibling groups. These males were maintained in a colony room that contained females. Based on data from several studies of hundreds of males reared in this way, we have observed that about 20% of these males respond to oestrous females on their first exposure.

9 Hormones and Oestrus Induction

Oestrogen primes various tissues responsible for reproduction including sites in the nervous system and uterus. We have shown that oestrogen induces behavioural oestrus, characterized by lordosis, in the female prairie vole (Dluzen and Carter 1979). As little as 1 μg or less of oestradiol benzoate in oil (EB) will induce lordosis in at least some percentage of ovariectomized female voles. In general, however, when testing an unselected group of females we obtain more reliable levels of receptivity with larger doses given in at least two injections. For example, in one experiment (Fig. 8) we found that a single injection of 13.2 μg EB did not induce lordosis (n = 9), and a single initial dose of 52.8 μg EB was effective in only 2 of 7 females. However, 6.6 μg EB given twice (total 13.2 μg EB) elicited lordosis in 7 of 10 females. One explanation for these findings is the possibility that the female vole is relatively unable to respond to her first exposure to oestrogen. To test this possibility we gave each female a second retest 2 to 3 weeks following the first test and using the same hormonal regimen to which they were exposed in the first test. The females that had received a single 13.2 μg EB injection during the initial trial again showed very little responsivity to a second single dose of that level. The females that had received multiple injections of EB on prior tests showed retest behaviour that was also relatively consistent with their initial test. The females that had received the massive 52.8 μg EB injection and were later given a second exposure to that dose of EB did, in fact, show high levels of responding (6 of 7 females) on the retest. These results, taken in conjunction with other experiments in this laboratory, have led us to hypothesize that the increased performance in the 52.8 μg EB retest may have been due, in part, to the presence of residual hormone from the first injection.

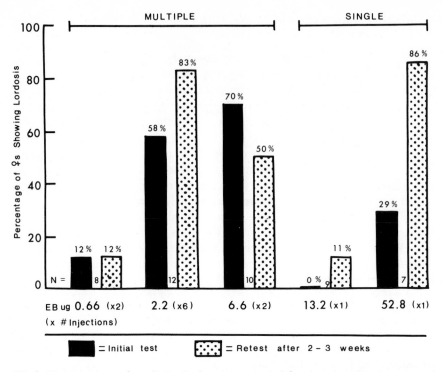

Fig. 8. The percentage of ovariectomized oestrogen-treated females responding to an experienced male with at least one lordosis. Tests shown here were given 48 h after the first oestradiol benzoate *(EB)* injection. Some females received a single injection (×*1*), some two injections, at 24 intervals, (×*2*), and some 6 injections, at 8-h intervals (×*6*). Each female received at least two consecutive 5-min tests. All females were retested 2–3 weeks later using the same dose, number of injections and test schedule they had received in initial testing

Thus, the 52.8 μg EB retest may have functionally reflected a multiple hormone treatment. Alternatively, the first hormone exposure may have produced a long-lasting change in the nervous system. However, the absence of significant or reliable increases in performance in the groups that received lower initial levels of EB (in single or multiple doses) does not support the latter hypothesis. There is evidence for rats that multiple pulses of *free* oestradiol are more effective in priming the nervous system than are single exposures. However, in other species injections of oestradiol benzoate (which is a slowly released form of hormone treatment) are generally adequate to elicit female sexual behaviour in females that subsequently receive progesterone (reviewed Clark and Roy 1983). Additional studies are needed to assess the physiological correspondence or lack of correspondence, among these cross-species comparisons.

As mentioned above, sexual receptivity is most reliably elicited in many rodent species through paradigms that involve an initial exposure to oestrogen followed approximately 24–48 h later by progesterone. We have repeatedly tested female prairie voles in such paradigms (Dluzen and Carter 1979; Carter et al., manuscript in preparation) and have been able to find no evidence to suggest that progesterone is essential for the induction of female sexual behaviour in the prairie vole. In our most recent experiments we primed female voles with suboptimal doses of EB (given twice). These treatments produced low levels of lordosis and should have permitted us to observe improvement, if any were possible, following progesterone treatment. Doses of 0.5 or 2.0 mg progesterone in oil were given to these animals following 48 h of EB priming (0.1, 0.35, or 0.65 μg given twice) and testing was conducted before and at about 4, 8, and 24 h after progesterone. Of 40 females that received progesterone 7 responded initially with lordosis, while 4 of the 23 that received oil showed lordosis. These results indicated that progesterone or oil did not differentially affect female sexual behaviour. In addition, the two doses of progesterone did not differ in their effectiveness.

Progesterone is apparently not essential for the induction of female sexual receptivity (lordosis) in the female prairie vole. However, we have previously observed (Dluzen and Carter 1979) that progesterone can inhibit the expression of lordosis in this species. The inhibitory effects of progesterone are pronounced within 24 h of exposure and there are indications that inhibitory effects of progesterone may appear even earlier in females treated with low doses of oestrogen. Recovery from the inhibitory effects of a single injection of progesterone (0.5 mg in oil) requires one or two days, assuming that oestrogen priming is continued.

Steroid hormones are synthesized in both the ovary and adrenal cortex. Therefore, experiments investigating the behavioural effects of progesterone or oestrogen must always take into account the possibility that adrenal steroids could influence any observed effects. We have also conducted experiments comparing the effectiveness of oestrogen, in both subthreshold and suprathreshold doses in ovariectomized and ovariectomized-adrenalectomized female prairie voles (Table 4). No behavioural differences were observed between groups of females with or without their adrenal glands. We have also examined the ability of adrenalectomized females with ovaries intact to respond to male-related stimuli and come into oestrus. The percentage of females showing oestrus was approximately the same in females following either adrenalectomy or sham-adrenalectomy and both groups were as likely to come into oestrus as unoperated females.

Table 4. The role of the adrenal gland in oestrus-induction in intact or ovariectomized female prairie voles

Treatment	% Oestrus induction	
1. Ovary intact	Male-exposed-natural oestrus	Uterine weight (mg)
Adrenalectomy	60% (9/15)	41 ± 6
SHAM-adrenalectomy	50% (7/14)	37 ± 3
2. Ovary removed	EB (10 μg × 2) induction[a]	Total lordosis duration/600 s
Adrenalectomy (+ OVX)	88% (16/18)	72 ± 13 (all Ss)
		81 ± 3 (+ Ss only)
SHAM-adrenalectomy (+ OVX)	68% (13/19)	57 ± 13 (all Ss)
		83 ± 4 (+ Ss only)

[a] Females selected for this study were ovariectomized and tested once prior to removal of the adrenal or SHAM operation. Only females that showed lordosis on this pretest were used in this study

Our experiments to date provide no evidence for a role for adrenal secretions in either the facilitation or inhibition of female sexual behaviour in this species.

There are reports in the female rat that the polypeptide hormone, luteinizing hormone-releasing hormone (LHRH) can act to enhance sexual receptivity in females primed with suboptimal doses of oestrogen. This facilitation occurs in the absence of progesterone (Moss and McCann 1973, Pfaff 1973). We have also injected (subcutaneously, in saline solution) doses of between 100 and 500 ng LHRH into ovariectomized, oestrogen-primed female voles. In comparison to saline treated females, no significant facilitation was observed following LHRH treatment. However, we have not shown that LHRH is biologically active in female voles treated in this manner. Therefore, we cannot discount the possibility that other doses or treatments of LHRH might have behavioural effects. However, doses of LHRH that are effective in rats are ineffective in prairie voles.

10 Oestrus Induction and Mating: Physiological Events

Exposure to male urine is followed rapidly by a series of physiological changes. For example, within 1 h, and in some cases within one minute following exposure to male urine, we have measured changes in norepinephrine and LHRH in the posterior (but not anterior) portion of the olfactory bulb. Serum levels of luteinizing hormone are also elevated within minutes of urine exposure, but return to unstimulated levels within 1 h following treatment (Dluzen et al. 1981). Preliminary studies of serum oestradiol suggest that a brief male exposure also produces transient increases in oestradiol levels. However, a more prolonged exposure to male pheromones is apparently necessary to initiate the physiological changes that lead to behavioural oestrus (Carter, Getz, and Cohen-Parsons, in press).

We have recently analyzed in greater detail some of the physiological correlates of behavioural oestrus in female prairie voles. Females were exposed to a male for 18 h and then maintained in male-soiled bedding for an additional 30 h to maximize the possibility of oestrus induction without permitting mating. A large number of females treated in this manner did not come into behavioural oestrus (Fig. 9, Activated, Non-oestrus). Females showing at least one lordosis were defined as oestrus (tested without permitting intromission and were then randomly assigned to one of the treatment groups shown in Table 5 and Fig. 9). Some females were left unmated, others were exposed to mating but separated from the male after he had achieved two ejaculations (less than 30 min) and others were permitted to interact and mate without restraint for 24 h. The latter, ad lib matings were monitored by time-lapse videotaping. Females from the unmated groups and from the groups that received two ejaculations were sacrificed at either 1 or 24 h after the onset of testing. The ad lib mating group was sacrificed 24 h from the onset of mating. A control group of inactivated (virgin, non-male-exposed) females was also run. Oestrogen levels (reported as pg mg^{-1} protein) and progesterone levels (reported as ng mg^{-1} protein) were measured by radioimmunoassay in the ovaries. Blood levels of progesterone (ng ml^{-1} serum) and various organ weights (standardized to 30 mg body weight) were also determined.

Ovarian oestrogen levels and uterine weights were lower in inactivated females than in those exposed to a male (Fig. 9). Of the male-exposed females, those that showed

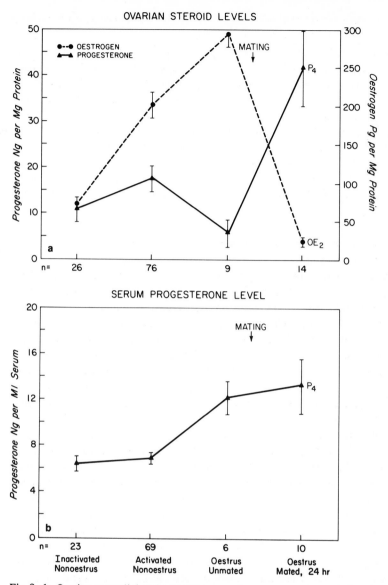

Fig. 9a, b. Ovarian oestradiol and progesterone and serum progesterone in females that were either reproductively inactive (inactivated); male-activated with (in most cases) increases in uterine weight, but not in behavioural oestrus (activated non-oestrus); male-activated, in behavioural oestrus (activated oestrus); or male-activated, in oestrus and then exposed for 24 h to ad lib mating

behavioural oestrus had significantly higher oestrogen levels and uterine weights than those that did not. Ovarian progesterone levels did not differ between inactivated females and nonoestrous (previously male-exposed) females; however, oestrous females had higher levels of serum progesterone and lower levels of ovarian progesterone than nonoestrous females. We cannot say, at present, whether the observed elevations in

Table 5. Steroid hormones, uterine weights, and ovulation in oestrous female prairie voles as a function of mating exposure and time from the onset of mating

Mating exposure	Time from mating onset	Ovarian oestrogen (ng mg^{-1} protein)	Ovarian progesterone (ng mg^{-1} protein)	Serum progesterone (ng ml^{-1})	Uterine weight (mg[a])	Ovulation frequency
None (unmated)	1 h	296 ± 37	6 ± 3	12 ± 2	40 ± 3	0/ 9
None (unmated)	24 h	207 ± 39	3 ± 4	11 ± 2	45 ± 4	0/10
2 Ejaculations	1 h	233 ± 25	5 ± 1	9 ± 1	40 ± 3	0/ 8
2 Ejaculations	24 h	165 ± 16	17 ± 7	7 ± 2	38 ± 4	0/13
Ad lib mating	24 h	25 ± 3	42 ± 9	13 ± 3	35 ± 2	11/14

[a]   Uterine weights were standardized to 30 mg body weight^{-1}

serum progesterone in intact oestrous females play a role in the facilitation of female sexual behaviour. However, in the prairie vole oestrogen alone induced high levels of receptivity (within 48 h). Even following ovariectomy and adrenalectomy, progesterone injections (at least in doses of 0.5 and 2.0 mg) did not produce reliable increases in receptivity (Dluzen and Carter 1979; Carter et al., manuscript in preparation). Our present results, therefore, suggest that any role that progesterone might play in the facilitation of female sexual behaviour in this species is either very minor or can readily be assumed by oestrogen.

These experiments also permitted us to examine the hormonal correlates of exposure to copulatory stimulation. Female prairie voles are reported to be reflex ovulators (Richmond and Conaway 1969) and the results of our experiment confirm this. Ovarian changes indicative of ovulation were observed in 11 of 14 females (Table 5) that remained with a male for 24 h on the day of behavioural oestrus (ad lib mating). For 2 of the 3 females that failed to ovulate, our videotape observations indicated that the mating bouts were unusually short in these pairs. Ovarian hormone levels were significantly different in the ad lib mating group (with or without the inclusion of the non-ovulating females). Ovarian oestrogens dropped and progesterone increased. Serum progesterone levels did not differ significantly from those observed in unmated oestrous females, but were higher than those of females exposed to two ejaculations and sacrificed at a comparable time.

The females exposed to only two ejaculations failed to ovulate. Hormone levels in these females were generally intermediate to those seen in ad lib mated and unmated, oestrous females. Previous research in the prairie vole has reported ovulation following relatively brief mating bouts and in some cases even following a single ejaculation (Gray et al. 1974). The females in our study apparently required more stimulation than those observed by Gray and associates. The reasons for these differences are not known at present, but could reflect the fact that the females used in that earlier study were older, were sexually experienced and/or had a prior history of breeding. Differential amounts of stimulation (intromissions or thrusts) provided by the males prior to ejaculation could have also influenced these results.

We were somewhat surprised to find relatively small increases in serum progesterone, even in those females that had ovulated. In *Microtus montanus*, serum progesterone levels are markedly elevated within one hour following the onset of mating (Gray et al. 1976). The absence of dramatic elevations in circulating progesterone at this time, however, may help to explain our observations of exceptionally long periods of sexual receptivity in female prairie voles, some of which continue to engage in lordosis bouts for periods longer than 24 h. Progesterone release is apparently somewhat slower in this species; perhaps the absence of a progesterone surge retards one of the inhibitory mechanisms thought to regulate the duration of sexual receptivity. In various other species, including the hamster (Carter et al. 1976), Mongolian gerbil (McDermott and Carter 1980), and brown lemming (Huck et al. 1982), the presence of progesterone synergizes with copulatory stimulation to abbreviate the duration of receptivity. Future studies of the prairie vole in our laboratory will examine this interaction in greater detail.

In summary, our results from coordinated field and laboratory studies indicate that many aspects of reproduction in the prairie vole, *Microtus ochrogaster*, show adaptations to a monogamous mating system. Reproduction in this species is regulated by social factors and often by pheromones. The reproductive behaviour of both males and females is suppressed by association with the parents. Physiological mechanisms regulating oestrus induction appear to rely on the continued production of ovarian oestrogens. Progesterone levels increase in oestrous females. However, progesterone is not essential for the induction of behavioural receptivity and may act primarily to inhibit oestrus in this species.

Acknowledgements. Supported by grants from the National Science Foundation (BNS 79-25713 to C.S.C.), the National Institutes of Health (HD 16679 to C.S.C. and HD 09328 to L.L.G.), and a Biomedical Support Grant, BRSG RR-07030. We wish to acknowledge the invaluable contributions of our collaborators and students including Drs. Joyce Hofmann, Janice Bahr, Dean Dluzen, Janet McDermott and Domingo Ramirez, and Diane Witt, Leah Gavish, Steve Manock, Kerry O'Banion, Sharon Spak, Matthew Smith, Julie Schneider, Lisa Casten, Daniel Volkening, James Gitzen, Cynthia Booth, Z. Leah Harris, Robert Chayer, Tiina Auksi, James Lindley, Joseph Balla, Anthony Indovina, Kenneth Adams, Stacie Bosnyak, Susie Davis, Kara Micetich, Reneé Kalinski, Linnea Read, and Jaye Nichols.

References

Batzli GO, Lowell LG, Hurley SS (1977) Suppression of growth and reproduction of microtine rodents by social factors. J Mammal 58:583–591

Carter CS, Landauer MR, Tierney BH, Jones T (1976) Regulation of female sexual behavior in the golden hamster: behavioral effects of mating and ovarian hormones. J Comp Physiol Psychol 90:839–950

Carter CS, Getz LL, Gavish L, McDermott JL, Arnold P (1980) Male-related pheromones and the activation of female reproduction in the prairie vole *(Microtus ochrogaster)*. Biol Reprod 23: 1038–1045

Carter CS, Getz LL, Cohen-Parsons M (in press) Social organization and behavioral endocrinology in a monogamous mammal. Advances in the Study of Behavior

Carter CS, Witt DM, Schneider J, Harris ZL, Volkening D (submitted for publication) Natural estrus induction in the prairie vole *(Microtus ochrogaster)*

Clark AS, Roy EJ (1983) Behavioral and cellular responses to pulses of low doses of estradiol-17B. Physiol Behav 30:561–565

Dluzen DE, Carter CS (1979) Ovarian hormones regulating sexual and social behaviors in female prairie voles, *Microtus ochrogaster*. Physiol Behav 23:597–600

Dluzen DE, Ramirez VD, Carter CS, Getz LL (1981) Male vole urine changes luteinizing hormone-releasing hormone and norepinephrine in female olfactory bulb. Science (Wash DC) 212:573–575

Fuentes SM, Dewsbury DA (1984) Copulatory behavior in voles (*Microtus montanus* and *M. ochrogaster*) in multiple-female test situations. J Comp Physiol Psychol 98:45–53

Gavish L, Carter CS, Getz LL (1981) Further evidence for monogamy in the prairie vole. Anim Behav 29:955–957

Gavish L, Carter CS, Getz LL (1983) Male-female interactions in prairie voles. Anim Behav 31:511–517

Gavish L, Hofmann JE, Getz LL (1984) Sibling recognition in the prairie vole, *Microtus ochrogaster*. Anim Behav 32:362–366

Getz LL (1978) Speculation on social structure and population cycles of microtine rodents. Biologist 60:134–147

Getz LL, Carter CS (1980) Social organization in *Microtus ochrogaster* populations. Biologist 62:56–69

Getz LL, Carter CS, Gavish L (1981) The mating system of the prairie vole, *Microtus ochrogaster*: field and laboratory evidence for pair-bonding. Behav Ecol Sociobiol 8:189–194

Getz LL, Dluzen D, McDermott JL (1983) Suppression of reproductive maturation in male-stimulated virgin female *Microtus* by a female urinary chemosignal. Behav Processes 8:59–64

Gray GD, Dewsbury DA (1973) A quantitative description of copulatory behavior in prairie voles *(Microtus ochrogaster)*. Brain Behav Evol 8:437–452

Gray GD, Zerylnick M, Davis HN, Dewsbury DA (1974) Effects of variations in male copulatory behavior on ovulation and implanation in prairie voles, *Microtus ochrogaster*. Horm Behav 5:389–396

Gray GD, Davis HN, Kenney AMCM, Dewsbury DA (1976) Effect of mating on plasma levels of LH and protesterone in montane voles *(Microtus montanus)*. J Reprod Fertil 47:89–91

Gruder-Adams S, Getz LL (1985) Comparison of the mating system and parental behavior in *Microtus ochrogaster* and *M. pennsylvanicus*. J Mammal 66:165–167

Hartung TG, Dewsbury DA (1979) Paternal behavior in six species of muroid rodents. Behav Neural Biol 26:466–478

Hasler MJ, Nalbandov AV (1974) The effect of weanling and adult males on sexual maturation in female voles *(Microtus ochrogaster)*. Gen Comp Endocrinol 23:237–238

Hofmann JE, Getz LL, Gavish L (1984) Home range overlap and nest cohabitation of male and female prairie voles. Am Midl Nat 112:314–319

Huck UW, Carter CS, Banks EM (1982) Natural or hormone induced sexual and social behaviors in the female brown lemming, *Lemmus trimucronatus*. Horm Behav 16:199–207

Kleiman D (1977) Monogamy in mammals. Q Rev Biol 52:39–69

Madison DM (1980) An integrated view of the social biology of *Microtus pennsylvanicus*. Biologist 62:20–33

McDermott JL, Carter CS (1980) Ovarian hormones, copulatory stimuli and female sexual behavior in the Mongolian gerbil. Horm Behav 14:211–223

McGuire MR, Getz LL (1981) Incest taboo between sibling *Microtus ochrogaster*. J Mammal 62:213–215

Moss RL, McCann SM (1973) Induction of mating behavior in rats by luteinizing hormone-releasing factor. Science (Wash DC) 181:177–179

Pfaff DW (1973) Luteinizing hormone-releasing factor potentiates lordosis behavior in hypophysectomized ovariectomized female rats. Science (Wash DC) 182:1148–1149

Richmond ME, Conaway CH (1969) Induced ovulation and oestrus in *Microtus ochrogaster*. J Reprod Fert Suppl 6:357–376

Richmond M, Stehn R (1976) Olfaction and reproductive behavior in microtine rodents. In: Doty RL (ed) Mammalian olfaction, reproductive processes and behavior. Academic, New York, pp 197–217

Thomas JA, Birney EC (1979) Parental care and mating system of the prairie vole, *Microtus ochrogaster*. Behav Ecol Sociobiol 5:171–186

Hormones and the Sexual Behaviour of Monkeys

E. B. KEVERNE[1]

1 Introduction

The sexual behaviour of monkeys is very different from that of non-primate species in that it is, to a large extent, emancipated from gonadal control. Female monkeys when paired daily in the laboratory with the male do not show true periodic oestrous behaviour but are prepared to receive the male throughout their menstrual cycle (Michael and Welegalla 1968), and for long periods even following ovariectomy (Michael and Zumpe 1970). Indeed, female solicitations to the males, an index of their willingness to mate, increase after ovariectomy (Zumpe and Michael 1970), a finding in marked contrast to many rodent species. Sexual interactions with the male do, however, vary during the menstrual cycle, being more frequent in the follicular phase especially around mid-cycle for a number of primate species (Talapoin – Scruton and Herbert 1970; Patas monkey – Rowell and Hartwell 1978; Pigtail macaque – Tokuda et al. 1968; Eaton and Resko 1974; Chacma baboon – Saayman 1970; Gelada baboon – Dunbar 1978; Gorilla – Nadler 1975a; Chimpanzee – Tutin 1980; Macaca fascicularis – Zumpe and Michael 1983). Paradoxically, the females solicitations to the male may be very low at this time, and most of the changes in sexual interactions in relationship to the menstrual cycle can be accounted for by changes in female attractiveness (Keverne 1976).

In the male monkey, castration has little effect on sexual behaviour in the short term. Males may continue to show sexual interest and mount females even years after castration (Phoenix 1976). Ejaculations cease within 5–10 weeks after castration, and likewise are restored after the same time period with testosterone replacement (Michael and Wilson 1973). It is difficult to reconcile these behavioural changes which take place over such a prolonged time period with an CNS action of testosterone (Resko and Phoenix 1972). A careful analysis of the behavioural data indicates that a major problem for the male following castration is intromission, and unintromitted thrusts increase dramatically some 5–10 weeks after castration (Michael and Wilson 1973). Moreover, this patterning of male behaviour has much in common with that of males that have received section of the dorsal nerve of the penis (Herbert 1973), a finding which is indicative of testosterone acting peripherally. Atrophy of sensory spines following castration may, therefore, be the principal way in which testosterone affects the behavioural interaction in male monkeys.

---

1 Department of Anatomy, University of Cambridge, Downing Street, Cambridge, CB2 3DY, United Kingdom

Neurobiology
(ed. by R. Gilles and J. Balthazart)
© Springer-Verlag Berlin Heidelberg 1985

The most significant influence on sexual behaviour in monkeys is the social environment. For the past 12 years our laboratory has focussed attention on the way in which the social status of an individual has consequences for both its behaviour and endocrine state. This we have achieved by studying social groups (3–5 males with 4–6 females) of Talapoin monkeys housed in large laboratory cages. The cages were partitioned in such a way that males and females could see each other, but were only given physical access twice daily for 50 min when behavioural interactions were scored (see Keverne et al. 1978a). Plasma and CSF samples were collected twice weekly for assay of hormone and amine transmitter metabolites (see Yodyingyuad et al. 1984).

2 Social Constraints on Mating

2.1 Males

Among such social groups, dominance was determined from the direction of aggressive interactions, and not the amount of aggression. More often than not, the dominant male in the group was not the most aggressive. However the dominant male in the group was always the most sexually active, often to the exclusion of all other males (Fig. 1). Intermediate ranking males often showed interest in the females but rarely overt sexual behaviour terminating in ejaculation, while subordinate males were totally excluded from females and never showed sexual interest, in groups once the hierarchy had been firmly established.

One endocrine consequence of social rank in males is differential changes in plasma testosterone. This increases some 200%–300% in dominant males on moving into the social group, while subordinate males show no such increases in testosterone, and in some cases it may decrease (Fig. 2) (Eberhart et al. 1980a). The question arises, therefore, as to whether these increases in testosterone may account for the differences seen

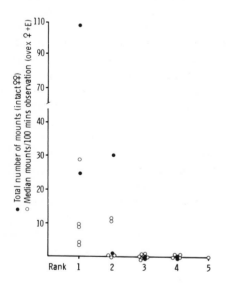

Fig. 1. Distribution of sexual behaviour according to male rank. *Closed circles* are total mounts during a 3-week period of observations for males grouped with intact females. *Open circles* are medians for intact males with ovariectomized females given oestrogen implants, hence ensuring a number of attractive females available to males

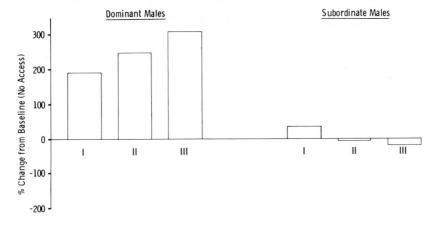

Fig. 2. Percentage changes in plasma testosterone in males of three different groups when they are given access to females. Only dominant, sexually active males show increases in plasma testosterone

in sexual behaviour of dominant males. Studies performed with castrate males would suggest this is not the case, since castrated dominant males continue to show sexual interest in females and remain dominant, and while administration of testosterone enhances the sexual behaviour of dominant males, it is without such effects in subordinates (Dixson and Herbert 1977; Eberhart et al. 1980b). Even supra-physiological doses of testosterone in subordinate males is without consequences for their sexual behaviour, although the aggression they receive may increase.

Aggressive behaviour, or at least the threat of potential aggression, may be of some importance for restricting the sexual behaviour of subordinates. As a consequence of their low status they show increased withdrawals, increased visual monitoring (Keverne et al. 1978b), and have restricted use of cage space (Keverne et al. 1978a). Moreover, the stress hormones cortisol and prolactin increase differentially in dominant and subordinate males (Eberhart et al. 1983). Whereas prolactin increases acutely in subordinates and remains high, cortisol may increase acutely in all males during group formation, but when groups are established, cortisol decreases in dominant males and increases in subordinates (Fig. 3). Moreover these high levels of cortisol persist for some weeks in subordinates, even after they are removed from the group. Hence the chronic effects of social subordination appear to carry over into other non-social situations. This not only applies to the so called "stress" hormones, but also to sexual behaviour itself. Males that have experienced chronic social subordination, when given the opportunity to interact with females in the absence of other more dominant males fail to do so at all adequately (Keverne et al. 1982b). Out of six social groups studied, only one subordinate male was sexually active, and all of this males sexual behaviour was initiated by females. Not all males were tested for sexual behaviour prior to group formation, but of those that were, sexual behaviour was high prior to their becoming subordinate. This would suggest there is no obvious predisposition for subordinance to be correlated with sexual inactivity. Males that became dominant showed enhancement of their sexual behaviour in the social group, and while removing subordinates reduced the sexual interactions of dominant males with females, they still continued to show sexual behaviour, unlike those males that had experienced social subordination.

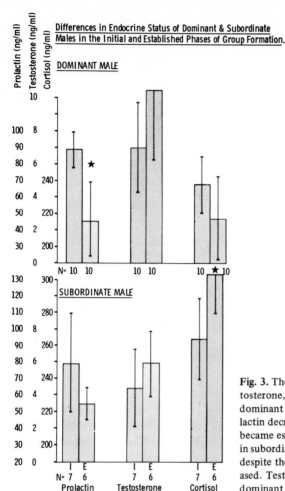

Fig. 3. The changes which occur in plasma testosterone, cortisol, and prolactin differ between dominant and subordinate males over time. Prolactin decreased in dominant males as the group became established (*E*) while cortisol increased in subordinates as the group became established, despite the fact that aggressive behaviour decreased. Testosterone was significantly higher in dominant than subordinate males. * P < 0.01

Although testosterone levels increased in subordinates when they were with females in the absence of other males, so too did their stress hormones, cortisol, and prolactin (Keverne et al. 1982a). These hormones increased when males that had experienced social subordination were housed with females, despite the fact that aggression they received was substantially and significantly reduced, and was no different from that of males that had experienced social dominance in the same situation (Eberhart et al. 1984).

Clearly then, learning or the behavioural experiences associated with social subordination play a large part, at least in the short term, in determining the sexual inactivity of males. Because of mortality and the greater incidence of mobility among dominant males, subordination may only be a transient phase in the life of these monkeys in their natural habitat. Nevertheless, the restrictions on sexual activity in subordinates seen in these captive studies would, by reducing their competition with dominant males, decrease the constant need for overt violence and aggression. Subordinates themselves would, by remaining in the social group, gain the benefits of food and protection against predators but only, at a cost in the short term to their reproductive potential.

A question that remains unanswered, however, is the neuroendocrine mechanism by which subordinates become sexually inhibited. The changes in testosterone associated with social status are not in themselves causally related to these events, nor are the elevated levels of prolactin, since reducing these levels of prolactin by treatment with bromocriptine is without effect on the sexual behaviour of subordinates. Recent studies would implicate the β-endorphin system of the limbic brain. This has a well-recognized inhibitory action on sexual behaviour in rodents and in the subordinate Talapoin monkey CSF levels of this transmitter are significantly elevated. Moreover, treatment of dominant males with the μ-receptor agonist, morphine, in low doses ($2\ \mu\mathrm{g\ kg}^{-1}$), inhibits their sexual behaviour, decreases testosterone and increases prolactin giving them a similar endocrine as well as the behavioural profile, to that of subordinates.

2.2 Females

Among female Talapoin monkeys the social hierarchy also has consequences for sexual behaviour, although these are not so marked as among the males. Low ranking females may not engage in as much sexual activity as dominant females, but they are not totally excluded (Fig. 4), and have potential to conceive. This difference seen in the sexual behaviour of subordinate females compared with its complete absence in subordinate males is related to different behavioural strategies shown by the sexes.

Males display very high levels of intrasexual aggression, while intrasexual aggression among females is very low (Fig. 5). Affiliative behaviours such as huddling and grooming are comparatively low among males but are observed frequently among females. Moreover, when males are allowed to interact with females, male intrasexual aggression

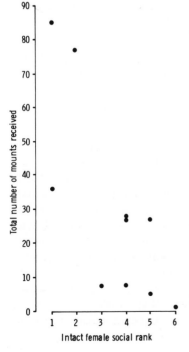

Fig. 4. Distribution of sexual behaviour according to female rank. All females with the exception of rank 6 received sexual mounts but the frequency was greater for higher ranking females

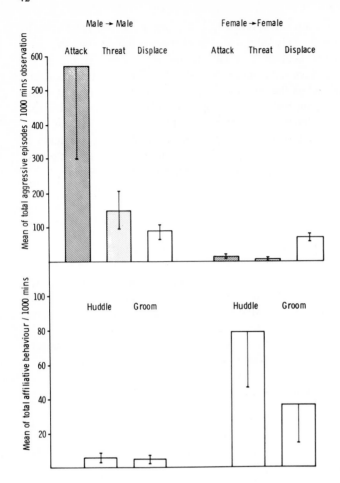

Fig. 5. Intrasexual aggressive behaviour, especially attacks and threats is significantly higher (P < 0.001) among males than among females. Displace, a mild form of assertiveness is not significantly different among males versus females. Affiliative behaviours are significantly higher among females than among males (P < 0.001)

increases, but decreases in females. Because affiliative behaviours are high and intense aggression (attacks, threats) is low among females, there is little physical restraint on the sexual behaviour of subordinate females. Indeed, the major strategy employed by dominant females to restrict the sexual activity of subordinates is quite different from that of males. When subordinates solicit males, the dominant female either distracts male attention by counter soliciting or, occasionally disrupts the interaction by threatening or mounting the female (Fig. 6). Hence, when subordinate females are removed from the influence of dominant females there is no carry over effect. Their soliciting behaviour followed by inspects and mounts received from males is no different from that of females that have experienced social dominance (Fig. 7). Moreover, they now initiate and receive high levels of sexual interaction without concomitant increases in the so called "stress hormones".

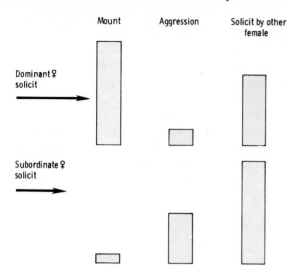

Fig. 6. Frequency of behaviours most likely to follow soliciting behaviour (number reflected by length of *arrow*) by the females differs according to rank. When dominant females solicit the most likely behaviour to follow is a mount. When subordinate females solicit, the most likely behaviour to follow is competitive soliciting from other females

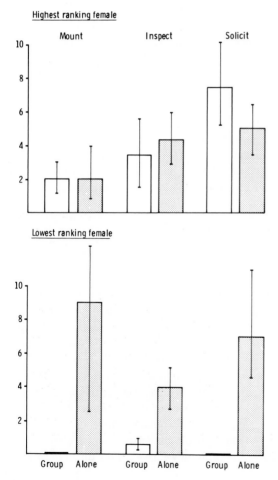

Fig. 7. Distribution of sexual behaviour (mean ± S.D.) of dominant (*above*) and subordinate (*below*) females in the social group (*group*) and in the absence of other females (*alone*) when oestrogen treated. Although subordinates do not solicit and are not attractive to males in the group, no "carry over" of this inhibition occurs in the absence of other females when sexual behaviour is no different from that of dominant females in the same situation

3 Brain Mechanisms Underlying Social Constraints

It would appear that many of the behavioural differences that we observe among males with respect to the social hierarchy cannot be accounted for purely in terms of changing gonadal hormone secretion. Neural mechanisms have to be invoked. Although at the present time little can be said as to what these neural mechanisms are which underlie these differences in behaviour brought about by the social environment, we have started to focus attention on the brains opiate system. We have therefore begun to investigate drugs which act on these neural systems and consider the consequences for behaviour and endocrine state in social groups of monkeys. High ranking males treated with the opiate antagonist naltrexone show a significant inhibition of sexual behaviour, a deficit that does not recover rapidly after withdrawal of the drug (Meller et al. 1980). Low ranking males do not show enhancement of sexual behaviour on treatment with naltrexone. Opiate receptor blockade does not alter aggression, but a consistent effect of the drug is to cause a marked increase in grooming invitations, and hence grooming behaviour, irrespective of rank and in both males and females (Fabre-Nys et al. 1982).

In addition to its behavioural effects, naltrexone has marked effects on hormone levels, which occurs independently of social rank and is consistent even among animals living in social isolation. In most males, cortisol, LH, testosterone, and prolactin increase on administration of opiate receptor blockers. This happens independently of the behavioural effects of opiate blockade, which require higher drugs dosage. Such a separation of endocrine and behavioural effects of opiate receptor blockade is essential to our interpretation of how the endogenous opiates may influence or be influenced by behaviour. Clearly, the behavioural effects are not secondary to endocrine changes since sex behaviour declines when testosterone increases.

We have recently been measuring in the CSF, 5HIAA (a metabolite of 5HT) and HVA (a metabolite of dopamine). A consistent finding has been the increased levels of 5HIAA but not HVA seen in those male monkeys which on moving into the group become socially subordinate (Yodyingyuad et al. 1984). Interestingly, a similar increase in CSF 5HIAA can be induced in non-subordinate monkeys living in social isolation by treatment with the opiate receptor blocker, naltrexone.

Hence, the data we have collected from monkeys living socially suggests that subordination has much in common at the behavioural, neuroendocrine, and neural levels with non-subordinate monkeys treated with the opiate receptor blockers naloxone or naltrexone. In many respects this finding is counter-intuitive since the prediction might be for increased opiate activity in monkeys under social stress. Indeed our studies on the CSF of subordinate monkeys show them to have higher levels of β-endorphin than their dominant cage mates. Moreover, the opiate agonist, morphine has many actions in common with the drug naloxone when given to grouped monkeys. It too increases prolactin, and decreases sexual behaviour in dominant males. This similarity in the action of opiate agonists and antagonists is difficult to understand at the present time without involving changes in receptors as a consequence of drug treatment, or mixed antagonist/agonist actions of the drug naloxone. Unfortunately these drugs are not specific to one receptor type and hence their systemic administration will effect both the β-endorphin and enkephalin systems. Hence, until we have a more direct means of manipulating specific parts of these opiate systems, the current interpretations of these data are plagued with problems.

4 Conclusions

In many primate groups, high ranking males are sexually more active (Carpenter 1942; Kaufman 1965; Bernstein 1976; Harcourt and Stewart 1977) and may leave more offspring than low ranking males (Smith 1981). The experiments reviewed here also show that in social groups of talapoin monkeys, sexual behaviour is not evenly distributed among all members of the group, but is related to the status of that individual in the groups aggressive hierarchy (Eberhart et al. 1980a). Moreover, this status has consequences for plasma levels of gonadal hormones. The teasing apart of the significance of gonadal factors from social factors in determining the sexual behaviour of monkeys in their social groups is, therefore, a difficult task. It is clear from laboratory studies involving heterosexual pairs of monkeys that gonadal steroids are necessary for normal levels of sexual behaviour to occur (Michael 1972; Keverne 1976). However, in the social context the role of the sex hormones is less obvious and an individuals position in the social hierarchy is all important. Even castrate males may be dominant and show some sexual behaviour (Dixson and Herbert 1977), while treating subordinate castrates with high doses of testosterone does not restore their sexual behaviour. Indeed, social subordination inhibits the sexual behaviour of males more rapidly and profoundly than does castration of males in heterosexual pair tests. A question of some importance is, therefore, the biological significance of changes in gonadal steroids in relationship to the social hierarchy. In dominant males with marked increases in plasma testosterone we observe high levels of sexual performance, and dominant males receive the highest levels of sexual invitations from females (Keverne 1979). It is possible, therefore, that the high testosterone of dominant males may enhance their arousal and perception of females, as well as attractiveness to females, while subordinates would remain unattractive and so reduce the aggression they might otherwise provoke from the dominant males. Such endocrine differences in responsiveness might be viewed as part of the subordinate males adaptation to minimise the cost of staying in a social group, while maintaining the potential for reproduction should the opportunity arise.

What emerges most clearly from these studies is the finding that chronic social stress may have marked consequences for plasma cortisol, prolactin, and sexual behaviour which carry over to situations lacking in social restraints. The linking of this behaviour to some neural mechanism which brings about subsequent endocrine changes is currently under investigation and appears to involve the brain's endogenous opiate system.

Acknowledgements. I am grateful to Helen Shiers and Kathy Batty for their excellent technical assistance with radioimmunoassays, and to the help and constructive criticism of my colleague Joe Herbert. The LH for iodination were prepared by Dr. L.E. Reichert and obtained through NIAMDD. The LH antiserum was supplied by Dr. G.D. Niswender. The prolactin standard was obtained from the MRC and the prolactin for iodination from Dr. P.S. Lowry. The prolactin antiserum was a gift from Dr. H.Friesen. These studies form part of a 5-year programme of research supported by MRC and would not have been possible without the help of Dave Abbott, Usannee Yodyingyuad, Claude Fabre-Nys, Jerry Eberhart and Rachel Meller.

References

Bernstein IS (1976) Dominance, aggression and reproduction in primate societies. J Theor Biol 60: 459–472

Carpenter CR (1942) Social behaviour of free-ranging rhesus monkeys *(Macaca mulatta)* I. Specimens, procedures and behavioural characteristics of estrus. J Comp Physiol Psychol 33:133–142

Dixson AF, Herbert J (1977) Gonadal hormones and sexual behaviour in groups of adult talapoin monkeys *(Miopithecus talapoin)*. Horm Behav 8:141–154

Dunbar RIM (1978) Sexual behaviour and social relationships among gelada baboons. Anim Behav 26:167–178

Eaton GG, Resko JA (1974) Ovarian hormones and sexual behaviour of *Macaca nemestrina*. J Comp Physiol Psychol 86:919–925

Eberhart JA, Keverne EB, Meller RE (1980a) Social influences on plasma testosterone levels in male talapoin monkeys. Horm Behav 14:247–266

Eberhart JA, Herbert J, Keverne EB, Meller RE (1980b) Some hormonal aspects of primate social behaviour. In: Endocrinology. Australian Academy of Sciences, Melbourne, pp 622–625

Eberhart JA, Keverne EB, Meller RE (1983) Social influences on circulating levels of cortisol and prolactin in male talapoin monkeys. Physiol Behav 30:361–369

Eberhart JA, Yodyingyuad U, Keverne EB (1984, in press) Subordination in male talapoin monkeys has consequences for sexual behaviour that persist in the absence of dominants. Physiol Behav

Fabre-Nys C, Meller RE, Keverne EB (1982) Opiate antagonists stimulate affiliative behaviour in monkeys. Pharmacol Biochem Behav 16:653–660

Harcourt SA, Stewart KJ (1977) Apes, sex and societies. New Sci 76:160–162

Herbert J (1973) The role of the dorsal nerves of the penis in the sexual behaviour of the male rhesus monkey. Physiol Behav 10:293–300

Kaufman JH (1965) A three year study of mating behaviour in a free-ranging band of rhesus monkeys. Ecology 46:500–512

Keverne EB (1976) Sexual receptivity and attractiveness in the female rhesus monkey. Adv Study Behav 7:155–200

Keverne EB (1979) Sexual and aggressive behaviour in social groups of talapoin monkeys. In: Sex, hormones and behaviour. CIBA Symp 62 (new series). Excerpta Medica, Amsterdam, pp 271–286

Keverne EB, Meller RE, Martinez-Arias AM (1978a) Dominance, aggression and sexual behaviour in social groups of talapoin monkeys. In: Chivers DJ, Herbert J (eds) Recent advances in primatology, vol 1. Academic, New York, pp 533–548

Keverne EB, Leonard RA, Scruton DM, Young SK (1978b) Visual monitoring in social groups of talapoin monkeys *(Miopithecus talapoin)*. Anim Behav 26:933–944

Keverne EB, Eberhart JA, Meller RE (1982a) Dominance and subordination concepts or physiological states? In: Advanced views in primate biology. Springer, Berlin Heidelberg New York, pp 81–94

Keverne EB, Meller RE, Eberhart JA (1982b) Social influences on behaviour and neuroendocrine responsiveness in Talapoin monkeys. Scand J Psychol Suppl 1:37–47

Meller RE, Keverne EB, Herbert J (1980) Behavioural and endocrine effects of naltrexone in male talapoin monkeys. Pharmacol Biochem Behav 13:663–672

Michael RP (1972) Determinants of primate reproductive behaviour. In: Diczfalusy E, Standley CC (eds) The use of non-human primates in research in human reproduction. WHO publication, Karolinska Institute, pp 322–362

Michael RP, Wellegalla J (1968) Ovarian hormones and the sexual behaviour of the female rhesus monkey *(Macaca mulatta)* under laboratory conditions. J Endocrinol 41:407–420

Michael RP, Wilson M (1973) Effects of castration and hormone replacement in fully adult male rhesus monkeys *(Macaca mulatta)*. Endocrinology 95:150–159

Michael RP, Zumpe D (1970) Sexual initiating behaviour by female rhesus monkeys *(Macaca mulatta)* under laboratory conditions. Behaviour 36:168–186

Nadler RD (1975a) Sexual cyclicity in captive lowland gorillas. Sciences (NY) 189:813–814

Phoenix CH (1976) Sexual behaviour of castrated male rhesus monkeys treated with 19-hydroxy-testosterone. Physiol Behav 16:305–310

Phoenix CH, Slob AK, Goy RW (1973) Effects of castration and replacement therapy on sexual behaviour of adult male rhesuses. J Comp Physiol Psychol 84:472–481

Resko JA, Phoenix CH (1972) Sexual behaviour and testosterone concentrations in the plasma of the rhesus monkey before and after castration. Endocrinology 91:499–503

Rowell TE, Hartwell KM (1978) The interaction of behaviour and reproductive cycles in patas monkeys. Behav Biol 24:141–167

Saayman GS (1970) The menstrual cycle and sexual behaviour in a troop of free-ranging Chacma baboons (Papio ursinus). Folia Primatol 12:81–110

Scruton DM, Herbert J (1970) The menstrual cycle and its effect upon behaviour in the talapoin monkey *(Miopithecus talapoin)*. J Zool (Lond) 162:419–436

Smith DG (1981) The association between rank and reproductive success of male rhesus monkeys. J Endocrinol 52:ii (abstract)

Tokuda K, Simms RC, Jensen JD (1968) Sexual behaviour in a captive group of pigtail macaques *(Macaca nemestrina)*. Primates 9:283–294

Tutin CEG (1980) Reproductive behaviour of wild chimpanzees in the Gombe National Park, Tanzania. J Reprod Fertil Suppl 28:43–57

Wilson M, Plant TM, Michael RP (1972) Androgens and the sexual behaviour of male rhesus monkeys. J Endocrinol 52:ii (abstract)

Yodyingyuad U, de la Riva C, Abbott DH, Herbert J, Keverne EB (1984) Relationship between dominance hierarchy, CSF levels of amine transmitter metabolites (5 HIAA and HVA) and plasma control in monkeys. Neuroscience (in press)

Zumpe D, Michael RP (1970) Ovarian hormones and female sexual invitations in captive rhesus monkeys. Anim Behav 18:293–301

Zumpe D, Michael RP (1979) Relation between the hormonal status of the female and direct aggression by male rhesus monkeys *(Macaca mulatta)*. Horm Behav 12:269–279

Zumpe D, Michael RP (1983) A comparison of the behaviour of *M. fascicularis* and *M. mulatta* in relation to the menstrual cycle. Am J Primatol 4:55–72

Mechanisms of Androgen-Activated Sexual Behaviour in Rats

P. SÖDERSTEN[1], P. ENEROTH[2], A. MODE[3], and J.-Å. GUSTAFSSON[3]

1 Introduction

The normal pattern of androgen secretion by the rat testis and its relationship to the display of sexual behaviour will be described here. The influence of some androgen metabolites and inhibitors of androgen metabolism on behavioural responses will be discussed. An alternative to the popular view that oestradiol-17β(OE) is the physiological stimulator of sexual behaviour will be presented.

2 Androgenic Control of Sexual Behaviour

Testosterone (T) is the main androgen produced by the testis (Nieschlag 1979). Due to the episodic pattern of T secretion by the testis the concentration of androgen in the blood of male mammals varies considerably during the day (Lincoln and Short 1980). Thus, the level of androgen in the serum of intact male rats can increase several-fold within a short period of time (Fig. 1; Ellis and Desjardins 1982; Södersten and Eneroth 1980, 1983; Södersten et al. 1983). Pulses of androgen in the blood of male rats are invariably preceded by one or more pulses of luteinizing hormone (LH) (Fig. 1; Ellis and Desjardins 1982; Södersten et al. 1983). Castration of male rats is followed by a T-reversible increase in both the frequency and amplitude of the LH pulses and it

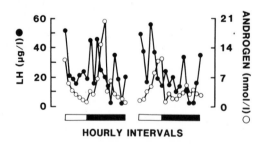

Fig. 1. Pulsatile secretion of *LH* and androgen in two male rats bled at hourly intervals. *Black bars* on the abscissa indicate the dark part of the LD cycle

1 Department of Psychiatry, Karolinska Institutet, 141 86 Huddinge, Sweden
2 Research and Development Laboratories, Karolinska Institutet, 104 01 Stockholm, Sweden
3 Department of Medical Nutrition, Karolinska Institutet, 141 86 Huddinge, Sweden

Neurobiology
(ed. by R. Gilles and J. Balthazart)
© Springer-Verlag Berlin Heidelberg 1985

seems likely that T acts both on the brain and pituitary gland to reduce LH pulse frequency and amplitude in the intact male (Steiner et al. 1982). Since LH pulsatility is a reflection of the episodic secretion of LH-releasing hormone (LHRH) by the brain (Ellis et al. 1983) it must be assumed that T acts on the LHRH producing neurons in the brain to control the episodic secretion of LH by the pituitary gland. We do not know what influence, if any, the episodic secretion of T by the rat testis has on the LHRH pulse generator in the brain.

Similarly, the possible influence of the episodic secretion of T on sexual behaviour is unknown. Although short-latency effects of T on sexual behaviour have been demonstrated (Malmnäs 1977), maintenance of constant levels of serum T, through implantation of T-filled constant-release implants, maintains the sexual behaviour of castrated rats at a normal level (Damassa et al. 1977) and injections of T into castrated, T-implanted rats have no effects on their sexual behaviour (Södersten et al. 1980). A remarkably low level of serum T (somewhat less than 10% of intact levels) is sufficient for maintenance of the behaviour for at least 2 months after castration (Damassa et al. 1977). Furthermore, T implants which produce serum androgen levels of about 15% of the intact level, activate the sexual behaviour of sexually inactive castrated rats within 2 days (Södersten et al. 1985). This contrasts to the comparative behavioural inefficacy of conventional injections of free or esterified T. Injections of T in doses which are required for activation of behavioural responses in castrated rats produce extremely high levels of serum T (several 1,000% of intact levels), but these rapidly decline to low levels (Södersten et al. 1980). The rapid fall and disappearance of androgen from the circulation following T injections is the reason for the inefficacy of such injections in inducing sexual behaviour (Södersten et al. 1980). Thus, continuous maintenance of a basal, lower than normal, level of serum androgen is sufficient for display of a normal pattern of sexual behaviour in male rats (Södersten et al. 1980).

T is taken up by passive diffusion across the membranes of nerve cells and is extensively and rapidly metabolized by neurons (McEwen 1981). The rat has no peripheral sex steroid-binding protein (Murphy 1968) and it seems likely therefore, that the brain of both intact and castrated T-injected animals is exposed to very high levels of androgen within short periods of time. Intraneuronal androgen metabolism may serve two purposes: formation of behaviourally active metabolites such as OE, and formation of inactive metabolites such as 17β-hydroxy-5α-androstan-3-one (5α-dihydrotestosterone, DHT). Formation of DHT in the brain may not be required for display of sexual behaviour by rats (Luttge 1979) but, considering the absence of a peripheral sex steroid-binding protein (Murphy 1968), 5α-reduction of T may serve to protect the brain from exposure to excessive amounts of androgen. The possible behavioural consequences of stimulation with high, supra-physiological doses of T are unknown.

Some problems with the current view that intracerebral aromatization is required for display of sexual behaviour by male rats and that 5α-reduction is not utilized by the rat brain in the control of the behaviour (Luttge 1979) will be considered here. Procedures for the measurement of hormones and behaviour and for hormone treatments have been described in the original papers.

3 Induction of Sexual Behaviour in Castrated Rats
by Combined Oestradiol-Dihydrotestosterone Treatment

Initial attempts to induce sexual behaviour in castrated rats with OE used unreasonably high, in all probability unphysiological, doses of oestradiol benzoate (OB, 50–100 μg; Davidson 1969; Södersten 1973). In view of the possible involvement of adrenal or other, androgens in the effects of high OB doses on male sexual behaviour (Luttge 1979) and the fact that OE interacts with the androgen receptor in the brain (Sheridan 1983) these results may be of limited interest. However, OE can control the sexual behaviour of rats in other ways than by acting as a direct stimulator.

Figure 2 shows that in prepuberally castrated rats, injections of T propionate (TP) induced sexual behaviour in a proportion of animals which was comparable to that of a group of intact vehicle-treated rats. Injections of DHT had no significant behavioural effect and low doses of OB (0.05–0.5 μg) also had no effect on the behaviour. However, when these low OB doses were combined with DHT the majority of the animals ejaculated (Fig. 2). Thus, injection of as little as 0.05 μg OB in combination with 1 mg DHT stimulated ejaculatory behaviour in 60% of the rats. Thus, OE and DHT act synergistically to control the behaviour of castrated rats. Since T acts on the brain to induce sexual behaviour in castrated rats (Smith et al. 1977) it must be assumed that the behavioural effect of the combined OE and DHT treatment resulted from a synergistic action of the OE and DHT in the brain (Baum and Vreeburg 1973; Larsson et al. 1973). Interestingly, implants of OB into the anterior hypothalamic – medial preoptic area (MPOA), the neural site at which T acts to control male sexual behaviour (Johnston and Davidson 1972) are considerably more potent in activating the sexual behaviour of castrated rats if given in combination with DHT injections (Davis and Barfield 1979) than if given alone (Christensen and Clemens 1974). Equally interesting, intracerebral implants of DHT, while being behaviourally inert if given alone (Johnston and Davidson 1972) stimulate sexual behaviour in castrated rats treated with OE systemically (Baum et al. 1982).

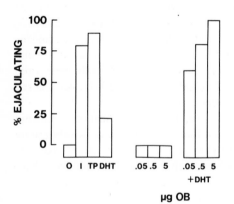

Fig. 2. Number of intact (*I*) and castrated rats ejaculating (%) after treatment with vehicle (*O*), testosterone propionate (*TP* 1 mg day^{-1}), 5α-dihydrotestosterone (*DHT* 1 mg day^{-1}) or various doses of oestradiol benzoate (*OB*) alone or in combination with 1 mg *DHT*

4 Female Sexual Behaviour in Male Rats

The possibility that there may be sufficient OE present in an intact male rat to affect his behaviour was supported by the finding that a considerable number of males of our strain showed female sexual behaviour, i.e. lordosis behaviour, as intacts without hormone treatment (Fig. 3; Södersten and Larsson 1974, 1975, Södersten et al. 1974).

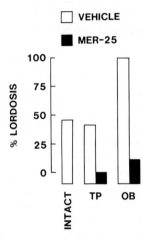

Fig. 3. Number of intact and castrated rats showing lordosis (%). The castrated rats were treated with testosterone propionate (*TP* 1 mg day^{-1}) or oestradiol benzoate (*OB* 15 μg day^{-1}) alone or in combination with the antioestrogen *MER-25* (10 mg day^{-1})

Lordosis is an oestrogen-dependent response in the rat (Pfaff and McEwen 1983) but oestradiol is present only in minute amounts in the blood of intact males (Södersten et al. 1974). However, since treatment with an oestrogen antagonist blocked lordosis in the intact rats which showed the behaviour spontaneously (Södersten and Larsson 1974) it seems likely that the display of lordosis by intact males is dependent upon an oestrogenic metabolite formed in the brain from T in the circulation. Similarly, treatment with TP or OB induced lordosis in castrated rats and these effects were blocked by anti-oestrogen treatment (Fig. 3; Södersten and Larsson 1974).

While these data support the notion that neural aromatization may be physiologically important in male rats their implications for the neuroendocrine control of male behaviour is unclear. For example, no correlations were found between the intensity of masculine behaviour and either the concentration of OE in the peripheral circulation or the intensity of feminine behaviour in intact males (Södersten et al. 1974). Also, a large group of male rats (n = 35) showed normal masculine behaviour but none of these rats showed lordosis after castration and treatment with T implants which reduced serum androgen concentrations to 30% of the intact level. Raising the concentration of serum androgen to the normal level, by implantation of another T implant, had no effect on male behaviour and induced female sexual behaviour in only 4 (11%) of the rats (Forsberg et al. 1985). Obviously, T can maintain male sexual behaviour after castration in male rats without stimulating female sexual behaviour.

5 Activation of Sexual Behaviour in Castrated Rats
by Androgens in the Absence of Oestrogenic Stimulation

Attempts to activate sexual behaviour in castrated rats by androgens in the absence of oestrogenic stimulation have usually been made using DHT, a T metabolite in the rat brain which is not aromatized (see Martini 1982). In the rat, contrary to some other mammalian species (Luttge 1979) peripheral or central neural administration of DHT does not stimulate behavioural responses (see Martini 1982, for a complete list of references). The interpretation of the failure of DHT to stimulate sexual behaviour in rats is, however, obscured by the fact that DHT is rapidly metabolized in the brain to 5α-androstane-$3\alpha,17\beta$-diol (3α-diol) and 5α-androstane-$3\beta,17\beta$-diol (3β-diol) Gustafsson et al. 1976; Naess 1976; Whalen and Rezek 1972). The 3α- and 3β-diols are weak androgens, only the 3β-diol has been found to stimulate male sexual behaviour (Baum and Vreeburg 1976). However, since the 3β-diol binds to the hypothalamic OE receptor (Vreeburg et al. 1975) we cannot be sure that behavioural responses induced by this or other 5α-reduced androgens (Paup et al. 1975; Södersten 1975) are, in fact, androgen-dependent. The demonstration that long-term treatment with DHT facilitates female sexual behaviour in ovariectomized rats (Beyer et al. 1971) would argue against this possibility.

These problems with DHT can be avoided by using the synthetic androgen 17β-hydroxy-17α-methyl-estra-4,9,11-trien-3-one (methyltrienolone, R 1881), which is not metabolized by androgen-sensitive target tissues and binds with high affinity to androgen receptors but does not interact with OE receptors (Asselin et al. 1976; Bonne and Raynaud 1976a, b; Dubé et al. 1976; Martini 1982; Raynaud et al. 1980).

Figure 4 shows that treatment with R 1881 was as effective as T in stimulating sexual behaviour in castrated, sexually inactive rats (Södersten and Gustafsson 1980a). Interestingly, the latency to the display of sexual behaviour by the R 1881-treated animals was shorter than that of the T-treated rats. A less pronounced effect of R 1881, was reported by Baum (1979). DHT, on the other hand, had a negligible effect on the behaviour. Injections of 2 μg OB induced sexual behaviour in 60% of a group of castrated rats (Fig. 4). These results suggest that sexual behaviour can be induced by an androgen as such, oestrogenic stimulation may not be required. The possible involvement of androgens in the control of sexual behaviour by T is also supported by the demonstra-

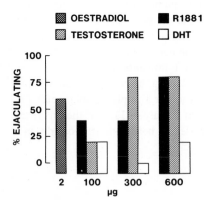

Fig. 4. Number of castrated rats ejaculating (%) after treatment with oestradiol, testosterone, methyltrienolone (R 1881), or 5α-dihydrotestosterone (DHT)

tion that treatment with the antiandrogen flutamide can inhibit T-activated sexual behaviour in castrated rats (Gladue and Clemens 1980). However, the results also show
that OB can induce all aspects of copulatory behaviour in what may be a reasonably
low dose, a finding which has been confirmed several times (Baum and Vreeburg 1973;
Södersten 1978; Södersten and Larsson 1974). However, it seems unlikely that androgen
aromatization is required for induction of sexual behaviour in castrated rats.

6 Sex Differences in Behavioural Androgen Sensitivity

Gonadectomized male and female rats differ in behavioural sensitivity to T. Thus, males
show higher levels of male behaviour than females after treatment with T. Figure 5 (top)
shows that all of a group of castrated males treated with T-filled constant-release implants mounted whereas only 50% of a group of ovariectomized females mounted after
the same T treatment (Mode et al. 1984). Also, the frequency of mounts/min was higher
in the males than in the females in a test where the males were prevented from intro-
mitting by occlusion of the vaginae of the stimulus females (Fig. 5 bottom). The concentration of androgen in the serum produced by the implants was identical in both
sexes (5.8 ± 0.9 nmol l^{-1}). Figure 5 (top) also shows that all of a group of five ovariectomized females treated with the same T implants showed lordosis behaviour after
progesterone treatment whereas only one of five castrated T-treated males displayed
lordosis. Despite the absence of measurable amounts of OE in the circulation all females
showed lordosis to all mounts by stimulus males but the one castrated male which
showed lordosis did so in response to only 50% of the mounts (Fig. 5 bottom).

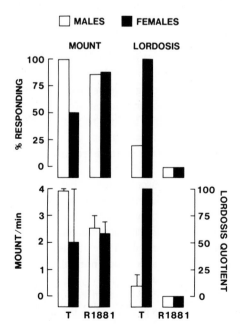

Fig. 5. Number of gonadectomized male and female rats showing mounts and lordosis (%, *top*)
after treatment with testosterone-filled constant-
release implants (*T*) or injections of methyltrienolone (*R 1881* 600 μg day^{-1}). The mean $\pm$
S.E.M. frequency of mounts and lordosis quotients are shown at the *bottom*

Sex differences in behavioural sensitivities to gonadal steroids such as those shown in Fig. 5 have traditionally been thought of as reflections of sex differences in brain function and genital anatomy which, in turn, are caused by perinatal androgen stimulation in the male and absence of androgen stimulation in the female (Södersten 1984). One sexually dimorphic brain function which may be relevant for the sex difference in behavioural androgen sensitivity is the sex difference in neural androgen metabolism (Gustafsson et al. 1976). Thus, when [^{3}H]T is injected into gonadectomized rats, considerably more radioactive T is recovered from the hypothalamus of the male than from that of the female rat brain whereas more radioactive 3α- and 3β-diols are found in the female hypothalamus (Gustafsson et al. 1976). Thus, more behaviourally inert T metabolites are formed from T in the circulation in the female than in the male hypothalamus.

When gonadectomized rats were treated with R 1881 no sex difference in behavioural androgen sensitivity was found (Fig. 5; Mode et al. 1984). An equal proportion of R 1881-treated male and female rats mounted when tested with sexually receptive stimulus females and no difference was found in the frequency of mounts in tests with stimulus females with occluded vaginae (Fig. 5; Mode et al. 1984). Interestingly, no R 1881-treated rat, male or female, showed lordosis (Fig. 5). Thus, the sex difference in behavioural androgen sensitivity was eliminated by treatment with an androgen which resists metabolism. Sex differences also exist in peripheral, hepatic, androgen metabolism, but these play no role in the sex difference in behavioural androgen sensitivity (Mode et al. 1984).

The data offer additional support for the suggestion that male sexual behaviour in the rat can be activated in the absence of oestrogenic stimulation.

7 A Possible Mechanism of Action of Oestradiol in the Neuroendocrine Control of Male Sexual Behaviour

There are several problems with the theory that OE is the stimulator of sexual behaviour in male rats (McEwen 1981). For example: an androgen such as 4-androstene-3,17-dione (androstenedione) is less potent than T in inducing male behaviour (Luttge 1979), yet androstenedione is a more effective precursor for neural aromatization (Selmanoff et al. 1977). Furthermore, OE has been found to bind to the androgen receptor in the rat brain (Sheridan 1983) and the very small amount of OE formed in the brain from T in the circulation may not be sufficient for sustaining sexual behaviour by itself (Selmanoff et al. 1977).

The effects of combined OB and DHT treatment on masculine sexual behaviour in castrated rats (see above) and the finding that R 1881 induced male, but not female, sexual behaviour, allow formulation of an alternative hypothesis of the role of OE in the neuroendocrine control of male behaviour. Thus, OE may act, not directly by stimulating the behaviour but indirectly, by modifying androgen metabolism, more specifically, by preventing the rapid metabolism of androgens which normally occurs via the 5α-reductase $- 3\alpha$- and 3β-hydroxysteroid-oxidoreductase pathways in the brain (Martini 1982). This hypothesis explains the synergistic behavioural effect of OB and DHT. Thus, in the presence of small amounts of OE, perhaps equivalent to the amounts normally formed in the brain, the rapid metabolism of DHT to 3α- and 3β-diols is prevented and DHT binds to the androgen receptor in the brain and activates the behaviour (Södersten and Gustafsson 1980b).

8 Is Oestradiol a 5α-reductase Inhibitor in the Male Rat Brain?

The hypothesis that OE modifies neural androgen metabolism (Södersten and Gustafsson 1980b) has lead us to reinterpret the results of previous experiments in which treatment with the aromatization inhibitor androst-1,4,6-triene-3,17-dione (ATD) prevented T from inducing sexual behaviour (Christensen and Clemens 1975; Morali et al. 1977). The absence of behavioural responses in the T+ATD-treated rats was interpreted as due to the absence of oestrogenic metabolites in the brain but it seems likely that, by preventing androgen aromatization, ATD directs androgen metabolism mainly via the 5α-reduction pathway and, therefore, only behaviourally inactive metabolites are formed and consequently no behavioural responses are induced by the treatment (Södersten et al. 1985). On this hypothesis it was predicted that treatment with a 5α-reductase inhibitor should stimulate sexual behaviour in castrated rats treated with T+ATD.

Figure 6 shows that castrated rats given empty implants did not copulate whereas OE- or T-filled implants induced the behaviour in groups of castrated rats. The T implants produced lower than normal or normal concentrations of serum androgen. The OE implants, which stimulated the behaviour, i.e. 100 μg OE ml^{-1} implants, did not increase the level of androgen above that of castrated untreated rats, showing that sexual behaviour can be displayed by castrated rats in the absence of androgen in the circulation. Treatment with the 5α-reductase inhibitor 17β-N,N-diethylcarbamoyl-4-methyl-4-aza-5α-androstan-3-one (4-MA; Brooks et al. 1981, 1982) had no effect, either stimulatory or inhibitory, on sexual behaviour induced by a threshold amount of T, as would be predicted on the basis of the work of others (Bradshaw et al. 1981). ATD, however, completely prevented the induction of sexual behaviour by T (Fig. 6). Interestingly, concurrent treatment with 4-MA induced sexual behaviour in castrated rats given combined T+ATD treatment and equally interesting, treatment with a dose of OE that had no behavioural effect in itself, i.e. 50 μg OE ml^{-1} implants, also stimulated the behaviour in the T+ATD-treated rats (Fig. 6; Södersten et al. 1985).

Control experiments were performed on female rats. Figure 7 shows that treatment of ovariectomized rats with T-filled constant-release implants and progesterone induced high levels of female sexual behaviour (see also Fig. 5). The response was completely blocked by treatment with ATD and could not be reactivated by the 4-MA treatment that restored male sexual behaviour in the castrated T+ATD-treated males (Fig. 6). OE implants, however, induced female sexual behaviour in the T+ATD-treated ovariectomized females. Figure 7 also shows that ATD-treatment had no effect on female sexual behaviour induced in ovariectomized rats by OE only. Thus, ATD has no anti-oestrogenic effect on female sexual behaviour. Since display of female sexual behaviour in response to mounts by male rats requires oestrogenic stimulation (Pfaff and McEwen 1983) it can be concluded that aromatization is necessary for T-induced female sexual

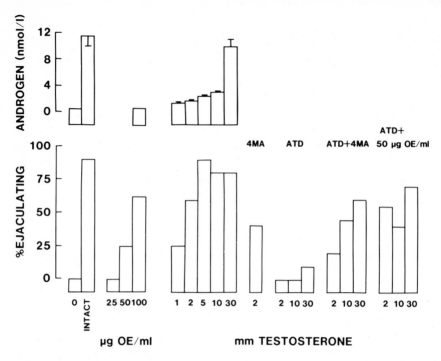

Fig. 6. Mean ± S.E.M. concentration of serum androgen (*top*) and number of castrated and intact rats ejaculating (%) after treatment with constant-release implants filled with oil solutions of oestradiol (*OE*) of various concentrations or crystalline testosterone. Testosterone-implanted rats were treated with a 5α-reductase inhibitor (*4MA* 16.7 mg day^{-1}) or an aromatization inhibitor (*ATD* 10 mg day^{-1}) or *ATD* in combination with *4MA* or *OE* implants

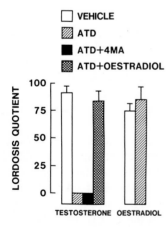

Fig. 7. Mean ± S.E.M. lordosis quotients in ovariectomized rats treated with constant-release implants filled with crystalline testosterone or oil solution of oestradiol in combination with an aromatization inhibitor (*ATD* 10 mg day^{-1}), *ATD* + a 5α-reductase inhibitor (*4MA*, 16.7 mg day^{-1}) or *ATD* + oestradiol-filled implants

behaviour and that 4-MA does not counteract the effect of ATD on neural aromatization.

The fact that treatment with a 5α-reductase inhibitor reactivated male but not female sexual behaviour in gonadectomized rats given combined treatment with T and an aromatization inhibitor and the reported absence of a sex difference in neural aromatization (Lieberburg and McEwen 1977) permit the conclusion that while aromatization is necessary for T-induced female sexual behaviour it is not required for T-induced male behaviour.

The finding that a low dose of OE, in itself without behavioural effect, induced male sexual behaviour in the castrated T-+ATD-treated rats in a manner comparable to that of a 5α-reductase inhibitor supports the hypothesis that OE acts by modifying neural androgen metabolism. Evidence already exists that OE can affect the 5α-,5β-reductase of 3α- and 3β-hydroxysteroid-oxidoreductase activity in the rat (Martini et al. 1978) and bird (Hutchison and Steimer 1981) brain.

Intracranial T implants are most effective in stimulating sexual behaviour if placed in the MPOA of the brain (Johnston and Davidson 1972) the site where neural 5α-reductase and aromatase activity is maximal (Selmanoff et al. 1977). Hence the possibility that OE might influence neural androgen metabolism would be maximal in the MPOA. When T implants are placed outside the MPOA in adjacent hypothalamic structures, they become behaviourally less effective and, interestingly, the rate of neural aromatization, but not 5α-reduction, decreases (Selmanoff et al. 1977). In the absence of an oestrogen, T might be rapidly converted into inactive metabolites, i.e. 3α- and 3β-diols, and this may be one reason why T implants are ineffective in inducing sexual behaviour if placed outside the MPOA. If OE is supplied by peripheral administration, intracranial implants of DHT, by themselves without behavioural effects (Johnston and Davidson 1972), will stimulate sexual behaviour even if placed far away from the MPOA (Baum et al. 1982).

Rapid metabolism through 5α-reduction may be a mechanism whereby pulses of androgen of testicular origin are inactivated in the rat brain. Such a mechanism may be required under physiological conditions since the male rat lacks a peripheral sex steroid-binding protein (see Introduction).

Acknowledgements. This work was supported by the Swedish Council for Research in the Humanities and Social Sciences and the Swedish Medical Research Council (No. 13X-2819). We thank Mary Lundh for typing the manuscript and the Journal of Endocrinology Ltd, Academic Press, and the Williams and Wilkins Company for permission to use previously published material.

References

Asselin J, Labrie F, Gourdeau Y, Bonne C, Raynaud J-P (1976) Binding of [^{3}H]methyltrienolone (R 1881) in rat prostate and human benign prostatic hypertrophy. Steroids 28:449–459

Baum MJ (1979) A comparison of the effects of methyltrienolone (R 1881) and 5α-dihydrotestosterone on sexual behaviour of castrated male rats. Horm Behav 13:165–174

Baum MJ, Vreeburg JTM (1973) Copulation in castrated male rats following combined treatment with estradiol and dihydrotestosterone. Science (Wash DC) 182:283–285

Baum MJ, Vreeburg JTM (1976) Differential effects of the anti-estrogen MER-25 and of three 5α-reduced androgens on mounting and lordosis behavior in the rat. Horm Behav 7:87–104

Baum MJ, Tobet SA, Starr MS, Bradshaw WG (1982) Implantation of dihydrotestosterone propionate into the lateral septum on medial amygdala facilitates copulation in castrated male rats given estradiol systemically. Horm Behav 16:208–223

Beyer C, Morali G, Cruz ML (1971) Effects of 5α-dihydrotestosterone on gonadotropin secretion and estrous behavior in the female wistar rat. Endocrinology 89:1158–1161

Bonne C, Raynaud J-P (1976a) Methyltrienolone, a specific ligand for cellular androgen receptors. Steroids 26:227–232

Bonne C, Raynaud J-P (1976b) Assay of androgen binding sites by exchange with methyltrienolone (R 1881). Steroids 27:449–507

Bradshaw WG, Baum MJ, Awh CC (1981) Attenuation by a 5 α-reductase inhibitor of the activational effect of testosterone propionate on penile erections in castrated male rats. Endocrinology 109:1047–1051

Brooks JR, Baptista ER, Berman C, Ham EA, Hichens M, Johnston DBR, Primka RL, Rasmusson GH, Reynolds GF, Schmitt SR, Arth GE (1981) Response of rat ventral prostate to a novel 5 α-reductase inhibitor. Endocrinology 109:830–836

Brooks JR, Berman C, Hichens M, Primka RL, Reynolds GF, Rasmusson GH (1982) Biological activities of a new steroidal inhibitor of Δ^4-5 α-reductase (41309). Proc Soc Exp Biol Med 169: 67–73

Christensen LW, Clemens LG (1974) Intrahypothalamic implants of testosterone on estradiol and resumption of masculine sexual behavior in long-term castrated male rats. Endocrinology 95: 984–990

Christensen LW, Clemens LG (1975) Blockade of testosterone-induced mounting behavior in the male rat with intracranial application of the aromatization inhibitor androst-1,4,6-triene-3,17-dione. Endocrinology 97:1545–1551

Damassa DA, Smith ER, Tennet B, Davidson JM (1977) The relationship between circulating testosterone levels and male sexual behavior in rats. Horm Behav 8:275–286

Davidson JM (1969) Effects of estrogen on the sexual behavior of male rats. Endocrinology 84: 1365–1372

Davis PG, Barfield RJ (1979) Activation of masculine sexual behavior by intracranial estradiol benzoate implants in male rats. Neuroendocrinology 28:217–227

Dubé JY, Chapdelaine P, Tremblay RR, Bonne C, Raynaud J-P (1976) Comparative binding specificity of methyltrienolone in human and rat prostate. Horm Res (Basel) 7:341–347

Ellis GB, Desjardins C (1982) Male rats secrete luteinizing hormone and testosterone episodically. Endocrinology 110:1547–1554

Ellis GB, Desjardins C, Fraser HM (1983) Control of pulsatile LH release in male rats. Neuroendocrinology 37:177–183

Forsberg G, Abrahamsson K, Södersten P, Eneroth P (1985) Effects of restricted maternal contact in neonatal rats on sexual behaviour in the adult. J Endocrinol 104:427–731

Gladue BA, Clemens LG (1980) Flutamide inhibits testosterone-induced masculine sexual behavior in male and female rats. Endocrinology 106:1917–1922

Gustafsson J-A, Pousette A, Svensson E (1976) Sex specific occurence of androgen receptors in the rat. J Biol Chem 251:4047–4054

Hutchison JB, Steimer T (1981) Brain 5 β-reductase: a correlate of behavioral sensitivity to androgen. Science (Wash DC) 213:244–246

Johnston P, Davidson JM (1972) Intracerebral androgens and sexual behavior in the male rat. Horm Behav 3:345–357

Larsson K, Södersten P, Beyer C (1973) Sexual behavior in male rats treated with estrogen in combination with dihydrotestosterone. Horm Behav 4:289–299

Lieberburg I, McEwen BS (1977) Brain cell nuclear retention of testosterone metabolites, 5 α-dihydrotestosterone and estradiol-17β, in adult rats. Endocrinology 100:588–597

Lincoln GA, Short RV (1980) Seasonal reproduction: nature's contraception. Recent Prog Horm Res 36:1–51

Luttge WG (1979) Endocrine control of mammalian male sexual behavior: an analysis of the potential role of testosterone metabolites. In: Beyer C (ed) Endocrine control of sexual behavior. Raven, New York, pp 341–387

Malmnäs C-O (1977) Short-latency effect of testosterone on copulatory behaviour and ejaculation in sexually experienced intact male rats. J Reprod Fertil 51:351–354

Martini L (1982) The 5 α-reduction of testosterone in the neuroendocrine structures. Biochemical and physiological implications. Endoc Rev 3:1–25

Martini L, Celotti F, Massa R, Motta M (1978) Studies on the mode of action of androgens in neuroendocrine tissues. J Steroid Biochem 9:411–417

McEwen BS (1981) Neural gonadal steroid actions. Science (Wash DC) 211:1303–1311

Mode A, Gustafsson J-A, Södersten P, Eneroth P (1984) Sex differences in behavioural androgen sensitivity: possible role of androgen metabolism. J Endocrinol 100:245–248

Morali G, Larsson K, Beyer C (1977) Inhibition of testosterone-induced sexual behavior in the castrated male rat by aromatase blockers. Horm Behav 9:203–213

Murphy BEP (1968) Binding of testosterone and estradiol in plasma. Can J Biochem 46:299–311

Naess O (1976) Characterization of the androgen receptors in the hypothalamus, preoptic area and brain cortex of the rat. Steroids 27:167–185

Nieschlag E (1979) The endocrine function of the human testis in regard to sexuality. In: Sachar EJ (ed) Sex, hormones and behaviour. Ciba foundation symp. Elsevier, Amsterdam, pp 183–208

Paup DC, Mennin SP, Gorski RA (1975) Androgen- and estrogen-induced copulatory behavior and inhibition of luteinizing hormone (LH) secretion in the male rat. Horm Behav 6:35–46

Pfaff DW, McEwen BS (1983) Actions of estrogens and progestins on nerve cells. Science (Wash DC) 219:807–814

Raynaud J-P, Bouton MM, Moguilewsky M, Ojasoo T, Philibert D, Beck G, Labrie F, Mornon JP (1980) Steroid hormone receptors and pharmacology. J Steroid Biochem 12:143–157

Selmanoff MK, Brodkin LD, Weiner RI, Siiteri PK (1977) Aromatization and 5α-reduction in discrete hypothalamic and limbic regions of the male and female rat. Endocrinology 101:841–843

Sheridan P (1983) Androgen receptors in the brain: what are we measuring? Endoc Rev 4:171–178

Smith ER, Damassa DA, Davidson JM (1977) Plasma testosterone and sexual behavior following intracerebral implantation of testosterone propionate in the castrated male rat. Horm Behav 8: 77–85

Södersten P (1973) Estrogen-activated sexual behavior in male rats. Horm Behav 4:247–256

Södersten P (1975) Mounting behavior and lordosis behavior in castrated male rats treated with testosterone propionate or estradiol benzoate or dihydrotestosterone in combination with testosterone propionate. Horm Behav 6:105–126

Södersten P (1978) Effects of anti-oestrogen treatment of neonatal male rats on lordosis behaviour and mounting behaviour in the adult. J Endocrinol 76:241–249

Södersten P (1984) Sexual differentiation: do males differ from females in behavioral sensitivity to gonadal hormones? Prog Brain Res 61:257–270

Södersten P, Eneroth P (1980) Neonatal treatment with antioestiogen increases the diurnal rhythmicity in the sesonal behaviour of adult male rats. J Endocrinol 85:331–339

Södersten P, Eneroth P (1983) Reproductive neuroendocrine rhythms. In: Balthazart J, Pröve E, Gilles R (eds) Hormones and behaviour in higher vertebrates. Springer, Berlin Heidelberg New York, pp 178–193

Södersten P, Gustafsson J-A (1980a) Activation of sexual behaviour in castrated rats with the synthetic androgen 17β-hydroxy-17α-methyl-estra-4,9,11-triene-3-one (R1881). J Endocrinol 87:279–283

Södersten P, Gustafsson J-A (1980b) A way in which estradiol might play a role in the sexual behavior of male rats. Horm Behav 14:271–274

Södersten P, Larsson K (1974) Lordosis behavior in castrated male rats treated with estradiol benzoate or testosterone propionate in combination with an estrogen antagonist, MER-25, and in intact male rats. Horm Behav 5:13–18

Södersten P, Larsson K (1975) Lordosis behavior and mounting behavior in male rats: effects of castration and treatment with estradiol benzoate or testosterone propionate. Physiol Behav 14: 159–164

Södersten P, de Jong FH, Vreeburg JTM, Baum MJ (1974) Lordosis behavior in intact male rats: absence of correlation with mounting behavior on testicular secretion of estradiol-17β and testosterone. Physiol Behav 13:803–808

Södersten P, Eneroth P, Ekberg P-H (1980) Episodic fluctuations in concentrations of androgen in serum of male rats: possible relationship to sexual behaviour. J Endocrinol 87:463–471

Södersten P, Eneroth P, Pettersson A (1983) Episodic secretion of luteinizing hormone and androgen in male rats. J Endocrinol 97:145–153

Södersten P, Eneroth P, Mode A, Hansson T, Johansson D, Näslund B, Liang T, Gustafsson J-A (1985) Evidence that estradiol-17β can control masculine sexual behavior in male rats by modifying androgen metabolism. Endocrinol

Steiner RA, Bremner WJ, Clifton DK (1982) Regulation of luteinizing hormone pulse frequency and amplitude by testosterone in the adult male rat. Endocrinology 111:2055–2061

Vreeburg JTM, Schretlen PJM, Baum MJ (1975) Specific high affinity binding of 17β-estradiol in cystosols from several brain regions and pituitary of intact and castrated adult male rats. Endocrinology 97:969–977

Neural Progestin Receptors: Regulation of Progesterone-Facilitated Sexual Behaviour in Female Guinea Pigs

J.D. BLAUSTEIN and T.J. BROWN[1]

1 Introduction

Besides having influences on a variety of other aspects of behaviour and reproductive physiology, oestradiol and progesterone interact to regulate the display of sexual behaviours during the oestrous cycle of many vertebrate species (Young 1961). In oestrogen-primed female rodents, progesterone both facilitates the display of sexual behaviour and inhibits its further facilitation by progesterone (Morin 1977). The latter effect of progesterone has been called desensitization (Blaustein 1982a,b). Both of these influences of progesterone are due to actions within the brain. In fact, both effects are seen after intracranial implantation of progesterone within the ventromedial hypothalamic area (Rubin and Barfield 1983, 1984; Morin and Feder 1974a).

Although the evidence is mostly correlational, we have suggested that intracellular receptors for progesterone in the mediobasal hypothalamus mediate the behavioural effects of progesterone on sexual behaviour in female guinea pigs (Blaustein and Brown 1983). The concentration of cytosol progestin receptors in the hypothalamus (as well as in other target tissues) is increased dramatically by oestradiol (Blaustein and Feder 1979b; MacLusky and McEwen 1978). Doses of oestradiol that are effective in priming rats and guinea pigs to respond to progesterone also promote the induction of cytosol progestin receptors in the hypothalamus. The time course of the induction of cytosol progestin receptors after oestradiol injection parallels that for the induction of responsiveness to progesterone for facilitation of sexual behaviour (Blaustein and Feder 1979b; Parsons et al. 1980). Progesterone causes the apparent increase in the concentration of these receptors in cell nuclei, their suspected site of action. The elevation in the level of nuclear progestin receptors is transient, remaining elevated until the approximate time of heat termination in guinea pigs (Blaustein and Feder 1980). Doses of progesterone that decrease behavioural responsiveness of guinea pigs to progesterone also down-regulate the concentration of cytosol progestin receptors (Blaustein and Feder 1979a). In addition, supplemental oestradiol treatment at the time of progesterone treatment, a hormonal treatment that overcomes progesterone-desensitization, increases the concentration of cytosol progestin receptors and causes greater accumulation of hypothalamic nuclear progestin receptors (Blaustein 1982a). Another hormonal treatment that overcomes progesterone-desensitization, injection of a pharmacological dose

---

1 Division of Neuroscience and Behavior, Department of Psychology, University of Massachusetts, Amherst, MA 01003, USA

Neurobiology
(ed. by R. Gilles and J. Balthazart)
© Springer-Verlag Berlin Heidelberg 1985

of progesterone in animals refractory to a moderate dose of progesterone, also enhances accumulation of hypothalamic nuclear progestin receptors, even in the presence of depressed levels of cytosol progestin receptors (Blaustein 1982b).

In this paper, we will discuss extensions of the work described above. We have tested further the possible role of hypothalamic progestin receptors in sexual behaviour by using a progesterone antagonist to block progesterone's interaction with progestin receptors, we have studied the possible role of retention of nuclear progestin receptors in determining heat duration, and we have examined the regulation of these receptors by the noradrenergic system.

The intracellular receptor model of oestradiol-progesterone regulation of sexual behaviour discussed in this paper (Fig. 1) is based on that proposed for steroid hormone action in the chick oviduct (O'Malley and Means 1974) and rodent uterus (Gorski and Gannon 1975). Recently, alternatives to the classical model of steroid hormone mechanism of action have been proposed. It has been suggested that all steroid hormone receptors normally may be localized in cell nuclei, but they may be either tightly or loosely associated with nuclear components depending on whether receptor-ligand binding has occurred (King and Greene 1984; Welshons et al. 1984). Another possibility

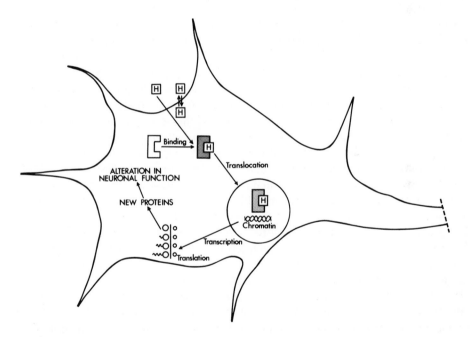

Fig. 1. Proposed model for steroid hormone mechanism of action in brain based on model originally developed for hormone action in the chick oviduct and rodent uterus. Steroid hormones may freely diffuse through the neuronal membrane. If there are intracellular receptors present in the neuron, the steroid hormone may bind, causing a conformational change. The hormone:receptor complex is then translocated into the cell nucleus where it may bind to acceptor sites on the chromatin. This may cause changes in gene expression, leading to the synthesis of new proteins, and ultimately to a change in function of the neuron. If one of the recently proposed model of steroid hormone action proves accurate, then the only substantive difference between it and the model depicted would be the intracellular location of the unoccupied receptors

is that intracellular receptors are present in equilibrium between the cytoplasm and nucleus of the cell (Sheridan et al. 1979). According to this scheme, steroid binding with consequent binding to chromatin acceptor sites causes an increase in the concentration of receptors in the cell nucleus as the receptors move from the cytoplasm to re-establish the initial equilibrium. Both of these models suggest that all or much of the apparent cytoplasmic localization of steroid hormone receptors in the absence of ligand is an artifact of homogenization.

Although the various models differ as to the subcellular compartment in which they claim unoccupied receptors reside, all three models are in agreement that the presence of hormone causes a greater or tighter association of receptors with nuclear components, presumably the chromatin. Because there are a number of questions to be answered regarding the alternative models of steroid hormone mechanism of action, it is premature to abandon the original model with its associated nomenclature. However, if one of the new models proves to be correct, then the nomenclature used in this and many other papers would require modification. The receptors that are referred to as cytosol receptors would be those receptors that are loosely associated with cell nuclei, while those that are called nuclear receptors would be those that are tightly associated.

2 Use of Progestin Antagonist

A recently developed progesterone antagonist, RU 486, has been shown to antagonize a variety of progesterone's effects in the mammalian uterus (Herrmann et al. 1982; Philibert et al. 1982). This drug also binds, in vitro, with high affinity to uterine cytosol progestin receptors (Philibert et al. 1982), suggesting that it may inhibit progesterone's action by inhibiting binding of progesterone to intracellular progestin receptors. We have found that RU 486 binds with high affinity to hypothalamic progestin receptors, in vitro, and therefore have used it to determine if progesterone's effect on sexual behaviour is mediated by intracellular neural progestin receptors.

In the first experiment, we tested the ability of RU 486 to block progesterone facilitation of sexual behaviour (Brown and Blaustein 1984a). Ovariectomized (OVX) guinea pigs pretreated with 10 μg oestradiol benzoate (40 h earlier) received either vehicle, 0.5 mg, or 5.0 mg RU 486 1 h prior to receiving 0.1 mg progesterone. Although the lower dose of the antagonist was ineffective in blocking the response to progesterone, the larger dose inhibited lordosis in nearly all of the animals (Table 1A).

Because RU 486 has also been reported to be a potent glucocorticoid antagonist (Moguilewsky and Philibert 1984), it is possible that in high doses the drug inhibits sexual behaviour by debilitating the animals. If the RU 486-induced inhibition of progesterone-facilitated lordosis is due to a debilitating effect of the drug, then it would be expected to inhibit lordosis regardless of the dose of progesterone used. To test this possibility, OVX, oestradiol benzoate-treated animals were injected with RU 486 prior to an injection of either 0.1 mg or 5 mg progesterone. As expected, a greater percentage of animals responded to the larger dose of progesterone (100% compared with 40%; Table 1B). In a separate experiment the effectiveness of progesterone in overcoming the inhibitory effect of RU 486 was compared with cortisol. If the inhibitory effect of RU 486 is due to an antiglucocorticoid action, then it would be expected that a large

Table 1A. RU 486 Inhibits progesterone-facilitated lordosis

−1 h	0 h	% Responding	Heat duration (H)	Heat duration (H) responders only	Latency to lordosis (H)
V	$P_{0.1}$	90%	7.30 (±0.90)	8.11 (±0.42)	4.44 (±0.63)
$RU_{0.5}$	$P_{0.1}$	100%	8.00 (±0.99)	8.00 (±0.99)	4.56 (±0.34)
RU_5	$P_{0.1}$	11%	0.56 (±0.56)	5.00 (−)	7.00 (−)
V	V	0%	−	−	−

Table 1B. A large dose of progesterone overcomes RU 486-induced inhibition of progesterone-facilitated lordosis

RU_5	$P_{0.1}$	40%	2.00 (±1.19)	5.00 (±2.38)	5.75 (±1.75)
RU_5	P_5	100%	9.33 (±0.77)	9.33 (±0.77)	3.67 (±0.50)

Table 1C. Failure of cortisol to overcome RU 486-induced inhibition of lordosis

RU_5	$P_{0.1}$	20%	2.00 (±2.00)	10.00 (−)	4.00 (−)
RU_5	P_5	100%	8.80 (±0.58)	8.80 (±0.58)	5.40 (±0.75)
RU_5	$P_{0.1}$ and $CORT_5$	0%	−	−	−
V	$P_{0.1}$	100%	7.40 (±1.63)	7.40 (±1.63)	4.60 (±1.03)

- All animals were primed with oestradiol benzoate at −40 h. Hourly tests for lordosis began at −1 h and continued until all animals were non-responsive. Values are mean (±SEM).
- V, vehicle; P, progesterone; RU, RU 486; CORT, cortisol
- Subscripts are doses in mg.

dose of cortisol would reverse the inhibitory effect of RU 486 as does a large dose of progesterone. Unlike progesterone, cortisol was ineffective in overcoming the RU 486-induced inhibition (Table 1C). The results of these two experiments suggest that the inhibition by RU 486 is specific to progesterone and is not due to the antiglucocorticoid action of RU 486.

In order to verify that RU 486 interacts in vivo with intracellular progestin receptors were assayed in OVX, oestrogen-treated guinea pigs injected prior to the assay with either the dose of RU 486 that results in behavioural inhibition (5 mg) or vehicle. RU 486 decreased the available cytosol progestin receptors by approximately 35% compared with oil-injected controls, a finding that has been confirmed by Scatchard analysis.

We are now interested in the mechanism by which RU 486 decreases the concentration of available progestin binding sites. It is possible that RU 486 decreases the availability of cytosol progestin receptors to progesterone either by causing a structural change in the cytosol progestin receptor, rendering it incapable of binding to progestins or by binding tightly and dissociating slowly from the receptor. It is also possible that RU 486 causes the accumulation of progestin receptors in cell nuclei without having the same genomic effects as progesterone-progestin receptor complexes. Evidence from this laboratory suggests that this last possibility is unlikely. We have been unable to observe any nuclear accumulation of progestin receptors under a variety of experimental conditions. It is therefore most likely that by one of the mechanisms listed, RU 486 decreases the availability of progestin receptors to progesterone, thus preventing the interaction of progesterone with progestin receptors and consequent nuclear accumulation.

3 Progestin Receptors and Heat Duration

The transient elevation in hypothalamic nuclear progestin receptor levels following progesterone injection correlates temporally with the expression of sexual receptivity. Nuclear progestin receptor levels increase prior to the initiation of sexual receptivity and decline to baseline levels as the receptive period terminates (Blaustein and Feder 1980). This correlation suggests that heat termination may result from the loss of progestin receptors from cell nuclei. We have tested this hypothesis by investigating how various oestradiol and progesterone treatments affect both heat duration and the retention of progestin receptors by hypothalamic cell nuclei. Based on our hypothesis, hormonal manipulations that delay heat termination should also delay the decline in nuclear progestin receptor levels.

To determine the effects of oestradiol on heat duration, OVX oestrogen-primed guinea pigs were given a supplemental oestradiol benzoate injection (10 μg) at the same time as a facilitatory injection of progesterone (Blaustein 1982a). Confirming earlier studies, these animals exhibited longer heat durations as compared to control animals that had received only the progesterone injection. Heat terminated in all of the control animals by 15 h after progesterone injection while 50% of the animals treated with supplemental oestradiol were still sexually receptive when the experiment was terminated at 16 h after progesterone injection. In a separate experiment, we found that supplemental oestradiol treatment increased the retention of nuclear progestin receptors. Twelve h after progesterone treatment, hypothalamic nuclear progestin receptor concentrations were 55% greater in animals treated with supplemental oestradiol as compared to animals receiving only progesterone.

In order to study progesterone's effect on heat duration and nuclear progestin receptor retention, we first attempted to increase heat duration by providing a continuous source of oestradiol and progesterone. This approach was based on a study by Lisk (1978) which demonstrated that in some circumstances, progesterone can maintain sexual receptivity in hamsters for an extended period of time. Lisk infused progesterone at three different rates into OVX hamsters implanted subcutaneously with an oestrogen pellet. Infusion of the low dose of progesterone failed to activate heat, while infusion of the high dose activated heats of normal duration. Infusion of the moderate dose, however, activated heats of extended duration. We reasoned that one possible explana-

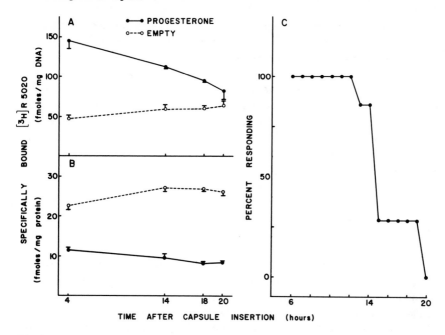

Fig. 2. A Nuclear progestin receptor levels in mediobasal hypothalamus-preopticarea of OVX guinea pigs implanted subcutaneously with a Silastic capsule containing oestradiol. Forty-eight h later, a 3-cm progesterone-filled or empty capsule was inserted and receptor levels measured 4, 14, 18, or 20 h later. **B** Cytosol progestin receptor levels of animals treated as in **A**. **C** Percent of guinea pigs, treated as in **A** (progesterone group only), responding during tests for lordosis

tion for these results is that, at an optimal dose of progesterone, nuclear progestin receptor levels remain elevated because of a balance between receptor induction (by oestradiol) and translocation of the receptors to cell nuclei (by progesterone). As long as such a balance is maintained, nuclear progestin receptor levels might remain elevated and the period of sexual receptivity might be extended. Therefore, in an attempt to increase heat duration, we implanted a wide range of lengths of Silastic capsules containing a variety of concentrations of progesterone into OVX guinea pigs which had received an oestradiol capsule 2 days earlier. We found that heat termination occurred at about the same time in all groups regardless of the size of progesterone capsule. Although small differences in heat duration were observed among the groups, these were caused by differences in latency to lordosis among the groups.

The finding, that heat termination occurs despite elevated blood levels of oestradiol and progesterone, introduced the possibility of a dissociation between nuclear progestin receptor retention and heat duration. Perhaps elevated blood levels of these hormones maintained elevated nuclear progestin receptor levels, even though they did not prolong sexual receptivity. Such a dissociation might suggest that some other process other than loss of nuclear progestin receptors is responsible for heat termination. Therefore, we investigated how long levels of progestin receptors in hypothalamic cell nuclei remain elevated following progesterone capsule insertion. Guinea pigs were treated as in the previous experiment except that only one size of progesterone-containing capsule

(3 cm), or an empty capsule was implanted, and hypothalamic progestin levels were measured at 4, 14, 18, and 20 h after capsule insertion. By 4 h after capsule insertion, nuclear progestin receptor levels were increased by approximately 200% and cytosol progestin receptor levels decreased by 50% as compared to control levels (Fig. 2). The level of cytosol receptors remained decreased over the duration of the experiment, and the concentration of nuclear receptors declined at a steady rate. By 20 h after capsule insertion, a time when similarly treated animals were no longer in heat, the level of nuclear progestin receptors had declined to a level only slightly above the control level. These results are consistent with our hypothesis that heat termination results from the decline in nuclear progestin receptor levels.

Morin and Feder (1973) reported that multiple progesterone injections administered at 3 h intervals prolong heat in OVX oestrogen-primed guinea pigs. In order to obtain a progesterone dependent delay in heat termination, we treated OVX, oestradiol-benzoate-treated guinea pigs with 50 μg progesterone (Brown and Blaustein 1984b). Animals were tested for lordosis, and 8 h after progesterone injection they received an additional 500 μg progesterone or the oil vehicle. Heat termination was delayed by more than 2 h in animals treated with supplemental progesterone as compared to control animals (Fig. 3). To determine the effect of this treatment on the retention of hypothalamic nuclear progestin receptors, animals were either treated as described above or were injected with oestradiol benzoate to establish baseline levels of progestin receptors. Animals were killed 8, 10, or 14 h after the initial progesterone injection (0, 2, or 6 h after

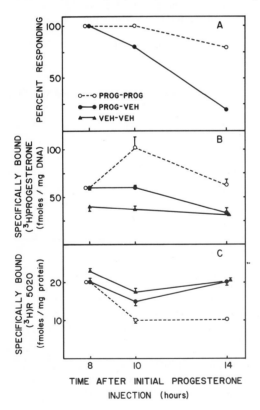

Fig. 3. A Percent of guinea pigs responding during tests for lordosis. Animals were treated with 50 μg progesterone 48 h after receiving 4 μg oestradiol benzoate. Eight h later, they received a supplemental injection of 500 μg progesterone or oil. B Mediobasal hypothalamus-preoptic area nuclear progestin receptor levels in guinea pigs treated as in A. Animals received 50 μg progesterone (*Prog*) or oil (*Veh*) 48 h after receiving 4 μg oestradiol benzoate. Eight h later, animals were killed or received 500 μg progesterone or oil and were killed 10 or 14 h after the initial progesterone injection. C Cytosol progestin receptor levels measured in animals described in B. (After Brown and Blaustein 1984b)

the second progesterone injection) and hypothalamic progestin receptor levels were measured. Hypothalamic nuclear progestin receptor levels were still elevated 8 h after the initial injection of progesterone. The injection of supplemental progesterone increased the level of nuclear progestin receptors measured at 10 h. At 14 h, a time when 80% of similarly treated animals were still sexually receptive, nuclear progestin receptor levels were still elevated in supplemental progesterone-treated guinea pigs. In contrast, nuclear progestin receptor levels in animals treated with only the initial injection of progesterone returned to baseline levels by 14 h, a time when 80% of similarly treated animals were no longer receptive.

To further investigate the relationship between heat duration and nuclear progestin receptor retention, OVX guinea pigs received a 1.0 cm progesterone capsule or an empty capsule 40 h after injection of 10 μg oestradiol benzoate. Two h later, the progesterone capsules were removed from one-half of the animals, and hypothalamic progestin receptor levels were measured 3, 6, 10, and 18 h after capsule insertion (1, 4, 8, and 16 h after capsule removal). By 3 h after capsule insertion cytosol progestin receptor levels were decreased in both groups (Fig. 4). Cytosol receptor concentrations remained at this level in the group exposed to capsules for only 2 h, but continued to decrease in the continuously exposed group. At 6 and 10 h after capsule insertion, nuclear progestin

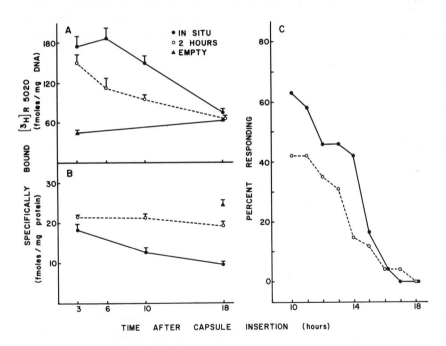

Fig. 4. A Nuclear progestin receptor levels in mediobasal hypothalamus-preopticarea of OVX guinea pigs injected with 10 μg oestradiol benzoate. Forty h later, they were implanted with either a 1-cm progesterone-filled or empty Silastic capsule. Two h later, the progesterone capsules were removed from one-half of the animals, and nuclear progestin receptor levels determined 3, 6, 10, and 18 h after capsule removal (nuclear receptors were measured only at 3 h and 18 h and cytosol receptors only at 18 h in the empty-capsule control group). **B** Cytosol progestin receptor levels of animals treated as described in A. **C** Percent of guinea pigs, treated as in A, responding during tests for lordosis

receptor levels were lower in animals exposed to capsules for 2 h as compared to levels measured in continuously exposed animals. By 18 h, nuclear receptor levels had declined to control levels in both groups.

In a separate experiment, similarly treated animals were tested for lordosis. Fewer animals responded in the group exposed to progesterone capsules for 2 h (42% vs 63%). However, of those animals that responded heat termination occurred at about the same time regardless of the amount of exposure to progesterone capsules. By 18 h after capsule insertion heat had terminated in all animals tested.

The data from these experiments are consistent with the hypothesis that heat termination results from the loss of progestin receptors from hypothalamic cell nuclei. Furthermore, they raise the question of which factors are responsible for the loss of nuclear progestin receptors. One such factor may be circulating progesterone levels. It seems likely that as the circulating level of progesterone declines, no further nuclear accumulation of progestin receptors would occur. Indeed, experiments in guinea pigs (Blaustein and Feder 1979a,b) and rats (McGinnis et al. 1981) show an apparent correlation between blood progesterone levels and nuclear retention of progestin receptors. However, our experiment demonstrating that nuclear progestin receptor levels decline in the presence of elevated blood progesterone levels indicates that circulating progesterone is not the only factor determining nuclear progestin receptor retention.

Another factor that may regulate nuclear progestin receptor retention is the availability of cytosol progestin receptors. As cytosol progestin receptor levels decrease because of translocation to cell nuclei and declining oestrogen-priming action, the level of nuclear progestin receptors decreases. We found that following supplemental progesterone injection, cytosol progestin receptor levels are further decreased. As nuclear progestin receptor levels returned to baseline, cytosol receptor levels were not replenished. This same relationship was observed in animals treated with oestradiol and progesterone-containing Silastic capsules. Following progesterone capsule insertion cytosol progestin receptor levels decreased and as nuclear progestin receptor levels declined toward baseline, cytosol receptor levels were not replenished. This is particularly interesting since these animals have elevated blood oestradiol levels and would be expected to have on-going progestin receptor induction. This raises the possibility that progesterone may act to inhibit progestin receptor induction by oestradiol. This possibility is currently being examined.

4 Noradrenergic Regulation of Progestin Receptors

Induction of sexual behaviour in female guinea pigs by oestradiol and progesterone involves a noradrenergic system. Blockade of noradrenergic transmission, either by inhibition of norepinephrine synthesis or by selective α-adrenergic receptor antagonists, inhibits sexual behaviour (Crowley et al. 1976, Nock and Feder 1979). In addition, noradrenergic agonists reverse the effect of noradrenergic antagonists.

Recently the hypothesis has been proposed that neurotransmitters influence the sensitivity of neural tissues to steroid hormones by modulation of the concentration of neural steroid hormone receptors (Nock et al. 1981). In a recent study of the interaction of the noradrenergic system with the progestin receptor system in the guinea pig brain, the observation was made that interference with noradrenergic transmission causes a decrease in the concentration of cytosol progestin receptors in the hypothalamus, but not other neuroanatomical areas. On the basis of this result the suggestion has been made that the decreased concentration of cytosol progestin receptors may be involved in the mechanism by which inhibitors of noradrenergic transmission block the induction of sexual receptivity by oestradiol and progesterone in female guinea pigs.

We attempted to test further the hypothesis that the inhibition of sexual behavior caused by an inhibitor of norepinephrine synthesis (U-14,624, a dopamine-β-hydroxylase inhibitor) is causally related to the drug-induced decrease in the concentration of hypothalamic cytosol progestin receptors (Blaustein 1984). A decreased concentration of cytosol progestin receptors would be expected to result in less accumulation of nuclear progestin receptors after progesterone injection. This decrease in nuclear progestin receptor concentration might, in turn, result in depressed lordosis responsiveness, as is seen under other conditions of attenuated accumulation of nuclear progestin receptors (Blaustein and Brown 1983).

In order to determine if U-14,624 results in a decrease in the accumulation of nuclear progestin receptors after progesterone injection as well as inhibition of progesterone-facilitated lordosis, guinea pigs were treated as follows (Blaustein 1984). Thirty-six h after injection of oestradiol benzoate, guinea pigs were injected with U-14,624 or vehicle. Twelve h later, they were either killed and hypothalamic and cerebral cortex progestin receptor levels assayed or injected with 500 μg progesterone, tested for lordosis and receptor assays performed 5 h later. By the time of the assay, 100% of the vehicle-injected guinea pigs were sexually receptive, while none of the drug-injected animals were. As was seen previously (Nock et al. 1981), cytosol progestin receptor levels were depressed by 24.4% at the time of progesterone injection (Fig. 5). To our surprise, we also observed an increase of 91.9 femtomoles mg^{-1} DNA in nuclear progestin receptors after U-14,624 treatment. These relationships did not persist 5 h after progesterone injection. At that time, neither nuclear nor cytosol progestin receptor concentrations differed significantly between drug-treated animals and controls, despite the expected inhibition of behavioural responsiveness. Therefore, we did not observe the anticipated decrease in the concentration of nuclear progestin receptors in response to progesterone in guinea pigs that were treated with U-14,624, and who did not respond behaviourally to the progesterone injection.

It is essential to determine if the nuclear receptors that accumulate after U-14,624 injection have the same characteristics as those that accumulate after progesterone. One characteristic of the drug-induced nuclear receptors that we would like to determine is whether or not the nuclear receptors are occupied by ligand. We cannot determine this in the progestin receptor system, because at present, we cannot distinguish between occupied and unoccupied receptors. However, we have also found that U-14,624 increases the concentration of nuclear oestrogen receptors in rat hypothalamus and anterior pituitary gland. In an attempt to determine if the receptors are occupied by an oestrogen-like compound (and perhaps are "functional" receptors), we performed the assay incubations at either 0 °C or 25 °C. If the receptors are occupied by an oestrogen-like substance, then they should require warming to 25 °C to be detected; however, because we found that they could be detected at 0 °C, the nuclear oestrogen receptors that ac-

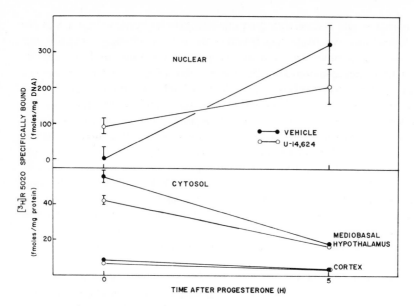

Fig. 5. Concentration of nuclear and cytosol progestin receptors in mediobasal hypothalamus and cerebral cortex from OVX guinea pigs injected with 10 μg oestradiol benzoate followed 36 h later with either U-14,624 or vehicle. Twelve h later, they were either killed (0 h or injected with 500 μg progesterone and killed 5 h later. Baseline levels of nuclear progestin receptors (the level of the control group at 0 h) have been subtracted from all values. (After Blaustein 1984)

cumulate after injection of U-14,624 appear to be unoccupied oestrogen receptors. Therefore, a consequence of U-14,624 injection in rats is to cause an apparent change in some cytosol oestrogen receptors, so that they are associated with cell nuclei. Although this experiment cannot be performed with nuclear progestin receptors in guinea pigs, it seems reasonable that the mechanism by which U-14,624 causes accumulation of nuclear oestrogen receptors in rats is the same or similar to the one by which it causes accumulation of nuclear progestin receptors in guinea pigs. When viewed from the perspective of the newly hypothesized models of steroid hormone action discussed above, it is possible that drug treatment alters the loosely associated receptors so that they become tightly associated with cell nuclei during homogenization.

It is not known if the nuclear progestin receptors that accumulate after U-14,624 treatment are functional nuclear progestin receptors. However, if the level that is present at the time of progesterone injection is considered as baseline, then the U-14,624-injected animals showed less of an increase in the concentration of nuclear progestin receptors after progesterone injection compared with the vehicle-injected guinea pigs (by 108 femtomoles mg^{-1} DNA). If, as is possible, the U-14,624-induced nuclear progestin receptors are nonfunctional receptors, then these results would support the hypothesis that the drug-related decrease in cytosol progestin receptors might cause a decrease in progesterone-facilitated lordosis, in part, by decreasing the concentration of "functional" nuclear progestin receptors that accumulate after progesterone treatment. Experiments are in progress to test this hypothesis.

We have also found that a variety of norepinephrine synthesis inhibitors seem to have a primary effect of causing a decrease in the concentration of cytosol oestrogen receptors in rat hypothalamus and pituitary gland without causing an increase in the concentration of nuclear oestrogen receptors. Although some nuclear accumulation of receptors occurs after treatment with some drugs (Blaustein 1984), the nuclear accumulation of the receptors may not be a necessary antecedent of the decrease in the concentration of cytosol receptors. Therefore the noradrenergic system seems to regulate either the concentration or the physicochemical characteristics of hypothalamic steroid hormone receptors. In this way, it could alter responsiveness of steroid-sensitive cells to specific steroid hormones.

In neuroanatomical studies, a subset of oestradiol-concentrating cells have been observed that appear to have noradrenergic neurons ending in close proximity (Heritage et al. 1977). It may be in this type of neuron that the noradrenergic system regulates the concentration of steroid hormone receptors. Such a relationship potentially provides the anatomical substrate for fine-tuning of steroid sensitivity within individual steroid-sensitive neurons.

5 Discussion

The experiments discussed here are consistent with the idea that neural progestin receptors are involved in mediating the behavioural effects of progesterone in guinea pigs. Perhaps the strongest evidence comes from the work with the progesterone antagonist, RU 486. Treatment of oestrogen-injected guinea pigs with RU 486 prior to progesterone injection blocks progesterone-facilitated sexual behaviour; this inhibition can be overcome by administration of a large dose of progesterone, but not cortisol, which suggests that RU 486 inhibits sexual behaviour by acting specifically on a progestin-sensitive system.

It has been argued that, because the polychlorinated insecticide o,p'-DDT induces responsiveness to progesterone in rats but does not increase the concentration of progestin receptors in the hypothalamus, oestradiol-induced progestin receptors are not necessary for progesterone facilitation of sexual behaviour (Etgen 1983). Because the induction of progestin receptors by oestradiol is of central importance to the model of oestradiol-progesterone regulation of sexual behaviour discussed here, we attempted to study this effect of DDT (Brown and Blaustein 1984c). Although we found the dose of DDT used in the previously study (200 mg kg^{-1} day^{-1} for 3 days) to be insufficient to prime rats to respond to progesterone, we found that twice the level used in the previous work (400 mg kg^{-1} day^{-1} for 3 days) was effective. This seems to be the threshold dose for behavioural responsiveness in our laboratory, because 50% of animals treated in this way responded to a progesterone injection. Contrary to the previous report, we found that a minimal behavioural effective dose of DDT does indeed induce hypothalamic progestin receptors. The most likely explanation for the discrepancy between our work and the previous work is that we used a slightly different technique to assay cytosol progestin receptors. Prior to incubation with (^{3}H)R 5020, we filtered the cytosol to remove any potentially competing DDT. This was necessitated by our finding, in contrast to Etgen's report, that DDT is an effective competitor for progestin receptors. In fact, its effectiveness as a competitor for progestin receptors is quite similar to its effectiveness as a competitor for oestrogen receptors. Therefore, it is necessary to remove the DDT from the cytosol prior to the receptor assay. In fact, this experiment provides additional support for the progestin receptor hypothesis. A minimal behaviourally effective dose of a drug that primes rats to respond to progesterone also induces cytosol progestin receptors in hypothalamus, pituitary gland, and uterus.

The evidence present in this paper suggests that progesterone interaction with progestin receptors not only facilitates sexual behaviour but also, under most circumstances, leads to its termination. Termination of heat seems to result from the loss of the previously elevated level of cell nuclear progestin receptors. Although in some cases, this loss may result, in part, from declining serum progesterone levels, it could occur in at least three other ways. As our data suggest, it is possible that the decline in the concentration of nuclear progestin receptors occurs secondarily to the down-regulation of cytosol progestin receptors. It is possible that there is a substance, perhaps regulated by progesterone, that inactivates directly nuclear progestin receptors. Finally, this loss of nuclear progestin receptors could be a consequence of inactivation following the uncoupling of progesterone from its receptor. Because of the apparent link between nuclear progestin receptor retention and heat duration, studying the mechanisms underlying the loss of nuclear progestin receptors may yield important new information about the regulation of heat duration.

We suggest that heat termination and progesterone-desensitization can be looked at as related phenomena. That is to say, progesterone's desensitization effect may be a consequence of the same cellular events that lead to heat termination. This parallel can be seen most clearly in Fig. 2. In the guinea pigs exposed to a continuous supply of progesterone, heat terminates by approximately 20 h. However, at the point that heat terminates, plasma progesterone levels are still elevated. Therefore, we can also say that, at that time, these guinea pigs are refractory to further stimulation by, or desensitized to, progesterone. The common underlying cause for heat termination and desensitization may be an inadequate level of nuclear progestin receptors. In the case of progesterone desensitization, as with heat termination, this may result from a diminished level of cytosol progestin receptors. We have postulated that this down-regulation of cytosol receptors, then prevents progesterone treatment from elevating sufficiently the level of nuclear progestin receptors. This may then result in refractoriness such that guinea pigs do not respond behaviourally to the second progesterone treatment.

If heat termination and progesterone desensitization are due to a common underlying mechanism, then treatments similar to those that delay heat termination might be expected to overcome progesterone's desensitization effect. This is true of either supplemental oestradiol treatment or supplemental progesterone treatment. Supplemental oestradiol results in an elevated level of nuclear progestin receptors in the heat extension paradigm and an increased accumulation of nuclear progestin receptors in response to a second progesterone injection in the progesterone desensitization paradigm. In both cases, this appears to be secondary to an elevated level of cytosol progestin receptors. Similarly, treatment with a large dose of progesterone results in a greater accumulation of nuclear progestin receptors even in the presence of low levels of cytosol progestin receptors in both procedures.

By this reasoning, then, progesterone desensitization may be looked at as an extension of heat termination. Heat may terminate because of a diminished concentration of progestin receptors in cell nuclei, and animals may remain refractory as long as an insufficient level of progestin receptors accumulates in cell nuclei.

The model for the mechanism of facilitation and desensitization of sexual behaviour by progesterone and of determination of heat duration presented here requires that progesterone's facilitatory and desensitization effects occur in the same cells. It has been shown in rats, that oestradiol and progesterone both act to facilitate sexual behaviour in the ventromedial hypothalamus (Rubin and Barfield 1980, 1983), and progesterone's desensitization effect also occurs at this site (Rubin and Barfield 1984). This finding of a common neuroanatomical substrate is essential to the claim that these different effects on behaviour occur by action within the same neurons. Yet, in guinea pigs, it has been reported that the facilitatory action of oestradiol (Morin and Feder 1974c) and progesterone (Morin and Feder 1974a) may occur by action within the ventromedial hypothalamus-acurate region, while its inhibitory or desensitization effect may occur by action in the midbrain (Morin and Feder 1974b). It is important to discuss some of the findings of these experiments at this time.

Morin and Feder (1974b) implanted oestradiol benzoate-primed guinea pigs with progesterone-containing cannulae in the ventromedial hypothalamus-arcuate area. This treatment resulted in the expression of sexual behaviour, while implants in other areas or implants containing control substances did not. Although it was reported that these animals were not refractory to a subsequent progesterone injection, there are several points that must be made about their findings. It is clear that the lordosis-promoting and heat-terminating effects of progesterone both occur at the same neuroanatomical site – the ventromedial hypothalamus-arcuate area. When progesterone is implanted into this area in oestrogen-primed guinea pigs, lordosis is seen within an hour or two, but heat duration lasts only slightly longer than normal despite the continued presence of the intrahypothalamic progesterone cannula. Therefore, progesterone action at another site is not essential for heat termination to occur.

Contrary to their conclusions, the data seem to support in two ways the notion that intrahypothalamic progesterone implants result in refractoriness to subsequent progesterone administration. When progesterone was injected 8 h after intrahypothalamic progesterone implantation, no difference in heat duration was observed compared with animals that received only the implant without the injection. This was taken as evidence that the progesterone implant did not have an inhibitory influence on response to the systemic progesterone administration. However, in the absence of the progesterone implant, the progesterone injection would have been expected to result in a heat duration of approximately 6 h with a latency of 4.5 h. This would have prolonged heat duration by approximately 4–5 h. Because this extension did not occur, we can conclude that the animals implanted with progesterone in the ventromedial hypothalamic-arcuate area were, in fact, refractory to the systemic progesterone administration 8 h after implantation.

In the experiment that provides the most compelling evidence that intrahypothalamic progesterone induces desensitization to subsequent progesterone injection, animals that had not responded by 8 h after intrahypothalamic implantation of progesterone or cholesterol were injected with progesterone. Although 91% of the cholesterol controls responded to the progesterone injection, only 65% of the progesterone-implanted animals responded to the progesterone injection. This trend toward an inhibitory effect of the progesterone implant was not statistically significant ($p = 0.13$, Fisher's Exact Probability Test). The progesterone-implanted animals that responded to systemic progesterone administration also showed a trend toward shorter heat durations in the animals with control implants, but this was not statistically significant (heat duration = 4.80 h in progesterone-treated animals compared with 6.44 h in controls). We have reanalyzed the published data of Morin and Feder, factoring into their heat duration values, the scores of animals that did not respond to progesterone injection, and therefore had heat durations of 0 h. In this case, we found a mean heat duration of all animals in the progesterone-implanted group of 3.11 h ($\pm$ 0.84; mean + S.E.M.) compared with 5.86 h ($\pm$ 1.08) in the controls. This difference is statistically significant by Student's t-test [$t_{(26)} = 2.02$, $p < 0.05$, 1-tailed test]. In light of this analysis, our conclusions are opposite to those made by Morin and Feder. Progesterone action in the ventromedial hypothalamus-arcuate area is sufficient to cause desensitization to further stimulation by systemic progesterone injection.

In a follow-up experiment, the authors reported that progesterone implantation into the ventromedial hypothalamic-arcuate area was not sufficient to inhibit responsiveness to progesterone 24 h later. Only 33% of the guinea pigs responded to progesterone one day after cholesterol-control implantation compared with 38% for animals that had received progesterone implants. These values can both be compared with 100% of non-implanted controls responding to the progesterone injection. Taken together, the results of these studies and of oestradiol-implant studies (Morin and Feder 1974c) agree with work done in rats (Rubin and Barfield 1980, 1983, 1984). They suggest that oestradiol and progesterone action in cells of the ventromedial hypothalamus-arcuate area is sufficient to prime animals to respond to progesterone, facilitate the expression of sexual behaviour, result in heat termination, and subsequently result in refractoriness to further stimulation of sexual behaviour by progesterone.

Morin and Feder (1974b) also reported that cannula implants of progesterone in the zona compacta of the midbrain substantia nigra of oestrogen-primed guinea pigs resulted in failure to respond to a systemic progesterone injection 8 h later without facilitating sexual behaviour. It is essential to rule out the possibility of diffusion of progesterone to a hypothalamic site. Before this can be considered a site for progesterone's desensitization effect discussed here, it is also necessary to show that this inhibition can be overcome by supplementary oestradiol or supplementary progesterone as can progesterone desensitization in other procedures.

A final question raised by the work presented here is the physiological or behavioural significance of the regulation of steroid hormone receptors by the noradrenergic system. Noradrenergic inhibitors cause the apparent decrease in the concentration of cytosol progestin receptors and increase the concentration of (probably unoccupied) nuclear progestin receptors. At present, we do not know how this process occurs, nor do we know what, if any, physiological function this regulation may have. We can only speculate, at this time, that this unique interaction may provide a means for the environmental modulation of steroid receptor concentrations, and hence sensitivity to particular hormones, in certain cells.

6 Conclusions

The data discussed here support the hypothesis that hypothalamic intracellular progestin receptors are involved in mediating the effects of progesterone on sexual behaviour of female guinea pigs, although they, in no way, exclude the possibility of alternative or complementary mechanisms. The cellular basis of the return to baseline levels of nuclear progestin receptors 12–20 h after progesterone treatment, along with the down-regulation of cytosol progestin receptors, is not certain. However, we suggest that these events lead in part to heat termination and subsequently to refractoriness to progesterone facilitation of lordosis. Although the mechanism and role of the regulation of hypothalamic progestin receptor levels by the noradrenergic system are unknown, it is possible that it is a means by which the environment may exert a modulatory role on hypothalamic responsiveness to sex steroid hormones.

Acknowledgements. The work conducted in the authors' laboratory was supported by grants BNS 13050 from the National Science Foundation, NS 19327 from the National Institutes of Health and Biomedical Research Support Grant 07048. We are grateful to Arnold Well for help with statistical analysis.

References

Blaustein JD (1982a) Alteration of sensitivity to progesterone facilitation of lordosis in guinea pigs by modulation of hypothalamic progestin receptors. Brain Res 243:287–300

Blaustein JD (1982b) Progesterone in high doses may overcome progesterone's desensitization effect on lordosis by translocation of hypothalamic progestin receptors. Horm Behav 16:175–190

Blaustein JD (1984) Noradrenergic inhibitors cause accumulation of nuclear progestin receptors in guinea pig hypothalamus. Brain Res 325:89–98

Blaustein JD, Brown TJ (1983) Mechanisms of oestrogen-progestin interactions in the regulation of lordosis in female guinea pigs. In: Balthazart J, Prove E, Gilles R (eds) Hormones and behaviour in higher vertebrates. Springer, Berlin Heidelberg New York, p 18

Blaustein JD, Feder HH (1979a) Cytoplasmic progestin receptors in female guinea pig brain and their relationship to refractoriness in expression of female sexual behavior. Brain Res 177:489–498

Blaustein JD, Feder HH (1979b) Cytoplasmic progestin receptors in guinea pig brain: characteristics and relationship to the induction of sexual behavior. Brain Res 169:481–497

Blaustein JD, Feder HH (1980) Nuclear progestin receptors in guinea pig brain measured by an in vitro exchange assay after hormonal treatments that affect lordosis. Endocrinology 106:1061–1069

Brown TJ, Blaustein JD (1984a) Inhibition of sexual behavior in female guinea pigs by a progestin receptor antagonist. Brain Res 301:343–349

Brown TJ, Blaustein JD (1984b) Supplemental progesterone delays heat termination and the loss of progestin receptors from hypothalamic cell nuclei in female guinea pigs. Neuroendocrinology 39:384–391

Brown TJ, Blaustein JD (1984c) o,p'-DDT induces functional progestin receptors in the rat hypothalamus and pituitary gland. Endocrinology 115:2052–2058

Crowley WR, Feder HH, Morin LP (1976) Role of monoamines in sexual behavior of the female guinea pig. Pharmacol Biochem Behav 4:67–71

Etgen A (1983) 1-(o-Chlorophenyl)-1-(p-chlorophenyl)2,2,2-trichloroethane: a probe for studying estrogen and progestin receptor mediation of female sexual behavior and neuroendocrine responses. Endocrinology 111:1498–1504

Gorski J, Gannon F (1975) Current models of steroid hormone action: a critique. Annu Rev Physiol 38:425–450

Heritage AS, Grant LD, Stumpf WE (1977) ^{3}H-Estradiol in catecholamine neurons of rat brain stem: combined localization by autoradiography and formaldehyde induced fluorescence. J Comp Neurol 176:607–630

Herrmann W, Wyss R, Riondel D, Teutsch G, Sakiz E, Baulieu EE (1982) Effet d'un stéroide anti-progestérone chez la femme: interruption du cycle menstruel et de la grossesse au début. CR Acad Sci Paris 294:933–938

King WJ, Greene GL (1984) Monoclonal antibodies localize oestrogen receptor in the nuclei of target cells. Nature (Lond) 307:745–747

Lisk RD (1978) The regulation of sexual "heat". In: Hutchison J (ed) Biological determinants of sexual behavior. Wiley, New York, p 425

MacLusky NJ, McEwen BS (1978) Oestrogen modulates progestin receptor concentrations in some rat brain regins, but not in others. Nature (Lond) 274:276–277

McGinnis M, Parsons B, Rainbow TC, Krey LC, McEwen BS (1981) Temporal relationship between cell nuclear progestin receptor levels and sexual receptivity following intravenous progesterone administration. Brain Res 218:365–371

Moguilewsky M, Philibert D (1984) RU 38486: potent antiglucococticoid activity correlated with strong binding to the cytosolic glucocorticoid receptor followed by an impaired activation. J Steroid Biochem 20:271–276

Morin LP (1977) Progesterone: inhibition of rodent behavior. Physiol Behav 18:701–715

Morin LP, Feder HH (1973) Multiple progesterone injections and the duration of estrus in ovariectomized guinea pigs. Physiol Behav 11:861–865

Morin LP, Feder HH (1974a) Hypothalamic progesterone implants and facilitation of lordosis behavior in estrogen-primed ovariectomized guinea pigs. Brain Res 70:81–93

Morin LP, Feder HH (1974b) Inhibition of lordosis behavior in ovariectomized guinea pigs by mesencephalic implants of progesterone. Brain Res 70:71–80

Morin LP, Feder HH (1974c) Intracranial estradiol benzoate implants and lordosis behavior of ovariectomized guinea pigs. Brain Res 70:95–102

Nock B, Feder HH (1979) Noradrenergic transmission and female sexual behavior of guinea pigs. Brain Res 166:369–380

Nock B, Blaustein JD, Feder HH (1981) Changes in noradrenergic transmission alter the concentration of cytoplasmic progestin receptors in hypothalamus. Brain Res 207:371–396

O'Malley BW, Means AR (1974) Female steroid hormones and target cell nuclei. Science (Wash DC) 183:610–624

Parsons B, MacLusky NJ, Krey L, Pfaff DW, McEwen BS (1980) The temporal relationship between estrogen-inducible progestin receptors in the female rat brain and the time course of estrogen activation of mating behavior. Endocrinology 107:774–779

Philibert D, Deraedt R, Teutsch G, Tournemine C, Sakiz E (1982) RU 38486 – a new lead for steroidal antihormones. In: 65th meeting endocrine society, abstract number 668

Rubin BS, Barfield RJ (1980) Priming of estrous responsiveness by implants of 17β-estradiol in the ventromedial hypothalamic nucleus of female rats. Endocrinology 106:504–509

Rubin BS, Barfield RJ (1983) Progesterone in the ventromedial hypothalamus facilitates estrous behavior in ovariectomized, estrogen-primed rats. Endocrinology 113:797–804

Rubin BS, Barfield RJ (1984) Progesterone in the ventromedial hypothalamus of ovariectomized estrogen-primed rats inhibits subsequent facilitation of estrous behavior by systemic progesterone. Brain Res 294:1–8

Sheridan P, Buchanan JM, Anselmo VC, Martin PM (1979) Equilibrium: the intracellular distribution of steroid receptors. Nature (Lond) 282:579–582

Welshons WV, Lieberman ME, Gorski J (1984) Nuclear localization of unoccupied oestrogen receptors. Nature (Lond) 307:747–749

Young WC (1961) The hormones and mating behavior. In: Young WC (ed) Sex and internal secretions. Williams and Wilkins, Baltimore, p 1173

Strategies for Determining the Molecular Mechanisms of Oestrogen Regulation of Female Reproductive Behaviour

A.M. ETGEN[1]

1 Introduction

1.1 Hormonal Regulation of Oestrous Behaviour

Steroid hormones secreted by the gonads play a pivotal role in regulating a variety of behavioural and neuroendocrine functions in vertebrates presumably via direct interactions of the steroids with specific target cells in the brain. One of the best studied examples of hormonal regulation of behaviour is the facilitation of mating behaviour in female mammals by the ovarian steroids oestradiol (OE_2) and progesterone (P). In rats, for example, the display of female sexual behaviour during the oestrous cycle is associated with endogenous fluctuations of plasma OE_2 and P levels (Powers 1970; Feder 1981). The behaviour is abolished following ovariectomy and can be restored in a dose-dependent fashion by replacement therapy with OE_2 and P given in the appropriate sequence (Boling and Blandau 1939, Beach 1942; Edwards et al. 1968). That brain cells are the site of action of ovarian steroids in controlling the expression of copulatory behaviour is supported by observations that application of minute amounts of OE_2 and P directly to restricted brain regions can activate the full complement of oestrous behaviours in female rats (Rubin and Barfield 1983; Barfield et al. 1984).

An important characteristic of ovarian steroid regulation of female sexual behaviour is the sequential nature of oestrogen and progestin action. In rats undergoing normal oestrous cycles, serum OE_2 levels rise 24 h or more before the rise in P (Goodman 1978; Feder 1981). This initial period of oestrogen "priming" appears to be a prerequisite for behavioural activation since administration of P to ovariectomized rats which have not been primed with oestrogen fails to stimulate behavioural receptivity (Boling and Blandau 1939). The observation that OE_2 alone is capable of activating mating behaviour, especially in rats (Davidson et al. 1968), emphasizes the central role of OE_2 in the induction of oestrous responsiveness.

Significant progress has been made in establishing the precise neuroanatomical site(s) at which OE_2 acts to facilitate sexual receptivity, and there is general agreement that the ventromedial nucleus of the hypothalamus (VMN) is most sensitive to the oestrous behaviour-promoting action of oestrogens in rats (Rubin and Barfield 1980), guinea pigs (Morin and Feder 1974), and hamsters (DeBold et al. 1982). However, much less is known about the mechanisms by which brain cells translate the OE_2 signal into an increased probability that specific behavioural patterns will occur in response to ap-

1 Department of Biological Sciences, Rutgers University, New Brunswick, NJ 08903, USA

Neurobiology
(ed. by R. Gilles and J. Balthazart)
© Springer-Verlag Berlin Heidelberg 1985

propriate stimuli. The remainder of this paper will review the experimental strategies we have adopted in an attempt to identify the critical molecular events underlying OE_2 induction of oestrous behaviour, with a particular focus on oestrogen activation of lordosis behaviour.

1.2 The Steroid-Receptor Model

Steroid hormone target tissues such as the uterus and oviduct possess macromolecules known as "receptors." These receptors are believed to be cytoplasmic proteins which, following hormone entry into the cell by passive diffusion, bind the steroid with high affinity, limited capacity, and relative stereospecificity. Binding of the steroid to the receptor somehow "activates" the receptor, and the steroid-receptor complex then translocates to the cell nucleus where it binds to chromatin "acceptor sites" and initiates changes in gene transcription (i.e. RNA synthesis) and translation (i.e. protein synthesis). These alterations in gene expression are believed to mediate the physiological responses of target tissues to steroid hormones (for comprehensive reviews, see Agarwal 1983). While recent data suggest that steroid receptors may normally have an intranuclear rather than a cytoplasmic localization (King and Greene 1984; Welshon et al. 1984), in either case it is the interaction of the hormone-receptor complex with the chromatin which is believed to be responsible for the subsequent target cell response. Can such a mechanism account for the behavioural effects of OE_2 in the brain?

Autoradiographic (Stumpf 1968; Pfaff and Keiner 1973) and cell fractionation techniques (Luttge and Whalen 1972; McEwen et al. 1975) have demonstrated that radiolabelled OE_2 is taken up and retained by neuronal nuclei in several brain regions. The concept that oestrogens might exert their actions on neural target tissues by a molecular mechanism similar to the one described above is supported by the demonstration of specific, limited capacity, high affinity OE_2 receptors in the hypothalamus and other brain regions, including the VMN (Eisenfeld 1970; Kahwanago et al. 1970; Rainbow et al. 1982b). OE_2-receptor complexes have also been shown to bind to hypothalamic chromatin (Whalen and Olsen 1978; Perry and Lopez 1978). Furthermore, oestrogen facilitation of oestrous behaviour can be blocked by concurrent administration of drugs which interfere with brain RNA and protein synthesis (Whalen et al. 1974; Quadagno and Ho 1975; Rainbow et al. 1982a; reviewed by Meisel and Pfaff 1984). Thus it seems reasonable to propose that the activation of female sexual behaviour by OE_2 occurs by receptor-mediated interactions within hypothalamic cell nuclei.

We have adopted two major strategies to test the hypothesis that nuclear interactions of hypothalamic oestrogen binding proteins (receptors) are involved in OE_2 facilitation of lordosis behaviour. The first of these is to utilize oestrogen antagonists (antioestrogens) as tools to probe the mechanism of oestrogen action at the molecular level. The underlying rationale for this strategy is that if we can determine how an antagonist blocks the behavioural effect of OE_2, we will have learned something about how OE_2 must normally act to regulate the behaviour. Thus most of the studies to be discussed below summarize our observations on the effects of a series of antioestrogens on oestrogen-dependent lordosis behaviour and on hypothalamic oestrogen receptors. Once a potentially important step in oestrogen action has been identified, the physiological relevance of this step can be tested using a second strategy, the comparison of hormone action in males and females. Since normal adult male rats are quite refractory to be oestrous behaviour-promoting effects of ovarian steroids, it might be predicted that male brains would be deficient in those aspects of OE_2 interaction with neural receptors that are essential for the expression of lordosis.

2 Studies with Antioestrogens

2.1 Inhibition of Behaviour and Nuclear Oestrogen Binding

Many laboratories have reported that antioestrogens injected concurrently with or within a few hours of oestrogen treatment completely block the induction of lordosis responses in female rats (for reviews see Roy et al. 1979b; Fabre-Nys 1982). Early biochemical studies with the synthetic oestrogen antagonists CI-628 and nafoxidine also demonstrated that most antioestrogen treatments which reduced lordosis behaviour reduced cell nuclear uptake of radiolabeled OE_2 by hypothalamic and preoptic area (HPOA) tissue (Roy and Wade 1977; Landau 1977; Wade and Blaustein 1978). Our initial study correlated the effects of three antagonists, CI-628, nafoxidine, and tamoxifen, on mating behaviour and on HPOA cell nuclear binding of OE_2 (Etgen 1979). All three compounds blocked oestrogen-induced lordosis in a dose- and time-dependent manner. Figure 1 shows that there is a substantial ($r = 0.67$) and statistically significant $[t(14) = 3.40, P < 0.01$, linear regression] correlation between the magnitude of inhibition of lordosis behaviour and the reduction in binding of ^{3}H-OE_2 in HPOA cell nuclei. These results strongly point to the cell nucleus as the critical locus of oestrogen receptor-mediated interactions which are necessary for activation of female rat sexual responses.

A more recent study further strengthens this conclusion (Howard et al. 1984). Intracerebral implants of the antioestrogen tamoxifen directly into the ventromedial hypothalamus (and sometimes the POA) significantly attenuated both the quantity and quality of lordosis responses induced by systemic oestrogen administration in female rats. Furthermore, the behavioural inhibition was correlated with a reduction of ^{3}H-OE_2 binding in hypothalamic but not preoptic cell nuclei (see Table 1). These data support

Table 1. Effects of intracerebral implants of tamoxifen on OE_2-induced lordosis[a] and nuclear oestrogen binding in hypothalamus (HYP) and preoptic area (POA) of ovariectomized female rats. (Adapted from Howard et al. 1984)

Implant	$\overline{X}$LQ		Nuclear ^{3}H-OE_2 binding, % control	
Site(n)	Pretest	Tamoxifen	HYP	POA
VMN (6)	80	8	67	84
POA (3)	75	20	43	108

LQ, lordosis quotient (lordosis responses/mounts × 100)

[a] OE_2 was administered at 0 and 6 h (1–2 μg injection^{-1}), 500 μg of P was delivered at 19 h, and animals were tested for lordosis behaviour at 24 h

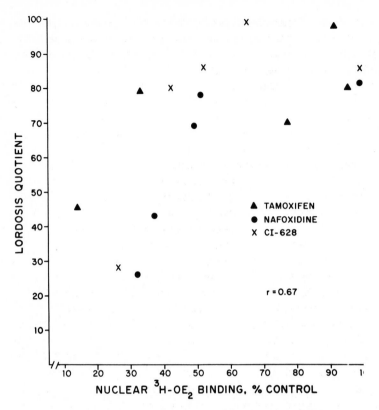

Fig. 1. Correlation between antioestrogen inhibition of lordosis behaviour and nuclear binding of
$^3H\text{-}OE_2$ in the HPOA of ovariectomized female rats. For behavioural studies, female rats received
antioestrogens 2, 24, 48, 96, or 168 h prior to 2 μg of OE_2B; behavioural tests were conducted
48 h after OE_2B administration and 4 h after injection of 500 μg of P. Lordosis quotient = lordosis
responses/mounts × 100. For biochemical studies, antioestrogens were injected at the same times
prior to intravenous injections of 40 μCi of $^3H\text{-}OE_2$, and rats were killed 1 h later. In both cases,
antioestrogen doses were 2 mg for *CI-628* and nafoxidine and 1 mg for tamoxifen. Control levels
of nuclear $^3H\text{-}OE_2$ binding were assessed in ovariectomized females given no prior hormonal treatment. (After Etgen 1979)

the hypothesis that nuclear binding of OE_2 by hypothalamic cells is a prerequisite for
oestrogen priming of oestrous behaviour.

2.2 Inhibition of OE_2-Receptor Binding by Antioestrogens

A simple interpretation of the evidence presented so far is that antioestrogens inhibit
OE_2 facilitation of reproductive behaviour by competing for OE_2 binding to cytosol
receptors and thus preventing receptor translocation into HPOA cell nuclei. Indeed we
and others have shown that antioestrogens compete for OE_2 binding to HPOA cytosol
receptors (Kurl and Morris 1978; Etgen and Whalen 1981/82). However, such a mechanism cannot account for the behavioural effects of oestrogen antagonists because these
agents are all capable of translocating oestrogen receptors to the nucleus where they

may be retained for prolonged periods of time (see Roy 1978 for review). This consideration has led to the hypothesis that antioestrogens form an abnormal ligand-receptor complex which (a) prevents OE_2-receptor complexes from interacting with behaviourally relevant chromatin binding sites, and (b) is itself unable to interact with the specific chromatin acceptor sites involved in the activation of lordosis behaviour (Etgen 1979; Etgen and Whalen 1981/82). This hypothesis would receive support from the demonstration that neural oestrogen receptors contain at least two interacting ligand binding sites. If this were the case, ligand binding at either site could produce unique conformational changes in the receptor protein which in turn would influence ligand binding at the other site and determine with which chromatin acceptor sites the ligand-receptor complex can interact. Kinetic data on the interactions of OE_2, nafoxidine, and tamoxifen with HPOA oestrogen receptors support the existence of multiple, interacting binding sites (Etgen and Whalen 1981/82). To investigate this possibility further we have looked in greater detail at the interactions of OE_2 and tamoxifen with HPOA oestrogen receptors.

The rationale for these studies is as follows. If there is only a single ligand binding site on the neural oestrogen receptor, radiolabeled OE_2 should dissociate from the receptor at the same rate in both the presence and absence of non-radioactive ligands (provided that reassociation with radioactive steroid is prevented). In contrast, if antioestrogen (or OE_2 itself) alter the rate of dissociation of ^3H-OE_2 from HPOA receptors, it may be inferred that multiple, interacting binding sites are present on the receptor such that ligand binding at one site influences ligand binding at other sites. Such long-range effects are likely to be mediated by ligand-induced conformational changes in the receptor protein.

Figure 2 presents the results of such an experiment. It is apparent that the antioestrogen tamoxifen accelerated the dissociation of ^3H-OE_2 from HPOA oestrogen receptors when compared to the dissociation rate observed with no added ligand or with nonradioactive OE_2 as the added ligand. Moreover, the enhanced dissociation rate was observed when either non-activated (+ molybdate) or activated (− molybdate) oestrogen-receptor complexes were used. Only activated receptors are believed to be capable of specifically binding to chromatin acceptor sites (see Grody et al. 1982 for recent review). These binding data are consistent with the hypothesis that brain oestrogen receptors possess more than one ligand binding site. They also support the notion that antioestrogens could interfere with OE_2 activation of lordosis behaviour by (a) accelerating the dissociation of OE_2 from nuclear receptors and/or (b) forming a ligand-receptor complex which is unable to interact with chromatin binding sites whose gene products are required for the expression of the behaviour.

2.3 Inhibition of Behaviour and Progestin Receptor Induction

Several laboratories have shown that oestrogen treatments which produce lordosis responding also induce cytosol progestin receptor synthesis in the HPOA of female rats. Therefore it has been proposed that the neural progestin receptor protein is a gene product which must be induced by OE_2 to prepare the neural substrate to respond to the behaviour-facilitating actions of P (for recent reviews see Etgen 1984; Feder 1984; McEwen and Krey 1984). In support of this proposal, Roy et al. (1979a) showed that

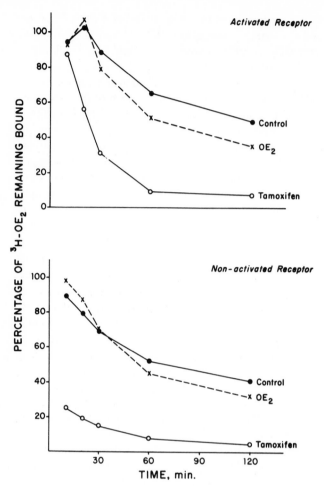

Fig. 2. Effects of 1,000-fold excess unlabelled OE_2 and tamoxifen on the dissociation of radio-labelled OE_2 from HPOA cytosol oestrogen receptors. Receptors were saturated with oestrogen and activated by incubating with 2 nM $^3H\text{-}OE_2$ for 10 min at 30 °C. In the *lower panel*, 10 mM sodium molybdate was included in all buffers to prevent activation. Free $^3H\text{-}OE_2$ concentration was reduced to approx. 0.02 nM prior to initiation of dissociation, and dissociation was carried out at 26 °C

OE_2 induction of HPOA progestin receptors was partially blocked (36%–66%) by the antioestrogen CI-628. However, the authors did not report behavioural data on animals treated with the CI-628 doses which were tested for antagonism of progestin receptor induction. In addition, it has been reported that many oestrogen antagonists fail to prevent OE_2 induction of uterine progestin receptors and/or are themselves capable of stimulating uterine and pituitary progestin receptor synthesis when given alone (Leavitt et al. 1977; Koseki et al. 1977; Jordan and Prestwich 1978; Kirchoff et al. 1983b). Thus we undertook a reexamination of the correlation between antioestrogen inhibition of lordosis behaviour and HPOA progestin receptor induction.

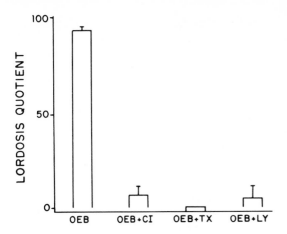

Fig. 3. Inhibition of oestrogen-dependent lordosis behaviour in ovariectomized female rats by antioestrogens. Control females received 2 μg of oestradiol benzoate (OEB) at 0 h, 500 μg of P at 48 h, and behaviour was evaluated at 52 h. Experimental animals received 2 mg of CI-628 (*CI*) 2 h before OEB, 2 mg of tamoxifen (*TX*) concurrently with OEB, or 4 mg of LY117018 (*LY*) concurrently with OEB and were tested 4 h following P injections. Values represent means ± SEM

Figure 3 shows that the oestrogen antagonists CI-628, tamoxifen and LY117018 virtually eliminate lordosis responses in female rats injected with 2 μg of OE_2 benzoate (OE_2B) 52 h prior to behavioural testing. We then administered the same doses of LY117018, CI-628, or tamoxifen, plus or minus 2 μg of OE_2B, to ovariectomized female rats of the same age (see Fig. 4). As expected, animals receiving 2 μg of OE_2B alone showed an approx. twofold elevation in HPOA cytosol progestin receptor levels. In agreement with Roy et al. (1979a), we also found that all 3 antagonists alone produced only a small rise in progestin binding activity and substantially attenuated the oestrogen-induced elevation. The antioestrogen LY117018 was the most effective antagonist of OE_2B-induced progestin receptor induction and the least effective inducer when given alone. These data seemed to indicate that progestin receptor induction might be a necessary step in OE_2 facilitation of lordosis.

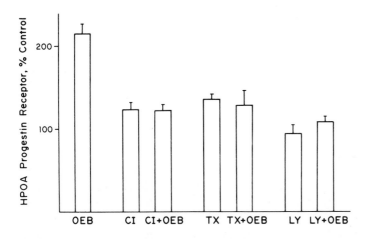

Fig. 4. Inhibition of oestrogen-induced HPOA progestin receptor synthesis in ovariectomized female rats treated with the same OEB and antioestrogen doses shown in Fig. 3. Tissue from two animals was combined for each point, and receptors were measured by incubating cytosols with 0.5 nM ^{3}H-R-5020. Each value represents the mean of three or four independent replications

This conclusion was questioned, however, when we measured HPOA progestin receptor induction in chronically antioestrogen-treated rats. After a pretest on week 1, animals received 2 μg of $OE_2 B$ plus CI-628 or tamoxifen on week 2. As expected, lordosis responses were suppressed. Control tests the next week demonstrated that the antioestrogens by themselves did not induce lordosis behaviour. A final test indicated that behavioural responsiveness to OE_2 had returned within a week following the last antioestrogen test. At least 2 weeks after their final antioestrogen test, rats which had previously been treated with CI-628 or tamoxifen were reinjected with vehicle, $OE_2 B$ alone, antioestrogen alone or $OE_2 B$ plus antioestrogen. As shown in Fig. 5, $OE_2 B$ combined with doses of CI-628 or tamoxifen known to inhibit behaviour usually elevated HPOA cytosol progestin receptors to slightly above control (non-oestrogen primed) levels, but the levels did not approach those normally seen in female rats given 2 μg of $OE_2 B$ alone (see Fig. 4). Animals given antioestrogen alone showed small, variable increases in brain progestin receptor content. However, we also observed that $OE_2 B$ itself produced only moderate (45%–50%) induction of HPOA progestin receptor in these chronically antioestrogen-treated animals rather than the expected twofold elevation despite the fact that the return of behavioral responsiveness to oestrogen treatment had been verified the previous week.

The combined results of the acute and chronic antioestrogen experiments imply that oestrogen induction of high levels of HPOA progestin receptors may not be obligatory for oestrogen priming of lordosis behaviour in female rats. The consistent attenuation of receptor induction by $OE_2 B$ in behaviourally responsive, chronically antioestrogen-treated rats suggests that stimulation of neural progestin receptor synthesis may not be

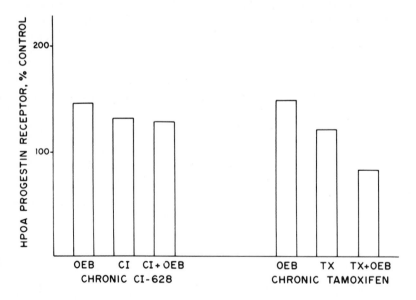

Fig. 5. Effects of chronic treatment with CI-628 (*CI*) or tamoxifen (*TX*) on *HPOA* progestin receptor levels. Animals which had received 2 weeks of behavioural testing with antioestrogens (see text for details) were used in these experiments. Other conditions are the same as in Fig. 4. Each value represents the mean of two to four independent replications

necessary for OE_2 activation of lordosis responding. However, this cannot be stated as a firm conclusion since receptor induction was not completely abolished and we have not measured progestin receptor levels in restricted hypothalamic nuclei such as the VMN.

3 Male-Female Comparisons

In contrast with adult females, adult male rats generally show little or no lordosis behaviour following OE_2 plus P treatment. The potential of the two sexes to express lordosis in adulthood can be reversed if neonatal males are castrated and neonatal females are exposed to androgens or oestrogens (Barraclough and Gorski 1962; Luttge and Whalen 1970). The ability to produce male and female rats which are either highly responsive or unresponsive to the behavioural effects of ovarian steroids has prompted investigators to compare receptor dynamics in male and female rat brains as a strategy to identify critical molecular events which mediate oestrous behaviour. This approach has provided evidence that sex differences in lordosis behaviour may be related to sex differences in the binding of OE_2 to nuclei and chromatin in the HPOA (Whalen and Massicci 1975; Whalen and Olsen 1978; Olsen and Whalen 1980; Nordeen and Yahr 1983). Similarly, reports of sex differences in oestrogen induction of neural progestin receptors have led to the hypothesis that the differential expression of oestrous behaviours in male and female rats might result from a deficiency of oestrogen induction of HPOA progestin receptors in males (Moguilewsky and Raynaud 1979; Rainbow et al. 1982c). Since our antioestrogen data did not unequivocally support the proposal that induction of progestin receptors is an essential intranuclear event underlying OE_2 activation of lordosis, we have also assessed the sensitivity of neural progestin receptors to oestrogen induction in male and female rats.

Our initial study (Etgen 1981) found that oestrogen priming produced comparable increases in HPOA progestin receptor levels in normal males, normal females, neonatally castrated males, and neonatally androgenized females. Of these four groups, only normal females and neonatally castrated males were behaviourally responsive to the same oestrogen treatments (Table 2). Similar data have since been reported by another laboratory

Table 2. Effect of oestrogen priming (two daily injections of 5 μg of OE_2 B) on HPOA progestin receptor (PR) levels and lordosis behaviour in male, female, neonatally castrated male, and neonatally androgenized female rats. (Adapted from Etgen 1981)

Sex	Neonatal Treatment[a]	Lordosis behaviour ($\overline{X}$LQ ± SEM)	% Increase in PR with OE_2B[b]
Female	Vehicle	95.3 ± 2.58	110
Female	500 μg TP	5.3 ± 1.51	106
Male	Vehicle	7.1 ± 2.81	105
Male	Castrated	80.0 ± 4.80	106

LQ, lordosis quotient (Lordosis responses/mounts × 100); TP, testosterone propionate

[a] Neonatal treatments were performed within 24 h of birth
[b] Compared to vehicle-treated controls

Table 3. Effects of OE_2 B priming on HPOA progestin receptor levels in weight-matched adult male and female rats

[a] OE_2 B priming regimen	Sex	[b,c] Progestin receptors % control
2 µg, 48 h pre-sacrifice	Female	181
	Male	179
8 µg, 48 h pre-sacrifice	Female	227
	Male	215
10 µg, 24, 48, 72 h pre-sacrifice	Female	318
	Male	208

[a] Indicated OE_2 B doses administered per 200 g body weight
[b] Controls received oil vehicle at same times pre-sacrifice
[c] Each value represents the mean of four to seven independent replications

(Ghraf et al. 1983; Kirchoff et al. 1983a). More recently, we have measured HPOA progestin receptor induction in weight-matched males and females as a function of oestrogen dose (see Table 3). The only condition which produced consistent, robust sex differences in HPOA cytosol progestin receptor content was the administration of high doses of oestrogen (10 µg of OE_2 B day^{-1} for 3 days prior to assay). Under this condition, females had consistently higher neural progestin receptor levels than their weight-matched male counterparts. This was the oestrogen priming regimen which was reported by Rainbow et al. (1982c) to produce significant sex differences in VMN progestin receptor levels. Comparable differences were never seen with lower doses of OE_2B (2 or 8 µg 48 h prior to assay) which are sufficient to facilitate oestrous behaviour in females (Whalen 1974).

Although we cannot rule out the possibility that sex differences in brain progestin receptors might have been detected with low dose oestrogen priming had we assayed microdissected hypothalamic nuclei (e.g. the VMN and periventricular POA), our data suggest that it may be premature to conclude that the refractoriness of male rats to the activation of oestrous behaviour by OE_2 is causally related to insensitivity of the male brain to oestrogen induction of progestin receptors. Similar conclusions have been reached in studies of progestin receptor induction in male and female guinea pigs (Blaustein et al. 1980). Present results do, however, indicate that under some circumstances the neural progestin receptor systems of males and females respond differently to oestrogen stimulation. Whether and how these differences relate to sexual dimorphisms in neuroendocrinology or behaviour remains to be established.

4 Summary and Conclusions

Evidence presented here provides strong support for the hypothesis that oestrogens regulate oestrous behaviour in female rats via receptor-mediated interactions within hypothalamic cell nuclei. The binding data are also consistent with the notion that both OE_2 and antioestrogens promote unique and different conformations of the neural oestrogen receptor protein such that the ligand-receptor complex formed when OE_2 is bound can interact with chromatin acceptor sites involved in lordosis facilitation while the antioestrogen-receptor complex cannot. However, the identity of the gene products which are induced by oestrogen to activate oestrous behaviour has yet to be established. One likely candidate, the neural progestin receptor, clearly is not sufficient for behavioural activation since the experiments with male rats demonstrate that animals with elevated HPOA progestin receptor levels do not necessarily exhibit lordosis responses. Further studies will be required to determine if progestin receptor induction is a necessary event. It seems likely that experiments utilizing oestrogen antagonists and capitalizing on sex differences in the potential to display steroid-dependent behaviour will continue to yield insights into the molecular mechanisms mediating oestrogen regulation of oestrous behaviour.

Acknowledgments. Supported by DHHS grants MH-34228, MH-36041 and BRSG PHS RR7058 and grants from the Charles and Johanna Busch Memorial Fund. The author acknowledges the important contributions of several collaborators to the studies reported here: Dr. Ronald Barfield, Dr. Richard Whalen, S. Beth Howard, Peter Shamamian, and Joan Sorenson. Appreciation is also extended to Alan Gerstein and Ellen Leiman for excellent technical assistance and to Jane Sherwood for typing the manuscript.

References

Agarwal MK (ed) (1983) Principles of receptorology. De Gruyter, Berlin

Barfield RJ, Glaser JH, Rubin BS, Etgen AM (1984) Behavioral effects of progestin in the brain. Psychoneuroendocrinology 9:217–231

Barraclough CA, Gorski RA (1962) Studies on mating behaviour in the androgen-sterilized female rat in relation to the hypothalamic regulation of sexual behaviour. J Endocrinol 25:175–182

Beach FA (1942) Importance of progesterone to induction of sexual receptivity in spayed female rats. Proc Soc Exp Biol Med 51:369–371

Blaustein JD, Ryer HI, Feder HH (1980) A sex difference in the progestin receptor system of guinea pig brain. Neuroendocrinology 31:403–409

Boling JL, Blandau RJ (1939) The estrogen-progesterone induction of mating responses in the spayed female rat. Endocrinology 25:359–364

Davidson JM, Rodgers CH, Smith ER, Bloch GJ (1968) Stimulation of female sex behavior in adrenalectomized rats with estrogen alone. Endocrinology 82:193–195

DeBold JF, Malsbury CW, Harris VS, Malenka R (1982) Sexual receptivity: brain sites of estrogen action in female hamsters. Physiol Behav 29:589–593

Edwards DA, Whalen RE, Nadler RD (1968) Induction of estrus: estrogen-progesterone interactions. Physiol Behav 3:29–33

Eisenfeld AJ (1970) Estradiol: in vitro binding to macromolecules from the hypothalamus, anterior pituitary and uterus. Endocrinology 86:1313–1318

Etgen AM (1979) Antiestrogens: effects of tamoxifen, nafoxidine, and CI-628 on sexual behavior, cytoplasmic receptors, and nuclear binding of estrogen. Horm Behav 13:97–112

Etgen AM (1981) Estrogen induction of progestin receptors in the hypothalamus of male and female rats which differ in their ability to exhibit cyclic gonadotropin secretion and female sexual behavior. Biol Reprod 25:307–313

Etgen AM (1984) Progestin receptors and the activation of female reproductive behavior: a critical review. Horm Behav 18:411–430

Etgen AM, Whalen RE (1981/82) Kinetic analysis of estrogen and antiestrogen competition for hypothalamic cytosol estrogen receptors. Evidence for noncompetitive ligand-receptor interactions. J Recept Res 2:531–553

Fabre-Nys C (1982) Anti-steroids and animal behaviour: a review. In: Agarwal MK (ed) Hormone antagonists. De Gruyter, Berlin, pp 77–88

Feder HH (1981) Estrous cyclicity in mammals. In: Adler NT (ed) Neuroendocrinology of reproduction. Plenum, New York, pp 279–349

Feder HH (1984) Hormones and sexual behavior. Annu Rev Psychol 35:165–200

Ghraf R, Kirchoff J, Grunke W, Reinhardt W, Ball P, Knuppen R (1983) Estrogen responsiveness of progestin receptor induction in the pituitary, preoptic-hypothalamic brain and uterus of neonatally estrogenized female rats. Brain Res 258:133–138

Goodman RL (1978) A quantitative analysis of the physiological role of estradiol and progesterone in the control of tonic and surge secretion of luteinizing hormone in the rat. Endocrinology 102: 142–150

Grody WW, Schrader WT, O'Malley BW (1982) Activation, transformation, and subunit structure of steroid hormone receptors. Endocr Rev 3:141–163

Howard SB, Etgen AM, Barfield RJ (1984) Antagonism of central estrogen action by intracerebral implants of tamoxifen. Horm Behav 18:256–266

Jordan VC, Prestwich G (1978) Effect of non-steroidal anti-oestrogens on the concentration of rat uterine progesterone receptors. J Endocrinol 76:363–364

Kahwanago I, Heinrichs WR, Herrmann WL (1970) Estradiol "receptors" in hypothalamus and anterior pituitary gland. Inhibition of estradiol binding by SH group blocking agents and clomiphene citrate. Endocrinology 86:1319–1326

King WJ, Greene GL (1984) Monoclonal antibodies localize oestrogen receptor in the nuclei of target cells. Nature (Lond) 307:745–747

Kirchoff J, Grunke W, Ghraf R (1983a) Estrogen induction of progestin receptors in pituitary, hypothalamic and uterine cytosol of androgenized female rats. Brain Res 275:173–177

Kirchoff J, Grunke W, Hoffmann B, Nagel W, Ghraf R (1983b) Estrogen agonistic and antagonistic action of 8 non-steroidal antiestrogens on progestin receptor induction in rat pituitary gland and uterus. Brain Res 289:380–384

Koseki Y, Zava DT, Chamness GC, McGuire WL (1977) Progesterone interaction with estrogen and antiestrogen in rat uterus-receptor effects. Steroids 30:169–177

Kurl RN, Morris ID (1978) Differential depletion of cytoplasmic high affinity oestrogen receptors after the in vivo administration of the antioestrogens, clomiphene, MER-25 and tamoxifen. Br J Pharmacol 62:487–493

Landau IT (1977) Relationships between the effects of the antiestrogen, CI-628, on sexual behavior, uterine growth, and cellular nuclear estrogen retention after estradiol-17β-benzoate administration in the ovariectomized rat. Brain Res 133:119–138

Leavitt WW, Chen TJ, Allen TC (1977) Regulation of progesterone receptor formation by estrogen action. Ann NY Acad Sci 286:210–225

Luttge WG, Whalen RE (1970) Dihydrotestosterone, androstenedione, testosterone: comparative effectiveness in masculinizing and defeminizing reproductive systems in male and female rats. Horm Behav 1:265–281

Luttge WG, Whalen RE (1972) The accumulation, retention and interaction of oestradiol and oestrone in central neural and peripheral tissues of gonadectomized female rats. J Endocrinol 52:379–395

McEwen BS, Krey LC (1984) Properties of estrogen-sensitive neurons: aromatization, progestin receptor induction and neuroendocrine effects. In: Celotti F, Naftolin F, Martini L (eds) Metabolism of hormonal steroids in the neuroendocrine structures. Serono symp publications, vol 13. Raven, New York, pp 117–128

McEwen BS, Pfaff DW, Chaptal C, Luine V (1975) Brain cell nuclear retention of 3H estradiol doses able to promote lordosis: temporal and regional aspects. Brain Res 86:155–161

Meisel RL, Pfaff DW (1984) RNA and protein synthesis inhibitors: effects on sexual behavior in female rats. Brain Res Bull 12:187–193

Moguilewsky M, Raynaud J-P (1979) The relevance of hypothalamic and hypophyseal progestin receptor regulation in the induction and inhibition of sexual behavior in the female rat. Endocrinology 105:516–522

Morin LP, Feder HH (1974) Intracranial estradiol benzoate implants and lordosis behavior of ovariectomized guinea pigs. Brain Res 70:95–102

Nordeen EJ, Yahr P (1983) A regional analysis of estrogen binding to hypothalamic cell nuclei in relation to masculinization and defeminization. J Neurosci 3:933–941

Olsen KL, Whalen RE (1980) Sexual differentiation of the brain: effects on mating behavior and [³H]estradiol binding by hypothalamic chromatin in rats. Biol Reprod 22:1068–1072

Perry BN, Lopez A (1978) The binding of ³H-labelled oestradiol- and progesterone-receptor complexes to hypothalamic chromatin of male and female sheep. Biochem J 176:873–883

Pfaff DW, Keiner M (1973) Atlas of estradiol-concentrating cells in the central nervous system of the female rat. J Comp Neurol 151:121–158

Powers JB (1970) Hormonal control of sexual receptivity during the estrous cycle of the rat. Physiol Behav 5:831–836

Quadagno DM, Ho GKW (1975) The reversible inhibition of steroid-induced sexual behavior by intracranial cycloheximide. Horm Behav 6:19–26

Rainbow TC, McGinnis MY, Davis PG, McEwen BS (1982a) Application of anisomycin to the lateral ventromedial nucleus of the hypothalamus inhibits the activation of sexual behavior by estradiol and progesterone. Brain Res 223:417–423

Rainbow TC, Parsons B, MacLusky NJ, McEwen BS (1982b) Estradiol receptor levels in rat hypothalamic and limbic nuclei. J Neurosci 2:1439–1445

Rainbow TC, Parsons B, McEwen BS (1982c) Sex differences in rat brain oestrogen and progestin receptors. Nature (Lond) 300:648–649

Roy EJ (1978) Antiestrogens and nuclear estrogen receptors in the brain. In: Lederis K, Veale WL (eds) Current studies of hypothalamic function, vol 1. Karger, Basel, pp 204–213

Roy EJ, Wade GN (1977) Binding of [³H]estradiol by brain cell nuclei and female rat sexual behavior: inhibition by antiestrogens. Brain Res 126:73–87

Roy EJ, MacLusky NJ, McEwen BS (1979a) Antiestrogen inhibits the induction of progestin receptors by estradiol in the hypothalamus-preoptic area and pituitary. Endocrinology 104:1333–1336

Roy EJ, Schmit E, McEwen BS, Wade GN (1979b) Antiestrogens in the central nervous system. In: Agarwal MK (ed) Antihormones. Elsevier, Amsterdam, pp 181–197

Rubin BS, Barfield RJ (1980) Priming of estrous responsiveness by implants of 17β-estradiol in the ventromedial hypothalamic nucleus of female rats. Endocrinology 106:504–509

Rubin BS, Barfield RJ (1983) Induction of estrous behavior in ovariectomized rats by sequential replacement of estrogen and progesterone to the ventromedial hypothalamus. Neuroendocrinology 37:218–224

Stumpf WE (1968) Estradiol-concentrating neurons: topography in the hypothalamus by dry mount autoradiography. Science (Wash DC) 162:1001–1003

Wade GN, Blaustein JD (1978) Effects of an anti-estrogen on neural estradiol binding and on behaviors in female rats. Endocrinology 102:245–251

Welshon WV, Lieberman ME, Gorski J (1984) Nuclear localization of unoccupied oestrogen receptors. Nature (Lond) 307:747–749

Whalen RE (1974) Estrogen-progesterone induction of mating in female rats. Horm Behav 5:157–162

Whalen RE, Massicci J (1975) Subcellular analysis of the accumulation of estrogen by the brain of male and female rats. Brain Res 89:255–264

Whalen RE, Olsen KL (1978) Chromatin binding of estradiol in the hypothalamus and cortex of male and female rats. Brain Res 152:121–131

Whalen RE, Gorzalka BB, DeBold JF, Quadagno DM, Ho GKW, Hough JC Jr (1974) Studies on the effects of intracerebral actinomycin-D implants on estrogen-induced receptivity in rats. Horm Behav 5:337–343

Symposium II

Behavioural Endocrinology of Birds

Organizer J. BALTHAZART

Testosterone and Aggressive Behaviour During the Reproductive Cycle of Male Birds

J.C. WINGFIELD and M.RAMENOFSKY [1]

1 Introduction

Over the last two decades, great advances have been made in our understanding of the endocrine control of aggression in both reproductive and non-reproductive contexts. These new insights stem primarily from work which has focused on endocrine, neuro-endocrine and enzymatic activity in the brain-gonad axis during the dramatic developmental periods of either puberty or seasonal breeding. Despite these sophisticated advances, simple correlations of circulating levels of hormones with either aggressive behaviour or social dominance have proved to be equivocal. Recent work on rodents (Schuurman 1980; Keverne et al. 1978; Brain 1983) and primates including man (e.g. Dixson 1980; Bernstein et al. 1983; Mazur 1983) suggest that such correlations depend to a great extent on taxonomic class, age, experience, social context, and other environmental influences. In primates, for example, simple correlations of plasma androgen and aggressive behaviour have been difficult to establish (Eaton and Resko 1974; Phoenix 1980). It is possible that the complex and diverse social systems, as typified by primates, may serve to obscure detection of any relationship (Dixson 1980; Bernstein et al. 1983). This, in addition, makes design of the critical experiment difficult, if not artificial. In rodents, with social systems that are generally less complex than primates, the evidence for correlations of circulating levels of hormones such as testosterone (T) with aggressive behaviour are more convincing, although not exclusively so. Once again, evidence suggests that these correlations are dependent upon age and social context, as well as environmental influences such as day length, presence of a mate, diet, and weather variables.

Although the endocrine control of aggressive behaviour in a variety of contexts is well established, the underlying mechanisms by which environmental factors influence endocrine secretion, hormone-behaviour interactions, and reproductive function are much less well known. In this communication we will focus specifically on the environmental and hormonal control of aggression during the reproductive cycle of male birds.

Long term changes in aggressive behaviour related to reproduction are most apparent in higher vertebrates that breed seasonally. Those at mid- to high-latitudes use the annual photocycle as proximate information to time reproductive development so that breeding commences at a time of year favourable for production and survival of young

---

[1] The Rockefeller University Field Research Centre, Tyrrel Road, Millbrook, NY 12545, USA, and Vassar College, Poughkeepsie, NY 12601, USA

Neurobiology
(ed. by R. Gilles and J. Balthazart)
© Springer-Verlag Berlin Heidelberg 1985

(e.g. Farner and Follett 1979; Farner and Gwinner 1980; Wingfield and Farner 1980; Wingfield 1980, 1983). Day length also regulates secretion of gonadotrophins and sex steroid hormones, such as T, that in turn influence aggressive behaviour. However, there are several types of aggressive behaviour associated with reproductive processes. For example, males of most avian species establish a territory for defence of food or other resources important for survival (e.g. Brown 1964). In addition, these males become aggressive toward conspecific males when females are sexually receptive, and this aggression, or mate-guarding behaviour, is thought to increase the probability of paternity of an individual male in the breeding pair or group. Thus, these distinct changes in aggressive context require that the neuroendocrine and endocrine control systems receive essential supplementary information from the environment. This type of information fine-tunes the regulation of aggressive behaviour and other reproductive functions (Wingfield 1980, 1983).

2 Hormonal Control of Aggressive Behaviour

The endocrine regulation of aggressive behaviour in birds, at least in reproductive contexts, is essentially very similar to that of mammals. In virtually all avian species studied to date, circulating levels of luteinizing hormone (LH) and T are elevated during the establishment of a breeding territory or during the mate-guarding period. These hormones are involved in, among other functions, the regulation of aggressive behaviour and sexual displays (e.g. of reviews and articles: Marler 1955, Pröve 1974; Silver et al. 1979; Harding 1981, 1983; Balthazart 1983; Adkins 1977, Cheng and Lehrman 1975; Adkins-Regan 1981).

The effects of sex steroid hormones on reproductive behaviour of males has been investigated in a variety of species and currently it appears that expression of aggressive behaviour in reproductive contexts may also depend upon metabolism of testosterone within the target cell to 5α- or 5β-dihydrotestosterone (for comprehensive reviews see Hutchison and Steimer 1983; Balthazart 1983; see also chapters by J. Hutchison and R.E. Hutchison and by J. Balthazart and M. Schumacher in this volume). In some species, however, aromatization of T to oestradiol-17β may also be important (Harding et al. 1984). Administration of T, or its metabolites, increases the occurrence, frequency and, in a few cases, intensity of aggressive displays of intact and castrated individuals (Bennett 1940; Kuo 1960; Adkins and Pniewski 1978; Rohwer and Rohwer 1978; Trobec and Oring 1972; Moore 1984; Wingfield 1984a, 1985a; Searcy and Wingfield 1980).

Recent investigations conducted on castrated Japanese quail, *Coturnix coturnix*, matched in dyadic encounters with an intact opponent (Ramenofsky 1982), indicate that T administered via subcutaneous implants in Silastic tubing promotes the following changes: (1) increased circulating levels of T from basal (0.1 ng ml^{-1}) to a physiological range for intact males (4.4 ng ml^{-1}), (2) increased frequency and duration of attack, and (3) occurrence of aggressive vocalization such as the "Growl" and "Kek" (Guyomarc'h 1974; Potash 1970) emitted during the attack, and (3) increased intensity of the "Strut" posture. If two castrates are paired, they will only approach one another, but never achieve physical contact. However, the administration of T to both individuals resulted in displays of the full repertoire of aggressive behaviours which included attack initiation, physical contact, and a high intensity component of the fight – neck to neck combat.

3 Testosterone Titre and Intensity of Aggressive Behaviour

In the light of these results it is logical to predict that individual differences in displays of aggressive behaviour would correspond with circulating levels of T. However, many investigations on diverse genera of both birds and mammals illustrate that such a clear-cut relationship is by no means universal (Table 1).

In Japanese quail, Balthazart et al. (1979) and Tsutsui and Ishii (1981) could find no relationship. However, in another investigation a positive relationship of aggressive displays with plasma T was found when naive subjects were used (Ramenofsky 1984). Quail, who had not previously interacted with one another, were paired for short-term dyadic encounters on 19 non-consecutive days of a round robin tournament. Plasma T was correlated positively with fighting success and individuals that won fights by initiating and consummating attacks had higher levels than individuals who attacked less frequently or those who failed to attack. This positive relationship, however, was apparent only prior (24 h) to the first fighting day and the following 3 days of the tournament. By day 5 and throughout the remainder of the study, the plasma levels of T measured in quail that won fights were identical to those who lost. Agonistic associations among the competitors were established during the early pairing days of the tournament, as determined by the infrequent occurrence of reversals of winner-loser status during the second match of specific pairs of opponents. Recently, Edens et al. (1983) have shown in male Japanese quail that aggressive behaviour over access to food drops once relationships between the pairs has stabilized. Together both sets of findings suggest that formation of social relationships reduces the level of aggressive activity and the degree to which the qualitative displays of aggression are coupled with the circulating levels of T.

To test this hypothesis further, studies were conducted on socially experienced quail who were paired frequently with the same opponent (Ramenofsky and Gorbman 1980). After repeated matches, it was possible for the observer to determine the agonistic (dominant – subordinate) relationships established within each pair. The criteria for dominance within a pair required that an individual win at least 60% of the matches within a period of 14 fights. Next, an implant of T was administered to the identified subordinate of the pair, while the dominant was given an empty implant to serve as a control. As expected, the increase in plasma T within the physiological range modified the aggressive behaviour of the subordinate. Both frequency of consummated attacks and percent of fights won were significantly increased over levels measured in the subordinates prior to implant. Additionally, the duration of high-intensity fighting (neck to neck combat) measured within the pair was enhanced. Nevertheless, the subordinates did not win a sufficient number of fights to be considered dominant, which suggests that T was not sufficient to alter the qualitative expression of aggressive displays to the point of overthrowing previously established agonistic relationships. Essentially similar

Table 1. Studies that have investigated the relationship between circulating levels of testosterone and aggressive behaviour or social dominance

Class/order	Species	Relationship positive (+) no (−)	Reference
Mammals			
Primates	Human		
	Homo sapiens	+	Ehrenkrantz et al. (1974)
		−	Dotson et al. (1974)
		+	Kreuz and Rose (1972)
		+	Persky et al. (1971)
		−	Buss et al. (1968)
	Non-human		
	Rhesus macaque	+	Rose et al. (1971)
	Macaca mulatta	+	Rose et al. (1972)
		+	Rose et al. (1975)
		−	Phoenix (1980)
	Japanese macaque	−	Eaton and Resko (1974)
	Macaca fuscata		
	Olive baboon	+	Sapolsky (1982)
	Papio anubis		
	Squirrel monkey	+	Mendoza et al. (1979)
	Saimiri sciureus		
Artiodactyls	Ram	−	Davant et al. (1974)
	Ovis aries		
	Deer	+	Bouissou (1983)
	Odocoileus virgianus		
Rodentia	Mouse	+	Machida et al. (1981)
	Mus musculus	−	Selmanoff et al. (1977)
		−	Barkley and Goldman (1977)
		−	Dessi-Fulgheri et al. (1976)
	Rat	+	Schuurman (1980)
	Rattus norvegicus		
	Guinea pig	+	Sachser and Pröve (1984)
	Cavia porsellus		
Aves	Japanese quail	−	Balthazart et al. (1979)
	Coturnix coturnix	−	Tsutui and Ishii (1981)
		+	Ramenofsky (1984)
	Red-winged blackbird	+	Harding (1981)
	Aegalius phoeniceus		
	White-crowned sparrow	−	Wingfield et al. (1982b)
	Zonotrichia l. gambelii		
	Song sparrow	+	Wingfield (1984a)
	Melospiza melodia		
	Harris' sparrow	−	Rohwer and Wingfield (1981)
	Zonotrichia querula		
	House sparrow	+	R. Hegner and J.C. Wingfield
	Passer domesticus		(unpublished)

results have been obtained in dominance hierarchies of California Quail, *Lophortyx californica*, and free-living Harris' Sparrows, *Zonotrichia querula* (Emlen and Lorenz 1942; Rohwer and Rohwer 1978) in which implants of T given to subordinate males increased rates of attack but did not necessarily result in more wins for the subordinates. In no case did a T-implanted quail or sparrow rise in status in the hierarchy.

In the sharp-tailed grouse, *Tympanuchus phasianellus*, implants of T given to subordinate males at the lek increased overt aggression but did not result in any change in territorial boundaries (Trobec and Oring 1972). In contrast, Searcy (1980) found that T-implanted male Red-winged Blackbirds, *Agelaius phoeniceus* did increase size of their territory but were not more aggressive than control males as assessed by their response to a simulated territorial intrusion. Red-winged Blackbirds are polygynous and males are constantly patrolling the territory. Thus it is possible that these males are maximally aggressive throughout the breeding season. On the other hand, in male Song Sparrows, *Melospiza melodia*, White-crowned Sparrows, *Zonotrichia leucophrys pugetensis*, and Pied Flycatchers, *Ficedula hypoleuca*, males feed young extensively and there is a pronounced decline in plasma levels of T as the parental phase ensues. If males of these species are given implants of T at this time they become more aggressive than controls (Wingfield 1984b,c; Moore 1984; Silverin 1980).

Another experiment illustrates well the rather transient relationship of endogenous levels of T and aggressive behaviour. Castrated adult male White-crowned Sparrows, *Z. l. gambelii*, were given implants of T that maintained circulating levels very similar to those observed in spring (see Wingfield and Farner 1978a,b). Controls were given empty implants. Each bird was housed one per cage and within each group cages were arranged so that birds could see and interact with one another without physical contact. The total frequencies of aggressive behaviours (songs and threat displays often seen during establishment of territories) were then recorded at intervals after implantation (Wingfield 1985a). There were no significant differences between controls and experimentals as aggressive behaviour increased, despite the wide differences in T levels between the groups, although controls did show a marked decline in aggressive behaviour by day 14. Thus, these data tend to contradict the hypothesis that there is a positive correlation of intensity of aggressive behaviour and plasma levels of T. However, these males had been housed together for almost 6 months and it is likely that social relationships between individuals had been established for some time. If a novel male was then introduced in a cage alongside, and frequencies of aggressive behaviours recorded in response to a bird that the subjects had never interacted with or seen before, then there was an immediate increase in total frequencies of aggression in both groups. However, males given the implants of T showed significantly more intense aggression toward the novel males than did controls (Wingfield 1985a). By day 2 of introduction of the novel male, levels of aggression had dropped dramatically illustrating how quickly social relationships can be established, and emphasizing the transient nature of the relationship between circulating levels of T and the intensity of aggressive behaviour.

In the light of the data discussed above it is of little surprise, therefore, that so few investigations have identified hormone-behaviour relationships (see Table 1), particularly since the social contexts (degree of social familiarity of the subjects) vary accross the studies. There is little doubt that T or other androgen metabolites are requisite for the complete expression of displays of aggressive behaviour. However, experiential factors such as the development of social (dominant – subordinate) relationships among individuals, as seen in laboratory studies, may intervene in such a manner as to influence the degree to which the circulating of T affects, or correlates with, frequency and intensity of aggressive behaviour.

4 Temporal Patterns of Circulating Levels of Testosterone and Aggressive Behaviour in Free-Living Birds

Many investigations establishing the role of T and its metabolites in the regulation of aggressive behaviour have been conducted in the laboratory. Until recently very few studies attempted to relate this relationship to changes in territorial and mate-guarding behaviour under natural conditions. The advent of techniques whereby plasma samples could be collected from free-living birds without disturbing the normal temporal progression of the breeding cycle (Wingfield and Farner 1976) allowed a very detailed correlation of circulating levels of T and changes in aggressive behaviour in the field. Typically, plasma levels of T are elevated in free-living males as they establish a breeding territory in spring, and when females are laying the first clutch (see Wingfield and Farner 1978a,b, 1980). This relationship of circulating T and intensity of aggressive behaviour is perhaps most well developed in the Song Sparrow (Wingfield 1984b). Males arrive in the breeding area in March with high plasma levels of T. Curiously, T levels then decline in April and increase for a second time in late April and early May coincident with the egg-laying period. Thus there are 2 peaks of T in plasma coincident with 2 periods of heightened aggressive behaviour. The first peak is correlated with establishment of a territory. Once the territories are defined and the pair bond formed, it may be over a month before the nesting phase begins and thus it is not surprising that T levels decline. Agonistic interactions over territories are much less intense at this time (Nice 1943; J.C. Wingfield, unpublished), but there follows a second period of heightened aggression in males accompanied by an increase in plasma levels of T when females are laying the first clutch of eggs (Wingfield 1984b). At this time males "guard" their sexually receptive mates from possible extra-pair copulations with neighbouring males.

Clearly there is a strong positive correlation of increased aggression and elevated levels of T in free-living male birds in agreement with many of the laboratory investigations discussed above. However, even under natural conditions this relationship is not universal. In the Western Gull, *Larus occidentalis wymani*, there is no increase in plasma levels of T in spring and no correlation of T and territorial behaviour (Wingfield et al. 1980, 1982b), although T levels do increase slightly in males during the mate-guarding period. In this species, pair bonds are usually formed for life and mates return to the same territory each year. Further, this species is sedentary around the breeding colony off the coast of southern California and thus pairs may return to their territories regularly throughout the year. In addition, Wingfield et al. (1982b) found that Western Gulls were very territorial after the breeding season had ended and also had plasma levels of T that were similar to those measured in March and April just before the egg-laying period. Thus, it appears that in this species which is territorial for most of year, there is no obvious correlation of plasma levels of T with territorial aggression, i.e. it is a stable system unlike many other species which establish a territory each year. On the other hand, it is possible that secretion of T would increase in Western Gulls when the pair bond and territory are formed for the first time during puberty. However, once the territory is established, T levels apparently decline and remain stable. Thus in birds, plasma levels of T are correlated with increased aggressive behaviour at times when territories are formed, when females are laying the first clutch, and when challenged by another male. Once agonistic relationships are established, frequencies of aggressive behaviour decline, and the relationship with plasma levels of T is no longer evident.

5 Timing and Organization of Temporal Patterns of Testosterone and Aggressive Behaviour

It is well known that the vernal increase in day length stimulates gonadal development and increases plasma levels of T (Farner and Follett 1979, Farner and Gwinner 1980; Wingfield and Farner 1980). Although photoperiodically induced gonadal development in the laboratory results in complete spermatogenesis accompanied by development of secondary sex characteristics, field investigations have shown that the temporal pattern of circulating levels of T under natural conditions are quite different from those of an artificially induced cycle in the laboratory, and the absolute levels of T are up to 10 fold higher in males sampled in the field (Wingfield and Farner 1980). These data suggest that environmental factors, in addition to day length, can influence the secretion of these hormones. This hypothesis was supported by Wingfield (1984b) who showed that in free-living male Song Sparrows, plasma levels of T are high in late March and early April when territories are established, and then decline during April when day length is increasing rapidly. Recent experiments have been conducted to try and identify the environmental cues that result in an increase in secretion of T over and above that induced solely by long days.

Since increased levels of T coincide with the period of territory establishment, it is reasonable to assume that stimuli associated with gaining and defending a territory directly increase secretion of T. To test this hypothesis adult male Song Sparrows were removed from their territories and the replacement males and their neighbours sampled (Wingfield 1985b). These removals were performed in April when most males had established territories and were mated, but had not begun the nesting phase. The resulting vacant territories were occupied by replacements within 12–72 h and all birds were captured for blood sampling within 1–3 days of arrival of a replacement. Controls were sampled and returned to their territories. Plasma levels of T were significantly higher in replacement males than in control males that already had a territory. In addition, the neighbours of a replacement also had elevated levels of T as they established a new territory boundary with the replacement male (Wingfield 1985b). These data suggest that a territory per se is not the stimulus for T secretion, but the interactions that occur between neighbouring males and the replacement as new boundaries are formed appear to be more important.

To test this further, territorial intrusions were simulated by placing a caged male Song Sparrow in the centre of a territory and playing tape-recorded conspecific song through a speaker placed adjacent to the caged decoy male (Wingfield 1985b). Territorial male Song Sparrows respond vigorously to these simulated territorial intrusions and attempt to attack and repel the intruder. Responding males were caught at intervals after onset of the intrusion and plasma levels of T measured. Control male Song Sparrows were captured in Potter traps baited with seeds. Circulating levels of T in all males exposed to simulated territorial intrusion were higher than those of controls supporting the hypothesis that interactions with an intruding, or novel, male can stimulate secretion of T. Further, Harding (1981) showed that in free-living Red-winged Blackbirds, plasma levels of T were highest in males that attacked a decoy male more intensely.

In a separate experiment, Wingfield (1984a) gave free-living and territorial male Song Sparrows subcutaneous implants of T in early spring. These implants maintain plasma T at high vernal levels and result in these males remaining more aggressive, and with larger territories, than controls (see also Wingfield 1984c). Plasma levels of T in males with territories neighbouring T-implanted males are higher than those with territories adjacent to less aggressive controls (Wingfield 1984a), thus confirming earlier suggestions that the aggressive behaviour of intruding males can stimulate secretion of T in the territory owners.

The functional significance of these relationships of environmental cues and temporal patterns of T secretion is unknown but it is suggested that these mechanisms ensure that high plasma levels of T, and thus aggression, are kept to a minimum because intense territorial behaviour is energetically expensive, exposes the individual to predation, and may even attract predators to the nest site. Continued high levels of territorial aggression including high rates of singing and frequent patrolling of the territory would also be redundant once territory boundaries are established thus reducing the need for continued high levels of T. As a result plasma levels peak only as the territory is established, or when the territorial male is seriously challenged by an intruder (Wingfield 1985a).

In the Song Sparrow there is a second peak of T as females become sexually receptive and begin laying the first clutch (Wingfield 1984b). Similarly in other species, plasma levels of T in males are maximal when females are in lay (e.g. Wingfield and Farner 1978a,b, 1980). It is also apparent that the stimulation for this increase of T, in addition to that induced by increasing day length, comes from the behaviour of the sexually receptive female. In the Ring Dove, *Streptopelia risoria* (Feder et al. 1977), and Rock Dove, *Columba livia* (Haase 1975; Haase et al. 1976) plasma levels of LH and T increased in males exposed to females. In addition, male White-crowned Sparrows show a further elevation in plasma levels T following pair formation (Wingfield and Farner 1978a,b) that appears to be precipitated by the sexually receptive female. If female White-crowned Sparrows are given subcutaneous implants of oestradiol to maintain sexual behaviour, particularly solicitation of copulation, then plasma levels of T rise in males paired with these females in the laboratory (Moore 1982). In the field, plasma levels of T are maximal during the egg-laying period and then decline as incubation ensues. However, if free-living female White-crowned Sparrows and Song Sparrows were given implants of oestradiol during the egg-laying period, thus maintaining sexual behaviour at high levels, then circulating T remained elevated in their male mates (Moore 1983; Runfeldt and Wingfield 1985). Males exposed to sexually receptive females also become aggressive toward conspecific males as they "mate-guard" to protect their paternity of the clutch by preventing extra-pair copulations with neighbouring males. Thus it can be suggested that the increase of T induced by the sexually receptive female results in an elevation in aggressive behaviour which in this context appears to centre on mate-guarding activity (Moore 1984). In untreated birds, the female is no longer receptive as soon as incubation begins. In males the stimulus for increased T secretion is lost, and plasma levels decline. This is important since males of many species show some form of parental behaviour. If plasma levels of T remained high, the resultant increase in aggression would interfere with normal parental behaviour thus reduce reproductive success. Silverin (1980) illustrated this point in the Pied Flycatcher by giving males implants of T during the parental phase when plasma levels of T are normally low (Silverin and Wingfield 1982). Implanted males became very aggressive and spent much time singing and patrolling the territory thus resulting in marked reduction of nesting success.

The effect of such interactions on endocrine state are, presumably, mediated by visual and auditory cues. Male Ring Doves that have been surgically deafened have lower plasma levels of T than control males after exposure to sexually receptive females. In addition, plasma levels of androgens in males separated from females by a glass partition were higher than those males held in isolation suggesting that visual cues are also important and physical contact less so (O'Connell et al. 1981).

It also appears that the behaviour of the female can fine-tune termination of reproduction in the male. Oestradiol treatment of free-ranging female Song Sparrows in July delays the normal late summer termination of reproductive activity in their otherwise untreated mates (Runfeldt and Wingfield 1985). Males mated to oestradiol-treated females continue to respond to simulated territorial intrusions (see previous Section) after control males have ceased territorial defence. Experimental birds remained paired on their territories for up to 2 months after controls had terminated reproductive activity, and also had higher plasma levels of T than controls. Once again these data suggest a major role for behavioural interactions in the temporal modulation of seasonal reproductive activity and associated aggressive behaviour.

6 Conclusions

Results from investigations on birds conducted in the laboratory as well as in the field offer new insight into the problem concerning the association of plasma testosterone with aggressive behaviour and its biological significance. These studies emphasize that an entire array of environmental influences contribute to the degree of coupling of plasma titres of T and the qualitative expression of aggressive behaviour. In theory, these ideas are not new, for the primate and rodent literature has discussed the impact of social influences upon this endocrine-behaviour axis for some time. However, environmental (including social) conditions have contributed variation that has resulted in controversy. This has proven to be a problem for investigations on mammals, many of which have extremely complex social systems, whereas in aves social systems tend to be less complex. In addition, the advent of field techniques that allow endocrinologic investigations under natural conditions, as well as parallel laboratory experimentation, could provide potentially unique insights into relationships of T and aggressive behaviour.

Acknowledgements. Preparation of this manuscript was supported by a Charles H. Revson Foundation Fellowship in Biomedical Research, and grant number PCM8316155 from the National Science Foundation to JCW.

References

Adkins EK (1977) Effects of diverse androgens on the sexual behaviour and morphology of castrated male quail. Horm Behav 8:201–207

Adkins EK, Pniewski EE (1978) Control of reproductive behaviour by sex steroids in male quail. J Comp Physiol Psychol 92:1169–1179

Adkins-Regan E (1981) Hormone specificity, androgen metabolism, and social behaviour. Am Zool 21:257–272

Balthazart J (1983) Hormonal correlates of behaviour. In: Farner DS, King JR, Parkes KS (eds) Avian Biology, vol 7. Academic, New York, pp 221–366

Balthazart J, Massa R, Negri-Cesi P (1979) Photoperiodic control of testosterone metabolism, plasma gonadotropins, cloacal gland growth, and reproductive behaviour in the Japanese quail. Gen Comp Endocrinol 39:222–235

Barkley MS, Goldman BD (1977) A quantitative study of serum testosterone, sex accessory organ growth, and the development of intermale aggression in the mouse. Horm Behav 8:208–218

Bennett MA (1940) The social hierarchy in ring doves II. The effect of treatment with testosterone propionate. Ecology 21:148–165

Bernstein IS, Gordon TP, Rose RM (1983) The interaction of hormones, behaviour, and social context in non-human primates. In: Svare B (ed) Hormones and aggressive behaviour. Plenum, New York, pp 535–562

Bouissou M-F (1983) Hormonal influences in ungulates. In: Svare B (ed) Hormones and aggressive behaviour. Plenum, New York, pp 507–533

Brain PF (1983) Pituitary gonadal influences on social aggression. In: Svare B (ed) Hormones and aggressive behaviour. Plenum, New York, pp 3–26

Brown JL (1964) The evolution of diversity in avian territorial systems. Wilson Bull 76:160–169

Buss A, Fischer H, Simmons A (1968) Aggression and hostility in psychiatric patients. J Consult Clin Psychol 32:21

Cheng M-F, Lehrman D (1975) Gonadal hormone specificity in the sexual behaviour of ring doves. Psychoneuroendocrinology 1:95–102

Davant J, Han DK, Moody EL (1974) Dominance in rams in relation to serum testosterone. J Anim Sci 38:1333–1334

Dessi-Fulgheri F, Lucarini N, Lupo di Prisco C (1976) Relationship between testosterone metabolism in the brain, other endocrine variables and intermale aggression in mice. Aggressive Behav 2:223–231

Dixson AF (1980) Androgens and aggressive behavior in primates: a review. Aggressive Behav 6:37–67

Dotson L, Robertson L, Tuchfeld B (1974) Some correlations among alcohols, cigarettes, hormones and hostility. Insurance Institute for Highway Safety Publication, Washington

Eaton GG, Resko JA (1974) Plasma testosterone and male dominance in Japanese macaque troops with repeated measures of testosterone in laboratory males. Horm Behav 5:251–259

Edens FW, Bursian SJ, Holladay SD (1983) Grouping in Japanese quail I. Agonistic behavior during feeding. Poult Sci 62:1647–1651

Ehrenkrantz J, Bliss E, Sheard M (1974) Plasma testosterone: correlations with aggressive behavior and social dominance in man. Psychosom Med 36:469–475

Emlen JT, Lorenz FW (1942) Pairing responses of free-living valley quail to sex-hormone pellets. Auk 59:369–378

Farner DS, Follett BK (1979) Reproductive periodicity in birds. In: Barrington EJW (ed) Hormones and evolution. Academic, New York, pp 829–872

Farner DS, Gwinner E (1980) Photoperiodicity, circannual and reproductive cycles. In: Epple A, Stetson MH (eds) Avian endocrinology. Academic, New York, pp 331–366

Feder HH, Storey A, Goodwin D, Reboulleau C, Silver R (1977) Testosterone and "5α-dihydrotestosterone" levels in peripheral plasma of male and female ring doves, *Streptopelia risoria*, during the reproductive cycle. Biol Reprod 16:666–677

Guyomarc'h JC (1974) Les vocalizations des gallinaces structure des sons et des repertoires ontogènes motrice et aquisition de leur semantique, vol 1. PhD Thésis, Univ Rennes, France

Haase E (1975) Zur Wirkung jahreszeitlicher und sozialer Faktoren auf Hoden und Hormonspiegel von Haustauben. Verh Dtsch Zool Ges 1975:137

Haase E, Paulke E, Sharp PJ (1976) Effects of seasonal and social factors on testicular activity and hormone levels in domestic pigeons. J Exp Zool 197:81–96

Harding CF (1981) Social modulation of circulating hormone levels in the male. Am Zool 21:223–232

Harding CF (1983) Hormonal influences on avian aggressive behaviour. In: Svare B (ed) Hormones and aggressive behaviour. Plenum, New York, pp 435–468

Harding CF, Sheridan K, Walters MJ (1984) Hormonal specificity and activation of sexual behaviour in male zebra finches. Horm Behav 17:111–133

Hutchison JB, Steimer TH (1983) Hormone – mediated behavioral transition: a role for brain aromatase. In: Balthazart J, Pröve E, Gilles R (eds) Hormones and behaviour in higher vertebrates. Springer, Berlin Heidelberg New York, pp 261–274

Keverne EB, Meller RE, Martinez-Arias AM (1978) Dominance, aggression and sexual behaviour in social groups of talapoin monkeys. In: Chivers DJ, Herbert J (eds) Recent advances in primatology, vol 1. Academic, New York, pp 553–547

Kreuz L, Rose RM (1972) Assessment of aggressive behavior and plasma testosterone in a young criminal population. Psychosom Med 34:321–332

Kuo ZY (1960) Studies on the basic factors in animal fighting III. Hormonal factors affecting fighting in quails. J Genet Psychol 96:217–223

Machida T, Yonezewa V, Noumura T (1981) Age-associated changes in plasma testosterone levels of male mice and their relation to social dominance or subordinance. Horm Behav 15:238–245

Marler P (1955) Studies of fighting in chaffinches I. Behaviour in relation to the social hierarchy. Br J Anim Behav 3:111–117

Mazur A (1983) Hormones, aggression, and dominance in humans. In: Svare B (ed) Hormones and aggressive behaviour. Plenum, New York, pp 563–576

Mendoza SP, Coe C, Loe EL, Levine S (1979) The physiological response to group formation in adult male squirrel monkeys. Psychoneuroendocrinology 3:221–229

Moore MC (1982) Hormonal response of free-living male white-crowned sparrows to experimental manipulation of female sexual behaviour. Horm Behav 16:323–329

Moore MC (1983) Effect of female sexual displays on the endocrine physiology and behaviour of male white-crowned sparrows, *Zonotrichia leucophrys gambelii*. J Zool (Lond) 199:137–148

Moore MC (1984) Changes in territorial defence produced by changes in circulating levels of testosterone: a possible hormonal basis for mate-guarding behaviour in white-crowned sparrows. Behaviour 88:215–226

Nice MM (1943) Studies in the life history of the song sparrow, vol 2. The behaviour of the song sparrow and other passerines. Dover, New York

O'Connell ME, Reboulleau C, Feder HH, Silver R (1981) Social interactions and androgen levels in birds I. Female characteristics associated with increased plasma androgen levels in the male ring dove *(Streptopelia risoria)*. Gen Comp Endocrinol 44:454–463

Persky H, Smith K, Basu G (1971) Relation of psychologic measures of aggression and hostility to testosterone production in man. Psychosom Med 33:265–277

Phoenix CH (1980) Copulation, dominance, and plasma androgen levels in adult Rhesus males born and reared in the laboratory. Arch Sex Behav 9:149–168

Potash LM (1970) Vocalizations elicited by electrical brain stimulation in *Coturnix coturnix japonica*. Behaviour 36:149–167

Pröve E (1974) Der Einfluß von Kastration und Testosteronsubstution auf das Sexualverhalten männlicher Zebrafinken *(Taeniopygia guttata castanotis* Gould). J Ornithol 115:338–347

Ramenofsky M (1982) Endogenous plasma hormones and agonistic behaviour in male Japanese quail, *Coturnix coturnix*. PhD Thesis, Univ Washington

Ramenofsky M (1984) Agonistic behaviour and endogenous plasma hormones in male Japanese quail. Anim Behav 32:698–708

Ramenofsky M, Gorbman A (1980) Plasma hormones and aggressive behavior in adult male Japanese quail. Am Zool 20:791

Rohwer W, Rohwer FC (1978) Status signalling in Harris' sparrows: experimental deceptions achieved. Anim Behav 26:1012–1022

Rohwer S, Wingfield JC (1981) A field study of social dominance, plasma levels of luteinizing hormone and steroid hormones in wintering Harris' sparrows. Z Tierpsychol 57:173–183

Rose RM, Holaday JW, Bernstein IS (1971) Plasma testosterone, dominance rank and aggressive behaviour in male Rhesus monkeys. Nature (Lond) 231:366–368

Rose RM, Gordon TP, Bernstein IS (1972) Plasma testosterone levels in male rhesus: influence of sexual and social stimuli. Science (Wash DC) 178:643–645

Rose RM, Bernstein IS, Gordon TP (1975) Consequences of social conflict on plasma testosterone levels in Rhesus monkeys. Psychosom Med 37:50–61

Runfeldt S, Wingfield JC (1985, in press) Experimentally prolonged sexual activity in female sparrows delays termination of reproductive activity in their untreated mates. Anim Behav

Sachser N, Pröve E (1984) Short-term effects of residence on the testosterone responses to fighting in alpha male guinea pigs. Aggressive Behav 10:285–292

Sapolsky RM (1982) The endocrine stress-response and social status in the wild baboon. Horm Behav 16:279–292

Schuurman T (1980) Hormonal correlates of agonistic behaviour in adult male rats. Prog Brain Res 53:415–520

Searcy WA (1980) Sexual selection and aggressiveness in male red-winged Blackbirds. Anim Behav 29:958–960

Searcy WA, Wingfield JC (1980) The effects of androgen and antiandrogen on dominance and aggressiveness in male red-winged blackbirds. Horm Behav 14:126–135

Selmanoff MK, Goldman BD, Ginsburg G (1977) Serum testosterone, agonistic behavior and dominance in inbred strains of mice. Horm Behav 8:107–119

Silver R, O'Connell M, Saad R (1979) Effect of androgens on the behaviour of birds. In: Beyer C (ed) Endocrine control of sexual behaviour. Raven, New York, pp 223–278

Silverin B (1980) Effect of long acting testosterone treatment on free-living pied flycatchers, *Ficedula hypoleuca*. Anim Behav 28:906–912

Silverin B, Wingfield JC (1982) Patterns of breeding behaviour and plasma levels of hormones in a free-living population of pied flycatchers, *Ficedula hypoleuca*. J Zool (Lond) 198:117–129

Trobec RJ, Oring LW (1972) Effects of testosterone propionate implantation on lek behaviour of sharp-tailed grouse. Am Midl Nat 87:531–536

Tsutsui K, Ishii S (1981) Effects of sex steroids on aggressive behaviour of adult male Japanese quail. Gen Comp Endocrinol 44:480–486

Wingfield JC (1980) Fine temporal adjustment of reproductive functions. In: Epple A, Stetson MH (eds) Avian endocrinology. Academic, New York, pp 367–389

Wingfield JC (1983) Environmental and endocrine control of reproduction: an ecological approach. In: Mikami S-I, Homma H, Wada M (eds) Avian endocrinology: environmental and ecological perspectives. Jpn Sci Soc Press. Springer, Berlin Heidelberg New York, pp 265–288

Wingfield JC (1984a) Environmental and endocrine control of reproduction in the song sparrow, *Melospiza melodia* II. Agonistic interactions as environmental information stimulating secretion of testosterone. Gen Comp Endocrinol 56:417–424

Wingfield JC (1984b) Environmental and endocrine control of reproduction in the song sparrow, *Melospiza melodia* I. Temporal organization of the breeding cycle. Gen Comp Endocrinol 56:406–416

Wingfield JC (1984c) Androgens and mating systems: testosterone-induced polgyny in normally monogamous birds. Auk 101:665–671

Wingfield JC (1985a) Environmental and hormonal control of territorial behaviour in birds. In: Follett BK, Ishii S, Chandola A (eds) Hormones and the environment. Jpn Sci Soc Press. Springer, Berlin Heidelberg New York, pp 265–277

Wingfield JC (1985b, in press) Short term changes in plasma hormones levels during establishment and defence of a breeding territory in male song sparrows, *Melospiza melodia*. Horm Behav

Wingfield JC, Farner DS (1976) Avian endocrinology – field investigations and methods. Condor 78:570–573

Wingfield JC, Farner DS (1978a) The endocrinology of a natural population of the white-crowned sparrow, *Zonotrichia leucophrys pugetensis*. Physiol Zool 51:188–205

Wingfield JC, Farner DS (1978b) The annual cycle of plasma irLH and steroid hormones in feral populations of white-crowned sparrows, *Zonotrichia leucophrys gambelii*. Biol Reprod 19:1046–1056

Wingfield JC, Farner DS (1980) Control of seasonal reproduction in temperate zone birds. Prog Reprod Biol 5:62–101

Wingfield JC, Martin A, Hunt GL Jr, Farner DS (1980) The origin of homosexual pairing of female western gulls *(Larus occidentalis wymani)* on Santa Barbara Island. In: Power D (ed) The california islands. Santa Barbara Mus Nat Hist, Santa Barbara, pp 461–466

Wingfield JC, Newman A, Hunt GL Jr, Farner DS (1982a) Endocrine aspects of female-female pairing in the western gull, *Larus occidentalis wymani*. Anim Behav 30:9–22

Wingfield JC, Smith JP, Farner DS (1982b) Endocrine responses of white-crowned sparrows to environmental stress. Condor 84:399–409

Phasic Effects of Hormones in the Avian Brain During Behavioural Development

J.B. HUTCHISON and R.E. HUTCHISON [1]

1 Introduction

Steroid hormones have been implicated in the sexual differentiation of behaviour in both birds and mammals (Beach 1974; Goy and McEwen 1980; Adkins-Regan 1983). Studies of the developing rodent brain, particularly in the rat, suggest that androgens irreversibly "organize" mechanisms of male sexual behaviour by direct action on the brain during a "critical" perinatal period (MacLusky and Naftolin 1981). The neural substrate of sexual behaviour in the male is differentiated in two ways. First, androgens masculinize by enhancement of systems underlying male behaviour and, second, defeminize by suppression of behavioural systems underlying female behaviour (Goy and McEwen 1980). Whether these processes operate independently or as a result of the action of different hormones is still unknown, but evidence has accumulated to support the view that an oestrogen, oestradiol-17β(E_2), formed from testosterone within the brain, is important for the sexual differentiation of male behaviour (Plapinger and McEwen 1978; Olsen 1979; Martini 1982). The mechanisms involved in sexual differentiation of avian behaviour appear at first sight to be the reverse of those in mammals. Oestrogens result in the differentiation (or demasculinization) of behaviour in female Japanese quail during early development, whereas the behaviour of the male develops without hormonal intervention (Adkins 1975; Hutchison RE 1978; Adkins-Regan 1983; Schumacher and Balthazart 1983). The generalization has been made that behavioural mechanisms of the heterogametic sex (female in birds, male in mammals) require the differentiating effects of steroids, the homogametic sex is "neutral" (Adkins 1975). However, this has been questioned with respect to birds (Konishi and Gurney 1982), because song is differentiated by early hormone action in the male of at least one avian species, the zebra finch *(Poephila guttata)*.

Irrespective of whether the developmental effects of steroids on brain mechanisms of behaviour occur in the male or the female, the actual neurones involved have not been identified except in one remarkable instance discovered recently by Gurney and Konishi (1980) in the zebra finch. In females of this species, exogenous E_2 initiates differentiation of neurones in telencephalic song control nuclei during the first few days after hatching. This treatment also induces females which do not normally sing, to respond to testosterone treatment in adulthood with the production of male-like song

1 MRC Unit on the Development and Integration of Behaviour, University Sub-Department, Madingley, Cambridge, United Kingdom

(Gurney and Konishi 1980; Gurney 1982). Therefore, an initial organizing action of oestrogen appears to be required for the later behavioural action of androgen in adulthood. Since it is well known that androgens can be converted to oestrogens within the brain of many vertebrate species (Naftolin et al. 1975; Callard et al. 1978; Hutchison and Steimer 1984), the required E_2 is thought to be derived by aromatization of testosterone within target brain areas (Gurney and Konishi 1980; Konishi and Gurney 1982).

The validity of the hypothesis that E_2 has an organizing action on brain neurones of the song control system depends on whether aromatizable androgens are available for conversion, or E_2 itself is available specifically in the male during the sensitive period of development. Unless this can be demonstrated, neuronal effects of exogenous E_2 in the developing brain are of pharmacological rather than physiological interest. The aim of this paper is primarily, therefore, to reassess the endocrinological aspects of brain differentiation in birds with particular emphasis on the song control system in the zebra finch.

2 Sexual Differentiation of Song Control

2.1 Characteristics of Zebra Finch Song and Vocalizations

Male and female zebra finches share a repertoire of calls (Silcox 1979). Calls have a simpler structure than song and are usually repeated, but not at fixed time intervals (Fig. 1b). Only the male sings, and the song is accompanied by courtship behaviour (directed song) or in situations characterized by low activity when no other bird is addressed (undirected song) (Morris 1954; Immelmann 1962; Sossinka and Böhner 1980). The song consists of a number of repeated introductory elements and song units or motifs (Price 1979) (see Fig. 1a). Directed song differs from undirected song in that the latter contains fewer introductory elements and song units per bout. Many males share similar introductory elements, and it has been suggested (Sossinka and Böhner 1980) that the introductory elements are characteristic of the species. The elements within the song units vary in number and type, with the result that each male has an individual song.

2.2 Sexual Dimorphism in Song Control

This topic has been the subject of intensive research over the past few years, and we do not intend to provide a comprehensive review here (see reviews by Konishi and Gurney 1982; Bottjer and Arnold 1984; Arnold and Gorski 1984, for detailed discussion). The vocal control system in song birds was discovered by Nottebohm (reviewed by Nottebohm et al. 1976) in the canary. This system, which is thought to control both song learning and motor production, consists of well-defined brain nuclei and fibre tracts. The major efferent components are the telencephalic nucleus, hyperstriatum ventrale pars caudale, (HVc) which projects to n. robustus archistriatalis (RA) and finally to the hypoglossal motorneurones (XIIts) which control vocal musculature. Certain other brain nuclei, magnocellular nucleus (MAN), nucleus intercollicularis (ICO) and area X of the

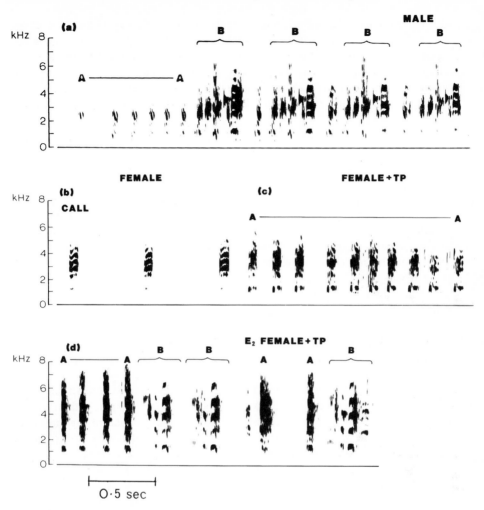

Fig. 1. a Sonagram of an adult male zebra finch song. Consisting of introductory elements $(A-A)$ and repeated song units (B). **b** Calls of an adult female zebra finch. **c** "Clumps" of introductory-type vocalizations of adult female zebra finch with a silastic implant of testosterone. **d** Song-like vocalizations of an adult female which received a unilateral implant of E_2 near HVc on day 1 after hatching and a silastic implant containing testosterone as an adult. The song consists of introductory elements $(A-A)$ and repeated units (B)

lobus parolfactorius (see also Gurney 1982; Arnold and Gorski 1984) are monosynaptically connected to HVc and are considered to be part of the vocal control system. There are marked sexual dimorphisms in size of these nuclei in which HVc, RA, and area X are larger in the male than the female brain of both canaries and zebra finches (Nottebohm and Arnold 1976). Autoradiographic studies have also shown that both HVc and RA in the male take up more radioactivity following systemic treatment with isotopically labelled testosterone than equivalent female nuclei (Arnold and Saltiel 1979). Uptake of labelled DHT is increased in the female HVc and RA by post-hatching treatment with E_2 (Arnold, pers. comm.), suggesting that neonatal E_2 masculinizes the pattern of steroid accumulation in these nuclei (Nordeen et al. 1984). Therefore, these male nuclei differ from those of the female in both size and number of steroid concentrating cells. Initially, it appeared that both the connecting fibre tracts and vocal control nuclei were present in the female zebra finch brain (Gurney 1982). However, recent work suggests that there is little connection between HVc and RA in the female brain (Konishi and Akutagawa 1985).

2.3 Differentiating Effects of Steroids

Androgen treatment of adult females has no effect on the volumes of brain nuclei, except for enlarging XIIts (Arnold 1980). However, using silastic pellets which sustain the release of testosterone, Gurney (1981, 1982) demonstrated a positive relationship between dosage and the degree of masculinization of RA. With low testosterone concentrations, this nucleus contains both large cells typical of the male and smaller cells of the female type. This appears to be a true early organizational effect, because testosterone administered to adult females which had not received early oestrogen treatment is ineffective in inducing song (Gurney 1982). Studies in mammals, rat (Gorski 1984), and gerbil (Yahr 1985, this volume) have revealed a similar organizing effect of androgen on the development of a component of the preoptic nucleus (sexually dimorphic nucleus, SDN) of the male, indicating that sexual dimorphism of target nuclei for steroids is not unique to the avian brain.

Formation of active metabolites of testosterone, E_2 and the non-aromatizable androgen, 5α-dihydrotestosterone (DHT), within target areas of the brain is thought to be important in steroid-dependent processes of sexual differentiation of the mammalian brain (reviewed in McEwen 1983). Similarly, presumed metabolites of testosterone influence neural development of the zebra finch. Briefly, (see Gurney 1981; Arnold and Gorski 1984, for a detailed account) E_2 administered at hatching was more effective in increasing the volumes of HVc and RA measured in adulthood (Gurney 1981) than DHT. However, the effects of these steroids show marked differences. Oestradiol increases the size of the cell soma and spacing between neurones, whereas DHT increases the number of cells, but has little effect on either somal size or spacing. Further development of both RA and HVc is apparent in adult females given testosterone which were also treated with E_2 at hatching. Therefore, sexual differentiation of the vocal control system appears to be a two-stage process and depends on the actions of both DHT and E_2 during the neonatal period. Gurney (1982) has also suggested that E_2, effective in early development, alters the sensitivity of the song control system to subsequent effects of androgen in adulthood. This follows from the experimental observation that DHT and testosterone are only effective in adult females that were pretreated at hatching with E_2.

Two important questions arising from this work are whether first, the anatomical effects match those on vocal behaviour and second, steroid effects are exerted directly on target cells in the vocal control nuclei associated with song. The earlier studies of Gurney (1982) provided an answer to the first question. Some females treated with E_2 just after hatching and subsequently with testosterone in adulthood, produced vocalizations which exhibited the stereotypy and acoustic characteristics of the male zebra finch song. The non-aromatizable androgen, DHT, was without effect on song differentiation, suggesting that masculinization is E_2 specific. Since zebra finch chicks in this study were reared with Bengalese finch parents, it is surprising that these E_2-treated female chicks learnt the characteristics of zebra finch song. Although cross-fostered, the female presumably used zebra finch males as tutors. An answer has also been obtained to the second question. Using minute "floating" implants of E_2 ($1-2$ μg) positioned stereotaxically near HVc on day 1 after hatching, we have shown (in a study carried out with F. Nottebohm, Rockefeller University, N.Y.) that some female zebra finches which had received intracerebral E_2 on day 1 after hatching, and were treated with testosterone as adults, developed new vocalizations which resembled male song. In 80% of these females, the initial phase of the song consisted of $4-15$ "clumps" of type A elements (Fig. 1) with an average interval between A vocalizations of $0.02-0.05$ s. The sibling males from the same nest were characterized by $4-17$ "A" type elements with an average interval of $0.02-0.14$ s. However, 40% of untreated females, and females with control implants placed subcutaneously, also emitted "clumps" of $5-10$ "A" type vocalizations ranging between $0.05-0.07$ s when treated as adults with testosterone. Intact females which had not been treated with testosterone generally made soft calls which were not clumped and had varying intervals between $0.07-0.17$ s (Fig. 1). Testosterone does, therefore, influence female vocal behaviour when given in adulthood. This effect is possibly related to the known action of androgen in increasing number of cells in vocal control nuclei (Gurney 1981). However, 30% of E_2 females also developed song units or motifs (Fig. 1) which were individually different and repeated consistently – a characteristic of male song. Oestradiol evidently can act directly on the vocal control system in the brain. Why this occurs in some females, but not others is still unknown. The reasons for the difference in effectiveness of E_2 implants will not be clarified until the cellular action of the implanted oestrogen has been analysed in these brains.

Analysis of the song characteristics of females which had been treated with E_2 after hatching and with testosterone in adulthood, and which had been reared with zebra finch parents, confirmed that the song of some individuals closely matches that of males in its "rich modulation, frequency bands and temporal organization" (Pohl-Apel and Sossinka 1982). The song elements were copies of the father's song in some cases, as is known to occur normally in zebra finches (Böhner 1983). This indicates that specific learning of the correct song model had taken place. However, a second type of song was also obtained which had a rudimentary structure similar to juvenile males. The variability in song structure was attributed to duration of post-natal E_2 treatment and exposure of vocal control nuclei to hormone (Pohl-Apel and Sossinka 1982). Similarly in our experiments with intracerebral implants, variability in song structure could be due to varying concentrations of steroid reaching the target areas of the brain. The conclusion can be drawn that differentiation of the song is not an "all or none" event.

Recently Konishi and Akutagawa (1985) has obtained evidence suggesting that E_2 does not only induce cell growth in the female song control system as was originally supposed (Gurney 1981). Female RA and possibly HVc and MAN cells appear to undergo neuronal atrophy and death between days 25 and 35, whereas their male counterparts do not. Exogenous oestrogen after hatching evidently prevents neuronal atrophy and death in experimental females. One of the possible consequences of E_2 action in females

is innervation of RA by the HVc axons (Konishi and Akutagawa 1985). A study
of the ontogeny of the HVc and RA (Bottjer et al. 1984) indicates that the volumes of
the male HVc and RA increase rapidly between days 12 to 25 of age. Since enlargement
of HVc precedes RA, these authors suggest that hormone action initiates development
of HVc which in turn has a trophic effect on RA. Whether E_2 has a neurotrophic effect
in preserving certain neurones in the male song control nuclei, or a growth promoting
effect, as demonstrated in organotype cultures of mouse preoptic tissue (reviewed in
Toran-Allerand 1984), is not known.

3 Peripheral or Central Origin of the Active Steroid?

For the hypothesis that E_2 has an organizational role in the brain, either aromatizable
androgen or E_2 should be available to target cells during the sensitive period. Circulating
levels of androgen are detectable during the post-hatching period in many avian species.
But this consists mainly of DHT (Wingfield et al. 1980), at least in nidiculous species
such as the white-crowned sparrow *(Zonotrichia leucophrys)* in which chromatographic
separation of steroids has been carried out. Evidence for oestrogens in the circulating
plasma of very young birds is sparse, but the embryonic chicken gonad is capable of
synthesizing E_2 (Woods and Erton 1978).

Circulating levels of steroids in plasma of zebra finch chicks have been measured
after hatching using a sensitive radioimmunoassay (Wingfield and Farner 1975) which
includes partial purification of each steroid fraction. Significant concentrations of
aromatizable androgens were found to be present in the plasma during the sensitive
period for the differentiation of the song control system (Hutchison et al. 1984). Testosterone levels were higher on day 1 than day 10 of age after hatching (Fig. 2). Androstenedione was also identified and levels of the non-aromatizable androgen, DHT,
were also relatively high. If differentiation of the song control system requires aromatization of androgens, as suggested previously (Gurney 1982), neither testosterone nor
androstenedione would be expected to occur in the plasma of female chicks during the
post-hatching period when the female brain is clearly sensitive to E_2. In fact, female
chicks had substantial levels of both androgens which were fully equivalent to those of
male chicks (Fig. 2). Therefore, the steroid requirements for masculinization of the
neural substrate of the vocal control system, aromatizable androgen and DHT, are
present in the female during the period when exogenous E_2 is maximally effective in
differentiating the female brain. Since adrenal concentrations of testosterone are known
to be high immediately before and after hatching (Tanabe et al. 1979) in chickens, the
adrenal could be the source of androgen in both male and female zebra finch chicks.

Although the plasma androgen profile appears to support the original view that E_2
could be formed locally in the brain, the lack of a sex difference in androgen level is
difficult to accommodate with the aromatization hypothesis. The position with regard
to plasma steroids is, however, more complex than was originally suspected. Oestradiol
levels, which are negligible in male chicks on days 1 and 2 post-hatching, show a pronounced increase on days 3 and 4 (Fig. 2; Hutchison et al. 1984). By day 10, E_2 has
again fallen to basal levels. Therefore, there is a peak in E_2 which occurs within the

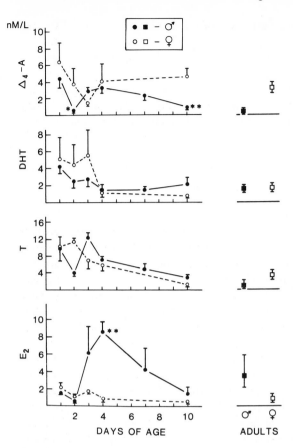

Fig. 2. Plasma levels of androstenedione (*4–A*), dihydrotestosterone (*DHT*), testosterone (*T*), and Oestradiol-17β (*E₂*) in male and female chicks. Adult plasma levels are indicated for comparison. (** *P* < 0.01 ANOVA, Genstat; sexes compared). (After Hutchison et al. 1984)

sensitive period for brain differentiation. During this peak, male E_2 levels are significantly higher than those of adult males. By contrast, E_2 levels in female chicks did not show any comparable elevation (Fig. 2). There is little doubt that the compound measured by RIA is E_2, because it has the same mobility in both conventional chromatography systems and HPLC. Since both male and female chicks show the same growth curve, the sex difference in E_2 level is unlikely to reflect a difference in growth rate. The source of E_2 in zebra finch chicks is still unknown, but E_2 has been detected in males of this species from days 10–74 (Pröve 1983), canaries (Güttinger et al. 1984) and in plasma from male chick embryos (Tanabe et al. 1979). Irrespective of its origin, the fact that E_2 is present in male chicks and not in females during the sensitive period for differentiation of the brain implies not only that there is a physiological role for E_2, but also that the timing of differentiation may depend on when this hormone appears in the plasma of the male. The latter point will be taken up in the final section of this paper.

4 Role of Steroid Metabolizing Pathways in the Brain

4.1 Active Metabolites

In view of the high concentrations of E_2 in the circulating plasma of male zebra finch chicks, it seems unlikely that local aromatization of testosterone in the brain is the primary source of E_2 for differentiation of the brain. Yields of oestrogen in the brain of mammals such as the rat ($< 1.0\%$ of substrate converted in vitro, Reddy et al. 1974) are extremely small and lower than 5α-reduced androgens (Selmanoff et al. 1977). Higher aromatase activity has been reported in the preoptic area of the Barbary dove *(Streptopelia risoria)* where levels of activity are similar to those of the 5α-reduction pathway (Steimer and Hutchison 1980). But this source cannot compare with amounts available in the male zebra finch for nuclear uptake in target cells of the brain from the high plasma concentrations of E_2. It follows from the aromatization hypothesis that brain aromatase activity must be specifically active in the male during the sensitive period, and inhibited or absent from the female brain. Both are unlikely, because sex differences in aromatase activity have not been seen in hypothalamic areas where enzyme activity has been detected in the early development of other species of birds (Barbary dove and quail; Hutchison and Steimer, in preparation). Conversion of testosterone to E_2 in nuclei of the vocal control system is likely to occur at low levels. However, no studies of brain aromatization in adult or juvenile zebra finches have been published yet. In other species, such as the Barbary dove (Steimer and Hutchison 1980; Hutchison and Steimer 1983) and quail (Schumacher and Balthazart 1983b) aromatase activity is concentrated in preoptic and posterior hypothalamic areas rather than the telencephalon where activity is minimal.

Are there mechanisms which could increase aromatase activity selectively within target areas of the male brain associated with song control? Measurement of basal levels of aromatase activity in tissue homogenates prepared from whole brain or large hypothalamic samples is unlikely to be productive approach in answering this question. Ideally, only target brain areas containing cells where the differentiating of E_2 are thought to occur should be examined. In practice, this is almost impossible using the microdissection and assay techniques available with a brain as small as that of the zebra finch chick (whole chick weighs approximately 0.7 g on day 1). Knowledge of enzyme kinetics will also be required to establish properties such as the affinity of the aromatase for its substrate (for review, see Hutchison and Steimer 1984) to obtain a valid model of androgen metabolism in the developing zebra finch brain. However, activity of the aromatase can be induced specifically in the preoptic area by increased plasma concentrations of either androgen or oestrogen. The induction effect has been identified in adult doves (Steimer and Hutchison 1981a; Hutchison and Steimer 1984). Thus elevated testosterone seen in zebra finch chicks after hatching could, in theory, induce aromatase activity in the brain of males after hatching. Developmental studies of quail chicks, which have partially characterized the hypothalamic aromatase (Hutchison and Schumacher, in preparation) indicate that enzyme activity is induced by exogenous testosterone. However, there appears to be no sex difference in the inductive effect (Schumacher and Hutchison, in preparation). Given that plasma testosterone levels are elevated in female chicks, a similar induction of the aromatase by testosterone would also be expected in target areas of the female brain. There is no reason to believe, therefore, that yields of E_2 might be increased specifically in the male by this means.

In view of the high plasma levels of aromatizable androgen in females, an important question to consider is why the female brain is not masculinized either by the direct effects of testosterone or by oestrogen formed from androgen. There seems little doubt that, as in other species of birds (Hutchison and Steimer 1983), some basal aromatase activity is present within the zebra finch telencephalon which could raise E_2 levels in target areas of both male and female brains. It could be suggested that the developing vocal control system in the female brain is insensitive to oestrogenic products of aromatase activity, or actively protected against them. The alpha-foetoprotein system which is thought to prevent masculinization of the female brain in species of rodents (e.g. rat, mouse reviewed in McEwen 1983) and has been discovered intraneuronally in the mouse (Toran-Allerand 1984), provides an example of a protective mechanism in the developing mammalian brain. Similarly, the lack of appropriate receptors for E_2 in the female zebra finch could confer insensitivity to the hormone during the sensitive period for differentiation of the vocal control system. This latter mechanism seems unlikely, however, because E_2 receptors occur in the developing brain of both sexes (Siegel et al. 1983).

4.2 Inactive Metabolites

Enzyme catalyzing reactions which result in the formation of active metabolites of testosterone, such as DHT and E_2, form only a part of the complex spectrum of enzymatic conversions in the brain (Hutchison and Steimer 1984). Studies of steroid metabolism in the adult brain, particularly in the dove (Steimer and Hutchison 1981b), where a detailed study of enzyme activity in different brain areas has been undertaken, have shown that conversion of testosterone to 5β-dihydrotestosterone (5β-DHT) and its corresponding $3\alpha/\beta,17\beta$-diols is the major pathway of androgen metabolism in all regions of the brain studied so far. But there are pronounced differences in level of 5β-reductase activity between brain areas in which hypothalamic and preoptic areas have lower activity than other regions examined so far. Predominance of 5β-reductase activity has also been recorded in the brain of quail (Balthazart and Schumacher 1983) and starlings (Massa 1980). The 5β-reductase is cytosolic (high-speed supernatant of brain cell homogenates. It is likely to occur at an early stage in the cellular action of testosterone in the brain. Both in vivo and in vitro metabolic studies suggest that 5β-reductase interacts preferentially with the substrate (testosterone) entering brain cells and competes effectively with alternative pathways of androgen metabolism (Hutchison and Steimer 1981). A number of lines of evidence (reviewed in Hutchison and Steimer 1984) indicate that the 5β-reduction of testosterone represents a major steroid inactivation pathway in brain cells (Fig. 3).

In view of the markedly higher levels of 5β-reductase activity in non-target striatal, septal, and parolfactory areas of the adult brain than in the hypothalamus, it has been suggested (Steimer and Hutchison 1981b) that brain areas not directly implicated in androgen action are "protected" from androgenic effects by selective 5β-reductase activity. Inactivation of testosterone by 5β-reduction could well be involved in maintaining the brain in a differentiated functional state in adulthood. The question arising from

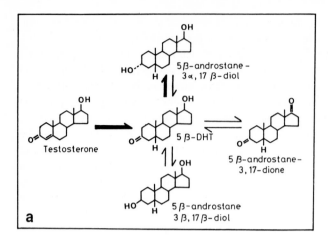

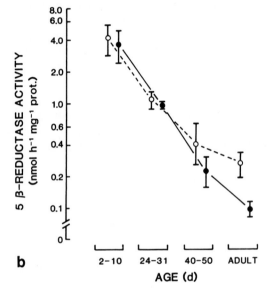

Fig. 3. a Pathways of 5β-reduction in the male dove brain. (After Steimer and Hutchison 1981b)
b Total 5β-reduction measured in the pre-optic (●) and septal areas (○) in developing male doves compared to the adult. The activity of 5β-reductase is significantly higher in early development, and there is no separation between septal and preoptic areas as in the adult brain

this, which is of immediate relevance to the developmental effects of steroids on song control, is whether metabolic inactivation of testosterone in brain cells plays any part in early brain differentiation.

The anatomical separation between brain areas in 5β-reductase activity, which is a feature of the adult brain in species of birds examined so far, does not occur in the developing brain (Hutchison and Steimer 1984; Hutchison and Schumacher, in prep.). The activity of 5β-reductase in male and female dove chicks is higher by an order of magnitude than adult enzyme activity and, therefore, the half-life of testosterone in the preoptic area of the newly hatched chick is considerably shorter than in the adult (Hutchison and Steimer 1984). Similar findings have been made in the cockerel (Massa and Sharp 1981) and quail chicks (Balthazart et al. 1984). Does 5β-reduction serve as a steroid inactivation mechanism in the brain of young birds? There is some evidence that 5β-DHT given alone, or in combination with E_2, stimulates juvenile copulatory activity in domesticated chicks (Balthazart and Hirschberg 1979). However, more recent work shows that testosterone is far less effective than 5α-DHT in inducing crowing in quail chicks (Balthazart et al. 1984). Since 5α-DHT cannot be 5β-reduced, it has been suggested (Balthazart et al. 1984) that the greater behavioural effectiveness of the α-reduced androgen in comparison with testosterone is due to the fact that testosterone is inactivated rapidly by 5β-reduction. As in other avian species studied so far, 5β-reduction should be a major pathway of testosterone metabolism in the developing zebra finch brain. This enzymatic pathway could, therefore, have a role in the sexual differentiation of the vocal control system. As described above, there is no sex difference in plasma testosterone levels during post-hatching development of the zebra finch. Both sexes have relatively high concentrations which are likely to be inactivated rapidly by 5β-reductase activity. Androstenedione would also be 5β-reduced. Following the argument presented above that the female song control system is potentially prone to differentiation by circulating androgens, known to be present in the circulating plasma, we suggest that inactivation by 5β-reduction could have a protective role in the developing female zebra finch brain (Fig. 4). Following this hypothesis, the surge in plasma E_2 during days 3 and 4 after hatching would not be affected by 5β-reductase activity, but testosterone would be inactivated in both male and female target areas. Similarly, DHT which is also present in the circulating plasma, would avoid inactivation and be available to initiate developmental changes in vocal control nuclei. This hypothesis must remain speculative until the 5β-reduction pathway has been studied experimentally in the developing zebra finch brain. However, there is some preliminary evidence to support it. In all areas of the zebra finch brain examined so far (hypothalamus, telen-

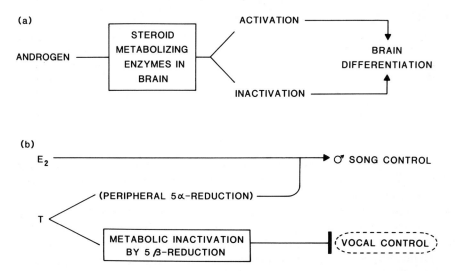

Fig. 4a,b. Scheme showing the suggested role of steroid metabolizing enzymes in development of the zebra finch song control system. **a** Both activating (aromatase) and inactivating (5β-reductase) enzymes are potentially available in the brain to influence differentiation. **b** Plasma oestradiol may initiate differentiation of the male song control system. Inactivation of testosterone and other aromatizable androgens in the brain could prevent differentiation of the female brain

cephalon including HVc, optic lobes, cerebellum), 5β-reductase activity was high 6 to 12 days after hatching and was lower by day 15–32 (Schumacher, Pröve, and Balthazart, pers. commun.). This appears to match the metabolic pattern found in other avian species.

5 What Determines the Sensitive Period for Brain Differentiation?

Current theory, based mainly on work in rodents, suggests that there are successive periods of sensitivity to steroids which depend on particular maturational stages of the brain. These studies (reviewed by McEwen 1983) will not be discussed in detail here. However, both secretion of the differentiating hormone and the state of differentiation of target neurones play an important part in determining the onset and duration of the sensitive periods. Elaboration of receptors for the effective steroid is likely to be important in the timing of the sexual differentiation of brain cells (Vito and Fox 1979). The perinatal increase in E_2 receptors measured in rats (McEwen 1983) is likely to be synchronized in time with the organizational effect of hormones on behavioural mechanisms.

An important question with regard to the sexual differentiation of the avian brain which needs to be examined is whether a strictly limited "critical" period exists for the effects of the active steroid. There is some evidence in female quail for an embryonic critical period in which E_2 eliminates development of male behaviour. Thus embryonic treatment of females with an anti-oestrogen (nitromifene citrate, CI-628) enhances male-type behaviour following androgen treatment in adulthood. Males are also behaviourally demasculinized by embryonic treatment with oestrogen (reviewed in Adkins-Regan 1983). Whether these hormonal or drug treatments act directly on the brain or via embryonic gonadal effects, has not been resolved (see R.E. Hutchison 1978 for review). A related factor is the plasticity in responsiveness to steroid hormones shown by the adult avian brain. Oestradiol does not necessarily act embryonically to differentiate mechanisms of behaviour. Demasculinization of female behaviour can be initiated by oestrogen in adult female quail that have been ovariectomized 6–12 h after hatching (R.E. Hutchison 1978; Schumacher and Balthazart 1983a). Therefore, in this case, the bipotentiality of the systems underlying sexual behaviour is maintained until the differentiating hormone, E_2, is available. The sensitivity of the brain to E_2 is evidently maintained despite an adult phenotype. In view of this prolonged oestrogen-sensitivity, the period during which plasma oestrogen levels normally rise becomes important in determining when sexual differentiation is initiated during development. Similarly, in the zebra finch, an important question is whether the post-hatching surge in E_2 determines the timing of brain differentiation, or whether factors associated with the brain neurones themselves restrict capacity for change during development. Arnold has pointed out (Arnold and Gorski 1984) that in the zebra finch "the brain of females given estradiol at hatching is surprisingly plastic in adulthood, since testosterone can cause significant morphological changes, which imply functional alterations." Nottebohm (1980) has also demonstrated convincingly that testosterone treatment increases the volumes of RA and HVc and dendritic fields in RA neurones of the adult female canary brain.

Therefore in a number of avian species, morphological changes in the brain can occur as a consequence of hormone action in adulthood. Sensitivity of the brain to steroid action does not appear to be restricted to embryonic or perinatal development.

Although there have been few studies of this problem published yet on the zebra finch, there appears to be a correlation between ability to sing and the period when E_2 treatment is initiated after hatching. Females treated from days 2–4 post-hatching until day 18 produce song that is similar in some cases to that of males; treatment after this period has no effect (Pohl-Apel and Sossinka 1984). Neurones of RA remain sensitive to the masculinizing effects of E_2 for a prolonged period from the day of hatching until day 40, though the response declines exponentially with age (Gurney 1981). Therefore, at the time of the peak in plasma E_2, the capacity for differentiation of the song control system is maximal. Although the song control system remains sensitive to the differentiating effects of exogenous E_2 for much of the developmental period, exposure of the male brain to the surge in E_2 between days 3 and 7 could trigger neuronal organization. In this case, maturational condition of the brain may not be a rigidly limiting factor in determining when brain differentiation is initiated. Appearance of specific receptors for E_2 in target brain cells could theoretically coincide with the surge in plasma E_2, and determine the onset of the sensitive period. It seems more likely to us, however, that neuroendocrine events controlling peripheral secretion of E_2 may ultimately determine when sexual differentiation of the song control system begins.

6 Conclusions

Hormones have an organizational role in brain development with respect to mechanism underlying behaviour. Peaks in gonadal steroid levels occur at developmental stages which coincide with sensitive periods for the differentiation of both the brain and behaviour. But the physiological factors which control the timing and action of hormones on the brain during development are poorly understood. Information is required both on the pattern of secretion of hormones by the developing gonads and what determines the sensitivity of target neurones in the brain to these hormones. Few studies have been made using the avian brain to answer these problems. However, the zebra finch provides the only example where steroid hormones have a sexually differentiating effect on brain cells unequivocally involved in behaviour. In the zebra finch, androgens initiate differentiation of telencephalic brain nuclei known to be involved in the control of song. The effect appears to be mediated by oestradiol-17β which is thought to be formed as an aromatization product within the brain. There is, however, no difference between the sexes in circulating levels of aromatizable androgens during early development, and oestradiol is elevated specifically in the male. The oestradiol surge coincides with the period when capacity for differentiation is maximal, indicating that brain aromatization is not a necessary requirements for male differentiation. Neuroendocrine events controlling the secretion of oestradiol are likely to determine the timing of the differentiation of the song control system. However, steroid metabolizing enzymes in brain cells are also likely to influence when and to what extent androgens are effective. Both in vitro and in vivo studies in avian species suggest that testosterone is rapidly converted to 5β-reduced metabolites within the avian brain. During early development, brain 5β-reductase activity is considerably higher than in adulthood. In view of the high plasma levels of aromatizable androgens in the developing zebra finch female, metabolic inactivation of androgen by 5β-reduction in brain target cells may prevent masculinization of the female brain.

Acknowledgements. We are grateful to A. Arnold and J. Balthazart for allowing us to quote unpublished work. We also thank M. Konishi for his comments on a first draft of the manuscript. Finally, P. Marler helped us considerably by providing space for some of the experimental work carried out at Rockefeller University, and discussing the analysis of song.

References

Adkins EK (1975) Hormonal basis of sexual differentiation in the Japanese quail. J Comp Physiol Psychol 89:61–71

Adkins-Regan E (1983) Sex steroids and the differentiation and activation of avian reproductive behaviour. In: Balthazart E, Pröve E, Gilles R (eds) Hormones and behaviour in higher vertebrates. Springer, Berlin Heidelberg New York, pp 218–230

Arnold AP (1980) Effects of androgens on volumes of sexually dimorphic brain regions in the zebra finch. Brain Res 185:441–444

Arnold AP, Gorski RA (1984) Gonadal steroid induction of structural sex differences in the central nervous system. Annu Rev Neurosci 7:413–442

Arnold AP, Saltiel A (1979) Sexual differentiation in pattern of hormone accumulation in the brain of a songbird. Science (Wash DC) 205:702–705

Balthazart J, Hirschberg D (1979) Testosterone metabolism and sexual behavior in the chick. Horm Behav 12:253–263

Balthazart J, Schumacher M (1983) Testosterone metabolism and sexual differentiation in quail. In: Balthazart J, Pröve E, Gilles R (eds) Hormones and higher vertebrates. Springer, Berlin Heidelberg New York, pp 261–274

Balthazart J, Schumacher M, Malacarne G (1984) Relative potencies of testosterone and 5α-dihydrotestosterone on crowing and cloacal gland growth in the Japanese quail *(Coturnix coturnix japonica)*. J Endocrinol 100:19–23

Beach FA (1974) Behavioral endocrinology and the study of reproduction. Biol Reprod 10:2–18

Böhner J (1983) Song learning in the zebra finch *Taeniopygia guttata*: selectivity in the choice of tutor and accuracy of song copies. Anim Behav 31:231–237

Bottjer SW, Arnold AP (1984, in press) The ontogeny of vocal learning in songbirds. In: Blass E (ed) Developmental processes in psychobiology and neurobiology. Plenum, New York

Bottjer SW, Glaessner SL, Arnold AP (1984) Development of the neural network controlling song behavior in zebra finches. Soc Neurosci Abstracts, vol 10

Callard GV, Petro Z, Ryan KJ (1978) Phylogenetic distribution of aromatase and other androgen-converting enzymes in the central nervous system. Endocrinology 103:2283–2290

Gorski RA (1984) Critical role for the medial preoptic area in the sexual differentiation of the brain. In: deVries GJ, de Bruin JPC, Uylings HBM, Corner MA (eds) Sex differences in the brain. The relation between structure and function. Prog Brain Res 61:129–146. Elsevier, Amsterdam

Goy RW, McEwen BS (1980) Sexual differentiation of the brain. MIT Press, Cambridge

Gurney ME (1981) Hormonal control of cell form and number in the zebra finch song system. J Neurosci 1:658–873

Gurney ME (1982) Behavioral correlates of sexual differentiation in the zebra finch song system. Brain Res 231:153–172

Gurney ME, Konishi M (1980) Hormone induced sexual differentiation of brain and behaviour in zebra finches. Science (Wash DC) 208:1380–1382

Güttinger HR, Pröve E, Weichel K, Pesch A (1984) Kurzberichte aus der laufenden Forschung. J Ornithol 125:245–247

Hutchison JB, Schumacher M (in preparation) Localization and partial characterization of testosterone metabolizing enzymes in the avian brain during early development

Hutchison JB, Steimer T (1981) Brain 5β-reductase: a correlate of behavioral sensitivity to androgen. Science (Wash DC) 213:244–246

Hutchison JB, Steimer T (1983) Hormone-mediated behavioural transitions: a role for brain aromatase. In: Balthazart J, Pröve E, Gilles R (eds) Hormones and behavior in higher vertebrates. Springer, Berlin Heidelberg New York, pp 261–274

Hutchison JB, Steimer T (1984) Androgen metabolism in the brain: behavioural correlates. In: de Vries GJ, de Bruin JPC, Uylings HBM, Corner MA (eds) Sex differences in the brain. The relation between structure and function. Prog Brain Res 61:23–51. Elsevier, Amsterdam

Hutchison JB, Wingfield JC, Hutchison RE (1984) Sex differences in plasma concentrations of steroids during the sensitive period for brain differentiation in the zebra finch. J Endocrinol 103:363–369

Hutchison RE (1978) Hormonal differentiation of sexual behavior in Japanese quail. Horm Behav 11:363–387

Immelmann K (1962) Beiträge zu einer vergleichenden Biologie australischer Prachtfinken (Spermestidae). Zool Jahrb Abt Syst Dekol Geogr Tierl 90:1–96

Konishi M, Akutagawa E (1985) Neuronal growth, atrophy and death in a sexually dimorphic song nucleus in the zebra finch brain. Nature (Lond) 315:145–147

Konishi M, Gurney ME (1982) Sexual differentiation of brain and behavior. Trends Neurosci 5: 20–23

MacLusky NJ, Naftolin F (1981) Sexual differentiation of the central nervous system. Science (Wash DC) 211:1294–1303

Martini L (1982) The 5α-reduction of testosterone in the neuroendocrine structures. Biochemical and biophysical implications. Endocr Rev 3:1–25

Massa R (1980) The role of androgens in male birds' reproduction. In: Delvio G, Brachet J (eds) Steroids and their mechanism of action in the nonmammalian vertebrates. Raven, New York, pp 148–159

Massa R, Sharp J (1981) Conversion of testosterone to 5β-reductase metabolites in the neuro-endocrine tissues of the maturing cockerel. J Endocrinol 88:263–269

McEwen BS (1983) Gonadal steroid influence on brain development and sexual differentiation. In: Greep RO (ed) Reproductive physiology IV. International review of physiology. University Park Press, Baltimore, pp 99–145

Morris D (1954) The reproductive behaviour of the zebra finch *(Poephilia guttata)* with special reference to pseudofemale behaviour and displacement activities. Behaviour 6:271–322

Naftolin F, Ryan KJ, Davies IJ, Reddy VV, Flores F, Petro D, Kuhn M, White RJ, Takaoka Y, Wolin L (1975) The formation of estrogens by central neuroendocrine tissue. Recent Prog Horm Res 31:295–316

Nordeen KW, Nordeen EJ, Arnold AP (1984) Estrogen masculinizes the pattern of androgen accumulation in the brain of a songbird. Soc Neurosci Abstracts, vol 10:454

Nottebohm F (1980) Testosterone triggers growth of brain vocal control nuclei in adult female canaries. Brain Res 189:429–436

Nottebohm F, Arnold AP (1976) Sexual dimorphism in vocal control areas of the song bird brain. Science (Wash DC) 194:211–213

Nottebohm F, Stokes TM, Leonard CM (1976) Central control of song in the canary *(Serinus canarius)*. J Comp Neurol 165:457–486

Olsen KL (1979) Androgen insensitive rats are defeminized by their testes. Nature (Lond) 279: 238–239

Plapinger L, McEwen BS (1978) Gonadal steroid and brain interaction in sexual differentiation. In: Hutchison JB (ed) Biological determinants of sexual behaviour. Wiley, Chichester, pp 153–219

Pohl-Apel G, Sossinka R (1982) Männchentypischer Gesang bei weiblichen Zebrafinken *(Taeniopygia guttata castenotis)*. J Ornithol 123:211–214

Pohl-Apel G, Sossinka R (1984) Hormonal determination of song capacity in females of the zebra finch: critical phase of treatment. Z Tierpsychol 64:330–336

Price PH (1979) Developmental determinants of structure in zebra finch song. J Comp Physiol Psychol 93:26–277

Pröve E (1983) Hormonal correlates of behavioural development in male zebra finches. In: Balthazart J, Pröve E, Gilles R (eds) Hormones and behaviour in higher vertebrates. Springer, Berlin Heidelberg New York, pp 368–374

Reddy VVR, Naftolin F, Ryan KJ (1974) Conversion of androstenedione to estrone by neural tissues from fetal and neonatal rat. Endocrinology 94:117–121

Schumacher M, Balthazart J (1983a) Effects of castration on postnatal differentiation in the Japanese quail *(Coturnix coturnix japonica)*. IRCS Med Sci Kibr Compend 11:102–103

Schumacher M, Balthazart J (1983b) Testosterone metabolism in discrete areas of the hypothalamus and adjacent brain regions of male and female Japanese quail *(Coturnix coturnix japonica)*. Brain Res 278:337–340

Schumacher M, Hutchison JB (in preparation) Testosterone induces hypothalamic aromatase during early development in quail

Selmanoff MK, Brodkin LD, Weiner RI, Siiteri PK (1977) Aromatization and 5α-reduction of androgens in discrete hypothalamic and limbic regions of the male and female rat. Endocrinology 101:841–848

Siegel LI, Fox TO, Konishi M (1983) Androgen and estrogen receptors in zebra finch brain. Soc Neurosci Abstr 9:1078

Silcox A (1979) The pair bonding in the zebra finch. PhD Thesis Newcastle-upon-Tyne

Sossinka R, Böhner J (1980) Song types in the zebra finch *(Poephilia guttata castenotis)*. Z Tierpsychol 53:123–132

Steimer T, Hutchison JB (1980) Aromatization of testosterone within a discrete hypothalamic area associated with the behavioural action of androgen in the male dove. Brain Res 192:586–591

Steimer T, Hutchison JB (1981a) Androgen increases formation of behaviourally effective androgen on the dove brain. Nature (Lond) 292:345–347

Steimer T, Hutchison JB (1981b) Metabolic control of the behavioural action of androgens in the dove brain: testosterone inactivation by 5β-reduction. Brain Res 209:189–204

Tanabe Y, Nakamura T, Fujioka K, Doi (1979) Production and secretion of sex steroid hormones by the testes, the ovary and the adrenal glands of embryonic and young chickens *(Gallus domesticus)*. Gen Comp Endocrinol 39:26–33

Toran-Allerand CD (1984) On the genesis of sexual differentiation of the central nervous system: morphogenetic consequences of steroidal exposure and possible role of alpha-fetoprotein. In: de Vries GJ, de Bruin JPC, Uylings HBM, Corner MA (eds) Sex differences in the brain. The relation between structure and function. Prog Brain Res 61:63–98. Elsevier, Amsterdam

Vito CC, Fox TO (1979) Embryonic rodent brain contains estrogen receptors. Science (Wash DC) 204:517–519

Wingfield JC, Farner DS (1975) The determination of five steroids in avian plasma by radioimmunoassay and competitive protein binding. Steroids 26:311–327

Wingfield JC, Smith JP, Farner DS (1980) Changes in plasma levels of luteinizing hormone, steroid and thyroid hormones during the post-fledgling development of white-crowned sparrows, *Zonotrichia leucophrys*. Gen Comp Endocrinol 41:372–377

Woods JE, Erton LH (1978) Plasma testosterone levels in the chick embryo. Gen Comp Endocrinol 27:543–547

Yahr P (1985) See this volume

Role of Testosterone Metabolism in the Activation of Sexual Behaviour in Birds

J. BALTHAZART and M.SCHUMACHER [1]

1 Introduction

As early as 1849, Berthold demonstrated that castration abolishes and testicular grafts restore sexual behaviour in the cockerel. This conclusion has since been verified by many independent researchers and has been extended to a large number of species belonging to all vertebrate classes. It has also been demonstrated that the steroid, testosterone (T) was responsible for the behavioural effects of the testes but we had to wait for the advent of radioimmunoassays in the early seventies before this hormone could repeatedly be measured in small animals such as the rat, mice, guinea pig, or quail used in laboratory studies and before plasma levels of the steroids could be related to the behaviour of the animals.

From that time on, it became possible to meet the three criteria which make it possible to claim that a selected hormone is responsible for a given behaviour, namely:

— removal of the endocrine gland secreting the hormone should abolish behaviour.
— replacement therapy either by a graft of endocrine gland or by administration of purified hormone should restore behaviour in castrates.
— and, finally, variations in hormone concentration and behaviour should be correlated and the doses of hormones that must be injected to restore behaviour in castrates should produce plasma levels of the hormone similar to those seen in intact animals.

During the seventies, data were accumulated that showed this kind of correlation between plasma hormones and behaviour (for reviews of the avian literature see Silver et al. 1979; Balthazart 1983) but at the same time numerous discrepancies were observed (see also Wingfield and Ramenovsky, this volume). In a long term study of the endocrine control of duck behaviour, we showed for example that the annual changes in plasma testosterone were positively correlated to the frequency of sexual behaviour (Balthazart and Hendrick 1976). This behaviour was suppressed by castration and restored by testosterone injections (Balthazart 1978; Deviche 1979) which confirmed its androgen dependence, but no relationship could be found between the individual levels of testosterone and the individual variations in behavioural activity (Balthazart et al. 1977). This and other data reviewed previously (see Balthazart 1983) suggested that the behavioural action of the hormone could be regulated at the level of the target

1 Laboratoire de Biochimie Générale et Comparée, Université de Liège, 17 place Delcour, 4020 Liège, Belgium

Neurobiology
(ed. by R. Gilles and J. Balthazart)
© Springer-Verlag Berlin Heidelberg 1985

organ, in this case the brain and essentially the anterior hypothalamus and preoptic area (Barfield 1969, 1971; Hutchison 1971, 1978).

In the last 5 years, our research has focussed on the brain mechanisms of testosterone action and on the respective roles played in the control of behaviour by the changes in plasma hormone levels on one hand and the changes in sensitivity to the hormone of the target organs on the other hand. The Japanese quail *(Coturnix coturnix japonica)* has been choosen as subject of these studies for a number of practical reasons including adequate size, fast breeding cycle, and easily quantifiable behaviour. The studies have concentrated on the testosterone metabolism in the target organs as it appeared that this is probably a critical step in the hormone action.

2 Brain Mechanisms in Testosterone Action

It is generally accepted that the behavioural action of testosterone at the brain level depends on a genomic action of the hormone very similar (identical?) to that responsible for the trophic effects of the hormone in peripheral structures such as the rat prostate, the chicken comb or the quail cloacal gland (e.g. McEwen 1981). The free hormone enters the cells probably by passive diffusion and then binds to specific receptors located in the cytosol (see Martin and Sheridan 1982; or Blaustein and Brown, this Vol. for a possible revision of this notion). The hormone-receptor complex is then translocated to the cell nucleus where it interacts with the DNA to generate the synthesis of new proteins which are responsible for the changes in cell physiology. Before it binds to the cytosolic receptors, testosterone can be metabolized into a number of compounds which eventually will also bind to specific receptors. In many cases, it has thus been proposed that testosterone only acts a prohormone but that its action at the brain levels is due to some of its metabolites.

In the avian brain, testosterone can be aromatized into oestradiol (E_2) or oestrone (E_1) (Callard et al. 1978; Steimer and Hutchison 1980; Schumacher et al. 1984) and this process is thought to play a critical role in the activation of copulation. In quail, for example, copulation can be activated by T as well as by E_2 (Adkins and Adler 1972), T induced copulation is blocked by the antiestrogen, CI-628 (Adkins and Nock 1976) and the aromatase inhibitor, ATD blocks T-induced but not E_2-induced copulatory behaviour (Adkins et al. 1980). It is thus likely that E_2 derived from T aromatization is somehow involved in the control of copulation but its precise mode of action remains to be uncovered. In addition it must be mentioned that androgens per se are capable of activating copulatory behaviour in quail (Balthazart et al. 1984a) so that the hormonal determinants of this behaviour probably include both androgen- and oestrogen-sensitive mechanisms.

In the bird brain, T is also 5α-reduced into 5α-dihydrotestosterone (5α-DHT) (Balthazart et al. 1984b; Schumacher et al. 1984) which is a behaviourally active steroid. In castrated quail, 5α-DHT stimulates crowing and strutting (Adkins and Pniewski 1978; Deviche and Schumacher 1982) and activates copulation either alone (Deviche and Schumacher 1982; Deviche, unpublished) or in synergy with E_2 (Adkins and Pniewski 1978; Balthazart et al. 1984a).

In all birds species studied so far, the brain also reduces T in position 5β to produce 5β-dihydrotestosterone (5β-DHT) and the corresponding diols (5β-androstane-3α or 3β, 17β-diol) (European starling: Massa et al. 1977; chicken: Nakamura and Tanabe 1974; Balthazart and Hirschberg 1982; Japanese quail: Balthazart et al. 1979; ring dove: Steimer and Hutchison 1981; zebra finch: Schumacher et al., unpublished; domestic duck: Willems 1978). Quantitatively, 5β-androstanes are the main metabolites of testosterone produced by the avian brain: more than 80% of the metabolites produced during the in vitro incubation of ^{14}C-testosterone with brain homogenates are 5β-reduced compounds. It is thus interesting to note that these compounds are almost completely devoid of androgenic activity. Indeed, 5β-DHT does not depress plasma LH (Davies et al. 1980; Balthazart and Hirschberg 1979), does not promote the growth of secondary sexual characteristics such as the chicken comb (Mori et al. 1974) or cloacal gland in quail (Adkins 1977; Massa et al. 1980) or does it only slightly when injected in very large doses (Chicken comb: Balthazart and Hirschberg 1979; Balthazart et al. 1981; quail cloacal gland: Deviche et al. 1982). Finally 5β-DHT seems devoid of any behavioral activity. In adult castrated quail or ring dove, 5β-DHT has no clear stimulatory effect on sexual behaviour (Adkins 1977; Steimer and Hutchison 1981) although marginal effects were observed when large doses of 5β-DHT were injected in quail in association with subthreshold doses of T (Deviche et al. 1982).

Altogether, these data suggest that T metabolism could regulate the action of T at the cellular level by changing the amounts of active (e.g. E_2 or 5α-DHT) versus inactive (e.g. 5β-DHT) metabolites which are produced when the hormone reaches its target cells and before it interacts with its receptors. The present paper will review a few physiological situations in quail where this mode of regulation has been demonstrated.

3 Assay Characteristics

The activity of testosterone metabolizing enzymes was estimated by two in vitro radioenzymatic assays in which homogenates of specific brain areas (or minced pieces of nervous tissue in the first studies) were incubated in the presence of radioactive testosterone labelled with ^{14}C or ^{3}H. The metabolites formed during these incubations were subsequently extracted by organic solvents and when appropriate, oestrogens were separated from androgens by phenolic partition. The metabolites were then purified by thin layer chromatography on silicagel and quantified by β-scintillation (see Schumacher et al. 1983, 1984 for the detail of methods). Their formal identity has been confirmed by recrystallization to constant specific activity or constant isotopic ratio and by chromatography in different systems of various derivatives (propionates and acetates) (Balthazart et al. 1979; Davies et al. 1980; Schumacher et al. 1984; Balthazart et al. 1984b).

In the assay using ^{14}C-testosterone, brain homogenates were incubated in the presence of relatively large amounts of substrate (final concentration around 1 μM i.e. 100 to 200 ng of T for an homogenate corresponding to 2–4 mg of brain tissue). This high substrate concentration permits to evaluate the rate of enzymatic transformation of testosterone without the interference of endogenous steroids or of binding proteins which would respectively dilute or sequester the radioactive substrate and thus change the apparent kinetics. Unfortunately the relatively low specific activity of this substrate (around 50 mCi mmole^{-1}) permits to measure only high enzymatic activities (5β-reductase) and the assay is not sensitive enough to measure precisely the aromatase or the 5α-reductase in the brain (the latter can nevertheless be evaluated in peripheral structures such as the cloacal gland).

On the contrary the ^{3}H-testosterone based assay uses physiological levels of tracer which has some advantages at the level of data interpretation (it can for example be ascertained that enzymatic activities truly reflects physiological processes and have not been altered by the very high level of substrate) but presents the disadvantage that results are potentially influenced by the endogenous steroids and binding proteins. This factor must be taken into account in the interpretation of the results. In addition, this assay is extremely sensitive due to the high specific activity of the substrate (60 Ci/mmole) and thus permits an easy detection of enzymes with low activity such as the aromatase and 5α-reductase (production of a few fmol mg^{-1} fresh weight can be detected).

Preliminary experiments permitted to select assay conditions in which the production of metabolites was linear with respect to duration of incubation and substrate concentrations. Kinetic studies were also performed which demonstrated that the 5α-reductase and the aromatase have kinetics which follow the Michaelis-Menten model and that these enzymes are not regulated in our assay conditions. By contrast, the 5β-reductase seems to be subjected to complex regulations. Results suggest the presence of two enzyme forms, one with low capacity and high affinity which has a sigmoid kinetics, the other with a larger capacity and lower affinity whose activity is inhibited at very high substrate concentrations. The maximum velocity of the 5β-reductase is much higher than that of the 5α-reductase or the aromatase (1940, 220, and 148 fmol mg^{-1} fresh weight h^{-1} respectively and the apparent affinities of the enzymes are also very different (Km = 47.3×10^{-8}, 11.4×10^{-8}, and 1.5×10^{-8} M for 5β-, 5α-reductase and aromatase respectively). This fits in well with the proposed role of the metabolites. At low substrate concentrations, the high affinity of the 5α-reductase and aromatase makes that active metabolites are formed predominantly while at higher concentrations, the inactivation of testosterone into 5β-reduced compounds (behaviourally inactive) would become more important and thus possibly regulate the hormonal activation through this inactivation process.

4 Physiological Studies

4.1 Research Strategy

In all studies presented below, the sexual behaviour of male Japanese quail was studied and quantified in selected physiological situations. Birds were also bled in association with the behavioural tests and plasma testosterone was measured by radioimmunoassay in these samples. This permitted the selection of a number of situations where a discrepancy existed between the behavioural performance of the animals and their expected plasma testosterone levels. In these cases, the T metabolism in a discrete part of the hypothalamus was studied by the in vitro assays. It was hoped that the previously mentioned discrepancies originated in a central regulation of hormone sensitivity and that this would involve specific shifts in the activity of testosterone-metabolizing enzymes. Two notes of caution must, however, be placed here:

— the absence of correlation between plasma testosterone and behaviour could have other interpretations than the one proposed here. These have been discussed previously (Balthazart 1983) and include rapid variations in the plasma hormone levels, absence of distinction between bound, and free hormone in the classical radioimmunoassays and effects of previous experience of the animals on their behaviour.
— the data presented in the following are correlative in nature. They show related changes in behaviour and in enzyme activities in the brain. We shall present causal interpretation of these correlations on the basis of additional experiments reviewed elsewhere (Adkins-Regan 1983; Balthazart 1983) which imply procedures such as castration and replacement therapy with testosterone or its metabolites, treatment with anti-oestrogens and anti-androgens, and with drugs which inhibit the metabolism of testosterone. In most cases, the interpretation of the correlations that we present here, if it makes sense from a biological point of view, should nevertheless be considered as tentative before we have more data on the in vivo effects of specific drugs inhibiting testosterone metabolism.

4.2 Individual Differences in Behaviour

Individual differences in reproductive function have been poorly studied and as a consequence their hormonal control is far from being understood. Quite frequently, it has been impossible to relate the individual levels of reproductive behaviour and of organs or properties which are known to be androgen-dependent (based on castration and replacement therapy) to the plasma levels of testosterone (e.g. in quail: Tsutsui and Ishii 1981; in domestic ducks: Balthazart 1978; Balthazart et al. 1977; in rats: Damassa et al. 1977; in mice: Dessi-Fulgheri et al. 1976; in guinea pigs: Harding and Feder 1976; in monkeys: Michael and Wilson 1975; see also Wingfield and Ramenovsky, this Vol.). As mentioned previously, this lack of correlation could have several origins but we decided to research whether it could be related to differences in brain metabolism of testosterone on the basis of a study by Dessi-Fulgheri et al. (1976) who showed that in mice aggressive behaviour was correlated to the androstenedione production by the brain but not to plasma testosterone.

Some support for this idea was found in a first experiment performed in collaboration with the group of R. Massa at the University of Milano (Balthazart et al. 1979). In this study, a group of 20 adult male quail was maintained for 20 days in short days to cause gonadal regression and then returned to the long photoperiod which induced a rapid testicular growth and an increase in plasma LH, FSH, and testosterone. Throughout the experiment males were kept in groups of four in five visually isolated cages. Sexual (neck grab, mount, copulation, and strutting) and aggressive (peck and chase) behaviour of these birds was recorded by introducing the four males from the same cage in a test arena with one adult receptive female for 5 min on days 4, 6, and 8 after transfer to long days (test A). Aggressive interactions between males were also recorded in the home cages for 5 min on days 5 and 7 (test B). On day 12, birds were killed, plasma were collected for later assay of testosterone and the hypothalamus and a small piece of hyperstriatum were incubated with ^{14}C-testosterone to study its in vitro metabolism. Testes weight and cloacal gland area (an androgen-dependent structure) were also recorded.

No relationship (significant Spearman rank correlation coefficient) could be detected between any of the behavioural measures and plasma testosterone. By contrast, testes weight and cloacal gland area were very good predictors of the behavioural performance, these variables being significantly higher in those birds who strutted during the test than in those which were inactive (Fig. 1). Significant relationships were also observed between the behaviour and the brain testosterone metabolism. Aggressive actions were more frequent in birds having a low 5β-reductase in their hypothalamus and a high production of androstenedione (probably reflecting indirectly a low 5β-reductase as both enzymes compete for the same substrate) was associated with a higher frequency of pecks, chases, and struts (see Fig. 1).

More recent studies tend to confirm the existence of relationships between individual variations in behaviour and in brain testosterone metabolism. During two independent experiments, groups of 22 (Expt. I) or 16 (Expt. II) young male Japanese quail were observed for behaviour and various endocrine variables during their sexual maturation (around 6 weeks of age). Blood samples were collected and assayed for LH, testosterone, and corticosterone, the body weight and cloacal gland area were repeatedly measured and the behaviour was recorded in three standardized situations namely:

— introduction for 5 min of each male individually in a test arena containing a receptive female (type A test).
— dyadic encounters of males for 1 min during which each male met with every other opponent in a random order [for N birds, N(N-1)/2 encounters]. During each of these tests (type B), the behaviour of the males was scored on the following ordinal scale. A score of + 1 was given if the male pecked, chased or performed neck grabs or mount attempts on the other male, he had a score of – 1 if he received these behaviours passively or while trying to escape. A score of 0 was attributed to both birds if none of these behaviours was observed and finally both birds had a score of + 1 if they both showed aggressive or sexual behaviour. The points of each bird were added at the end of the encounters and this was called their dominance index [scores ranging from – (N-1) to (N-1) with N = number of birds tested].
— quantitative recordings of the number of crows emitted by each bird in its home cage (type C test) for five 10 min periods.

At the end of the experiments, birds were killed and their anterior and posterior hypothalamus were incubated with ^{14}C-testosterone. Testes weight and cloacal gland area were also measured.

The three types of behavioural tests measured various aspects of the reproductive behaviour (sexual and aggressive) and all these measures were found to be strongly correlated (see Delville et al. 1984). We shall thus only present the relationships of the dominance index with the endocrine variables keeping in mind that these are representative for the relationships that were observed with the other behavioural measures. In both experiments, the dominance index was positively related to the testes weight and cloacal gland (Significant Spearman correlation coefficient; see Fig. 2). When the most dominant birds were compared to those having the lowest dominance scores, it was found that testes weight and cloacal gland area were significantly larger in the former.

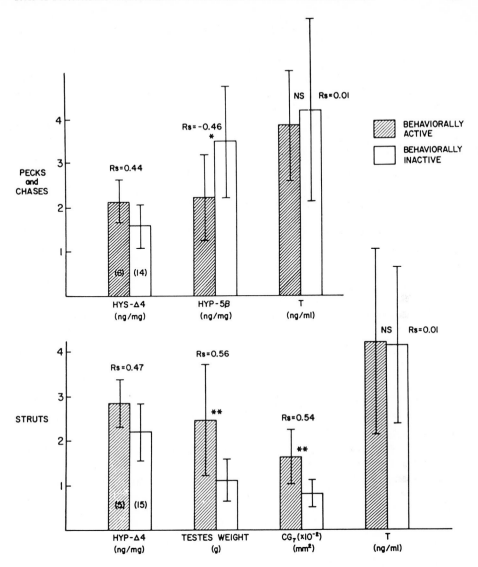

Fig. 1. Relationships between reproductive behaviour, testes weight, cloacal gland area (*CG*), plasma testosterone (*T*), and brain testosterone metabolism in a group of adult male quail. The Fig. 1 shows the significant correlation coefficients (*Rs* Spearman rank correlation coefficient) and the mean levels (+ SD) of the endocrine variables in sexually active and inactive birds. These levels are compared by the t-test (* = $P < 0.05$; ** = $P < 0.01$). *HYS* hyperstriatum; *HYP* hypothalamus; Δ4 production of androstenedione; 5β production of 5β-androstanes (DHT + diol)

The correlation of behaviour with plasma testosterone and brain testosterone metabolism were less consistent. In Expt. II, no relationship between behaviour and plasma testosterone was detected while brain 5β-reductase (specifically in the anterior hypothalamus) was negatively correlated to the dominance index. This confirmed the finding of the previous experiment. By contrast an opposite pattern of correlations was

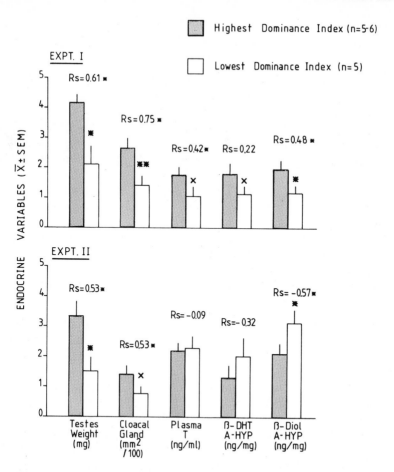

Fig. 2. Correlations between the dominance index (see text), testes weight, cloacal gland area, plasma testosterone (*T*), and 5 β-reduction of testosterone in the anterior hypothalamus (*A-HYP*) in groups of adult male quail. Presentation of data is as in Fig. 1 except that mean levels of endocrine variables are calculated using only the extreme birds in the dominance index scale (N = 5–6 birds). *β-DHT* production of 5 β-dihydrotestosterone; *β-diol* production of 5 β-androstane-3 α,17 β-diol

found in Expt. I where plasma testosterone was positively related to the behaviour but the latter showed no relationship with 5 β-DHT production and showed a positive correlation (as opposed to a negative one in the other 2 experiments) with the 5 β-diol production. All these correlations were probably specific in nature because no significant relationship was observed between the same behavioural measures and testosterone metabolism in the adjacent posterior hypothalamus which was studied as a control area.

The three independent experiments presented here have revealed consistent relationships between individual differences in reproductive behaviour on one hand and testes weight and cloacal gland area on the other hand. These morphological variables are reliable predictors of the behavioural performance of the animals. In only one experiment out of three, could we find a positive correlation between plasma testosterone and reproductive behaviour. The absence of correlation in two cases could have many explanations such as:

— our assay did not distinguish between testosterone and dihydrotestosterone which could have obscured the existing relationship.
— our assay did not measure specifically the free testosterone but rather gave a level for the total hormone which is only partly available to the brain and it has been shown at least in one species that better correlation between testosterone and sexual behaviour are found when only the free testosterone is measured (Chambers et al. 1981).
— the androgen requirement for behavioural stimulation is less than the amount normally present in an intact animal and the individual differences bear no relationship with the plasma levels of the hormone.
— plasma levels of testosterone changes very quickly so that levels measured in one sample are not a stable individual characteristics.
— or finally relationships between plasma testosterone and behaviour are obscured by the previous experience of the birds as elegantly shown for aggressive behaviour by the recent study of Ramenovsky (1984).

In two of the three studies negative correlations could also be found between measures of reproductive behaviour and 5β-reductase activity in the hypothalamus. These are biologically relevant as 5β-reduced metabolites are behaviourally inactive. These metabolic differences could be a causal explanation for the behavioural differences: birds which would not differ in their plasma testosterone levels would inactivate more or less the hormone in their brain which would result in different levels of behavioural activation. The interpretation of the data is however complicated by the finding that in one experiment (precisely the one in which behaviour was related to plasma testosterone) a positive relationship between dominance index and brain 5β-reductase was observed. With the available data, it can thus only by stated that individual differences in behaviour are always realted to aspects of testosterone metabolism in the brain. The direction of this relationship is however variable and the origins of this variability have not been identified so far. The recent work of Ramenovsky (1984) clearly points to the possible role of previous experience and further studies are needed to clarify this question.

4.3 Aging of the Reproductive System

Aging of the reproductive system is a rapid phenomenon in quail. Already at the age of one year the fertility of the eggs has declined and it has been established that this is at least partly related to a decline in the copulatory behaviour of the male (Ottinger et al. 1983). Considering that plasma testosterone is highly correlated with the initiation and increase in sexual behaviour during maturation (Ottinger and Brinkley 1979) and that testosterone restores copulation in castrated quail (Adkins 1977; Schumacher and Balthazart 1983) it had been expected that the reproductive decline in aging birds would be associated with decreased plasma testosterone levels. A detailed study revealed, however, that this was not the case and that the behavioural regression was not associated at least in its early phases with a decrease in plasma testosterone (Ottinger et al. 1983).

During a stay at the university of Maryland, we thus studied in collaboration with M.A. Ottinger whether the decline of sexual behaviour in aging birds was related to changes in sensitivity of the hypothalamus to testosterone which would involved modifications of the testosterone metabolism by this structure (Balthazart et al. 1984b).

Sexually experienced male quail from three different age groups (20, 76, and 147 weeks) were thus selected during preliminary tests on the basis of their sexual behaviour: 5–7 sexually active and inactive birds were taken from each age group. Their sexual behaviour was then quantified during two tests in an observation arena by presenting them for 5 min each time to two receptive females. Some of the previously inactive birds showed weak sexual behaviour (neck grabs) on these occasions but the activity was significantly different in active (+) and inactive (−) birds (see Table 1). All quail were then killed, their testes weight and cloacal gland area were measured, serum was collected for testosterone assay and several tissues including anterior and posterior hypothalamus and cloacal gland area were dissected and used in the in vitro assay for testosterone metabolism.

As shown in Table 1, testes weight, cloacal gland area, and serum testosterone were all affected by age (significantly lower in older animals by ANOVAS). This effect was also much more pronounced in those birds which were behaviourally inactive: all these variables decreased very much in old inactive birds but were hardly affected by age in the sexually active quail.

Major changes in testosterone metabolism by the anterior hypothalamus and cloacal gland were also observed as a function of age and sexual activity of the birds (see Fig. 3). In the anterior hypothalamus, the 5β-reductase (production of 5β-DHT and 5β-diol) steadily decreased with age in active as well as inactive birds while the 5α-reductase increased in older birds but this time specifically in the sexually active ones. A completely different pattern of changes was detected in the cloacal gland. In this tissue, 5β-reduction of testosterone increased with age and was significantly higher in inactive than in active birds (at least in older birds; there was thus a significant interaction between the effects of age and behavioural activity). The production of 5α-DHT increased with age while the production of 5α-diol was decreasing especially in inactive birds, all this resulting in a total 5α-reduction (production of 5α-DHT + 5α-diol) which was not affected by age nor behavioural activity.

If we accept the view that 5β-reduction is an inactivation pathway for testosterone while 5α-reduction produces compounds (5α-DHT) which are involved in the activation of the copulation, then the altered enzyme function observed in the anterior hypothalamus of old active males could explain their sexual activity inspite of a substantial though not significant decrease in serum testosterone and in testes weight. Indeed in these birds, the inactivation of testosterone was reduced while the production of active metabolites was enhanced. It can thus be considered that a similar level of behavioural activation was obtained at the cellular level through a more efficient use of the substrate which was present in reduced amounts.

It is, however, also possible that the sexual activity by itself maintained moderate levels of serum testosterone and directly or indirectly influenced the brain enzymatic activities. The direction of the causal links suggested by this study thus cannot be ascertained without additional studies. It is nevertheless interesting to note that 5α-reductase was increased in the brain of birds which had reduced serum testosterone. In

Table 1. Sexual behaviour, morphological variables, and serum testosterone levels (T) in six groups of male quail of three different ages which showed (+) or did not show (−) sexual behaviour during preliminary tests

Age of birds	20 weeks		76 weeks		147 weeks	
	+	−	+	−	+	−
% Copulating	71	0	40	0	50	0
Neck grab latency (s)	123 + 132	251 + 70	186 + 155	253 + 115	111 + 127	300
Testes weight (g)	3.38 + 0.40	3.19 + 0.69	3.10 + 0.75	2.11 + 1.46	2.32 + 0.96	0.53 + 0.76
Cloacal gland area (mm^2)	278 + 44	216 + 47	203 + 27	132 + 80	240 + 26	80 + 32
Serum T (ng ml^{-1})	3.05 + 1.48	2.44 + 1.93	1.95 + 0.72	0.83 + 0.68	1.79 + 0.54	0.64 + 0.39

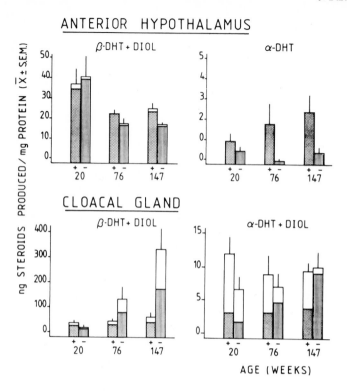

Fig. 3. Testosterone metabolism in the anterior hypothalamus and cloacal gland of male Japanese quail from three age groups (20, 76, and 147 weeks) selected for showing (+) or not showing (−) sexual behaviour. *Shaded areas* dihydrotestosterone *(DHT)* production; *open areas* androstane-diols productions

other studies (Balthazart et al. 1979; Balthazart et al. 1983; Section 4.4 in this Chap.) we have shown that 5α-reductase activity is increased in the cloacal gland when birds are exposed to elevated levels of testosterone. In these cases, the enzymatic changes amplify at the cellular level (through increased production of active metabolites) a hormonal signal transported by the blood (increased testosterone level). In the present study, we have indentified an independent enzymatic change (increased 5α-DHT production in the hypothalamus) which is expected to have opposite effects of those resulting from the alteration of circulating hormones (small decrease in testosterone level). This is to our knowledge the first demonstration of an independent enzymatic change which potentially induces a behavioral effect by itself rather than just amplifying the response to a peripheral stimulation by the hormone. These causal relationships remain to be established with more certitude.

Changes in testosterone metabolism by the cloacal gland also support the idea that the action of testosterone is regulated at the cellular level. In this gland, the 5β-reductase was significantly increased with age and more so in inactive birds whose gland was dramatically decreased in size. These birds thus has a decreased level of testosterone and in addition inactivated the hormone more at the cellular level. It can thus be considered that the increased 5β-reductase served as a chemical amplifier of the changes in serum testosterone. No obvious interpretation can be given to the change in production of 5α-reduced compounds as total 5α-reduction was not affected and both 5α-DHT (which increased with age) and 5α-diol (which decreased with age) have trophic effects on the structure.

4.4 Sexual Dimorphism in the Sensitivity to Testosterone

In quail the behavioural and morphological responses to testosterone are sexually differentiated. Testosterone treatment restores copulatory behaviour in castrated males to the level that was seen before castration but the same treatment is nearly without effect in females. Furthermore, a same testosterone treatment promotes a larger growth of the cloacal gland in gonadectomized males than in females (Balthazart et al. 1983).

Even treatment of females with very high doses of testosterone fails to elicit sexual behaviour in the birds which suggest that their behavioural insensitivity to the hormone does not result from an increased peripheral catabolism but rather reflects a central mechanism (Balthazart and Schumacher 1983, Balthazart et al. 1984b). Considering the important role played by testosterone metabolism in the induction of its behavioural effects, it was hypothesized that the insensitivity to androgens observed in females could be related to a different testosterone metabolism in their brain producing insufficient amounts of active metabolites or alternatively inactivating the active hormone too quickly.

A first study supported this idea by showing that testosterone metabolism is sexually dimorphic in peripheral structures such as the cloacal gland and the sternotracheal muscles (Balthazart et al. 1983) but revealed no such difference in the hypothalamus. The whole hypothalamic area (from the tractus septomesencephalicus to the level of the occulomotor nerves) had, however, been analyzed in this study and potential sexual differences in metabolism could have been diluted in a large mass of sexually non-differentiated nervous tissue. In addition, this study had been performed with ^{14}C-testosterone so that only 5β-reductase had been measured accurately and no information had been collected on the aromatase and 5α-reductase.

A microdissection of the hypothalamic area was thus designed using a procedure similar to that of Steimer and Hutchison (1981) for the ring dove and additional experiments were undertaken. The radioenzymatic assay based on ^{14}C-testosterone showed that the 5β-reductase activity is not evenly distributed in the hypothalamus. This enzymatic activity was decreasing following the rostro-caudal axis in both males and females (Schumacher et al. 1983). There was also some suggestion that the 5β-reductase was more active in females than in males at least in limitted portions of the hypothalamus. The same dissection procedure was then used in all subsequent experiments but this time the ^{3}H-labelled testosterone was used as substrate to gain information on all major testosterone metabolizing enzymes.

In intact males and females, this revealed that not only the 5β-reductase but also the 5α-reductase and the aromatase were showing precise neuroanatomical distributions (Schumacher and Balthazart 1984). We confirmed the rostro-caudal decrease in 5β-reductase activity. The 5α-reductase showed an opposite pattern of changes (highest levels in the tuberal hypothalamus) while the aromatase was much more active in all samples originating from the hypothalamus itself than from the adjacent more anterior areas (mainly lobus parolfactorius; see Fig. 4). Several cases of marked sexual dimorphism were also revealed: the aromatase was more active in males than females throughout the hypothalamus (significant only in the most posterior areas) while the 5β-reductase was more active in females (significant only in the preoptic area and adjacent lobus parolfactorius).

These sexual differences in enzymatic activities are obviously related to the differential sensitivity to testosterone of male and female quail. Male brains indeed produce in larger quantities metabolites which are involved in the activation of copulation (E_2) while female brains inactivate more quickly the hormone (higher 5β-reductase). It is thus possible that the insensitivity of females to testosterone is causally related to an inadequate metabolism of the hormone.

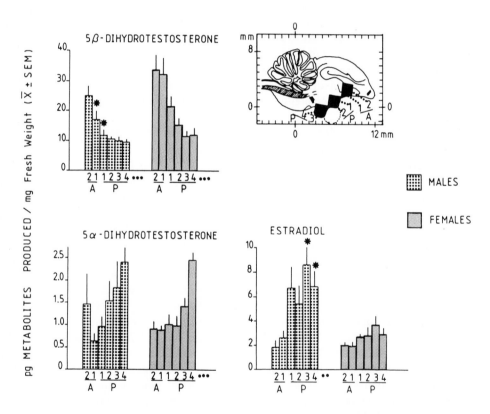

Fig. 4. Testosterone metabolism in limited parts of the hypothalamus and adjacent telencephalic areas (*see inset*) in male and female quail as measured with the in vitro radioenzymatic assay using ^{3}H-testosterone. Productions in the different brain areas within one sex were compared by ANOVAS (*asterisks under the graphs next to the label of columns*) and productions in corresponding areas of males and females were compared by t-tests (*asterisks above columns*). * = $P < 0.05$; ** = $P < 0.01$; *** = $P < 0.001$

However, all these studies had been performed on gonadally intact birds so that the observed differences could have been due to the different hormonal conditions to which the birds were exposed. In other words the enzymatic differences could have been induced by the circulating gonadal hormones rather than being true stable sexual differences. The same type of experiment was thus repeated to look for similar enzymatic differences not only in intact but also in gonadectomized males and females and also in birds treated with testosterone at doses which restore sexual behaviour in males but not in females. The results are shown in Figs. 5–7. This study of intact birds largely confirmed the previous results and these will thus not be described in detail (see Figs.).

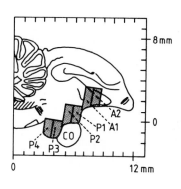

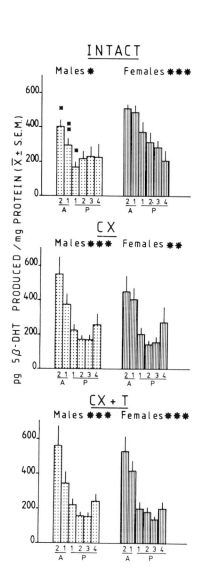

Fig. 5. In vitro production of 5β-dihydrotestosterone (5β-DHT) in different brain areas of intact, castrated (CX), and testosterone-treated castrated (CX + T) male and female quail. See Fig. 4 for additional comments

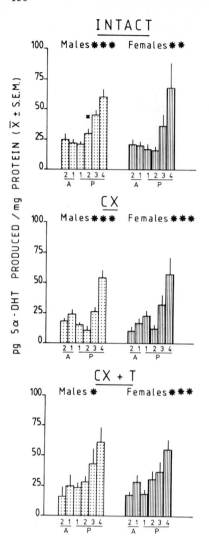

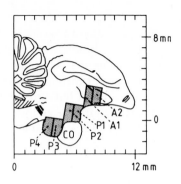

Fig. 6. In vitro production of 5 α-dihydrotestosterone *(5 α-DHT)* in different brain regions of male and
female quail. See Figs. 4 and 5 for additional comments

The reaction to castration and replacement by testosterone was extremely different
from one enzymatic activity to the other.

The sexual differences in 5β-reductase dissapeared in gonadectomized birds and were
not restored by testosterone treatment although the neuroanatomical pattern of enzyme
distribution was conserved in all physiological situations. In fact castration slightly increased the production of 5β-DHT in males (samples A2 and A1 mainly but effects far
from significant) and decreased it in females (effect significant for samples P1, P2, and
P3). It was not restored to the intact level by the exogenous testosterone neither in
males nor in females. The male-female differences observed in intact animals were thus
only induced by the endogenous hormones and essentially by an ovary-induced increase
in enzyme activity.

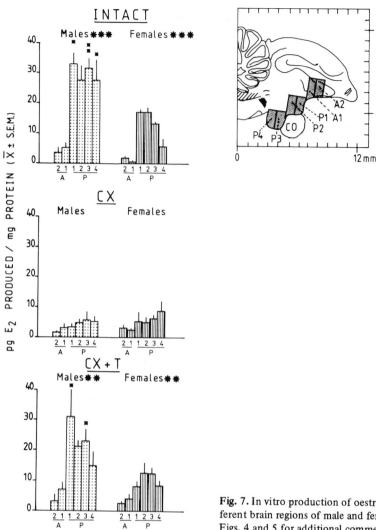

Fig. 7. In vitro production of oestradiol (E_2) in different brain regions of male and female quail. See Figs. 4 and 5 for additional comments

Only one sex-related difference in 5α-DHT production was present in intact birds (in sample P2 corresponding to the posterior paraventricular nucleus) and a similar trend (though not significant) had been detected in the previous experiment (see Fig. 4). Interestingly 5α-reductase in both males and females was not affected by castration and testosterone treatment except in sample P2. 5α-DHT production in P2 was reduced by castration and restored to the precastration level by testosterone in males. It was not affected by gonadectomy in females but was induced by testosterone to the male level ($p < 0.05$ by Neuman-Keuls tests). The 5α-reductase activity in some nuclei contained in sample P2 (perhaps the paraventricular nucleus) is thus inducible by testosterone in both males and females. The sexual difference seen in intact birds only results from the presence of higher testosterone levels in males.

The study of aromatase however revealed true sexual differences in enzyme activities. As seen in the previous experiment, the aromatase activity was much higher in intact males than females. This sexual dimorphism dissapeared in castrated birds. The enzymatic activity was then induced in both sexes by testosterone but the extend of this induction was significantly different in the two sexes. In males testosterone treatment restored the aromatase to its precastration levels in all parts of the hypothalamus while the same treatment in females resulted in a smaller induction producing enzymatic levels similar to those seen in intact females.

In summary, peripheral hormones control testosterone metabolism in the brain in a complex way depending on the enzyme considered, the neuroanatomical site and the sex of the birds. The 5β-reductase is hardly affected by testosterone in the physiological range of concentrations (marginal increase, not significant following castration in males) but is stimulated by one ovarian hormone in the preoptic area and anterior hypothalamus (significant decrase in P1, P2, and P3 following ovariectomy). The 5α-reductase is not controlled by peripheral hormones except in sample P2 where it is strongly inducible by testosterone in both males and females. Finally the aromatase is inducible by testosterone in the whole the hypothalamus (effect is however more dramatic in the preoptic area) but this induction is sexually differentiated so that enzymatic activities in intact birds and in testosterone-treated birds are different. The neuroanatomical and sexual specificity of the enzymatic controls strongly suggest that they play some biological role. In particular, the sexual dimorphism in aromatase activity in the preoptic area and its differential induction by testosterone in males and females support the notion that these enzymatic differences play a role in the differential sensitivity to testosterone. If the induction of copulation by testosterone requires its aromatization into oestradiol as suggested by numerous experimental studies (Adkins and Pniewski 1978; Adkins et al. 1980; Balthazart et al. 1984b), the enzymatic differences observed here represent a molecular correlate (cause?) for this behavioural phenomenon.

5 Conclusion

The study of testosterone metabolism in the quail brain has revealed many physiological situations in which changes in the behavioural activity of the birds was closely paralled by changes in enzymatic activities in specific areas of the hypothalamus. Considering that the metabolites produced by these enzymes are important in the induction of behaviour, it can be expected that in many cases the observed correlations have a causal meaning and reflect a control of the hormone action through its metabolism in the target organ. It is also quite possible that the performance of one behaviour could either directly or indirectly via changes in plasma hormones, alter enzyme activities in the brain. Future research will thus have to uncover whether these changes in testosterone metabolism are causes or consequences of the behavioural activity of the birds.

Acknowledgments. We are indebted to Professor E. Schoffeniels for his continued interest in our work. The studies presented in this review were supported by a grant nbr. 2.4518.80 from the F.R.F.C. to Professor Schoffeniels and grants from the belgian F.N.R.S. (credits aux chercheurs) to J. Balthazart. M. Schumacher was supported by a grant from the I.R.S.I.A. and is presently Aspirant du F.N.R.S.

References

Adkins EK (1977) Effects of diverse androgens on the sexual behavior and morphology of castrated male quail. Horm Behav 8:201–207

Adkins EK, Adler NT (1972) Hormonal control of behavior in the Japanese quail. J Comp Physiol Psychol 81:27–36

Adkins EK, Nock BL (1976) The effects of the antiestrogen CI-628 on sexual behavior activated by androgen or estrogen in quail. Horm Behav 7:417–429

Adkins EK, Pniewski EE (1978) Control of reproductive behavior by sex steroids in male quail. J Comp Physiol Psychol 92:1169–1178

Adkins EK, Boop JJ, Koutnik DL, Morris JB, Pniewski EE (1980) Further evidence that androgen aromatization is essential for the activation of copulation in male quail. Physiol Behav 24:441–446

Adkins-Regan EK (1983) Sex steroids and the differentiation and activation of avian reproductive behaviour. In: Balthazart J, Pröve E, Gilles R (eds) Hormones and behaviour in higher vertebrates. Springer, Berlin Heidelberg New York, pp 218–228

Balthazart J (1978) Behavioural and physiological effects of testosterone propionate and cyproterone acetate in immature male domestic ducks, Anas platyrhynchos. Z Tierpsychol 47:410–421

Balthazart J (1983) Hormonal correlates of behavior. In: Farner DS, King JR, Parkes KC (eds) Avian biology, vol 7. Academic, New York, pp 221–365

Balthazart J, Hendrick JC (1976) Annual variations in reproductive behavior, testosterone, and plasma FSH levels in the Rouen duck, Anas.platyrhynchos. Gen Comp Endocrinol 28:171–183

Balthazart J, Hirschberg D (1979) Testosterone metabolism and sexual behavior in the chick. Horm Behav 12:253–263

Balthazart J, Hirschberg D (1982) Effect of several androgens on testosterone metabolism in the brain and crest of male chicks. IRCS Med Sci Libr Compend 10:377–378

Balthazart J, Schumacher M (1983) Testosterone metabolism and sexual differentiation in quail. In: Balthazart J, Pröve E, Gilles R (eds) Hormones and behaviour in higher vertebrates. Springer, Berlin Heidelberg New York, pp 237–260

Balthazart J, Deviche P, Hendrick JC (1977) Effects of exogenous hormones on the reproductive behaviour of adult male domestic ducks II. Correlation with morphology and hormone plasma levels. Behav Proc 2:147–161

Balthazart J, Massa R, Negri-Cesi P (1979) Photoperiodic control of testosterone metabolism, plasma gonadotrophins, cloacal gland growth and reproductive behaviour in the Japanese quail. Gen Comp Endocrinol 39:222–235

Balthazart J, Malacarne G, Deviche P (1981) Stimulatory effects of 5β-dihydrotestosterone on the sexual behavior in domestic chicks. Horm Behav 15:246–258

Balthazart J, Schumacher M, Ottinger MA (1983) Sexual differences in the Japanese quail: behavior, morphology and intracellular metabolism of testosterone. Gen Comp Endocrinol 51:191–207

Balthazart J, Schumacher M, Malacarne G (1984a) Interaction of androgens and estrogens in the control of sexual behavior in male Japanese quail. Physiol Behav (in press)

Balthazart J, Turek R, Ottinger MA (1984b) Altered brain metabolism of testosterone is correlated with reproductive decline in aging quail. Horm Behav 18:330–345

Barfield RJ (1969) Activation of copulatory behavior by androgen implanted into the preoptic area of the male fowl. Horm Behav 1:37–52

Barfield RJ (1971) Activation of sexual and aggressive behavior by androgen implanted into the male ring dove brain. Endocrinology 89:1470–1476

Berthold AD (1849) Transplantation der Hoden. Arch Anat Physiol 16:42–46

Callard GV, Petro Z, Ryan KJ (1978) Conversion of androgen to estrogen and other steroids in the vertebrate brain. Am Zool 18:511–523

Chambers KC, Hess DL, Phoenix CH (1981) Relationship of free and bound testosterone to sexual behavior in old rhesus males. Physiol Behav 27:615–620

Damassa DA, Smith ER, Tennet B, Davidson JM (1977) The relationship between circulating testosterone levels and male sexual behavior in rats. Horm Behav 8:275–286

Davies DT, Massa R, James R (1980) Role of testosterone and of its metabolites in regulating gonadotrophin secretion in the Japanese quail. J Endocrinol 84:211–222

Delville Y, Hendrick JC, Sulon J, Balthazart J (1984, in press) Testosterone metabolism and testosterone-dependent characteristics in Japanese quail. Physiol Behav

Dessi-Fulgheri F, Lucarini N, Lupo di Prisco C (1976) Relationships between testosterone metabolism in the brain, other endocrine variables and intermale aggression in mice. Aggressive Behav 2:223–231

Deviche P (1979) Behavioral effects of castration and testosterone propionate replacement combined with ACTH in the male domestic duck (Anas platyrhynchos L.) J Exp Zool 207:471–480

Deviche P, Schumacher M (1982) Behavioural and morphological dose-responses to testosterone and 5α-dihydrotestosterone in the castrated male Japanese quail. Behav Processes 7:107–121

Deviche P, Bottoni L, Balthazart J (1982) 5β-dihydrotestosterone is weakly androgenic in the adult Japanese quail (Coturnix coturnix japonica). Gen Comp Endocrinol 48:421–424

Harding CF, Feder HH (1976) Relation between individual differences in sexual behavior and plasma testosterone levels in the guinea pig. Endocrinology 98:1198–1205

Hutchison JB (1971) Effects of hypothalamic implants of gonadal steroids on courtship behaviour in Barbary doves (Streptopelia risoria). J Endocrinol 50:97–113

Hutchison JB (1978) Hypothalamic regulation of male sexual responsiveness to androgen. In: Hutchison JB (ed) Biological determinants of sexual behaviour. Wiley, Chichester, pp 277–317

Martin PM, Sheridan P (1982) Towards a new model for the mechanism of action of steroids. J Steroid Biochem 16:215–229

Massa R, Cresti L, Martini L (1977) Metabolism of testosterone in the anterior pituitary gland and the central nervous system of the European starling (Sturnus vulgaris). J Endocrinol 75:347–354

Massa R, Davies DT, Bottoni L (1980) Cloacal gland of the Japanese quail: androgen dependence and metabolism of testosterone. J Endocrinol 84:223–230

McEwen BS (1981) Cellular biochemistry of hormone action in brain and pituitary. In: Adler NT (ed) Neuroendocrinology of reproduction, physiology and behavior. Plenum, New York, pp 485–518

Michael RP, Wilson MI (1975) Mating seasonality in castrated male rhesus monkeys. J Reprod Fertil 43:325–328

Mori M, Suzuki K, Tamaoki B (1974) Testosterone metabolism in rooster comb. Biochim Biophys Acta 337:118–128

Nakamura T, Tanabe Y (1974) In vitro metabolism of steroid hormones by chicken brain. Acta Endocrinol 75:410–416

Ottinger MA, Brinkley HJ (1979) Testosterone and sex-related physical characteristics during maturation of the male Japanese quail (Coturnix coturnix japonica). Biol Reprod 20:905–909

Ottinger MA, Duchala CS, Masson M (1983) Age-related reproductive decline in the male Japanese quail. Horm Behav 17:197–207

Ramenovsky M (1984) Agonistic behaviour and endogenous plasma hormones in male Japanese quail. Anim Behav 32:698–708

Schumacher M, Balthazart J (1983) The effects of testosterone and its metabolites on sexual behavior and morphology in male and female Japanese quail. Physiol Behav 30:335–339

Schumacher M, Balthazart J (1984) Sexual dimorphism and the hypothalamic metabolism of testosterone in male and female Japanese quail (Coturnix coturnix japonica). Prog Brain Res 61:51–61

Schumacher M, Contenti E, Balthazart J (1983) Testosterone metabolism in discrete areas of the hypothalamus and adjacent brain regions of male and female Japanese quail (Coturnix coturnix japonica). Brain Res 278:337–340

Schumacher M, Contenti E, Balthazart J (1984) Partial characterisation of testosterone metabolizing enzymes in the quail brain. Brain Res 305:51–59

Silver R, O'Connell M, Saad R (1979) Effect of androgen on the behavior of birds. In: Beyer C (ed) Endocrine control of sexual behavior. Raven, New York, pp 223–278

Steimer T, Hutchison JB (1980) Aromatization of testosterone within a discrete hypothalamic area associated with the behavioral action of androgen in the male dove. Brain Res 192:586–591

Steimer T, Hutchison JB (1981) Metabolic control of the behavioral action of androgens in the dove brain: testosterone inactivation by 5β-reduction. Brain Res 209:189–204

Tsutsui K, Ishii S (1981) Effects of sex steroids on aggressive behavior of adult male Japanese quail. Gen Comp Endocrinol 44:480–486

Willems J (1978) Le controle de la secretion des hormones gonadotropes chez le canard domestique (Anas platyrhynchos L.). Memoire de Licence, Univ Liege, Belgium

Symposium III

Sexual Differentiation

Organizer J. BALTHAZART

Endocrine Control of Behavioural Sexual Differentiation in the Male Ferret

M.J. BAUM [2], M.S. ERSKINE, E.R. STOCKMAN, and L.A. LUNDELL [1]

1 Introduction

Over the past 25 years much evidence has accumulated (reviewed in Baum 1979) to show that sexual dimorphisms in mammalian social behaviour ultimately derive from dimorphic patterns of sex steroid hormone secretion and brain action during critical perinatal periods of development. It is well established that a primary source (in the view of many investigators, the only source) of this perinatal sex difference in steroidal environment results from the presence of testes in the male. Over the past 13 years we have explored the contribution of testicular secretions to the process of brain and behavioural sexual differentiation in the male ferret (Mustela furo), a carnivorous mammal in which gestation lasts approx. 42 days. The results of an initial experiment (Baum 1976) showed that prenatal administration of testosterone propionate (TP) to female ferrets caused extensive masculinization of the external genital organs, whereas this treatment had no effect on the females' ability to display either feminine or masculine coital behaviour in adulthood, following gonadectomy and concurrent treatment with either oestradiol benzoate (OB) or TP. By contrast, females which received TP over the first 10 postnatal days of life later displayed high levels of masculine coital behaviour, when tested with concurrent OB or TP stimulation. These findings focussed our attention on the late gestational and early postnatal ages of development as potentially important periods for the process of brain sexual differentiation in ferrets.

2 Masculinization

We (Erskine and Baum 1982) measured plasma concentrations of testosterone (T), as well as dihydrotestosterone (DHT) in samples collected from male and female ferrets between the ages of day − 5 (5 days prior to expected parturition) and postnatal day 40. Since then, additional data have been collected on plasma androgen concentrations extending out to postnatal week 10. These data are all summarized in Fig. 1. It will be seen that plasma concentrations of T were most dramatically elevated in males at the

1 Department of Biology, Boston University, Boston, MA 02215, USA
2 Address for all correspondence: Dr. M.J. Baum, Dept. of Biology, Boston University,
   2 Cummington Dt. Boston, MA 02215, USA

Neurobiology
(ed. by R. Gilles and J. Balthazart)
© Springer-Verlag Berlin Heidelberg 1985

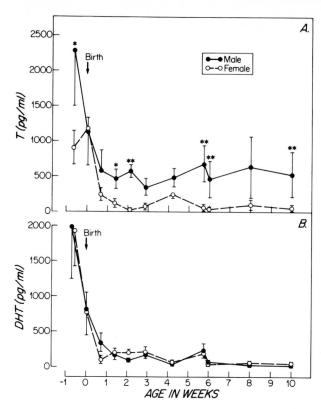

Fig. 1. A Concentration of testosterone (*T*) and **B** dihydrotestosterone (*DHT*) in plasma of male and female ferrets killed at different perinatal ages. Some of the results are taken from Erskine and Baum (1982)

prenatal age sampled, although mean concentrations were persistently higher (significantly so at several ages) in males than in females at all of the early postnatal ages sampled. By contrast, plasma concentrations of DHT were equivalent in the two sexes at all ages.

As stated above, our initial results (Baum 1976) suggested that the critical period during which testicular hormone causes coital masculinization in ferrets is neonatal. This conclusion was strengthened by the results of an additional study (Baum et al. 1982) in which administration of T via Silastic capsules to female ferrets over postnatal days 0–15 increased their capacity to display neck grip, mount, and pelvic thrusting behaviours up to the level of control males, which had been left gonadally intact until the eleventh postnatal week. Additional studies (Baum and Erskine 1984) have recently been completed which establish clearly that the period between postnatal days 5 and 20 is a crucial one for the masculinizing action of testicular hormone on coital behaviour, although this period may not be the only perinatal period during which hormones influence the developing brain mechanisms which ultimately control the expression of this behaviour. The postulated importance of days 5–20 for coital masculinization stems from the observation that castration of male ferrets at postnatal day 5 completely prevented the display of neck grip, mount, and pelvic thrusting behaviour above the level displayed by control females, following adult administration of T and tests with oestrous females. Males castrated at postnatal days 20 or 35, however, displayed equivalent, high levels of masculine behaviour.

Despite the unambiguous demonstration of the importance of the early postnatal period in the process of coital masculinization, additional results suggest that the action in male ferrets of some hormone prior to postnatal day 5 may also play a critical role in enhancing the "sensitivity" of the developing CNS to the action of T between days 5 and 20. Data supporting this view derive from observations made on groups of female ferrets which were ovariectomized on postnatal day 5 and implanted subcutaneously over days 5–20 with either of 2 different dosages of T, delivered subcutaneously from Silastic capsules containing different dilutions of T with cholesterol. Two additional groups of females were gonadectomized on day 5 and later implanted with either of 2 different dosages of T over postnatal days 20–35. Plasma concentrations of T which were achieved in these various female groups are shown in Fig. 2, along with data for gonadally intact male ferrets at comparable ages (redrawn from Fig. 1). Groups of male and female ferrets (sexes combined) were gonadectomized on day 5 and implanted with one of the two different T dosages in Silastic capsules on day 5 and later killed on day 6, 10, or 15. As shown in part A of Fig. 2, resultant plasma T levels in ferrets given the higher dosage of T were considerably higher than in gonadally intact males on day 6, and subsequently declined by day 15 to concentrations which were still slightly above those of gonadally intact males. Other female ferrets, gonadectomized on day 5 and given this high dosage of T over days 5–20 later displayed levels of neck

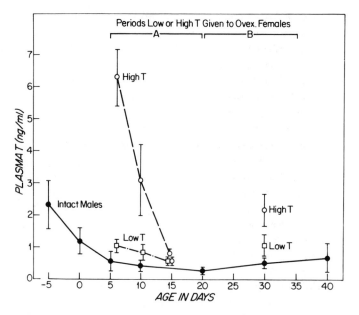

Fig. 2. Concentration of testosterone (*T*) in plasma of ferrets of both sexes gonadectomized on postnatal day 5. Some animals (*A*) received SC Silastic capsules containing T diluted with cholesterol (1:5 = low dosage; 1:1 = high dosage; 2-mm length) on day 5 and were then killed on postnatal days 6, 10, or 15. Other ferrets (*B*) received SC Silastic capsules containing T diluted with cholesterol (1:5 = low dosage; 1:1 = high dosage; 10-mm length) on day 20 and were killed on day 30. Plasma T concentrations in gonadally intact male ferrets killed at various perinatal ages are reproduced for comparison from Fig. 1. (After Baum and Erskine 1984; Erskine and Baum 1982)

grip and mounting behaviour when given T in adulthood which were equivalent to that of males castrated on postnatal day 35. These latter (control) males, however, displayed significantly higher levels of pelvic thrusting behavior than the females given the high dosage of T neonatally. Interestingly, females implanted with capsules releasing the lower dosage of T on day 5, and killed on days 6, 10, or 15 (Fig. 2), had plasma T concentrations which were considerably lower than the levels achieved in females given the higher dosage of T, but which were still slightly higher than the levels present in gonadally intact males across the ages of 5–20 days. Despite the male-like concentrations of T achieved in females implanted with the lower dosage of T, only a marginal degree of coital masculinization was achieved: Females gonadectomized on day 5 and implanted over days 5–20 with the lower dosage of T later displayed a slight elevation in neck grip behaviour after adult T treatment, but showed no significant enhancement of either mount or pelvic thrusting behaviours. As shown in Fig. 2, part B, administration of either of 2 dosages of T to gonadectomized ferrets of either sex on day 20 resulted in plasma concentrations of T by day 30 which were both significantly higher than those present in gonadally intact males over this period. Despite this elevation in plasma T, other females which were ovariectomized on day 5 and implanted with these dosages of T over days 20–35 displayed levels of masculine coital behaviour in adult tests which were indistinguishable from the low levels shown by females which were simply ovariectomized on days 5 or 35 and given no early steroid treatment.

Our results show that male and female ferrets respond differentially to the masculinizing action of T between postnatal days 5 and 20, with males being considerably more responsive than females. Previous work by Weisz and Ward (1980) points to a similar phenomenon in the rat. As in the ferret, a prenatal period (days 18–19 of gestation) exists in the rat during which plasma T concentrations are higher in males than in females. This difference disappears at the end of gestation, but then reappears immediately after birth, and persists for more than 1 week postnatally. Several lines of evidence suggest that in the rat, as in ferrets, prenatal exposure to heightened levels of T sensitizes the male to the subsequent action of T neonatally. Thus, female rats treated both pre- and neonatally with TP showed a higher degree of coital masculinization than females treated only neonatally (Ward 1969). Also, prenatal administration of antiandrogen to male rats reduced the degree of coital masculinization which otherwise resulted from the neonatal action of endogenous testicular secretions in these rats (Ward and Renz 1972).

3 Sexual Preferences

In addition to studying the masculine coital behaviour of male ferrets castrated at different neonatal ages, and of females given different dosages of T over postnatal days 5–20 or 20–35, we have examined the sexual partner preferences of these animals in a free choice situation (Stockman et al. 1985). In adulthood, groups of ferrets were tested in a T-maze under several different concurrent endocrine conditions to determine whether they preferred to approach and interact with either an oestrous female or a sexually active stud male. When tested in the absence of any endogenous or exogenous sex steroids, male and female ferrets in the various treatment groups chose to approach the stimulus male and female on approx. an equal number of trials. The same was true when T was given to all ferrets in adulthood. When OB was injected, however, males castrated on day 35 preferred to approach oestrous females whereas females ovariec-tomized on day 35 preferred to approach stud males. Neonatal manipulation of sex steroid availability caused intermediate patterns of partner preference in other groups of ferrets. Thus, castration of male ferrets on postnatal day 5 caused a significant shift in partner preference, away from an oestrus female. This shift was not, however, suf-ficient to duplicate completely the preference pattern displayed by control females. Likewise, female ferrets given the high dosage of T over postnatal days 5–20 chose to approach a stud male in the T-maze tests significantly less often than control females, although this neonatal treatment did not come close to causing a complete reversal in partner preference to the control male pattern. Thus, although manipulation of T con-centrations over days 5–20 had significant effects on animals' partner preferences, just as it had affected ferrets' masculine copulatory potential, it could not account for the complete male pattern of response. It seems likely that the typical male pattern of sexual partner preference depends, in addition, on the action of a sex steroid at some period prior to postnatal day 5.

4 Defeminization

In rodents, dogs, pigs, and sheep perinatal exposure of the male to testicular steroids reduces the capacity to display the typical feminine pattern of sexual behaviour, in response to adult treatment with ovarian steroids (reviewed in Baum 1979; Ford 1982). To date, this defeminizing action of testicular steroids has been best documented for the receptive components of the feminine sexual pattern, i.e. behaviours such as lordosis, standing immobile, and tail deviation, which enable the mounting male to achieve penile intromission and intravaginal ejaculation. Surprisingly, the male ferret seems not to undergo any significant degree of receptive defeminization as a result of its exposure perinatally to male-typical concentrations of T. Thus, male and female ferrets gonad-ectomized in adulthood and given increasing dosages of OB displayed equivalent incre-ments in acceptance quotients (ratio 100 of the duration of acceptance posturing/dura-tion of neck grip by stud male) (Baum and Gallagher 1981). Previous studies using several different rodent species (Fadem and Barfield 1981), dogs (Beach et al. 1977), pigs (Ford 1983), and rhesus monkeys (Thornton 1983) have shown that the proceptive, or appetitive components of the feminine sexual response are also attenuated in males as a consequence of the perinatal action of testicular hormone. We explored this issue in our ferrets by studying the approach latencies of different groups of animals to a sexually active stud male, which was restrained behind a wire-mesh screen in the goal area of an L-shaped runway (Baum et al. 1985). All ferrets were tested for approach latencies in this apparatus and also in separate tests for acceptance behaviour, both after adult treatment with increasing dosages (0, 5, 10, and 15 μg kg^{-1}) of OB. Females ovariectomized on days 35 or 5 and given no further treatment until adulthood dis-played a striking, dose-related reduction in approach latencies to the stud male following OB. By contrast, males castrated on day 35 showed progressively longer approach latencies to a stud male, as the dosage of OB and the number of repeated exposures to the test situation increased. Males castrated at postnatal days 20 or 5 later had approach latencies in response to these same adult dosages of OB which appeared progressively more similar to that of control females. Castration of males on day 5 failed, however, to cause a complete overlap in approach latency function with the control females. Administration of T (in either a high or a low dosage) over days 5–20 or 20–35 failed to defeminize the proceptive approach function of groups of females. The acceptance quotients of all ferrets, regardless of sex or neonatal treatment, as expected, showed equivalent increments in response to increasing dosages of OB given in adulthood.

Our results strongly imply that proceptive defeminization occurs in ferrets, just as in all of the other mammalian species studied to date. Again, the results point to a crucial contribution of male sex steroids, acting prior to postnatal day 5, to promote this process. No trace of defeminization (either proceptive or receptive) was seen in females given either a high or low dosage of T between days 5–20 or 20–35. Yet, castration of males at day 20 or day 5 caused significant attenuation in the defeminization of proceptive behavior compared with control males castrated on postnatal day 35. These observations imply that exposure of the developing male brain to steroids prior to day 5 somehow plays an obligatory role in sensitizing the CNS to the action of testicular hormone acting as late as days 20–35.

5 Conclusions

The studies described here concerning coital masculinization, the masculinization of sexual partner preference, and proceptive defeminization all point to a prolonged sequence of steroidal effects (beginning 1–2 weeks prior to birth and extending out 4–5 weeks postnatally) on the developing CNS in the male, to create the masculine phenotype. One obvious potential determinant of this male pattern of response is the increased concentrations of T, which are consistently present perinatally in males of this species (see Fig. 1). Much evidence obtained primarily in rodents suggests, however, that the normal process of masculine brain and behavioural sexual differentiation depends, at least in part, on the action of oestradiol formed from circulating androgen in subcortical brain regions during perinatal development (reviewed in Baum 1979). Earlier studies on the ferret (Baum et al. 1982; Baum et al. 1983) suggested that the process of coital masculinization is caused solely by the action of T itself, and cannot be attributed to the action of oestradiol formed directly in the male brain from circulating precursor. Extensive work has shown that the ferret hypothalamus, preoptic area, and temporal lobe is capable of aromatizing androgen as early as 8 days prior to parturition, with the level of aromatase activity being significantly higher in males than in females (Tobet et al. 1985). Additional research suggests that this prenatal sex difference in neural aromatase activity is not caused by the heightened concentration of T present in males, although the activation of neural androgen receptors in adult brain may under some circumstances promote aromatase activity. In addition to the capacity to form oestrogen, subcortical neural tissues of ferrets contain adult-like concentrations of oestrogen as well as androgen receptors both prenatally and neonatally (Vito et al. 1985). Thus the mechanism which would enable developing neurons to respond at the genomic level to circulating androgen or to oestrogen formed locally is present perinatally in the male ferret. More work is now needed to specify precisely which sex steroid acts prior to day 5 to initiate the process of brain "sensitization," which seems to be a prerequisite for the neonatal completion of brain and behaviour sexual differentiation in male ferrets.

Acknowledgment. The research described here was supported by U.S. Public Health Service grant HD13634 and by Research Career Development Award MH000392 (M.J.B.) and by National Service Award F32 MH08579 (E.R.S.).

References

Baum MJ (1976) Effects of testosterone propionate administered perinatally on sexual behavior of female ferrets. J Comp Physiol Psychol 90:399–410

Baum MJ (1979) Differentiation of coital behavior in mammals: A comparative analysis. Neurosci Biobehav Rev 3:265–284

Baum MJ, Erskine MS (1984) Effect of neonatal gonadectomy and administration of testosterone on coital masculinization in the ferret. Endocrinology 115:2440–2444

Baum MJ, Gallagher CA (1981) Increasing dosages of estradiol benzoate activate equivalent degrees of sexual receptivity in gonadectomized male and female ferrets. Physiol Behav 26:751–753

Baum MJ, Gallagher CH, Martin JT, Damassa DA (1982) Effect of testosterone, dihydrotestosterone, or estradiol administered neonatally on sexual behavior of female ferrets. Endocrinology 111:773–780

Baum MJ, Gallagher CA, Shim JH, Canick JA (1983) Normal differentiation of masculine sexual behavior in male ferrets despite neonatal inhibition of brain aromatase or 5α-reductase activity. Neuroendocrinology 36:277–284

Baum MJ, Stockman ER, Lundell LA (1985, in press) Evidence of proceptive without receptive defeminization in male ferrets. Behavioral Neuroscience

Beach FA, Johnson AI, Anisko JJ, Dunbar IF (1977) Hormonal control of sexual attraction in pseudohermaphroditic female dogs. J Comp Physiol Psychol 91:711–715

Erskine MS, Baum MJ (1982) Plasma concentrations of testosterone and dihydrotestosterone during perinatal development in male and female ferrets. Endocrinology 111:767–772

Fadem BH, Barfield RJ (1981) Neonatal hormonal influences on the development of proceptive and receptive feminine sexual behavior in rats. Horm Behav 15:282–288

Ford JJ (1982) Testicular control of defeminization in male pigs. Biol Reprod 27:425–430

Ford JJ (1983) Postnatal differentiation of sexual preference in male pigs. Horm Behav 17:152–162

Stockman ER, Callaghan RS, Baum MJ (1985, in press) Effect of neonatal castration and testosterone treatment on sexual partner preference in the ferret. Physiol Behav

Thornton JE (1983) Effects of prenatal androgen on adult ovarian cyclicity and female sexual behavior in the rhesus monkey. Doctoral dissertation, Univ Wisconsin

Tobet SA, Shim JH, Osiecki ST, Baum MJ, Canick JA (1985, in press) Androgen aromatization and 5 α-reduction in ferret brain during perinatal development: effects of sex and testosterone manipulation. Endocrinology

Vito CC, Baum MJ, Bloom C, Fox TO (1985) Androgen and estrogen receptors in perinatal ferret brain. J Neurosci 5:268–274

Ward IL (1969) Differential effect of pre- and postnatal androgen on the sexual behavior of intact and spayed female rats. Horm Behav 1:25–36

Ward IL, Renz FJ (1972) Consequences of perinatal hormone manipulation on the adult sexual behavior of female rats. J Comp Physiol Psychol 78:349–355

Weisz J, Ward IL (1980) Plasma testosterone and progesterone titers of pregnant rats, their male and female fetuses, and neonatal offspring. Endocrinology 106:306–316

Aromatization: Is It Critical for the Differentiation of Sexually Dimorphic Behaviours?

K.L. OLSEN[1]

1 Introduction

While it is readily accepted that exposure to testicular secretions during a limited, sensitive stage of perinatal development permanently alters an organism's behavioural responsivity to gonadal hormones in adulthood, it is unclear which hormone(s) mediates the events. Identity of the hormone or combination of hormones that bring about behavioural defeminization (suppression of female-typical responses) and behavioural masculinization (enhancement of male-typical responses) is critical for our eventual understanding of the neural mechanisms underlying sexual differentiation. Testosterone, the major secretory product of the developing testes (Resko et al. 1968; Corbier et al. 1978) is a likely candidate for the differentiating hormone. Indeed testosterone or testosterone propionate mimics the action of the testes when given to neonatally castrated males or females during perinatal development (Harris and Levine 1965; Whalen and Edwards 1967; Thomas et al. 1982 and others). However, this androgen is readily metabolized in peripheral and neural tissues (Mainwaring 1977) and one of its metabolites is oestrogen (Reddy et al. 1974). Moreover, oestrogens can also cause defeminization in rats (Wilson 1943; Feder and Whalen 1965). Since oestrogen is formed from circulating androgens within specific neural tissues, it has been postulated that oestrogens mediate sexual differentiation (Naftolin et al. 1975; Naftolin and MacLusky 1984).

To determine whether an androgen or an oestrogen is the differentiating hormone has proved to be quite difficult. Administering oestrogens to neonatally castrated males or female rats is confounded by the presence of an α-foetoprotein in the serum during development (Raynaud et al. 1971; Plapinger et al. 1973; McEwen et al. 1975; Whalen and Olsen 1978). Given that this protein preferentially binds oestrogens, administering testosterone to newborn rats could result in higher oestrogen accumulation in neural tissue than when oestrogen is given itself. Since the identity of the differentiating substance can not be defined by simply administering the specific hormone, other strategies had to be developed to separate the action of androgens from that of oestrogens. These studies have relied extensively on the use of various compounds that can dissect the natural role of hormones (see reviews: Plapinger and McEwen 1978; Baum 1979a; Whalen 1982; Olsen 1983a).

Research has mainly concentrated on blocking or interfering with the action of a specific hormone. For example, cyproterone acetate (Ward and Renz 1972) or flut-

---

1 Department of Psychiatry and Behavioural Science, State University of New York, Stony Brook, Stony Brook, NY 11794, USA

Neurobiology
(ed. by R. Gilles and J. Balthazart)
© Springer-Verlag Berlin Heidelberg 1985

amide (Clemens et al. 1978; Gladue and Clemens 1978) was administered during perinatal development to examine the contribution of androgens. Along the same line, oestrogen antagonists have been given to determine whether these agents can block the differentiating action of testes or of exogenous testosterone (McEwen et al. 1977; Booth 1977a; Södersten 1978; Etgen and Whalen 1979). Another strategy is to prevent the formation of oestrogen from either circulating or exogenous testosterone through perinatal exposure to aromatase inhibitors (Vreeburg et al. 1977; McEwen et al. 1977; Booth 1978, Clemens and Gladue 1978; Whalen and Olsen 1981; Whalen et al. 1985). Results from these studies have provided important information about the role of androgen and oestrogen in the behavioural differentiation process.

A different approach has capitalized on administering synthetic compounds which mimic the action of androgens or oestrogens while overcoming some of the inherent problems found when using the natural hormones. For example, oestradiol but not the synthetic oestrogens, diethylstilbestrol (DES) or RU5828, is sequestered by the presence of an α-foetoprotein. By administering either DES or RU5828, an oestrogen can now interact with specific neural tissues during perinatal development (Fox 1975; MacLusky et al. 1976). Findings indicate that oestrogenic compounds not bound by the serum α-foetoprotein are potent defeminizing agents (Doughty et al. 1975; Tilson and Lamartiniere 1979) and thus, has provided valuable information on oestrogen's role in behavioural differentiation.

The aim of this chapter is to discuss the behavioural and biochemical actions of a synthetic steroid, methyltrienolone (R1881 = 17β-hydroxy-17α-methyl-estra-4,9,11-triene-3-one), that overcomes many of the problems associated with administering androgens during development. As mentioned earlier, perinatal exposure to testosterone is comfounded by its ability to be metabolized into oestrogens. An alternative approach has been to give androgens, such as dihydrotestosterone (DHT) or androsterone, that are presumably not aromatized in neural tissue. Results from these studies indicate that DHT does not defeminize or masculinize (as defined by the ejaculatory response) the neural substrates underlying behaviour in rats (Whalen and Rezek 1974; McDonald and Doughty 1974; Hart 1977; Booth 1977b; Södersten and Hansen 1978; Van der Schoot 1980). Although DHT is presumably not converted into oestrogens, it is rapidly metabolized into other androgens (Mainwaring 1977). (Testosterone is also metabolized into androgens by peripheral and neural tissue but the pattern of recovered metabolites differs.) Some investigators have proposed that the rapid conversion of DHT into other less behaviourally potent androgens, and not its inability to be converted into oestrogens underlie the behavioural ineffectiveness of the steroid (Gay 1976). Similar to the synthetic oestrogens which overcame the problems associated with the presence of the α-foetoprotein, R1881, made available through the generousity of J.P. Raynaud, provides a excellent tool to address the direct involvement of androgens in the processes of sexual differentiation.

2 Properties of Methyltrienolone (R1881)

R1881 is a potent synthetic steroid which binds with high affinity to putative androgen receptors in both peripheral (Bonne and Raynaud 1975) and neural tissues (Olsen and

Etgen 1983). Moreover, it does not compete for oestrogen receptors in hypothalamus (Raynaud and Moguilewsky 1977). Unlike testosterone and DHT, R1881 is presumably not metabolized into other androgens (Bonne and Raynaud 1976). Unlike testosterone, R1881 is presumably not metabolized into oestrogens (Salmon et al. 1971; Doering and Leyra 1984a,b). This inability of R1881 to be aromatized into oestrogens has been demonstrated in both human placenta microsomes, a tissue that possesses a high level of aromatase activity, and in the hypothalamic-preoptic area, an area of brain thought to be involved in the differentiation of sexual behaviours (Doering and Leyra 1984a,b). Behavioural findings also suggest that R1881 is presumably not being converted into oestrogens. When R1881 is given in lieu of oestrogen followed 48 h by progesterone, neither ovariectomized rats (Doering and Leyra 1984b; Mode et al. 1984) nor hamsters (DeBold, pers. commun.) exhibit lordotic behaviour.

While R1881 may not mimic oestrogen's action in activating female-typical responses, it will induce masculine mating responses, presumably acting solely as an androgen. Baum (1979b) reported that treatment with R1881 facilitated intromissions but it was more behaviourally effective when given in combination with oestrogen benzoate. (These results suggest that R1881 is not being metabolized into oestrogens.) Södersten and Gustafsson (1980), using a different strain of rats and hormonal regime, reported that R1881 treatment stimulated all components of male copulatory behaviour, including ejaculation. These results were replicated in a later study (Mode et al. 1984). Recently, it has been reported that administration of R1881 induces mating behavior in castrated male hamsters (Lisciotto and DeBold 1984), common marmosets (Callithrix Jacchus) (Harris and Dixson 1984), and quail (Deviche 1984). Thus, the androgenic properties of R1881 is capable of inducing male-typical behaviours in a variety of species.

Given that R1881 has potent behavioural effects and it is not readily metabolized into either androgens or oestrogens, this synthetic steroid could be a powerful tool in elucidating the role of androgens and oestrogens in the differentiation of sexual behaviours.

3 R1881 Effects upon the Development of Mating Behaviours

3.1 Defeminization

Much evidence indicates that oestrogen, derived from the intracellular conversion of testicular androgens, acts solely to induce defeminization (see reviews: Baum 1979a; Plapinger and McEwen 1978; Olsen 1983a). This conclusion is based upon results from a number of studies. Consistent with the theory that oestrogen is the defeminizing hormone are the findings that the aromatizable androgens, testosterone and androstenedione, but not DHT can suppress the development of female-typical behaviours when given to female rats shortly after birth (Brown-Grant et al. 1971; Whalen and Rezek 1974). Moreover, oestrogens (e.g. 17β-oestradiol, oestradiol benzoate, RU 2858) can mimic the defeminizing action of the perinatal testes (Wilson 1943; Doughty et al. 1975). It has also been reported that oestrogen-antagonists given to intact males or androgen-treated females during postnatal development attenuate the inhibition of lordotic behavior (McEwen et al. 1977; Booth 1977a; Södersten 1978). Another line of evidence which supports the importance of aromatization in the defeminization process comes from work with the androgen-insensitive *(tfm)* male rats. These males have a genetic mutation than render them resistant to androgens but not to oestrogens (Stanley et al. 1973; Bardin and Catterall 1981; Fox et al. 1982). Like wild-type males, androgen-resistant rats do not exhibit lordotic behaviour following ovarian hormone treatment in adulthood, unless they are castrated shortly after birth (Olsen 1979; Olsen and Whalen 1981). Given their inherited resistance to androgens in combination with the presence of aromatase activity in brain tissue (Naftolin et al. 1975), suggest that oestrogen derived from circulating testicular androgens are mediating behavioural defeminization.

Based on the plethora of evidence indicating that oestrogen is the active differentiating hormone, it was predicted that the non-aromatizable androgen, R1881, would be ineffective in suppressing the development of female-typical behaviours. This, however, was not the case (Olsen 1983b). R1881 administered neonatally either via implants (first ten days) or injections (first 5 days/100 μg day^{-1}) inhibited the capacity of female rats to display receptive and proceptive behaviours following ovarian hormones in adulthood. As can be seen in Fig. 1, both implants and injections of R1881 caused a similar reduction in lordotic behavior. Testosterone, given as implants, caused almost complete defeminization, while injecting the hormone caused a partial inhibition similar to that found following exposure to R1881 treatment. DHT as well as the control vehicles had no appreciable effect upon the development of behaviour.

Given the intrinsic properties of R1881, the present results suggest that R1881 is causing a partial defeminization by direct androgenic involvement. Although R1881 has progestin-like properties (see Sect. 4), there is no compelling evidence implicating a role for progesterone in the defeminization process (Hull 1981). Indeed a proposed function of progesterone during development involves its ability to protect against the

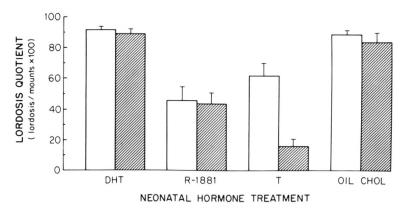

Fig. 1. The *open bars* represent the mean lordosis quotient (± S.E.M.) of female rats injected daily with 100 μg of 17β-hydroxy-17α-methylestra-4,9,11-triene-3-one *(R1881)*, 5α-dihydrotestosterone *(DHT)*, testosterone *(T)*, or *oil* for the first 5 postnatal days. The *hatched bars* represent the mean lordosis quotient (± S.E.M.) of female rats implanted with Silastic capsules containing *R1881, DHT, T,* or cholesterol *(Chol)* on the day of birth. The capsules were removed 10 days later. In adulthood, all rats were ovariectomized and given 2 μg of oestradiol benzoate 48 h and 24 h before 500 μg of progesterone. Behavioural testing began 3.5 h after the last injection. (Olsen 1983b, reproduced by permission of *The Journal of Endocrinology*.)

masculinizing properties of endogenous androgens and oestrogens, which in this case is not relevant. The present data do not eliminate oestrogen involvement in the defeminization process. As can be seen in Fig. 1, testosterone administered via implants caused almost complete defeminization while R1881 was only partially effective. This behavioural difference is probably attributed to testosterone being converted into oestrogens. Indeed during normal development, aromatization of androgens may play a critical role in the defeminization process. However, the present data indicate that this may not be the only mechanism by which androgens mediate the differentiation of sexual behaviours.

Given these unexpected results with rats, R. Whalen and I decided to determine whether R1881 was also effective in suppressing the development of lordotic behaviour in female hamsters. Hamsters, as a species are extremely sensitive to the defeminizing and masculinizing properties of oestrogen (Paup et al. 1972; Coniglio et al. 1973). As little as 50 ng of oestradiol benzoate or 50 pg of the synthetic oestrogen RU-2858 given to newborn female hamsters could defeminize hamsters (Whalen and Etgen 1978; Etgen and Whalen 1979). Much higher doses of testosterone propionate are required to cause a similar suppression of behaviour (DeBold and Whalen 1975), suggesting that aromatization must occur for androgens to be effective. Based on the compeling evidence that oestrogen mediates defeminization in hamsters (see Baum 1979a; Etgen 1981; Ruppert and Clemens 1981; Whalen 1982; Olsen 1983a), it was predicted that hamsters, unlike rats, would not be defeminized by neonatal exposure to R1881 treatment.

A paradigm similar to the rat study was used. At birth, female hamsters received either Silastic implants (removed 7 days later) or injections (5 days/100 μg day^{-1}) of R1881, testosterone, DHT, or cholesterol/oil. In adulthood, hamsters were ovariectomized and tested for their potential to exhibit the lordotic posture following ovarian hormone treatment. Males from liters receiving oil treatment were castrated in adulthood and tested under the same hormonal conditions. Several weeks after the final female mating test, hamsters received injections of testosterone propionate and were tested for their potential to display male behaviour. These results are discussed in Section 3.2.

The results from this study are found in Fig. 2. Neonatal exposure to the synthetic androgen R1881 (via implant or injections) caused a slight but significant reduction in lordotic behaviour. On the other hand, postnatal testosterone treatment suppressed lordotic behavior of female hamsters to that exhibited by normal males (see Fig. 2). DHT, when administered through implants but not injections, also had a slight inhibitory effect upon the development of behaviour. These results are consistent with the findings recently reported by Pleim and DeBold (1983) and by DeBold (1984) that non-aromatizable androgens, although not as effective as testosterone, can cause a partial defeminization of behaviour in hamsters.

While the present findings indicate that R1881 can cause a partial defeminization in both species, a strong statement supporting or eliminating a direct involvement of androgens can not be made until parallel biochemical studies are carried out. The assumption in these studies is that R1881 is not being converted by neural tissues into oestrogens but is acting solely as an androgen. The possibility exists that R1881 could be interacting with the oestrogen system independent of the aromatization process. In

154

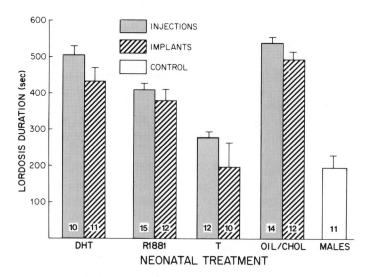

Fig. 2. The *solid bars* represent the mean lordosis duration (± S.E.M.) of female hamsters injected daily with 100 μg of 17β-hydroxy-17α-methylestra-4,9,11-triene-3-one (*R1881*), 5α-dihydrotestosterone (*DHT*), testosterone (*T*), or *oil* for the first 5 postnatal days. The *hatched bars* represent the mean lordosis duration (± S.E.M.) of female hamsters implanted at birth with Silastic capsules containing *R1881, DHT, T,* or cholesterol (*CHOL*). Implants were removed 7 days later. The *open bar* represents male hamsters given oil injections for the first five postnatal days. In adulthood, all hamsters were gonadectomized and treated with 10 μg of oestradiol benzoate 48 h before 500 μg of progesterone. Testing began 4 h after the progesterone injection. (After Olsen and Whalen, in prep.)

peripheral system, DHT, an non-aromatizable androgen, has been shown to translocate cytoplasmic oestrogen receptors into the nucleus (Rochefort et al. 1972; Ruh et al. 1975; Rochefort and Garcia 1976; Schmidt et al. 1976; Schmidt and Katzenellenbogen 1979). At high doses, DHT caused a similar accumulation of oestrogen into the nuclear compartment as found following the administration of oestrogen itself (Ruh et al. 1975). Moreover, oestrogen translocated into the nucleus via DHT, induced physiological changes normally associated with oestrogen stimulation. Possibly, the high levels of R1881 used in the present studies are sufficient to translocate oestrogen into the nucleus. Thus, R1881 is causing defeminization by an indirect oestrogen action and not via its androgenic properties. These biochemical studies are critical for the interpretation of the present data.

In conclusion, the present results (Figs. 1, 2) indicate that non-aromatizable androgens can have a defeminizing action. Thus, in both rats and hamsters, defeminization can occur via direct androgen stimulation. This conclusion is based on the properties of R1881 and makes the assumption that R1881 exposure during development does not cause a translocation of oestrogen receptors into the nucleus. Biochemical studies are now in process to access the intracellular effects of R1881 treatment in perinatal brain. It should be noted that in both species, testosterone was more effective than R1881 in suppressing the development of female mating behaviours. The defeminizing action of testosterone, in rats but not in hamsters, depended upon its route of administration; female rats exposed neonatally to testosterone via implants exhibited significantly lower levels of lordotic behaviour than when testosterone was given through injections. Given that the high exposure to R1881 was not as effective as testosterone, suggests that during normal development, aromatization may play an important role in behavioural defeminization.

3.2 Masculinization

While most evidence indicates that oestrogens are acting solely to cause defeminization, they may not be sufficient to masculinize all aspects of copulatory behaviour, including ejaculation. Indeed studies have reported that high levels of oestrogens are disruptive to the development of ejaculatory behaviour (Whalen 1964; Harris and Levine 1965; Feder 1967 and others). Given that masculinization and defeminization are independent processes (Whalen 1974, 1982), it is not unreasonable to believe that different mechanisms may be operating during their differentiation. For example, the timing of the sensitive periods may overlap but still be separate events. In addition, masculinization and defeminization may be mediated by different hormonal regimes.

Increasing evidence is accumulating that, in rats, masculinization is induced by either testosterone alone or androgens in combination with oestrogen. Moreover, the ejaculatory component of male mating behaviour may be differentiated by different steroid(s) than are the mounting and intromission components. For example, male rats castrated and treated with testosterone propionate at birth will show consistent ejaculatory behaviour following the appropriate hormone treatment in adulthood. Males castrated and given either DHT propionate or oestradiol benzoate will mount and intromit but do not ejaculate in adulthood. However, if DHT propionate is combined with oestradiol benzoate, than the behaviour is indistinquishable from rats receiving testosterone propionate (Booth 1977b; Hart 1977; Södersten and Hansen 1978; Van der Schoot 1980). These data suggest that either an androgen or an oestrogen can induce mounts with intromission but the expression of the ejaculatory component in adulthood requires either testosterone itself or a combination of androgens and oestrogens during development.

Given the properties of R1881 (see Sect. 2), it is an ideal compound to examine whether an androgen alone is sufficient or both androgens and oestrogens are required for masculinization of ejaculatory component of masculine behaviour. Experiments were carried out to determine whether perinatal exposure to androgens, independent of oestrogen stimulation, could mimic the differentiating action of the testes. In these studies, rats exposed prenatally to the aromatase inhibitor, ATD, were castrated and given R1881 either via implants or injections at birth, the rationale being that oestrogen stimulation would be insignificant following these perinatal hormonal manipulations.

As can be seen in Table 1, neonatal exposure to R1881, irrespective of the perinatal treatment, enhanced the ability of the rats to display masculine behaviour as measured by an increase in both the percentage and in the number of intromissions. However, neonatally castrated rats given R1881 treatment did not ejaculate following testosterone propionate treatment in adulthood. In contrast, rats exposed prenatally to either ATD or vehicle and castrated after the developmental period (in this case at 60 days of age), exhibited all aspects of copulatory behaviour following the appropriate stimulation in adulthood. Males castrated at birth and given vehicle did not show high levels of mating

Table 1. Effects of perinatal hormonal manipulations on the development of male-typical behaviours in rats

Perinatal treatments				Mating responses		
Prenatal + Postnatal		Mounting		Intromissions		Ejaculation
		%	Frequency[a]	%	Frequency[a]	%
ATD[b]	+ Intact	100%	7.3 ± 1.5	100%	13.3 ± 0.5	100%
ATD	+ D1[c]-Oil injections[d]	91%	22.1 ± 5.6	73%	4.2 ± 1.1	0%
ATD	+ D1-Cholesterol implant[e]	90%	31.2 ± 4.4	70%	6.5 ± 5.1	0%
ATD	+ D1-R1881 injection	100%	9.8 ± 2.6	90%	10.6 ± 2.0	0%
ATD	+ D1-R1881 implant	100%	16.1 ± 4.3	100%	17.2 ± 4.9	0%
Vehicle (PG)	+ Intact	89%	9.6 ± 2.0	100%	11.0 ± 1.5	100%
PG	+ D1-Oil injections	75%	24.2 ± 5.7	50%	2.2 ± 1.2	0%
PG	+ D1-Cholesterol implant	100%	34.8 ± 8.6	80%	8.2 ± 2.5	0%
PG	+ D1-R1881 injection	90%	16.2 ± 2.8	90%	13.7 ± 2.8	0%
PG	+ D1-R1881 implants	100%	28.8 ± 5.0	100%	17.1 ± 3.2	0%

[a] Frequency scores represent the mean ± S.E.M. of only the rats that responded on the fourth (last) mating test. Rats received daily injections of 200 μg of testosterone propionate and were tested 10 days, 17 days, 24 days, and 31 days after the first injection

[b] ATD: Aromatase blocker which was administered from day 10 of gestation until parturation

[c] D1: Day of castration; all male rats were castrated within 24 h of birth

[d] injections: Rats received 5 daily injections of either oil (0.05 μl) or R1881 (100 μg 0.05 μl^{-1}) beginning at birth

[e] implants: Rats were implanted as birth with Silastic capsules containing either cholesterol or R1881; they were removed 10 days later. (After Olsen, in prep.)

behaviour when tested as adults. These later findings replicate our previously reported study on ATD effects in combination with neonatal castration (Whalen and Olsen 1981).

As illustrated in Table 1, R1881 was not sufficient to masculinize the ejaculatory component of male mating behaviour. Possibly, in rats, oestrogen stimulation in combination with androgens is necessary for the development of all aspects of copulatory behaviour. These data are consistent with results from other studies using different strategies to identify the masculinizing hormones (Hart 1977; Booth 1977b; Van der Schoot 1980). The critical question now becomes whether males, castrated and given R1881 and oestrogen at birth, will ejaculate following androgen treatment in adulthood. This studies are now in progress.

Table 2 shows the effects of neonatal exposure to R1881 on the development of mounting behaviour in hamsters. The rationale is that since this species is extremely sensitive to the differentiating properties of oestrogens, exposure to the non-aromatizable androgen, R1881, should be ineffective in masculinizing behaviour. Since behavioural differentiation occurs postnatally in hamsters, a new experiment was not neces-

Table 2. Effects of postnatal exposure to R1881, testosterone, dihydrotestosterone or control vehicles on the development of mounting behavior in female hamsters

Postnatal treatments	Masculine mating behaviour	
	Precent Mounting (Rear only)	Mount Frequency Scores[a]
Controls:		
Oil injections[b]	8%	0.08 ± 0.28
Cholesterol implants[c]	17%	2.0 ± 1.9[d]
Males	100%	8.7 ± 2.6
R1881:		
Injections	67%	0.58 ± 0.20
Implants	81%	1.82 ± 0.90
Testosterone:		
Injections	83%	2.2 ± 0.75
Implants	89%	2.2 ± 1.2
Dihydrotestosterone:		
Injections	60%	0.50 ± 0.62
Implants	9%	0.09 ± 0.30

[a] Mount Frequency Scores: Hamsters were gonadectomized at 60 days of age. Ten days following the last female mating test, all hamsters began receiving daily injections of 500 μg of testosterone propionate. Mating tests were given 10 and 17 days after the first injection. Each hamster received a mean score for the two mating tests. The "mount frequency scores" represent mean ± SEM of each group. Zero scores are included in the averages

[b] injections: Hamsters received 5 daily injections of hormone (100 μg 0.05 μl^{-1}) or oil beginning at birth

[c] implants: Hamsters were implanted at birth with Silastic capsules containing hormone; they were removed 7 days later

[d] One hamster received a mean mount score of 22. (After Olsen and Whalen, in prep.)

sary. Following the last female mating test, the hamsters, described in the previous Section, were treated with testosterone propionate and tested for their ability to display male-typical behaviours. When administered androgen in adulthood, 67% of the R1881-treated hamsters showed mounting, although the frequency of response was very low. Several of the hamsters only mounted once in one of the two mating tests and only 17% exhibited mounts with thrusts. Treatment with R1881 did influence mating behaviour since only 3 of 24 control hamsters exhibited mounting when given androgen treatment in adulthood. However, the masculine behaviour of the R1881-treated males was not equivalent to that of other males or females neonatally exposed to testosterone. As seen in Table 2, androgen treatment in adulthood induced 100% of the males and 85% of the testosterone-treated females to mount. Both mount frequency and the percent of hamsters showing mount with thrusts were enhanced as compared with the R1881 treated hamsters. The findings that hamsters exposed neonatally to R1881 are only slightly masculinized are consistent with hypothesis that in this species, oestrogens indeed play a major role in the masculinization process.

4 Specificity of R1881 Binding in Neural Tissue

In the above discussion, only the androgenic properties of R1881 were considered. This steroid has provided a means to dissect the contribution of androgens from oestrogens in both the development and regulation of mating behaviours. In addition, since R1881 is not readily metabolized, it is becoming a preferred ligand in biochemical studies assessing androgen binding activity within target tissues (Max 1981; McGinnis et al. 1983; Perez-Palacio et al. 1983). While R1881 could be a very powerful tool in understanding androgen action, caution is needed. A potential problem is that R1881 is not only a potent androgen but has progestin-like properties. For example, this synthetic hormone binds with high affinity to both peripheral (Dube et al. 1976, 1978; Zava et al. 1979) and neural (Olsen and Etgen 1983) progestin receptors. Moreover, R1881 when given 48 h after oestrogen stimulation will facilitate the display of lordosis in both rats and hamsters. As compared with progesterone, R1881-treated animals exhibited lordotic behaviour earlier and, in rats, the dose required for maximal receptivity was lower (Olsen et al. 1984). While interaction with the progestin system may not be critical for interpreting R1881 action in the defeminization process, progesterone exposure is known to interfere with behavioural masculinization (Diamond et al. 1973; Hull 1981). Possibly the inability of R1881 to masculinize all aspects of male mating behavior (see Table 1) results from its progestin-like components and not its inability to be aromatized into oestrogens.

Given the importance of R1881 as a tool in both behavioural and biochemical studies, A. Etgen and I decided to assess the specificity of R1881 binding in preoptic-hypothalamic area isolated from male and female gonadectomized rats. As shown in Table 3, competition experiments found that 100-fold excess of progesterone or the synthetic progestin, R5020, was 60%–70% as effective as unlabelled DHT or R1881 in displacing radiolabelled ligand (3H-R1881). Thus, a significant component of 3H-R1881 binding in neural tissue can be contributed progestins. Since it well known that oestrogen treatment elevates progestin binding levels, competition experiments were also carried out in rats primed 48 h before sacrifice with 10 μg of oestradiol benzoate. Results using a one point assay with 2 nM 3H-R1881 indicated that oestrogen priming increased total

Table 3. Competition by androgens and progestins for radiolabelled methyltrienolone (R1881) binding in preoptic-hypothalamic cytosols

Ligand	Relative binding affinity					
	Males		Females		tfm	
	Oil	EB[a]	Oil	EB	Oil	EB
R1881	1.00	1.00	1.00	1.00	1.00	1.00
Dihydrotestosterone	0.86	0.90	0.98	0.85	0.90	0.80
R5020	0.62	0.71	0.81	0.79	0.76	0.98
Progesterone	0.62	0.65	0.94	1.08	0.78	0.98

[a] Gonadectomized male, female, and androgen-insensitive (tfm) rats were injected with 10 μg of oestradiol benzoate 48 h before sacrifice

[b] By definition, competition with R1881 = 1.00. (After Olsen and Etgen, in prep.)

Table 4. Competition by various steroids for radiolabelled R5020 binding in preoptic-hypothalamic cytosols

Ligand	Relative binding affinity	
	Oil	EB[a]
R5020 (50 nM)[b]	1.00	1.00
Progesterone (50 nM)	0.83	0.95
Methyltrienolone (R1881; 50 nM)	0.86	0.85
Dihydrotestosterone (50 nM)	0.29	0.23
Dihydrotestosterone (200 nM)	0.65	0.39

[a] Ovariectomized female rats were injected with 10 μg of oestradiol benzoate 48 h before they were killed

[b] By definition R5020 binding = 1.00. (After Olsen and Etgen, in prep.)

binding activity without altering the pattern of competition by the unlabelled steroids. Scatchard analysis of 3H-R1881 binding suggested the presence of two binding components, possibly androgen and progestin.

Similar competition experiments were performed with the androgen-resistant *(tfm)* rats, a mutant deficient in number of putative androgen receptor proteins (see reviews, Fox et al. 1982; Bardin and Catterall 1981). In preoptic-hypothalamic tissue, R5020 and progesterone were more effective in displacing 3H-R1881 binding than seen for wild-type rats (see Table 3). Not surprising, unlabelled progestins were better inhibitors than DHT in cytosols from oestrogen primed *tfm* rats; approximately 98% of the binding was displaced by progestin as compared with R1881 as the ligand. Recently, investigators have used 3H-R1881 to assess androgenic properties in target tissues from *tfm* rats (Max 1981). Given the major progestin component in R1881 binding activity in these mutants, caution is needed interpreting results obtained with this ligand.

Since progestins are good competitors for R1881 binding in neural tissue, A. Etgen and I assessed the ability of R1881 to compete for radiolabelled progestin (R5020) binding in preoptic-hypothalamic tissue of ovariectomized female rats. These results are found in Table 4. R1881 was an effective inhibitor; relative binding activity was similar to that seen when progesterone was used as the ligand.

These data indicate that progestins, as well as androgens, contribute significantly to R1881 binding in the brain. Given the multiplicity of actions of R1881, caution is needed in extrapoliting results using this synthetic steroid.

5 Summary and Conclusions

R1881 is a synthetic steroid which binds with high affinity to androgen receptors in target tissues. It is presumably not metabolized into oestrogens nor does it bind to oestrogen receptors in neural tissues. Moreover, R1881 is not readily converted to other androgens. Given these properties, R1881 was used to elucidate the differentiating roles of androgens and oestrogens in the development of sexually dimorphic behaviours.

It was found that neonatal exposure to R1881 caused a partial defeminization in rats and had a slight but significant suppression of behaviour in hamsters. These data suggest that androgens can have a direct influence on the development of female-typical behaviours, independent of the aromatization process. R1881 was not as effective as testosterone, suggesting that during normal differentiation oestrogens may be involved. Definitive conclusion on the direct role of androgens in the defeminization process can not be made until parallel biochemical studies are carried out to assess the intracellular effects resulting from perinatal R1881 treatment.

Studies were also carried out to determine whether androgens in the absence of oestrogen could mimic the differentiating action of the testes. To diminish oestrogen's contribution, postnatal exposure to R1881 was combined with prenatal ATD (aromatase inhibitor) and neonatal castration. Rats, castrated and given R1881 treatment at birth, mounted and intromitted but did not ejaculate following androgen treatment in adulthood. Moreover, hamsters, a species that is particularly sensitive to the masculinizing properties of oestrogen, are only slightly masculinized following perinatal exposure to R1881 treatment. These data suggest that masculinization (as defined by the ejaculatory system) is mediated by either testosterone alone or androgens in combination with oestrogens.

It must be noted that R1881 is not only a behaviourally (and biochemically) potent androgen, but also has progestin-like properties. Studies were carried out that examined the relative contribution of androgens and progestins to 3H-R1881 binding in preoptic-hypothalamic cytosols. The results indicated that progestins, as well as androgens, contribute significantly to R1881 binding in the brain. Thus, both the progestin and androgen properties should be considered when interpreting results from studies using R1881 as a ligand.

Acknowledgements. This research was supported by NIH Grant HD-15221. I thank Dr. J.-P. Raynaud of Roussel Uclaf for generously supplying our group with R1881. I wish to thank Dr. Richard Whalen and Dr. Anne Etgen who collaborated on some of the studies presented in this chapter. Expert technical assistance by Ms. Kathleen Hock and Ms. Donna Clark is greatly appreciated.

References

Bardin CW, Catterall JF (1981) Testosterone: a major determinant of extragenital sexual dimorphism. Science 211:1285—1294

Baum MJ (1979a) Differentiation of coital behavior in mammals: a comparative analysis. Neurosci Biobehav Rev 3:265—284

Baum MJ (1979b) A comparison of the effects of methyltrienolone (R1881) and 5α-dihydrotestosterone on sexual behavior of castrated male rats. Horm Behav 13:165—174

Bonne C, Raynaud J-P (1975) Methyltrienolone, a specific ligand for cellular androgen receptors. Steroids 26:227—232

Bonne C, Raynaud J-P (1976) Assay of androgen binding sites by exchange with methyltrienolone (R1881). Steroids 27:497—507

Booth JE (1977a) Sexual behavior of male rats injected with the anti-oestrogen MER-25 during infancy. Physiol Behav 19:35—39

Booth JE (1977b) Sexual behaviour of neonatally castrated rats injected during infancy with oestrogen and dihydrotestosterone. J Endocrinol 72:135—141

Booth JE (1978) Effects of the aromatization inhibitor androst-4-ene-3,6,17-trione on sexual differentiation induced by testosterone in the neonatally castrated rat. J. Endocrinol 79:69–79

Brown-Grant K, Munck A, Naftolin F, Sherwood MR (1971) The effects of the administration of testosterone propionate alone or with phenobarbitone and of testosterone metabolites to neonatal female rats. Horm Behav 2:173–182

Clemens LG, Gladue BA (1978) Feminine sexual behavior in rats enhanced by prenatal inhibition of androgen aromatization. Horm Behav 11:190–201

Clemens LG, Gladue BA, Coniglio LP (1978) Prenatal endogenous androgenic influences on masculine sexual behavior and genital morphology in male and female rats. Horm Behav 10:40–53

Coniglio LP, Paup DC, Clemens LG (1973) Hormonal specificity in the suppression of sexual receptivity of the female golden hamster. J Endocrinol 57:55–61

Corbier P, Kerdelhue B, Picon R, Roffi J (1978) Changes in testicular weight and serum gonadotropin and testosterone levels before during and after birth in the perinatal rats. Endocrinology 103:1985–1991

DeBold JF (1984) Androgenic and estrogenic control of sexual differentiation in hamsters (*Merocricetus auratus*). Abstr Comp Physiol Biochem, Liege

DeBold JF, Whalen RE (1975) Differential sensitivity of mounting and lordosis control systems to early androgen treatment in male and female hamsters. Horm Behav 6:197–209

Deviche P (1984) Steroid regulation of sexual behaviour in the male quail. Abstr Comp Physio Biochem, Liege

Diamond M, Llacuna A, Wong CL (1973) Sex behavior after neonatal progesterone, testosterone, estrogen and antiandrogens. Horm Behav 4:73–88

Doering CH, Leyra PT (1984a) Methyltrienolone (R1881) is not aromatized by placental microsomes or rat hypothalamic homogenates. J Steroid Biochem 20:1157–1162

Doering CH, Leyra PT (1984b) The lack of aromatization of methyltrienolone (R1881). In: Martini L (ed) Metabolism of steroids in neuronal structures. Raven, New York, pp 139–147

Doughty C, Booth JE, McDonald PG, Parrott RF (1975) Effects of oestradiol-17β, oestradiol benzoate and the synthetic oestrogen RU2858 on sexual differentiation in the neonatal female rat. J Endocrinol 67:419–424

Dube JY, Chapdelaine P, Tremblay RR, Bonne C, Raynaud J-P (1976) Comparative binding specificity of methyltrienolone in human rat prostate. Horm Res 7:341–347

Dube JY, Chapdelaine P, Dionne FT, Cloutier D, Tremblay RR (1978) Progestin binding in testes from three siblings with the syndrome of male pseudohermaphroditism with testicular feminization. J Clin Endocrinol Metab 157:547–558

Etgen AM (1981) Differential effects of two estrogen antagonists on the development of masculine and feminine sexual behavior in hamsters. Horm Behav 15:299–311

Etgen AM, Whalen RE (1979) Masculinization and defeminization induced in female hamsters by neonatal treatment with estradiol, RU-2858 and nafoxidine. Horm Behav 12:211–217

Feder HH (1967) Specificity of testosterone and estradiol in the differentiating neonatal rat. Anat Rec 157:79–86

Feder HH, Whalen RE (1965) Feminine behavior in neonatally castrated and estrogen-treated male rats. Science 147:306–307

Fox TO (1975) Oestradiol receptor of neonatal mouse brain. Nature (Lond) 258:441–444

Fox TO, Olsen KL, Vito CC, Wieland SJ (1982) Putative steroid receptors: genetics and development. In: Schmitt FO, Bloom FE, Bird S (eds) Molecular genetics and neurosciences: a new hybrid. Raven, New York, pp 289–306

Gay VL (1976) Species variation in the metabolism of dihydrotestosterone: correlation with reported variations in behavioral response. Abst 9th Annu Meet Soc Study Reprod, Philadelphia

Gladue BA, Clemens LG (1978) Androgenic influences on feminine sexual behavior in male and female rats: defeminization blocked by prenatal antiandrogen treatment. Endocrinology 103:1702–1709

Harris DHR, Dixson A (1984) Investigations into the restoration of sexual behaviour in castrate male *Callithrix Jacchus* common marmosets using a non-metabolisable synthetic androgen R1881 metribolone. Abstr Comp Physiol Biochem, Liege

Harris GW, Levine S (1965) Sexual differentiation of the brain and its experimental control. J Physiol (Lond) 181:379–400

Hart BL (1977) Neonatal dihydrotestosterone and estrogen stimulation: effects on sexual behavior of male rats. Horm Behav 8:193–200

Hull EM (1981) Effects of neonatal exposure to progesterone on sexual behavior of male and female rats. Physiol Behav 26:401–405

Lisciotti CA, DeBold JF (1984) Androgenic and estrogenic control of sexual and aggressive behavior in male hamsters (*Mercricetus auratus*). Abstr Comp Physiol Biochem, Liege

MacLusky NJ, Chaptal C, Lieberburg I, McEwen BS (1976) Properties and subcellular interrelationships of presumptive estrogen receptor macromolecules in the brains of neonatal and prepubertal female rats. Brain Res 114:158–165

Mainwaring WIP (1977) The mechanism of action of androgens. In: Gross F, Grumbach MM, Labhart A, Lipsett MB, Mann T, Samuels LT, Zander J (eds) Monographs on endocrinology, vol 10. Springer, Berlin Heidelberg New York, pp 1–178

Max SR (1981) Cytosolic androgen receptors in skeletal muscle from normal and testicular feminization mutant (Tfm) rats. Biochem Biophys Res Commun 101:792–799

McDonald PG, Doughty C (1974) Effects of neonatal administration of different androgens in the female rat: correlation between aromatization and the induction of sterilization. J Endocrinol 61:95–103

McEwen BS, Plapinger L, Chaptal C, Gerlach J, Wallach G (1975) Role of fetoneonatal estrogen binding proteins in the association of estrogen with neonatal brain cell nuclear receptors. Brain Res 96:400–406

McEwen BS, Lieberburg I, Chaptal C, Krey L (1977) Aromatization: important for sexual differentiation of the rat brain? Horm Behav 9:249–263

McGinnis MY, Davis PG, Meaney MJ, Singer M, McEwen BS (1983) In vitro measurement of cytosol and cell nuclear androgen receptors in male rat brain and pituitary. Brain Res 275:75–82

Mode A, Gustafsson J-A, Södersten P, Eneroth P (1984) Sex differences in behavioural androgen sensitivity: possible role of androgen metabolism. J Endocrinol 100:245–248

Naftolin F, MacLusky N (1984) Aromatization hypothesis revisited. In: Serio M, Motta M, Zanisis M, Martini L (eds) Sexual differentiation basic and clinical aspects. Serono Symp Publ, vol 11. Raven, New York, pp 79–91

Naftolin F, Ryan KJ, Davies J, Reddy VV, Flores F, Petro Z, Kuhn M, White RJ, Takaoka Y, Wolin L (1975) The formation of estrogen by central neuroendocrine tissues. In: Greep RO (ed) Recent progress in hormone research. Academic, New York, pp 295–319

Olsen KL (1979) Androgen-insensitive rats are defeminized by their testes. Nature (Lond) 279: 238–239

Olsen KL (1983a) Genetic determinants of sexual differentiation. In: Balthazart J, Prove E, Gilles R (eds) Hormones and behavior in higher vertebrates. Springer, Berlin Heidelberg New York, pp 138–158

Olsen KL (1983b) Effects of 17β-hydroxy-17α-methyl-estr-4,9,11-triene-3-one (R1881): evidence for direct involvement of androgens in the defeminization of behaviour in rats. J Endocrinol 98:431–438

Olsen KL, Etgen AM (1983) Specificity of methyltrienolone (R1881) binding in brain and pituitary. Abstr Soc Neurosci, Boston

Olsen KL, Whalen RE (1981) Hormonal control of the development of sexual behavior in androgen-insensitive (*tfm*) rats. Physiol Behav 27:883–886

Olsen KL, Pleim ET, Lisciotto CA, DeBold JF (1984) Methyltrienolone (R1881) facilitates female mating behavior in estrogen-primed ovariectomized rats and hamsters. Abstr Soc Neurosci, Anaheim

Paup DC, Coniglio LP, Clemens LG (1972) Masculinization of the female golden hamster by neonatal treatment with androgen or estrogen. Horm Behav 3:123–131

Perez-Palacios G, Chavez B, Vilchis F, Escobar N, Larrea F, Perex AE (1983) Interaction of medroxyprogesterone acetate with cytosol androgen receptors in the rat hypothalamus and pituitary. J Steroid Biochem 19:1729–1735

Plapinger L, McEwen BS (1978) Gonadal steroid-brain interactions in sexual differentiation. In: Hutchison JB (ed) Biological determinants of sexual behavior. Wiley, New York, pp 153–224

Plapinger L, McEwen BS, Clemens LE (1973) Ontogeny of estradiol binding sites in rat brain II. Characteristics of a neonatal binding macromolecule. Endocrinology 93:1129–1139

Pleim ET, DeBold JF (1983) Differentiation of sexual and aggressive behavior in hamsters by estrogen or non-aromatizable androgens. Abstr Soc Neurosci, Boston

Raynaud J-P, Moguilewsky M (1977) Steroid competition for estrogen receptors in the central nervous system. Prog Reprod Biol 2:78–87

Raynaud J-P, Mercier-Bodard C, Baulieu EE (1971) Rat estradiol binding plasma protein (EBP). Steroids 18:767–788

Reddy VVR, Naftolin F, Ryan KJ (1974) Conversion of androstenedione to estrone by neural tissues from fetal and neonatal rats. Endocrinology 94:117–121

Resko JA, Feder HH, Goy RW (1968) Androgen concentrations in plasma and testis of developing rats. J Endocrinol 40:485–491

Rochefort H, Garcia M (1976) Androgen on the estrogen receptor I-binding and in vivo nuclear translocation. Steroids 28:549–561

Rochefort H, Ligon F, Capony F (1972) Formation of estrogen nuclear receptor in uterus: effect of androgens, estrone and nafoxidine. Biochem Biophys Res Commun 47:662–670

Ruh TS, Wassilak SG, Ruh MF (1975) Androgen-induced nuclear accumulation of the estrogen receptor. Steroids 25:257–273

Ruppert PH, Clemens LG (1981) The role of aromatization in the development of sexual behavior of the female hamster (*Mesocricetus auratus*). Horm Behav 15:68–76

Salmon J, Raynaud J-P, Pottier J (1971) Etude metabolique d'un steroide trienique: Le R1881. In: Valette G, Cohen Y (eds) Symp Prog Tech Nucl Pharmacodyn. Masson and Cie, Paris, pp 237–247

Schmidt WN, Katzenellenbogen BS (1979) Androgen-uterine interaction: an assessment of androgen interaction with the testosterone- and estrogen-receptor system and stimulation of uterine growth and progesterone receptor synthesis. Mol Cell Endocr 15:91–108

Schmidt WN, Sadler MA, Katzenellenbogen BS (1976) Androgen-uterine interaction: nuclear translocation of the estrogen receptor and induction of the synthesis of the uterine-induced protein (IP) by high concentrations of androgens "in utero" but not "in vivo". Endocrinology 98:702–716

Södersten P (1978) Effects of anti-oestrogen treatment of neonatal male rats on lordosis behaviour and mounting behaviour in the adult. J Endocrinol 76:241–249

Södersten P, Gustafsson J-A (1980) Activation of sexual behavior in castrated rats with the synthetic androgen 17β-hydroxy-17α-methyl-estra-4,9,11-triene-3-one (R1881). J Endocrinol 87:279–283

Södersten P, Hansen S (1978) Effects of castration and testosterone, dihydrotestosterone or oestradiol replacement treatment in neonatal rats on mounting behaviour in the adult. J Endocrinol 76:251–260

Stanley AJ, Gumbreck LG, Allison JE, Easley RB (1973) Part 1. Male pseudohermaphroditism in the laboratory Norway rat. Reckent Prog Horm Res 29:43–64

Thomas DA, Barfield RJ, Etgen AM (1982) Influence of androgen on the development of sexual behavior in rats I. Time of administration and masculine copulatory responses, penile reflexes, and androgen receptors in females. Horm Behav 16:443–454

Tilson HA, Lamartiniere CA (1979) Neonatal exposure to diethylstilbestrol affects the sexual differentiation of male rats. Neurobehav Toxicol 1:123–128

Van der Schoot P (1980) Effects of dihydrotestosterone and oestradiol on sexual differentiation in male rats. J Endocrinol 84:397–407

Vreeburg JTM, van der Vaart PDM, van der Schoot P (1977) Prevention of central defeminization but not masculinization in male rats by inhibition neonatally of oestrogen biosynthesis. J Endocrinol 74:375–382

Ward IL, Renz FJ (1972) Consequences of perinatal hormone manipulation on adult sexual behavior of female rats. J Comp Physiol Psychol 78:349–355

Whalen RE (1964) Hormone-induced changes in the organization of sexual behavior in the male rat. J Comp Physiol Psychol 57:175–182

Whalen RE (1974) Sexual differentiation: models, methods and mechanisms. In: Friedman RC, Richart RM, Van de Wiele RL (eds) Sex differences in behavior. Wiley, New York, pp 467–481

Whalen RE (1982) Current issues in the neurobiology of sexual differentiation. In: Vernadakis A, Timiras PS (eds) Hormones in development and aging. Spectrum, New York, pp 273–304

Whalen RE, Edwards DA (1967) Hormonal determinants of the development of masculine and feminine behavior in male and female rats. Anat Rec 157:173–180

Whalen RE, Etgen AM (1978) Masculinization and defeminization induced in female hamsters by neonatal treatment with estradiol benzoate and RU-2858. Horm Behav 10:170–177

Whalen RE, Olsen KL (1978) Prednisolone modified estrogen-induced sexual differentiation. Behav Biol 24:549–553

Whalen RE, Olsen KL (1981) Role of aromatization in sexual differentiation: effects of prenatal ATD treatment and neonatal castration. Horm Behav 15:107–122

Whalen RE, Rezek DL (1974) Inhibition of lordosis in female rats by subcutaneous implants of testosterone, androstendione or dihydrotestosterone in infancy. Horm Behav 5:125–128

Whalen RE, Gladue BA, Olsen KL (1985, in press) Genetic and temporal aspects in the perinatal development of feminine sexual behavior. Horm Behav

Wilson JG (1943) Reproductive capacity of adult female rats treated prepuberally with estrogenic hormone. Anat Rec 86:341–359

Zava DT, Landrum KB, Horwitz KB, McGuire WL (1979) Androgen receptor assay with (3H)-methyltrienolone (R1881) in the presence of progesterone receptors. Endocrinology 104:1007–1012

Prenatal Androgens in Female Rats and Adult Mounting Behaviour

A.K. SLOB and J.T.M. VREEBURG [1]

1 Introduction

Adult female rats given testosterone propionate (TP) will easily display mounting and intromission behaviour when placed with an oestrous female rat (e.g. Beach 1968; Ward and Sperr 1969; Södersten 1972). It has been suggested that such mounting behaviour, like that of normal male rats (e.g. Goy and McEwen 1980; Baum 1979; Feder 1984), required prenatal "androgenic organization" of neural tissues which mediate copulatory behaviour. This idea was derived from experiments with female fetuses in which the action of testosterone or its metabolites was suppressed by anti-androgens or anti-aromatase substances. As adults such females were found to display less (TP-induced) mounting behaviour (Stewart et al. 1971; Ward and Renz 1972) and/or more 'feminine' behaviour (Clemens and Gladue 1978; Clemens et al. 1978; Gladue and Clemens 1978).

The origin of androgens in female rat fetuses was somewhat puzzling. While it was known that in males the fetal gonads produced androgens, the fetal ovaries were supposed not to be active in steroidogenesis. Ward and Renz (1972), who were among the first investigators to suggest an endogenous prenatal androgenic modification of the nervous system ("masculinization") of female rats, postulated that the adrenals might be the source of the androgen(s). Another speculation about the origin of prenatal androgen came from the work of Clemens and collaborators. They were the first to suggest a prenatal morphological and behavioural "masculinization" of female rat fetuses through exposure to androgen secreted by the testes of male fetuses (Clemens and Coniglio 1971; Clemens 1974; Clemens et al. 1978). These investigators reported that female fetuses next to male fetuses had a longer ano-genital distance at birth and displayed more TP-induced mounting behaviour in adult life than did females that had not been in such close proximity to males in fetal life. Clemens and co-workers suggested that fetal male androgens may reach a female fetus by way of direct diffusion across the amniotic membranes late in gestation.

These reports prompted us to undertake the following two series of experiments. The first consisted of measurements of plasma levels of androgens in female and male rat fetuses. Once measurable amounts of testosterone (T) were found in female fetal plasma, more detailed experiments were done to find the origin of these androgens. The second series of experiments were concerned with TP-induced mounting behaviour in adult females stemming from litters with or without male fetal littermates.

---

1 Department of Endocrinology, Growth and Reproduction, Faculty of Medicine, Erasmus University, P.O. Box 1738, 3000 DR Rotterdam, The Netherlands

Neurobiology
(ed. by R. Gilles and J. Balthazart)
© Springer-Verlag Berlin Heidelberg 1985

In this chapter some of our earlier work will be summarized along with preliminary data from current investigations.

2 Testosterone Levels in Female and Male Rat Fetuses

A first experiment was undertaken to determine whether there was a sex difference in fetal plasma testosterone and whether plasma T levels in female fetuses were influenced by the total number of male 'womb-mates' (Slob et al. 1978). Hemihysterectomized females were time-mated (day after night of mating = day 0 of pregnancy) and anaesthetized with ether on day 20 of pregnancy: fetuses with their placentae were removed and fetal blood was collected. Blood from fetuses of same sex was pooled. Plasma T concentrations were later estimated by radioimmunoassay (method: Verjans et al. 1973). The results are shown in Table 1.

Two way ANOVA revealed a significant sex difference ($p < 0.01$), but females from litters with a majority of males did not have higher T levels than females from litters with a minority of males. Although this finding did not disprove Clemens' hypothesis, i.e. that female fetuses receive T through amniotic diffusion from their male "womb-mates", it did not support it either.

In a second series of experiments T levels were determined in the blood of female and male rats during the last days of fetal life and during the first day after birth (Slob et al. 1980). Also T levels in the ovaries and testes were measured before (day 20) or after birth. Intact females were time-mated and on days 19, 20, and 21 of pregnancy they were anaesthetized with ether and killed. Fetal blood was collected as described above. At various times after the onset of delivery one or two pups were removed from the litter and their blood was collected. Pooling of blood was done so that pups from different litters contributed to a single pool of blood.

Results can be seen in Table 2. Two factor ANOVA of the 1978a prenatal T-data revealed a significant effect of sex ($p < 0.01$) and of gestational age ($p < 0.01$). Further analysis showed that at day 19, T-levels were higher than at day 20 ($P < 0.01$) and day 21 ($P < 0.01$). Sex differences were also found in 1976 and in 1978b, but they

Table 1. Plasma concentrations (mean ± SE) of testosterone in male and female rat fetuses on day 20 of pregnancy. The small number of fetuses/litter is due to the hemihysterectomy of the mothers. In parentheses: number of pools

		Mean number, range in litter		Plasma testosterone (ng ml^{-1})	
Sex ratio	Mothers n	Male	Female	Male	Female
Male > female	11	4.5, 3–6	1.7, 0–3	0.62 ± 0.10 (5)	0.13 ± 0.03 (3)
Male = female	5	2.2, 1–3	2.2, 1–3	0.55 ± 0.15 (2)	0.06 ± 0.04 (2)
Male < female	14	1.8, 0–3	2.9, 1–6	0.89 ± 0.12 (4)	0.19 ± 0.07 (5)
Total	30			0.68 (11)	0.13 (10)

Table 2. Mean (±SE) levels of testosterone in the plasma and gonads of female and male rat fetuses at gestational ages of 19, 20, and 21 days, and at various times during 24 h after birth. In parentheses: number of pools

Date of experiment[a]	Fetal/newborn age	Male Testosterone Plasma (ng ml^{-1})	Testes (ng mg^{-1})	Female Testosterone Plasma (ng ml^{-1})	Ovaries (ng mg^{-1})
1976	19 days	0.94 (1)	—	0.41 (1)	—
	20 days	0.54 (1)	—	0.26 (1)	—
1978a	19 days	0.73 ± 0.06 (2)	—	0.31 ± 0.05 (2)	—
	20 days	0.47 ± 0.04 (6)	—	0.23 ± 0.04 (6)	—
	21 days	0.33 ± 0.04 (3)	—	0.08 ± 0.06 (3)	—
1978b	20 days	0.68 ± 0.04 (5)	1.23 ± 0.15 (5)	0.55 ± 0.22 (3)	0.04 ± 0.005 (2)
1979	1 h	3.03 ± 0.06 (3)	1.45 ± 0.03 (3)	0.31 ± 0.05 (3)	0.10 ± 0.005 (2)
	3 h	2.24 ± 0.24 (2)	1.67 ± 0.04 (3)	0.22 ± 0.06 (2)	0.11 ± 0.01 (2)
	6 h	1.31 ± 0.47 (3)	1.53 ± 0.21 (2)	0.33 ± 0.02 (3)	0.10 ± 0.05 (2)
	12 h	0.52 (1)	—	0.15 (1)	—
	18 h	0.50 (1)	—	0.19 (1)	—
	24 h	1.00 ± 0.27 (3)	0.81 (1)	0.11 ± 0.03 (2)	—

[a] Blood was collected during four experimental procedures. Although methods were similar, data are presented separately because hormone determinations were carried out independently of each other

were not statistically significant. ANOVA of the 1979 (day 1) T-data revealed effects of sex (P < 0.01), of neonatal age (P < 0.01) and an interaction (P < 0.01). Further analysis showed that T levels in females were not different at the various hours of the day, but that the levels in males were (P < 0.01). T levels appeared highest at 1 and 3 h after birth (P < 0.05), but at 6, 12, 18, and 24 h after birth the levels did not differ significantly. The sex difference was statistically significant at 1 h (P < 0.01), 3 h (P < 0.01), 6 h (P < 0.05), and 24 h (P ≈ 0.05). The T-concentration of the gonads was significantly higher in testes than in ovaries (P < 0.01).

The relatively high levels of testosterone in female rat fetuses (50% of the levels found in male littermates on days 19 and 20) was intriguing. Such data have also been reported by Weisz and Ward (1980). The origin of these high T levels in female fetuses was unknown. It seemed unlikely that the ovaries were the source, in view of the low T levels within ovaries.

3 Origin of Endogenous Androgens in Female Rat Fetuses

From the literature (Gibori and Sridaran 1981; Sridaran et al. 1981) as well as from work done in our department (de Greef et al. 1981) it seemed likely that the placenta secretes androgens into the maternal circulation. Whether this organ also supplies androgens to the fetuses was unknown. Therefore an experiment was carried out to investigate the possible secretion of testosterone and androsterone (A) into the fetal circulation (Vreeburg et al. 1983).

Time mated female rats were anaesthetized with urethane on day 20 or day 21 of their pregnancy. The fetuses were exposed in situ, injected with heparin and then peripheral or umbilical venous blood was collected. The placentae of 5 pregnant rats were removed on day 20, and placentae of one litter were pooled by sex.

Again, a clearcut sex difference in plasma testosterone of 20 day old rat fetuses was found. The concentrations were higher than those measured previously (see above) but similar to those reported by Weisz and Ward (1980). We have no explanation for these

Table 3. Testosterone (day 20) and androsterone (day 20 and 21) concentrations (ng ml^{-1}; mean±SE) in peripheral and umbilical venous plasma of male and female fetuses. Also androsterone concentrations (ng g^{-1}) in male and female placentas. In parentheses: number of pools

Sex of fetus		Testosterone		Androsterone[a]	
Male	Peripheral plasma	1.32 ± 0.19[b]	(5)	12.9 ± 1.3	(6)
	Umbilical vein plasma	0.37 ± 0.03	(5)	11.5 ± 1.0	(6)
	Placenta			33 ± 2.2	(5)
Female	Peripheral plasma	0.36 ± 0.04	(5)	13.3 ± 1.4	(6)
	Umbilical vein plasma	0.27 ± 0.02	(5)	12.3 ± 0.9	(6)
	Placenta			33 ± 1.8	(5)

[a] Androsterone levels are too high: adding alumina thin layer chromatography step to the androsterone assay of a number of samples resulted in about 24% lower values

[b] Different from other testosterone values (P < 0.01)

higher values. May be it had something to do with the manner in which blood was collected: the uterus was opened and the fetuses with their placentae remained in situ. It also took considerable time before all blood samples were collected. There were no sex differences in androsterone levels in peripheral plasma or in umbilical venous plasma.

The lower T concentrations in umbilical vein blood of male fetuses than in peripheral plasma show that a major part of the testosterone disappears from male fetal blood during circulation through the placenta. This might also explain why plasma T levels are high in newborn male rats during the first few hours after birth (Corbier et al. 1978; Pang et al. 1979; Slob et al. 1980). At birth the connection between fetus and placenta is disrupted so that the placental clearance of T stops abruptly and the plasma concentration of this androgen rises. In contrast to the males, in female fetuses the T-concentrations in umbilical vein and peripheral plasma were almost the same. Apparently in female fetuses T is not cleared from blood that circulates through the placenta. Since in female fetuses the ovaries do not secrete T, one could assume that the endogenous T in female fetuses is of placental origin. It had been shown that the placenta possesses the enzymes necessary to convert pregnenolone and progesterone into T (Chan and Leathem 1975). We hypothesized therefore that during circulation of fetal blood through the placenta, T will exchange between fetal blood and placental tissue, so that the concentration of unbound T in fetal umbilical vein blood will approach that in placental tissue. The high levels of androsterone both in the placenta and in the umbilical vein plasma strongly suggest that the placenta is the source of this 5α-reduced androgen compound in fetal plasma.

The significance of the placenta for steroidogenesis was further investigated in our department by P.E. Post and M. Houweling. Time-mated 18-day pregnant females were ovariectomized and adrenalectomized (n = 4) or sham operated under ether anaesthesia (n = 4). One day (24–28 h) later, blood was collected under ether anaesthesia from the orbital plexis, and then the animals were anaesthetized with urethane (i.p.) and the fetuses plus placentae were removed from the uterus. Fetal blood was collected in heparinized capillary tubes from the jugular and carotid vessels. Within each litter same sex fetal blood was pooled. Placentae were collected and pooled similarly. Samples were stored at – 20 °C. Later steroids were measured, using radioimmunoassays with alumina thin layer chromatography. Progesterone (P) assays were done with the method described by de Greef et al. (1981), androsterone and testosterone assays with the method described by Verjans et al. (1973). The antibody for A was given to us by S. Hillier; it had been raised in rabbits against androsterone-3-hemisuccinyl BSA-serum.

The results are shown in Table 4. In maternal plasma the (P) concentration was reduced by more than 90% after ovariectomy and adrenalectomy, whereas in placental tissue and in fetal plasma the decrease was about 35% and 75% respectively. Since the levels of P remained relatively high in placentae and fetuses (in comparison with that of maternal plasma) it would seem that the placenta itself may be an important source of progesterone. This corroborates recent data published by MacDonald and Matt (1984).

Plasma T levels were again higher in males than in females. Placental T concentrations were similar for male and female fetuses, a finding which is compatible with the lack of a sex difference in the concentration of umbilical venous plasma-T (see Table 3). The A-levels were higher both in male placental tissue (statistically significant in sham-

Table 4. Concentration of various steroids (mean ± SE) in maternal and fetal plasma and placental tissue at day 19 of pregnancy. The mothers were ovariectomized and adrenalectomized (n = 4) or sham operated (n = 4) 24–28 h earlier. Placentae and fetal plasma were pooled per sex per mother. In parentheses: number of pools

Steroid measured	Operation day 18 of pregnancy	Maternal plasma (4) (ng ml⁻¹)	Placental tissue (ng g⁻¹)		Fetal plasma (ng ml⁻¹)	
			male (4)	female (4)	male (2–4)	female (2–4)
Progesterone	ovex + adrenex	2.3 ± 0.15 [a]	51.4 ± 5.4 [b]	48.6 ± 0.5 [b]	12.4 ± 0.6 [b]	11.4 ± 0.5 [b]
	sham	113 ± 18	80.8 ± 8.1	75.6 ± 9.0	42.0 ± 2.0	46.1 ± 1.6
Testosterone	ovex + adrenex	0.26 ± 0.07	0.40 ± 0.07	0.33 ± 0.03	0.47 ± 0.01	0.13 ± 0.02 [c]
	sham	0.24 ± 0.03	0.32 ± 0.03	0.29 ± 0.03	0.44 ± 0.03	0.12 ± 0.02 [c]
Androsterone	ovex + adrenex	0.39 ± 0.10	21.0 ± 2.0	14.0 ± 2.7	2.3 ± 0.4	1.6 ± 0.5
	sham	0.37 ± 0.03	20.0 ± 1.2	14.0 ± 1.1 [c]	2.8 ± 0.8	2.2 ± 0.09 [c]

[a] $P < 0.01$ compared to sham controls
[b] $P < 0.05$ compared to sham controls
[c] $P < 0.05$ compared to male value

animals) and in male fetal plasma. This finding might be explained by the fact that in male fetuses placental A is formed both out of locally produced T and out of testicular T. The peripheral A-levels are considerably lower than those measured in the earlier experiment (see Table 3). The difference might be due to the use of a different (more specific?) antibody, and to the fact that no thin layer chromatography step was done in the earlier study (see legend, Table 3), and to the manner in which blood was collected.

In summary we can say that removal of ovaries and adrenals of pregnant rats does not significantly alter T and A contents in placentae and fetuses. This, again, strongly suggests that the placenta is a major source of androgens in female rat fetuses. Moreover, the placenta also seems to be a major source of androgens in the maternal circulation: ovariectomy plus adrenalectomy does not significantly alter T and A plasma levels. This agrees with recent data of MacDonald and Matt (1984) and Warshaw et al. (1984).

In a further study, androgen concentrations were estimated in maternal and fetal plasma and in placental and fetal tissue at various times during the second half of pregnancy. Female rats were time-mated and on each of days 11, 13, 15, 17, 19, and 21 of pregnancy four females were operated upon. First maternal plasma was collected (orbital plexus) under ether anaesthesia. Then urethane was injected i.p. and placentae and fetuses were obtained as described above. Also fetal blood collection and pooling of blood samples and organs was as described above. From day 17 of gestational age the fetuses were sexed by the appearance of the internal gonads. After storage at $-20\,^{\circ}$C, A and T were measured as before.

Table 5. Concentrations (mean ± SE) of testosterone and androsterone in maternal plasma, male and female placentae and male and female fetuses during the second half of pregnancy

Day of preg-nancy	Maternal plasma (pg ml⁻¹)	Placental tissue Male	Male + female	Female	Male	Fetal tissue Male + female	Female
			Testosterone (rg g⁻¹)				
11	154 ± 16		700 ± 78			108 ± 18	
13	378 ± 22		435 ± 61			ND [a]	
15	366 ± 34		151 ± 16			ND	
17	448 ± 9	190 ± 19		188 ± 14	365 ± 43 [b]		ND
19	342 ± 34	310 ± 13		264 ± 53	375 ± 43 [b]		76 ± 8
21	427 ± 29	313 ± 39 [c]		211 ± 25	185 ± 9 [b]		104 ± 10
	(ng ml⁻¹)		Androsterone (ng g⁻¹)				
11	0.32 ± 0.03		66.8 ± 6.7			9.3 ± 1.8	
13	0.66 ± 0.05		47.5 ± 3.6			3.7 ± 0.9	
15	0.44 ± 0.03		11.4 ± 1.1			2.0 ± 0.3	
17	0.21 ± 0.03	12.4 ± 2.0		10.5 ± 1.4	6.6 ± 0.7		4.2 ± 0.8
19	–	22.6 ± 1.2 [c]		15.5 ± 0.6	11.6 ± 0.3 [b]		5.9 ± 0.5
21	0.18 ± 0.01	14.8 ± 1.7		11.2 ± 1.2	7.4 ± 0.2		6.4 ± 0.9

[a] Non-detectable

Statistically significant sex difference:
[b] P < 0.01
[c] P < 0.05

The results are summarized in Table 5. From day 13 of pregnancy plasma T levels in maternal blood remained relatively constant at about 400 pg ml^{-1}. A levels were highest at day 13 of pregnancy. Placental tissue contained highest T levels and highest A levels on day 11 of pregnancy. Apparently the rate of placental steroidogenesis is high around day 11. This is supported by the finding of highest maternal plasma P-levels around day 12 of pregnancy in ovariectomized plus adrenalectomized females (Mac-Donald and Matt 1984). The T pattern is different from what has been described by Bridges et al. (1982), who found highest T concentrations (approximately 1,000 pg ml^{-1}) at days 18 and 20 of pregnancy.

The sex differences in placental androgen content were statistically significant (Student's t) only at day 21 for T, and day 19 for A. Also in whole fetuses the androgen concentrations were lower in females than in males; statistically significant at day 17, 19, and 21 for T, and at day 19 for A. This sex difference in androgen levels is probably due to the fact that male fetuses have two sources of T: the placenta and the testes.

The maternal plasma T-levels are similar to other recently published data from our department: a plasma T level of 440 pg ml^{-1} was found on day 21 of pregnancy in rats that were injected with 0.1 ml oil on days 16 through 20 (Slob et al. 1983). It may be noted that in our laboratory T values are lower than those reported by Weisz and Ward (1980), Bridges et al. (1982) and by Ward and Weisz (1984). We have no explanation for this discrepancy.

4 Litter Composition at Birth and Adult Female Mounting

A second line of research in our department is connected with behavioural experiments. These were done to test the Clemens' hypothesis described above. If the prenatal presence and/or proximity of male fetuses affects copulatory behaviour in female rats, then clear behavioural differences should be apparent between females stemming from all-female litters and females born in litters with an abundant number of male siblings (Slob and van der Schoot 1982).

In a large breeding colony (Department of Anatomy, Erasmus University Rotterdam; Wistar, Amsterdam R-strain) all litters born were checked immediately after delivery. During a 2 months' period four 'types' of litters were assigned to this experiment: 1. all-female litters (n=5; 23 females); 2. one male and 4–8 females (n=5; 9 females); 3. equal number of male and female siblings (n=8; 8 females); 4. one female and 3 to 8 males (n=4; 4 females). Animals were exposed to a reversed 14-h light: 10-h darkness/day regimen.

At the age of about 4 months all females were ovariectomized and subsequently injected with TP (the equivalent of 0.1 mg TP day^{-1}). The females were behaviourally tested in a semi-circular arena with an oestrogen and P-primed ovariectomized stimulus female (during dark period in red light, 15 min test^{-1}). Various behaviours were scored but for the analysis of the data only mounts with pelvic thrusts and intromission-like mounts were considered.

The results of three tests during the 7th and 8th week of TP injections are shown in Fig. 1. Virtually all females displayed mounting behaviour. Two-way ANOVA plus sub-

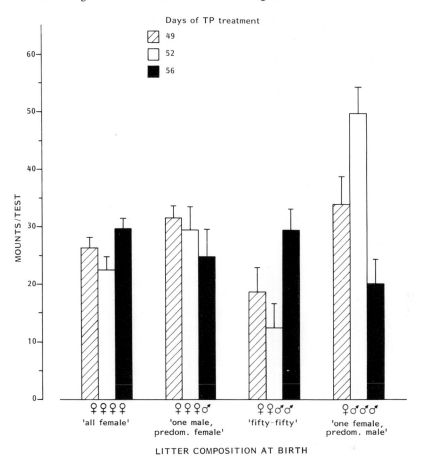

Fig. 1. Frequency (mean±SE) of TP-induced mounting behaviour (mounts with or without accompanying "intromission" behaviour towards hormonally primed oestrous female rats) of female rats during 15-min tests: effect of litter composition at birth. There were no consistent significant differences in mounting behaviour of female rats from "all female litters" and those from litters with predominantly male siblings

sequent analyses revealed that during the first test only the "fifty-fifty" females differed from all other females. During second test 'predominantly male' females and "fifty-fifty" females were different, higher and lower respectively, from all other females.

Although these results were rather convincing, and similar results were published by other investigators (van de Poll et al. 1982), we wanted to repeat this experiment because of the relatively small number of "predominantly male" females.

This was done in our department by T. Brand and H.C. van Os. Three types of litters were collected: 1. all-female litters (n=3; 17 females); 2. fifty-fifty female litters (n=6; 6 females); 3. predominantly male and one female litters (n=3; 3 females). Rearing and testing procedures were as described above. At a mean age of 111 days all females

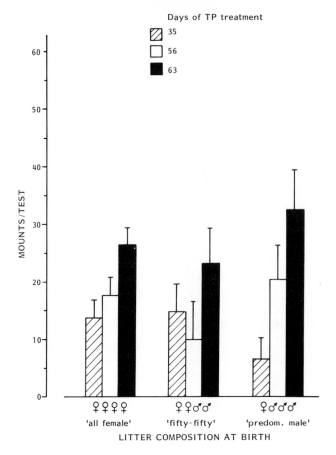

Fig. 2. Frequency (mean ± SE) of TP-induced mounting behaviour of female rats stemming from 3 types of litters at birth. See also legend of Fig. 1

were ovariectomized and thereafter regularly injected with TP (the equivalent of 0.1 mg day^{-1}). The experimental females were tested with oestrogen and P primed female partners, a total of 7 times. The initial four tests were used to let the experimental females adapt to the testing situation; these data will not be presented. The results of the last three tests (following 35, 56, and 63 days TP-treatment) are depicted in Fig. 2.

Two-way ANOVA revealed only an effect of days of testing [F(2/46) = 11.47; P < 0.01]. Further analysis (LSD-procedure) showed a significant increase in mounting with higher frequency in the last test than in the first two tests. The mount frequencies in the last test were very similar to what was found earlier (see Fig. 1).

During the tests for mounting behaviour, Brand and van Os noted the occurrence of proceptive behaviours (earwiggle and present) and occasionally the lordotic response when a stimulus female mounted the experimental female. Therefore receptive behaviour was tested with an experienced male partner. The first test was carried out after 77 days of TP injections, the second test the next day, about 3 h after an injection of 2.5 mg P. Lordosis quotient was calculated as the sum of lordoses divided by the sum (at least 10) of mounts, mounts with pelvic thrusts, intromissions and ejaculations, multiplied by 100. The results are shown in Fig. 3.

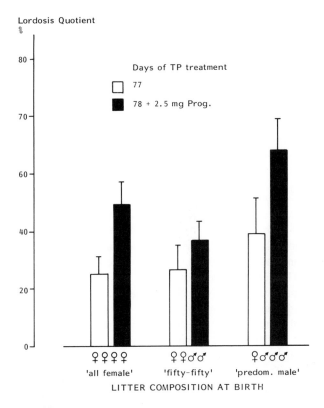

Fig. 3. Lordosis quotient (mean ± SE) of female rats from 3 types of litters at birth. Animals were tested after 77 days of TP treatment and the next day 3 h following an injection of 2.5 mg progesterone

Two-way ANOVA showed a significant stimulatory effect of P treatment [F(1/22) = 24.8; P < 0.01] on lordosis behaviour. There were no differences between females related to litter composition at birth, both with or without P injection. The lordosis quotient following 77 days of TP injections were similar to those reported by van de Poll et al. (1982) for ovariectomized females after 14 days of TP treatment (0.1 mg day^{-1}).

5 Prenatal Cyproterone Acetate and Adult Female Mounting

In order to investigate the significance of testosterone in female rat fetuses for adult TP-induced mounting behaviour, a second experiment was carried out by Brand and van Os. Female rats were exposed prenatally to cyproterone acetate (CA), a potent anti-androgen (Hamada et al. 1963). This study partly repeated experiments performed by Ward and Renz (1972).

From day 12 through day 22 of pregnancy female rats (unilaterally tubal-ligated) were daily injected with either 10 mg CA (0.1 ml injection; 23 females), or 0.1 ml sesame oil (n = 7). All pregnant females were delivered by caesarian sectio (day 21 for oil mothers, day 22 for CA mothers), and the offspring was cross-fostered to untreated mothers which had usually given birth the day before. It was impossible to ascertain

Table 6. Mean (± SE) frequencies of TP-induced mounting behaviour (mounts with pelvic thrusts plus intromissions) of prenatally oil- or CA-treated male and female rats

Sex	Prenatal treatment	N	Mean age at test (days of TP treatment)		
			45 (10)	49 (14)	54 (19)
Female	CA	16	27.8 ± 5.7[a]	33.5 ± 6.6	37.9 ± 5.6[a]
	oil	9	44.7 ± 2.6	42.3 ± 4.0	55.4 ± 3.4
Male	CA	14	32.4 ± 5.5	35.2 ± 5.6	51.6 ± 7.1
	oil	7	41.1 ± 11.3	39.1 ± 5.3	52.4 ± 4.5

[a] Significantly different from controls p < 0.05

the sex of the offspring of CA mothers: the ano-genital appearance was such that they all looked like females. The cross-fostering was not completely successful and resulted in a mortality of 11% in control animals and 68% in CA-treated animals.

The surviving animals were weaned at 30 days of age and gonadectomized at day 35. Gonadectomy was followed by TP-injections (see above). Ten, 14, and 19 days after the start of TP treatment all animals were tested with an oestrogen and P primed stimulus female. All procedures were identical as before.

During the last 15-min test all control males ejaculated twice with their partners, whereas in the first test only half of these males ejaculated only once. This illustrates the general increase in sexual activity between 45 and 54 days, a phenomenon that occurred in all groups. Besides a difference in ejaculatory behaviour, there was also a highly significant difference between CA-males and oil-males for intromission behaviour: mean (± SE) frequencies of 4.6 ± 1.1 and 31.3 ± 2.9 respectively. Females displayed low frequencies of intromission behaviour: CA-females 1.1 ± 0.4, oil-females 1.3 ± 0.3. Mounting behaviour (see Table 6) was significantly lower in 2/3 tests in prenatally CA-treated females than in their controls. This supports the idea that prenatal androgens are important for adult (TP-induced) mounting behaviour in female rats and male rats as well. The results of this experiment corroborate to those reported by Ward and Renz (1972).

6 Discussion

The results of these experiments confirm that there is a sex difference in endogenous blood and tissue levels of testosterone in male and female rat fetuses (Turkelson et al. 1977; Weisz and Ward 1980; Ward and Weisz 1984), and that the placenta is probably the major site for the production of androgens in female rat festuses (Rembiesa et al. 1972). The androgens (T and A) in maternal blood also seem to come from the placenta. In male fetuses there is also endogenous testicular T in the circulation (e.g. Warren et al. 1972).

The behavioural experiments have demonstrated that females without male womb-mates display the same TP-induced mounting frequencies as females that had male womb-mates. The cyproterone acetate study supported the idea that prenatal T was important for adult TP-induced mounting behaviour.

Thus, it seems unlikely that female rat fetuses receive significant amounts of T from their brothers as was suggested by L.G. Clemens. Although this theory seems to hold for the mouse (Gandelman et al. 1977; vom Saal and Bronson 1980; Rines and vom Saal 1984), no such evidence has accrued for the rat (Meisel and Ward 1981). The latter investigators suggested that only the presence of males on the caudal side of the females in the same uterine horn affected TP-induced mounting behaviour of such animals. In contrast to the idea of interamniotic diffusion they proposed that "masculinizing hormones secreted by fetal males may be carried via the uterine vasculature to female littermates located further downstream" (Meisel and Ward 1981). If this assumption is right, then T from males would go through the bloodstream to the placenta and then enter the female fetus. This seems unlikely, since we have recently shown that the placentae of guinea pigs and of rats are highly effective in metabolizing exogenous T to 5α-reduced substances (Vreeburg et al. 1981; Slob et al. 1983). Testosterone injected to the pregnant mother reaches the fetuses not as such, but mainly as androsterone. This 5α-reduced compound is thought not to be able to "androgenize" the central nervous system (CNS), an action which is attributed to the aromatase metabolite, oestradiol (e.g. Vreeburg et al. 1977; MacLusky and Naftolin 1981). Another recent study reported "no reliable contribution of littercomposition (...) with respect to differentiation of female sexual behaviour" (Tobet et al. 1982). It is interesting to note that these investigators monitored the natural birth of each pup from unilaterally ovariectomized mothers. This may be a much less stressful experimental design than delivery through caesarian section.

The hypothesis that female rats through their placentae produce androgens which could affect CNS development at the end of fetal life, is consistent with our findings. However, the consistency as such is no proof that androgens are required for organization of CNS systems involved in the display of mounting behaviour in adulthood. Such statement would require the analysis of behaviour in animals in which prenatal androgen production and/or exposure is diminished or inhibited. Present work addresses the latter question.

Acknowledgements. Thanks are due to Prof. J.J. van der Werff ten Bosch for critical reading of the manuscript and his continuous interest and support for this research.

References

Baum MJ (1979) Differentiation of coital behavior in mammals: a comparative analysis. Neurosci Biobehav Rev 3:265–284

Beach FA (1968) Factors involved in the control of mounting behavior by female mammals. In: Diamond M (ed) Perspectives in reproduction and sexual behavior. Indiana Univ Press, Bloomington, pp 83–131

Bridges RS, Todd RB, Logue CM (1982) Serum concentrations of testosterone throughout pregnancy in rats. J Endocrinol 94:21–27

Chan SWC, Leathem JH (1975) Placental steroidogenesis in the rat: progesterone production by tissue of the basal zone. Endocrinology 96:298–303

Clemens LG (1974) Neurohormonal control of male sexual behavior. In: Montagna W, Sadler WA (eds) Reproductive behavior. Plenum, New York, pp 23–54

Clemens LG, Coniglio L (1971) Influence of prenatal litter composition on mounting behavior of female rats. Am Zool 11:617–618

Clemens LG, Gladue BA (1978) Feminine sexual behavior in rats enhanced by prenatal inhibition of androgen aromatization. Horm Behav 11:190–201

Clemens LG, Gladue BA, Coniglio LP (1978) Prenatal endogenous androgenic influences on masculine sexual behavior and genital morphology in male and female rats. Horm Behav 10:40–53

Corbier P, Kerdelhue B, Picon R, Roffi J (1978) Changes in testicular weight and serum gonadotropin and testosterone levels before, during and after birth in the perinatal rat. Endocrinology 103:1985–1991

Feder HH (1984) Hormones and sexual behavior. Annu Rev Psychol 35:165–200

Gandelman R, vom Saal FS, Reinisch JM (1977) Contiguity to male foetuses affects morphology and behaviour of female mice. Nature (Lond) 266:722–724

Gibori G, Sridaran R (1981) Sites of androgen and estradiol production in the second half of pregnancy in the rat. Biol Reprod 24:249–256

Gladue BA, Clemens LG (1978) Androgenic influences on feminine sexual behavior in male and female rats: defeminization blocked by prenatal antiandrogen treatment. Endocrinology 103: 1702–1709

Goy RW, McEwen BS (1980) Sexual differentiation of the brain. MIT Press, Cambridge

Greef WJ de, Schenck PE, Vreeburg JTM, van der Vaart PDM, Baum MJ (1981) Evidence that a placental factor other than androsterone or dihydrotestosterone inhibits oestrogen-induced lordosis behaviour in pregnant rats. J Endocrinol 89:13–23

Hamada H, Neumann F, Junkmann K (1963) Intrauterine antimaskuline Beeinflussung von Rattenfeten durch ein stark Gestagen wirksames Steroid. Acta Endocrinol 44:380–388

MacDonald GJ, Matt DW (1984) Adrenal and placental steroid secretion during pregnancy in the rat. Endocrinology 114:2068–2073

MacLusky NJ, Naftolin F (1981) Sexual differentiation of the central nervous system. Science (Wash DC) 211:1294–1303

Meisel RL, Ward IL (1981) Fetal female rats are masculinized by male littermates located caudally in the uterus. Science (Wash DC) 213:239–242

Pang SF, Caggiula AR, Gay VL, Goodman RL, Pang CSF (1979) Serum concentrations of testosterone, oestrogens, luteinizing hormone and follicle-stimulation hormone in male and female rats during the critical period of neural sexual differentiation. J Endocrinol 80:103–110

Poll NE van de, van der Zwan SM, van Oyen HG, Pater JH (1982) Sexual behavior in female rats born in all-female litters. Behav Brain Res 4:103–109

Rembiesa R, Marchut M, Warchol A (1972) Ovarian-placental dependency in rat. Part I. Biotransformation of C_{21} steroids to androgens by rat placenta in vitro. Steroids 19:65–84

Rines JP, vom Saal FS (1984) Fetal effects on sexual behavior and aggression in young and old female mice treated with estrogen and testosterone. Horm Behav 18:117–129

Saal FS vom, Bronson FH (1980) Sexual characteristics of adult female mice are correlated with their blood testosterone levels during prenatal development. Science (Wash DC) 208:597–599

Slob AK, van der Schoot P (1982) Testosterone induced mounting behavior in adult female rats born in litters of different female to male ratios. Physiol Behav 28:1007–1010

Slob AK, Ooms MP, Vreeburg JTM (1978) Sex ratio in utero and the plasma concentration of testosterone in male and female rat foetuses. J Endocrinol 79:395–396

Slob AK, Ooms MP, Vreeburg JTM (1980) Prenatal and early postnatal sex differences in plasma and gonadal testosterone and plasma luteinizing hormone in female and male rats. J Endocrinol 87:81–87

Slob AK, den Hamer R, Woutersen PJA, van der Werff ten Bosch JJ (1983) Prenatal testosterone propionate and postnatal ovarian activity in the rat. Acta Endocrinol 103:420–427

Södersten P (1972) Mounting behaviour in the female rat during the estrous cycle, after ovariectomy, and after estrogen or testosterone administration. Horm Behav 3:307–320

Sridaran R, Basuray R, Gibori G (1981) Source and regulation of testosterone secretion in pregnant and pseudopregnant rats. Endocrinology 108:855–861

Stewart J, Pottier J, Kaczender-Henrik E (1971) Male copulatory behavior in the female rat after perinatal treatment with an anti-androgenic steroid. Horm Behav 2:247–254

Tobet SA, Dunlap JL, Gerall AA (1982) Influence of fetal position on neonatal androgen-induced sterility and sexual behavior in female rats. Horm Behav 16:251–258

Turkelson CM, Dunlap JL, MacPhee AA, Gerall AA (1977) Assay of perinatal testosterone and influence of antiprogesterone and theophylline on induction of sterility. Life Sci 21:1149–1158

Verjans HL, Cooke BA, de Jong FH, de Jong CMM, van der Molen HJ (1973) Evaluation of a radioimmunoassay for testosterone estimation. J Steroid Biochem 4:665–676

Vreeburg JTM, van der Vaart PDM, van der Schoot P (1977) Prevention of central defeminization but not masculinization in male rats by inhibition neonatally of oestrogen biosynthesis. J Endocrinol 74:375–382

Vreeburg JTM, Woutersen PJA, Ooms MP, van der Werff ten Bosch JJ (1981) Androgens in the fetal guinea-pig after maternal infusion of radioactive testosterone. J Endocrinol 88:9–16

Vreeburg JTM, Groeneveld JO, Post PE, Ooms MP (1983) Concentrations of testosterone and androsterone in peripheral and umbilical venous plasma of fetal rats. J Reprod Fertil 68:171–175

Ward IL, Renz FJ (1972) Consequences of perinatal hormone manipulation on the adult sexual behavior of female rats. J Comp Physiol Psychol 78:349–355

Ward IL, Sperr EV (1969) Effects of prolonged androgen on the sexual behaviour of intact and spayed female rats. Physiol Behav 4:765–768

Ward IL, Weisz J (1984) Differential effects of maternal stress on circulating levels of corticosterone, progesterone, and testosterone in male and female rat fetuses and their mothers. Endocrinology 114:1635–1644

Warren DW, Haltmeyer GC, Eik-Nes KB (1972) Synthesis and metabolism of testosterone in the fetal rat testis. Biol Reprod 7:94–99

Warshaw ML, Khan I, Gibori G (1984) Placental and luteal steroidogenesis in the pregnant rat. 7th Int Congr Endocrinol Abstr. Excerpta Medica, Amsterdam, p 1480

Weisz J, Ward IL (1980) Plasma testosterone and progesterone titers of pregnant rats, their male and female fetuses, and neonatal offspring. Endocrinology 106:306–316

Searching for Neural Correlates
of Sexual Differentiation in a Heterogeneous Tissue

P. YAHR[1]

1 Introduction

Nearly 20 years have passed since the hypothalamus-preoptic area (HPOA) was identified as a target tissue mediating the effects of gonadal steroids on male and female sexual behaviour (Davidson and Bloch 1969; Eisenfeld and Axelrod 1965; Lisk 1962, 1967; Harris and Michael 1964). Since then our knowledge of how HPOA cells accumulate and metabolize steroids has rapidly progressed. We know, for example, that HPOA cells that respond to testosterone (T) often convert it first to oestradiol (OE_2) and/or dihydrotestosterone (DHT; Luttge 1979, Martini 1982). These metabolites then bind to intracellular receptors. In this regard, T-sensitive cells in the HPOA resemble T-sensitive cells in the male reproductive tract. In females, HPOA cells that respond to progesterone (P) resemble P-sensitive cells in the female reproductive tract in that they synthesize most of their P receptors only after they have been exposed to OE_2 (Blaustein and Brown, this Vol.; Moguilewski and Raynaud 1979a,b; MacLusky and McEwen 1978, 1980). The receptors themselves are similar in the HPOA and peripheral targets (Barley et al. 1975; Feder et al. 1979; Moguilewsky and Raynaud 1979a), and in both tissues, the steroid eventually binds to acceptor sites on the chromatin (Fox and Johnston 1974; Whalen and Olsen 1978). Moreover, these processes are similar in adults and neonates (MacLusky and Naftolin 1981). These observations have encouraged the view that steroids activate mating behaviour in adulthood, and sexually differentiate the HPOA during early development, in the same way that they modify cellular functions in other parts of the body, i.e., by modifying synthesis of messenger RNA and protein.

Despite this progress we know little about what happens after steroid binding that changes sexual behaviour. Several laboratories have demonstrated hormone-induced changes in HPOA proteins, such as synthetic and degradative enzymes for neurotransmitters, and neurotransmitter receptors (Griffiths et al. 1975; Luine et al. 1974; Luine and McEwen 1983; Luine et al. 1977; Luine and Rhodes 1983; Rainbow et al. 1980b; Wallis and Luttge 1980). However, it is not clear which of these biochemical changes, if any, is related to male or female sexual behaviours. It has also been difficult to relate sex differences in the HPOA to specific sex differences in behaviour.

---

1 Department of Psychobiology, University of California, Irvine, CA 92717, USA

Neurobiology
(ed. by R. Gilles and J. Balthazart)
© Springer-Verlag Berlin Heidelberg 1985

2 Heterogeneity in the HPOA

This frustrating situation has probably developed because of a diversity of hormone-sensitive cell types in the HPOA. Heterogeneity does not pose problems for research on properties that are shared by all or nearly all cells that respond to a particular hormone, such as the presence of specific binding proteins or metabolic enzymes. For such analyses, diverse cell types can be combined and studied as a group. But when the focus shifts to analyses of cellular function, heterogeneity can hamper efforts to study hormone action. Even if steroids always affect cells by altering protein synthesis, the particular proteins affected will vary from one cell type to another. In one type of HPOA cell, the hormone may regulate production of an enzyme involved in neurotransmitter synthesis. In an adjacent or intermingled cell type, it may regulate production of a different neurotransmitter or alter the number of postsynaptic receptors. Thus the magnitude of the change in any one cell type may be too small to detect biochemically without large samples. Moreover when biochemical data are available, heterogeneity can complicate attempts to correlate them with specific behavioural functions. An even greater problem exists if the hormone affects the same protein in different cell types, but in opposite directions.

How heterogeneous is the HPOA? No one knows for sure because relatively little is known about the detailed anatomy of the HPOA. Yet if the diversity of peptides present there provides a clue (Grant et al. 1984; Swanson and Sawchenko 1983), it may be extensively subdivided by peptidergic transmitter type. Each of these subdivisions may be subdivided, in turn, based on neuronal connections. Swanson has demonstrated, for example, that the oxytocinergic cells of the paraventricular nucleus project to several sites besides the posterior pituitary (Sawchenko and Swanson 1982; Swanson 1977; Swanson and Kuypers 1980; Swanson and McKellar 1979). Yet even without details of HPOA anatomy, we know that this area is sufficiently heterogeneous in regard to sexual behaviour that either it or the behaviour, and preferably both, must be carefully dissected to obtain meaningful correlates between the two.

This understanding developed from behavioural analyses. Perhaps the most important contribution was the "orthogonal" model of sexual differentiation (Whalen 1974). This model points out that sexual behaviour does not differentiate along a continuum of masculinity-femininity. If it did, any change in the expression of masculine traits (i.e. traits that are usually better developed in males than in females) would be accompanied by an equal and opposite change in the expression of feminine traits (i.e. traits that are usually better developed in females than in males). This occurs when one primordial tissue gives rise to homologous structures in males and females, and possibly in other situations. The genitalia are an example (Feder 1981). The more the genital tubercle becomes a penis, the less it resembles a clitoris. The gonads of fish may be another. According to Atz (1964), the testes and the ovaries of fish develop from a single cell type. Thus for every cell that differentiates into a testicular cell, there is one less that can differentiate into an ovarian cell.

In contrast, masculine and feminine aspects of sexual behaviour differentiate independently of one another (Goy and Goldfoot 1975; Whalen 1974). Developmental events that enhance the expression of masculine behaviours do not necessarily cause any decrement, much less an equal or compensatory decrement, in the expression of

feminine behaviours. Similarly, events that suppress the development of feminine behaviours do not necessarily promote the development of masculine behaviours. Either,
neither or both patterns may develop. Normal males and females show predominantly
one pattern or the other, but these dimorphisms are not causally related. For example,
female rats that gestate between (Clemens et al. 1978) or downstream from (Meisel
and Ward 1981) males readily mount other females if given T in adulthood. Yet they
readily show lordosis when mounted if given OE_2 and P. The mechanisms underlying
the development of mounting behaviour in female rats are subject to debate (see Slob
and Vreeburg, this Vol.), but everyone agrees that, for whatever reason, some females
show high levels of both masculine and feminine sexual behaviours depending on the
type of hormone and/or stimulus partner available. Similar results are obtained when
newborn male rats are treated with androstenedione (Goldfoot et al. 1969; Stern 1969),
when they are treated with a drug that prevents metabolism of T to OE_2 (Davis et al.
1979a), or when newborn female hamsters are exposed to low doses of T (DeBold and
Whalen 1975). These data suggest that the critical period for enhancing masculine
sexual behaviour precedes the critical period for suppressing feminine sexual behaviour
and that the two processes are differentially sensitive to certain steroids.

      Male rats carrying the X-linked allele for testicular feminization *(tfm)* provide an
example of the opposite situation. They show neither mounting nor lordosis despite
appropriate hormonal stimulation in adulthood (Beach and Buehler 1977). They will
show lordosis as adults if they are castrated as neonates (Olsen 1979; Olsen and Whalen
1981). Thus *tfm* males normally become defeminized by their testes without becoming masculinized. This apparently reflects differential sensitivity of the two processes
to oestrogen. *Tfm* males have a normal complement of HPOA receptors for OE_2 (Fox
1975; Olsen, this Vol.). Defeminization of lordosis seems to proceed through the action
of this metabolite of T. In contrast, *tfm* males are deficient in HPOA receptors for
DHT. This deficit may underly the failure of masculinization. In other words, different
metabolites of T may be involved in enhancing masculine behaviour than in suppressing
feminine behaviour.

      The independent development of masculine and feminine sexual behaviour resembles
sexual differentiation of the reproductive tract. Rather than developing from a single,
bipotential anlage as the genitalia do, the male and female reproductive tracts develop
independently from two separate anlagen (Feder 1981; Wilson et al. 1981). Both are
initially present in both sexes and both are influenced by testicular secretions, but the
secretion that stimulates the Wolffian ducts to form a male reproductive tract is not
the same as the secretion that prevents the Mullerian ducts from forming a female reproductive tract. If one is present without the other, or if the individual can respond
to only one of them, the individual may have both types of internal reproductive organs
in adulthood or neither (Wilson et al. 1981).

      To emphasize that masculine and feminine sexual behaviours develop independent-
ly, Whalen (1974) suggested that different terms be used for the hormonal processes
affecting them. The terms masculinization and defeminization were selected because
they specify the directions in which gonadal steroids push sexual development in mammals. In mammals, feminine sexual patterns develop in both sexes, and masculine patterns in neither, if gonadal hormones are missing. In normal males, the potential for
showing feminine sexual behaviour is actively suppressed by T or its metabolite, OE_2.

Thus T and OE_2 defeminize males. T also enhances their potential to show masculine patterns of sexual behaviour, i.e., T masculinizes mammalian males. The degree to which these processes occur varies from one species to another (Baum 1979; Baum and Gallagher 1981), but among mammals the directions of T's effects are always the same. In other classes, the directions in which hormones push sexual differentiation can vary; therefore, different terms are appropriate (Adkins-Regan 1981). In birds, for example, masculine rather than feminine patterns of copulatory behaviour develop in both sexes in the absence of gonadal hormones. This masculine potential is actively suppressed in avian females by OE_2 which also enhances their potential to show female sexual behaviour. Thus OE_2 feminizes and demasculinizes female birds. The principle of independent development of masculine and feminine patterns of sexual behaviour is conserved.

3 Dissection of the HPOA

The fact that masculinization and defeminization occur independently suggests that they involve different target tissues. There is growing evidence to support this view. In rats, for example, the mediobasal hypothalamus (MBH), particularly the ventromedial nucleus (VMN), mediates stimulatory effects of OE_2 and P on the lordosis reflex (Davis and Barfield 1979b; Davis et al. 1979; Matthews and Edwards 1977; Rubin and Barfield 1980, 1983a,b) and appears to be the site at which this behaviour becomes defeminized in males during early development. Implanting T into the MBH of newborn female rats makes them less likely to show lordosis in adulthood (Christensen and Gorski 1978; Hayashi 1976). It does not make them more likely to mount. The POA, more specifically the medial POA (MPOA), mediates T's stimulatory effects on mounting behaviour (Davidson and Bloch 1969; Heimer and Larsson 1966/67; Kelley and Pfaff 1978) and appears to be the neural locus for masculinizing this response. Implanting T into the POA of newborn females increases their tendency to mount other females without suppressing their tendency to perform lordosis when mounted (Christensen and Gorski 1978). Implants of OE_2 mimic these masculinizing and defeminizing effects of T (Christensen and Gorski 1978; Nordeen and Yahr 1982).

Since mounting and lordosis are controlled by the POA and MBH, respectively, studying these subdivisions of the HPOA separately is a first step toward overcoming the heterogeneity of the HPOA. This is a fairly straightforward dissection and has been used many times. For example, E. Nordeen and I found this approach useful when we were attempting to resolve a paradox in the data on sex differences in oestrogen binding to cell nuclei. When the HPOA was studied as a whole, cell nuclear binding of OE_2 was either the same in males and females or showed a sex difference favouring females (DeBold 1978; Marrone and Feder 1977; Ogren et al. 1976; Olsen and Whalen 1980; Whalen and Massicci 1975; Whalen and Olsen 1978). The paradox was that while nuclear binding of OE_2 was thought to determine sensitivity to OE_2, sex differences in OE_2 binding were unidirectional, always favouring females when they occurred. In contrast, sex differences in sensitivity to OE_2 sometimes favour males.

Greater binding of OE_2 in the female than in the male HPOA made some sense in that female rats are more sensitive to OE_2 than males are in regard to lordosis (Pfaff

1970; Pfaff and Zigmond 1971; Whalen et al. 1971). They are also more sensitive to OE_2 in regard to the positive feedback control of gonadotropin secretion required for ovulation (Neill 1972). In other words, lower OE_2 binding by the male HPOA was a potential correlate of defeminized lordosis behaviour and/or defeminized gonadotropin secretion. Occassional failures to detect this sex difference in OE_2 binding could simply have meant that the difference was small and/or detectable only under certain assay conditions. What did not make sense was the consistent failure to detect any potential correlate for the masculinization of mounting. In regard to mounting, male rats are more sensitive to OE_2 than females are (Pfaff 1970, Pfaff and Zigmond 1971). Indeed, it is the most important metabolite of T for activating masculine sexual behaviour (Davis and Barfield 1979a; McEwen 1981). Thus underlying the sex difference in T's effects on mounting is a sex difference in sensitivity to OE_2 that favors males. If binding of OE_2 to target cell nuclei is a reliable correlate of sensitivity to oestrogen, then males should bind more OE_2 than females do in the POA cells that control mounting. Yet when cell nuclear binding was studied separately in the MBH and POA, sex differences were never seen (Lieberburg et al. 1980; Lieberburg and McEwen 1977; Maurer and Woolley 1974). A sex difference in "cytoplasmic" receptor number (King and Green 1984; Welshons et al. 1984) was detected in the MPOA (Rainbow et al. 1982), but this sex difference also favoured females.

To reexamine the hypothesis that greater sensitivity to OE_2 is accompanied by greater binding, we compared oestrogen binding in the POA of male and female rats (Nordeen and Yahr 1983), focussing on earlier timepoints than others had studied. Our data, which are summarized in Fig. 1, showed that males do bind more OE_2 than females in cell nuclei of the POA 30 min after the hormone is injected intravenously. This is not true in the MBH (see Fig. 2), and by 60 min after hormone injection, oestrogen binding favors females in both regions (see Figs. 1 and 2). Thus while sex differences in the MBH consistently favour females, sex differences in the POA can favour either sex depending on the timepoint analyzed.

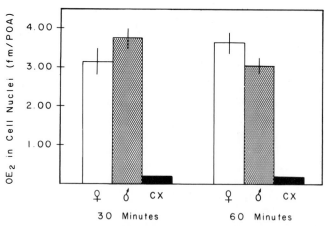

Fig. 1. Mean levels in femtomoles (fm) of OE_2 in cell nuclei of the POA and cortex (CX) of male and female rats 30 and 60 min after an intravenous injection of tritiated OE_2. *Vertical lines* indicate standard errors. (Nordeen and Yahr 1983)

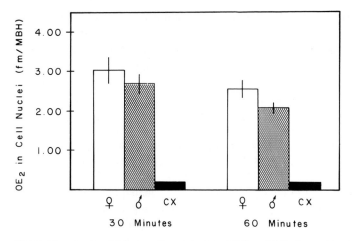

Fig. 2. Mean levels of OE_2 in cell nuclei of the MBH and CX of male and female rats 30 and 60 min after an intravenous injection of tritiated OE_2. *Vertical lines* indicate standard errors. (Nordeen and Yahr 1983)

This complexity in the POA was not surprising. While studying the MBH and POA separately should improve the probability that processes related to lordosis can be distinguished from those related to mounting, both the MBH and the POA are themselves heterogeneous tissues. In addition to mediating oestrogenic effects on mounting, the POA of rats is implicated in other effects of OE_2 including the induction of maternal behaviour (Numan et al. 1977), increased locomotor activity (Wade and Zucker 1970) and positive feedback control of gonadotropin secretion (Goodman 1978; Kalra and McCann 1975; Nance et al. 1977). The POA probably also mediates the effects of T and OE_2 on urinary scent marking (Brown 1977, 1978; Price 1975; Scouten et al. 1980), as it does in other species (Hart 1974; Hart and Voith 1978; Yahr 1977, 1983). Similarly, the MBH mediates other effects of OE_2 besides lordosis, such as suppression of food intake (Wade and Zucker 1970) and negative feedback control of gonadotropin secretion (Bishop et al. 1972). For some of these phenotypes, like scent marking (Brown 1978), sex differences in sensitivity to OE_2 seem to follow the pattern seen in mounting, i.e. males are more sensitive than females. But for others, such as increased locomotor activity (Gentry and Wade 1976) and negative feedback (Neill 1972), no sex differences exist. For still others, like positive feedback (Neill 1972), males are less sensitive to OE_2 than females are. The chances therefore seem good that each of these phenotypes involves a different group of oestrogen-sensitive cells.

Because the cells that control one of these functions can not yet be distinguished from the others, their steroid-binding properties and other responses to steroids can not be studied separately. Finer dissections, such as those achieved with the Palkovits (1973) punch technique, may be useful in approaching this goal. But even these dissections may not provide the resolution required to correlate biochemistry with behaviour because functionally distinct cell types may not be segregated into distinctive nuclear groupings. In the ventrolateral VMN, for example, oestrogen-accumulating cells that project to the dorsal midbrain, an area implicated in lordosis, are intermingled with oestrogen-accumulating cells that do not project there and with cells that project to the dorsal midbrain but that do not take up OE_2 (Morrell and Pfaff 1982). Moreover, cells of the first type are in the minority. Thus additional dissection techniques are needed.

4 Dissection of the Behavioural and Neuroendocrine Phenotypes

Dissecting behaviours and other neuroendocrine phenotypes is a complementary approach that is often overlooked. If the subjects' sensitivities to a hormone are assessed, biochemical analyses can be done on groups selected to differ on the phenotype of interest while potentially confounding variables can be equated or counterbalanced. In analyzing sex differences in the POA, for example, one might want to know if the differences covary with gonadotropin secretion, mounting behaviour, or neither. To address such questions, one cannot simply assess the biochemical parameter of interest in neonatally androgenized females and neonatally castrated males. Data from these groups provide clues about the role steroids play in sexual differentiation. However, by themselves, these manipulations provide few clues about functional correlates because they either reproduce too many of the sex differences or they reproduce them too variably. These problems can sometimes be overcome by using manipulations that produce variable results and then screening the potential subjects for the phenotypes that they display.

We used this approach to explore possible correlates of decreased oestrogen binding in the male POA, and MBH, 60 min after hormone injection (Nordeen and Yahr 1983). To generate our groups, we exposed female rats to T or OE_2 as neonates or capitalized on naturally occurring variations in sexual behaviours. Later we ovariectomized the females and tested them for their tendency to show lordosis when given OE_2 and P and to mount when given OE_2 and DHT. At ovariectomy, we also noted the number of corpora lutea (CL) in each ovary as an index of positive feedback. Then we selected two groups of females that differed substantially in both feminine sexual behaviour and ovarian function – one group virtually never showed lordosis (see Fig. 3) and had no CL; the other group showed lordosis 80% of the times they were mounted and averaged more than ten CL per ovary. In addition, we selected the subjects so that they were comparable in mounting behaviour (see Fig. 3). All of them had high mounting scores, i.e. they were masculinized in terms of this behaviour. When their brains were assayed for OE_2 binding, the two groups differed as much as males and females normally do (see Fig. 4). Thus the sex differences seen at this timepoint in the MBH and POA may indeed be related to defeminization of lordosis and gonadotropin secretion in males. Clearly neither is related to the sex difference in mounting. Thus we have eliminated one variable from consideration and have thereby strengthened the argument that nuclear binding of OE_2 correlates with responsiveness to this steroid.

We obtained essentially the same results when we repeated the analysis, this time comparing defeminized and normal females while holding mount frequency equal and low (see Fig. 5), i.e. none of the females in these two groups were masculinized in terms of this behaviour. A third group was both masculinized and defeminized. Again, low binding of OE_2 was associated with defeminization of gonadotropin secretion and fe-

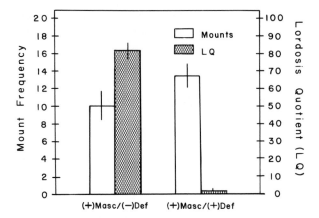

Fig. 3. Behavioural profiles of female rats used to study the effect of defeminization on cell nuclear binding of OE_2. Mount frequencies for three tests during treatment with OE_2 benzoate (OEB) and DHT propionate (DHTP) were averaged for each female. Similarly, LQ scores were averaged over two tests during treatment with OEB and P. The data shown are the means ± standard errors of these averages. Females that obtained high mounting scores were considered to be masculinized in regard to this behaviour and were designated (+)Masc. Females that obtained low LQ scores were considered to be defeminized in regard to this behaviour and were designated (+)Def. The (+)Def females were also anovulatory and were therefore also considered to be defeminized in regard to positive feedback control of gonadotropin secretion. The (−)Def females were not defeminized by either criterion. (Nordeen and Yahr 1983)

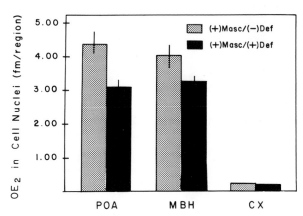

Fig. 4. Effect of defeminization on cell nuclear binding of OE_2. The data shown are the mean levels (± standard errors) of OE_2 in the cell nuclei of the POA, MBH, and CX 60 min after an intravenous injection of tritiated OE_2. The subjects were the ones whose behavioural profiles are shown in Fig. 3. (Nordeen and Yahr 1983)

male sexual behaviour (see Fig. 6). Masculinization of mounting behaviour added nothing to the response. By applying this phenotypic dissection technique again, we hope to determine if enhanced binding of OE_2 in the male POA 30 min after hormone injection is related to the masculinization of mounting behaviour.

The analysis we used was derived from the orthogonal model of sexual differentiation and sought to disentangle masculinizing and defeminizing aspects of sexual differentiation. However, many other phenotypic dissections can and should be used to study neural correlates of masculine and feminine behaviours. Lordosis, for example,

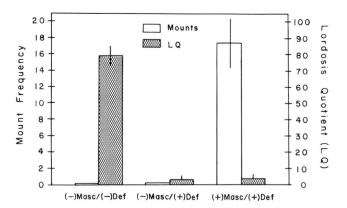

Fig. 5. Behavioural profiles of female rats used to study the effects of masculinization and defeminization on cell nuclear binding of OE_2. The subjects were categorized as $(+)$Def, $(-)$Def, and $(+)$Masc as described in the legend for Fig. 3. Females that rarely or never mounted were considered not to be masculinized in regard to this behaviour and were designated $(-)$Masc. The data are summarized as in Fig. 3. (Nordeen and Yahr 1983)

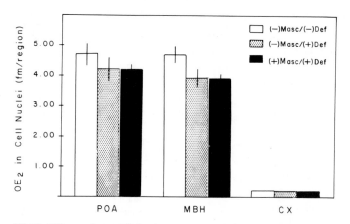

Fig. 6. Effects of masculinization and defeminization on cell nuclear binding of OE_2. The data shown are summarized as in Fig. 4 and represent OE_2 binding to cell nuclei 60 min after an intravenous injection of tritiated OE_2. The subjects were the ones whose behavioural profiles are shown in Fig. 5. (Nordeen and Yahr 1983)

is only one component of the feminine sexual behaviour of rodents. Beach's (1976) classification of feminine sexual behaviours has renewed awareness of this fact. He pointed out that a female's lordosis quotient (LQ), an index of her receptivity to the sexual advances of a male, can provide a very different view of her sexual behaviour than the one obtained by assessing her initiative in the sexual interaction. Under some hormonal conditions, for example, female rats actively solicit copulation by approaching the male, moving away from him, and then stopping abruptly. These "proceptive" behaviours increase the chance that the male will follow the female and assume the mounting position. Under other conditions, proceptivity does not occur. The important point here is that proceptive and receptive responses appear to be controlled independently by steroid hormone action on the HPOA. They often occur together, but each can be elicited without the other. For example, proceptivity seems to depend more heavily than lordosis does on the action of both OE_2 and P (Rainbow et al. 1980a). Much less is known about the neural basis of proceptivity than about the lordosis reflex, but both can be elicited by hormone implants into the VMN (Rubin and Barfield 1983b). The dissection of feminine sexual behaviours can only help in the search for neural correlates.

Masculine sexual behaviour can be similarly dissected. For example, Madlafousek has shown that under certain hormonal conditions male rats show no sexual initiative but are receptive to the advances of highly proceptive females (Hlinak et al. 1979; Madlafousek et al. 1976). In this case, the behavioural response, mounting, is the same whether it occurs as a proceptive or a receptive behaviour, so the dissection is based on the effective stimuli (e.g. pheromonal versus pheromonal plus behavioural cues). In principle, though, it is the same distinction that Beach (1976) proposed for feminine sexual behaviours. In other regards, masculine sexual behaviour has been dissected more than feminine sexual behaviour has. For example, the parameters that affect mounting are routinely distinguished from those that affect intromission and ejaculation. Yet neuroendocrine analyses of masculine responses have focussed almost entirely on copulatory behaviours. Particularly in rats, the species most often used for biochemical analyses, other masculine social behaviours are largely ignored, including those that are probably controlled by androgen action on the POA (Scouten et al. 1980). Androgen-dependent communication behaviours related to courtship and territorial defense are often controlled by the POA in other species (Hart 1974; Yahr 1977, 1983). Their inclusion in analyses of HPOA function may be useful, especially for understanding the effects of DHT.

Having raised the issue of dissecting masculine and feminine sexual behaviours into their component parts, I should express a caviat about masculinization and defeminization. While these terms are useful for specifying the directions in which various phenotypes are pushed by hormones during development, they should not be construed to imply that sexual differentiation involves two processes at the mechanistic level. The cellular mechanism by which one phenotype, such as lordosis, becomes defeminized may be different than the mechanism by which another, such as positive feedback, becomes defeminized. In this case, both phenotypes become less sensitive to OE_2; thus each may involve decreased oestrogen binding by neurons subserving that function. But in one case, the decrease may be caused by a decrease in the number of cells devoted to the function. In the other, it may be due to a decrease in the binding capacity of individual neurons, to name only two possibilities. Fewer cells could occur because the cells die or because they differentiate into another cell type. The latter could involve establishing a different set of connections, migrating to another site and/or changing transmitter type. A decreased binding capacity could result from decreased synthesis of intracellular receptors or from decreased access of receptors to chromatin acceptor sites. Moreover, one neuronal system may become masculinized by the same cellular mechanism by which another cell group becomes defeminized.

5 Anatomical and Histochemical Analysis of the HPOA

As useful as tissue dissection techniques can be, the most promising technique for identifying biochemical changes that subserve particular behaviours is histochemistry. Histochemical techniques are advantageous because they preserve anatomical detail and thus increase the probability that different cell types can be recognized and studied independently of one another. Granted, this approach also has limitations, but the possibility of dissecting the HPOA this way has become more feasible recently with the development of sensitive immunocytochemical assays and video-imaging technologies. This approach has also been encouraged by the discovery of structural sex differences in the brain.

The first report of neuroanatomical sex differences in the HPOA, a sex difference in synaptic organization (Raisman and Field 1971), was, of course, particularly exciting. This excitement was heightened when it was discovered that the synaptic connections developed under the influence of gonadal steroids (Raisman and Field 1973). Indeed, it appeared that these differences in connectivity would provide the first clear neural correlate of a sexually dimorphic function controlled by this area. The question was, which one? Unfortunately, that question is still unanswered, presumably due to the difficult and tedious nature of quantitative electron microscopy (EM).

In the meantime, several other sex differences in neuroanatomy have been observed at the light microscopic level. The HPOA of rats, for example, contains a sexually dimorphic nucleus (SDN) visible with a Nissl stain that is larger in males than females (Gorski et al. 1978; Gorski et al. 1980). In at least four species of rodents, the medial preoptic nucleus (MPON) is also larger in males and there are sex differences in the patterns of cellular density in the anterior hypothalamus (AH; Bleier et al. 1982). Interestingly, the VMN is also larger in male than in female rats (Matsumoto and Arai 1983). In hamsters (Greenough et al. 1977) and crab-eating macaques (Ayoub et al. 1983), the orientation of dendrites of POA neurons differs between the sexes. These anatomical analyses further reveal the heterogeneity of the HPOA.

At least two of these dimorphic traits, SDN size and VMN size, are influenced by gonadal hormones during early development (Dohler et al. 1982; Gorski et al. 1978; Matsumoto and Arai 1983), and others may be affected as well. Thus these systems have great potential for revealing the neural bases of sexually differentiated behaviours. It is therefore ironic that not one of these neuroanatomical sex differences has been associated yet with a function. In most cases, no functional correlates were sought. In fact, the SDN is the only one that has been studied under conditions where any potential correlates could be eliminated. Unfortunately, all of the ones studied were. In their original report, Gorski et al. (1978) showed that neonatally castrated males and normal females, both of which secrete gonadotropins cyclically, differ significantly in SDN size. The larger SND's of the neonatally castrated males were about the same size as the SDN's of neonatally androgenized females, which do not secrete gonadotropins cyclically. These two groups also differ in lordosis behaviour. Thus the large SDN size of males apparently does not reflect defeminization of either of these phenotypes. Moreover, it does not reflect masculinization of mounting. We found no differences in SDN volume between females that showed high levels of mounting behaviour and females that showed none (Nordeen and Yahr 1982). More recently, Arendash and Gorski

(1983) showed that SND lesions have no effect on the copulatory behaviour of male rats. Perhaps the SDN will turn out to be the signature of early hormonal effects on a behaviour pattern related to communication.

Communication is one of the sexually dimorphic functions that may be controlled by a sexually dimorphic area (SDA) that we have identified in the gerbil HPOA. The SDA is a group of cells extending 200–300 μm anterior-posterior at the border between the POA and AH. When visualized with a Nissl stain, the SDAs of male and female gerbils differ in shape and prominence (Commins and Yahr 1984a). This is particularly true in the posterior half of the SDA where, as shown in Fig. 7, the male SDA appears

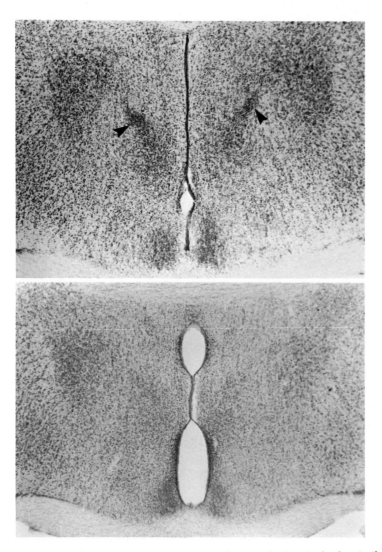

Fig. 7. The sexually dimorphic area (SDA) of a male (*top*) and of a female (*bottom*) gerbil. The photomicrographs shown are coronal sections through the posterior part of the SDA at the level of the suprachiasmatic nuclei. The *arrowheads* point out the SPApc of the male SDA

hooked or C-shaped and contains a dense subset of cells, the SDA *pars compacta* (SPApc). The male SDA appears hooked because a narrow band of cells extends between the prominent, ovoid cell group forming the lateral SDA and the more elongated midline group forming the medial SDA. The SDApc is on or near this connecting bridge of cells. In females, the lateral SDA is also distinct, although less so than in males, but the borders of the medial SDA are vague and the bridge is missing or faint. SDA cells of females appear to be distributed throughout the area that, in males, lies between the medial and lateral SDA and below the bridge. Also, most females lack the SDApc. Although we are just beginning to study the functions of SDA cells, we have been able to implicate the SDA in the control of two behaviours stimulated by gonadal steroids. Lesions of the male SDA disrupt both masculine copulatory behaviour and glandular scent marking (Commins and Yahr 1984c). For both behaviours, the deficits after SDA lesions are greater than after lesions placed elsewhere in the HPOA (see Figs. 8 and 9). Thus developmental analyses of these behaviours and of the SDA appear worthwhile. Preliminary data (Ulibarri and Yahr, unpublished) indicate that the sex differ-

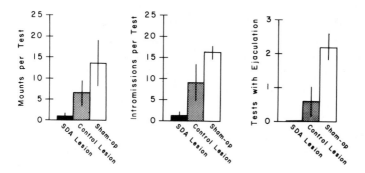

Fig. 8. Parameters of sexual behaviour for gonadally intact male gerbils that received bilateral lesions of the SDA, lesions of the HPOA anterior or posterior to the SDA (control lesion), or sham operations. The data shown are means ± standard errors. (Commins and Yahr 1984c)

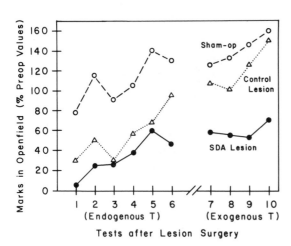

Fig. 9. Scent marking scores of male gerbils that received lesion surgeries as summarized in the legend to Fig. 8. The males were tested while they were gonadally intact (endogenous T) and after they were castrated and given subcutaneous implants of T (exogenous T). The data shown are group means expressed relative to the groups' scores before lesion surgery. (Commins and Yahr 1984c)

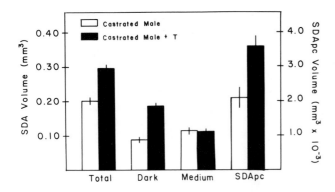

Fig. 10. Effects of T on the volume of the SDA and SDApc in male gerbils castrated in adulthood as measured in Nissl-stained sections. The data shown are means ± standard errors. (Commins and Yahr 1984a)

ences, at least in the SDApc, develop postnatally under the influence of testicular androgens. Tentatively it appears that both sexes have an SDApc at birth and that, over the next two weeks, it disappears in females and enlarges in males.

The SDA may also be a useful model system for histochemical analyses of hormone action in adulthood. SDA cells accumulate both of the major metabolites of T (Commins and Yahr 1985), with DHT uptake being particularly intense in the SDApc. More importantly, though, these structures provide visible, quantifiable markers of T's effects. In both sexes, the SDA fades after gonadectomy, but enlarges and stands out clearly again when the castrates receive T (Commins and Yahr 1984a). Data for males are shown in Fig. 10. In the other species discussed above, no adult hormonal effects have been detected on sexually dimorphic structures (Gorski et al. 1978; Matsumoto and Arai 1983; Raisman and Field 1973), although few of them have been studied from this perspective. Adult hormonal effects on neuroanatomy have been reported in the sexually dimorphic motor nuclei that control singing in songbirds (Nottebohm 1980, 1981; Nottebohm and Arnold 1976). In this system, T appears to influence nuclear size, at least in part, by increasing dendritic length (DeVoogd and Nottebohm 1981) and by stimulating neurogenesis (Goldman and Nottebohm 1983). However, we feel that hormone-induced changes in the gerbil SDA are more likely to reflect thionin's ability to function as a "metabolic" stain. The Nissl granules that incorporate the stain are the arrays of rough endoplasmic reticulum (ER; Palay and Palade 1955) on which cells synthesize proteins for export or for incorporation into cell membranes (Alberts et al. 1983). Thus decreased Nissl staining in castrated males may simply be due to decreased synthesis of such proteins and disaggregation of the rough ER (LaVelle 1951, 1956). Such disaggregation has been demonstrated by EM in the VMN of female rats after ovariectomy (Cohen and Pfaff 1981).

Synthesis of acetylcholinesterase (AChE) may be one metabolic process reflected in Nissl staining. Cells that synthesize AChE are scattered throughout the SDA, except in the SDApc, and the activity of this enzyme within the SDA varies with the animal's hormonal state (Commins and Yahr 1984b). Castration decreases AChE activity, but T can completely prevent this change (see Fig. 11). The AChE-containing cells of the gerbil SDA are probably not cholinergic since they apparently do not contain choline-acetyltransferase (Holets et al., unpublished), the essential enzyme for synthesizing acetylcholine; however, they may be cholinoceptive cells. This possibility is intriguing

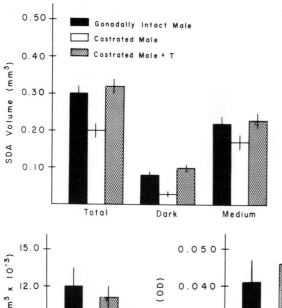

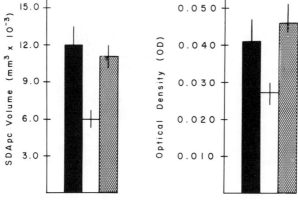

Fig. 11. Effects of castration and replacement of T on the volume of the gerbil SDA and SDApc as measured in sections stained for AChE activity. Also shown are data for optical density measurements of AChE activity within the SDA. The data shown are means ± standard errors. (Commins and Yahr 1984b)

because pharmacological analyses suggest that cholinoceptive cells in the gerbil HPOA are involved in androgenic control of scent marking (Yahr 1977).

Like the SDA as a whole, the SDApc is hormone-sensitive in adults. As shown in Figs. 10 and 11, its volume shrinks by 40%–50% after castration. Again, exposure to T prevents this change (Commins and Yahr 1984a,b). This effect cannot be explained by decreased stainability, since it is also detected by AChE histochemistry where the SDApc appears as an area uniquely devoid of AChE activity (Commins and Yahr 1984b). In this case, T may influence cell size, as it does in motor neurons of the spinal nucleus of the bulbocavernosus of rats (Breedlove and Arnold 1981), or cell number, as in the song control nuclei (Goldman and Nottebohm 1983). The function of this extremely dimorphic and hormone-sensitive cell group is still unknown.

6 Lateralization in the HPOA

The final heterogeneity of the HPOA that I will consider concerns differences between its left and right sides. Traditionally, hypothalamic systems are thought of as symmetric.

However, we have gathered data that challenge the assumption that the two sides of the HPOA participate equally in sexual differentiation. We studied sexual development in female rats that were exposed to OE_2 neonatally on only one side of the brain (Nordeen and Yahr 1982). To do this, we placed OE_2 pellets unilaterally into either the MBH or POA 24-48 h after the pup was born. Cholesterol was implanted on the other side, and controls received cholesterol bilaterally. (Implanting similar pellets of tritiated OE_2 showed that such implants effectively confine hormonal stimulation to the implanted side.) As adults, the females were examined for ovulation and were tested for male and female sexual behaviour in response to OE_2 plus DHT and OE_2 plus P, respectively. To our surprise, the effects of the neonatal implants varied with both location and side. MBH implants defeminized lordosis, when they were on the left. POA implants masculinized mounting, when they were on the right. Only left side implants defeminized gonadotropin secretion as reflected by failure to ovulate, although both the MBH and POA were involved in this response. These data are summarized in Figs. 12-14.

One way to explain these results is to hypothesize that the left HPOA matures slightly earlier than the right. Accelerated development on the left side of the brain has been postulated (Corballis and Morgan 1978) to account for left side dominance in other behaviours, e.g. bird song and human language. Since the critical periods for masculinization differ, asymmetric maturation rates imply that the two sides of the HPOA could pass through them at different times. In rats, defeminization occurs primarily after birth, but masculinization is well underway prenatally (Goy and McEwen 1980). Thus

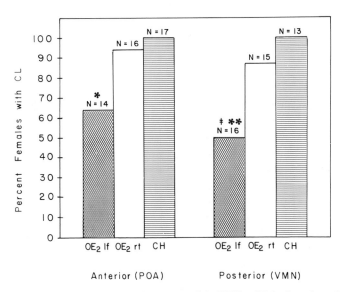

Fig. 12. Effects of unilateral exposure of the VMN or POA of newborn female rats to OE_2 on ovulation as assessed by the presence of corpora lutea (CL) in the ovaries. The females received the intracerebral implants of OE_2 on the left or right side and received an implant of cholesterol contralaterally. These groups are designated OE_2 lf and OE_2 rt, respectively. A third group, designated CH, received cholesterol implants bilaterally. From Nordeen and Yahr (1982). Copyright 1982 by the American Association for the Advancement of Science (AAAS)

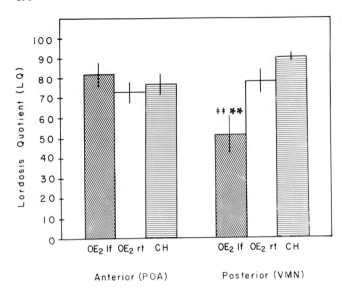

Fig. 13. Effects of unilateral exposure of the VMN or POA of newborn female rats to OE_2 on the tendency to show lordosis when mounted after receiving OEB and P. The subjects are the same ones used in the analysis summarized in Fig. 12. The data shown are means ± standard errors (Nordeen and Yahr 1982). Copyright 1982 by the AAAS

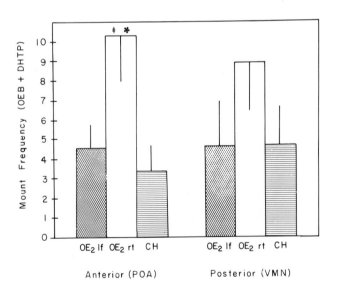

Fig. 14. Effects of unilateral exposure of the VMN or POA of newborn female rats to OE_2 on the tendency to mount a receptive female after receiving OEB and DHTP. The subjects are the same ones used in the analyses summarized in Figs. 12 and 13. The data shown are means ± standard errors. (Nordeen and Yahr 1982). Copyright 1982 by the AAAS

shortly after birth, left side neurons mediating lordosis or positive feedback may be susceptible to defeminization, while the corresponding neurons on the younger right side would not respond. By the same age, left side neurons that mediate mounting would be past the stage where they could be masculinized, but corresponding neurons on the right could still respond. A corollary to this hypothesis is that the side of the HPOA that becomes masculinized or defeminized will vary with the age of exposure to T or OE_2. For example, prenatal masculinization of females by male sibs (Clemens et al. 1978; Meisel and Ward 1981) should be limited to the left POA.

Published data that could be used to evaluate this question are scarce. This makes it particularly interesting that the one report that provides pertinent data provides data consistent with the asymmetric maturation hypothesis. In a series of three experiments, Davis et al. (1979) implanted OE_2 into the right MBH, left MBH or both to induce lordosis in adult female rats. They found that right side implants were as effective as bilateral ones and were twice as effective as implants on the left. One explanation for these results is that the left MBH is less sensitive to OE_2 than the right, i.e. that the left MBH is at least partially defeminized. If any defeminization occurs in normal female rats, it probably occurs prenatally, while the females are exposed to the steroids secreted by their male sibs and their mother. The hypothesis of earlier maturation of the left is consistent with the Davis et al. results in that it predicts that any defeminization occurring before birth would be confined to the left. If the defeminization is not severe, it may be camouflaged by retention of normal function on the right. In discussing their data, Davis et al. wondered why the effects of unilateral implants varied so much between experiments, but did not consider that side of implantation may have affected their results. This is a good example of how the *Zeitgeist* of hypothalamic symmetry has prevented researchers from exploring this aspect of heterogeneity in the HPOA. Recently, though, asymmetries have also been observed in hypothalamic content of luteinizing hormone releasing hormone (Gerendai et al. 1978) and in control of gonadotropin secretion after hemicastration (Nance and Moger 1972; Nance et al. 1983).

An alternative explanation for the apparent asymmetries that we and Davis et al. observed is that the left side of the HPOA dominates lordosis and positive feedback while the right side dominates mounting. Clearly both this hypothesis and the asymmetric maturation hypothesis may pertain. To explain our data, for example, we must postulate that the right HPOA cannot trigger ovulation or sustain female sexual behaviour after the left side has been severely defeminized, even though it may be able to do so if acting along, i.e. after the left side is destroyed. In future research, we will be testing both of these hypotheses. A third possibility is that the asymmetries lie outside the HPOA. For example, the two sides of the MBH may have been equally defeminized by our neonatal implants. The expression of defeminization could still be asymmetric if the MBH must interact with an asymmetric system to control behaviour. Initially, though, we plan to focus our efforts on the heterogeneous HPOA.

Acknowledgement. This review was prepared while P. Yahr was supported by Research Scientist Development Award MH00478 from the National Institute of Mental Health.

References

Adkins-Regan E (1981) Early organizational effects of hormones: an evolutionary perspective. In: Adler NT (ed) Neuroendocrinology of reproduction physiology and behavior. Plenum, New York London, p 159

Alberts B, Bray D, Lewis J, Roff M, Roberts K, Watson JD (1983) Molecular biology of the cell. Garland, New York

Arendash GW, Gorski RA (1983) Effects of discrete lesions of the sexually dimorphic nucleus of the preoptic area or other medial preoptic regions on the sexual behavior of male rats. Brain Res Bull 10:147–154

Atz JW (1964) Intersexuality in fishes. In: Armstrong CN, Marshall AJ (eds) Intersexuality in vertebrates including man. Academic, New York, p 145

Ayoub DM, Greenough WT, Juraska JM (1983) Sex differences in dendritic structure in the preoptic area of the juvenile macaque monkey brain. Science (Wash DC) 219:197–198

Barley J, Ginsburg M, Greenstein BD, MacLusky NJ, Thomas PJ (1975) An androgen receptor in rat brain and pituitary. Brain Res 100:383–393

Baum MJ (1979) Differentiation of coital behavior in mammals: a comparative analysis. Neurosci Biobehav Rev 3:265–284

Baum MJ, Gallagher CA (1981) Increasing dosages of estradiol benzoate activate equivalent degrees of sexual receptivity in gonadectomized male and female ferrets. Physiol Behav 26:751–753

Beach FA (1976) Sexual attractivity, proceptivity, and receptivity in female mammals. Horm Behav 7:105–138

Beach FA, Buehler MG (1977) Male rats with inherited insensitivity to androgen show reduced sexual behavior. Endocrinology 100:197–200

Bishop W, Kalra PS, Fawcett CP, Krulich L, McCann SM (1972) The effects of hypothalamic lesions on the release of gonadotropins and prolactin in response to estrogen and progesterone treatment in female rats. Endocrinology 91:1404–1410

Bleier R, Byne W, Siggelkow I (1982) Cytoarchitectonic sexual dimorphisms of the medial preoptic and anterior hypothalamic areas in guinea pig, rat, hamster, and mouse. J Comp Neurol 212: 118–130

Breedlove SM, Arnold AP (1981) Sexually dimorphic motor nucleus in the rat lumbar spinal cord: response to adult hormone manipulation, absence in androgen-insensitive rats. Brain Res 225: 297–307

Brown RE (1977) Odor preference and urine-marking scales in male and female rats: effects of gonadectomy and sexual experience on responses to conspecific odors. J Comp Physiol Psychol 91:1190–1206

Brown RE (1978) Hormonal control of odor preferences and urine-marking in male and female rats. Physiol Behav 20:21–24

Christensen LW, Gorski RA (1978) Independent masculinization of neuroendocrine systems by intracerebral implants of testosterone or estradiol in the neonatal female rat. Brain Res 146: 325–340

Clemens LG, Gladue BA, Coniglio LP (1978) Prenatal endogenous androgenic influences on masculine sexual behavior and genital morphology in male and female rats. Horm Behav 10:40–53

Cohen RS, Pfaff DW (1981) Ultrastructure of neurons in the ventromedial nucleus of the hypothalamus in ovariectomized rats with or without estrogen treatment. Cell Tissue Res 217:451–470

Commins D, Yahr P (1984a) Adult testosterone levels influence to the morphology of a sexually dimorphic area in the Mongolian gerbil brain. J Comp Neurol 224:132–140

Commins D, Yahr P (1984b) Acetylcholinesterase activity in the sexually dimorphic area of the gerbil brain: sex differences and influences of adult gonadal steroids. J Comp Neurol 224:123–131

Commins D, Yahr P (1984c) Lesions of the sexually dimorphic area disrupt mating and marking in male gerbils. Brain Res Bull 13:185–193

Commins D, Yahr P (1985) Autoradiographic localization of estrogen and androgen receptors in the sexually dimorphic area and other regions of the gerbil brain. J Comp Neurol 231:473–489

Corballis MC, Morgan JJ (1978) On the biological basis of human laterality I. Evidence for a maturational left-right gradient. Behav Brain Sci 2:261–336

Davidson JM, Bloch GJ (1969) Neuroendocrine aspects of male reproduction. Biol Reprod 1:67–92

Davis PG, Barfield RJ (1979a) Activation of masculine sexual behavior by intracranial estradiol benzoate implants in male rats. Neuroendocrinology 28:217–227

Davis PG, Barfield RJ (1979b) Activation of feminine sexual behavior in castrated male rats by intrahypothalamic implants of estradiol benzoate. Neuroendocrinology 28:228–233

Davis PG, Chaptal CV, McEwen BS (1979a) Independence of the differentiation of masculine and feminine sexual behavior in rats. Horm Behav 12:12–19

Davis PG, McEwen BS, Pfaff DW (1979b) Localized behavioral effects of tritiated estradiol implants in the ventromedial hypothalamus of female rats. Endocrinology 104:898–903

DeBold JF (1978) Modification of nuclear retention of [^{3}H]estradiol by cells of the hypothalamus as a function of early hormone experience. Brain Res 159:416–420

DeBold JF, Whalen RE (1975) Differential sensitivity of mounting and lordosis control systems to early androgen treatment in male and female hamsters. Horm Behav 6:197–209

DeVoogd T, Nottebohm F (1981) Gonadal hormones induce dendritic growth in the adult avian brain. Science (Wash DC) 214:202–204

Dohler KD, Coquelin A, Davis F, Hines M, Shryne JE, Gorski RA (1982) Differentiation of the sexually-dimorphic nucleus in the preoptic area of the rat brain is determined by the perinatal hormone environment. Neurosci Lett 33:295–298

Eisenfeld AJ, Axelrod J (1965) Selectivity of estrogen distribution in tissues. J Pharmacol Exp Ther 150:469–475

Feder HH (1981) Hormonal actions on the sexual differentiation of the genitalia and gonadotropin-regulating systems. In: Adler NT (ed) Neuroendocrinology of reproduction: physiology and behavior. Plenum, New York, p 89

Feder HH, Landau IT, Walker WA (1979) Anatomical and biochemical substrates of the actions of estrogens and antiestrogens on brain tissues that regulate female sex behavior of rodents. In: Beyer C (ed) Endocrine control of sexual behavior. Raven, New York, p 317

Fox TO (1975) Androgen- and estrogen-binding macromolecules in developing mouse brain: biochemical and genetic evidence. Proc Nat Acad Sci USA 72:4303–4307

Fox TO, Johnston C (1974) Estradiol receptors from mouse brain and uterus: binding to DNA. Brain Res 77:330–336

Gentry RT, Wade GN (1976) Sex differences in sensitivity of food intake, body weight, and running-wheel activity to ovarian steroids in rats. J Comp Physiol Psychol 90:747–754

Gerendai I, Rotsztejn W, Marchetti B, Kordon C, Scapagini U (1978) Unilateral ovariectomy-induced luteinizing hormone-releasing hormone content changes in the two halves of the mediobasal hypothalamus. Neurosci Lett 9:333–336

Goldfoot DA, Feder HH, Goy RW (1969) Development of bisexuality in the male rat treated neonatally with androstenedione. J Comp Physiol Psychol 67:41–45

Goldman SA, Nottebohm F (1983) Neuronal production, migration, and differentiation in a vocal control nucleus of the adult female canary brain. Proc Nat Acad Sci USA 80:2390–2394

Goodman RL (1978) The site of the positive feedback action of estradiol in the rat. Endocrinology 102:151–159

Gorski RA, Gordon JH, Shryne JE, Southam AM (1978) Evidence for a morphological sex difference within the medial preoptic area of the rat. Brain Res 148:333–346

Gorski RA, Harlan RE, Jacobson CD, Shryne JE, Southam M (1980) Evidence for the existence of a sexually dimorphic nucleus in the preoptic area of the rat. J Comp Neurol 193:529–539

Goy RW, Goldfoot DA (1975) Neuroendocrinology: animal models and problems of human sexuality. Arch Sex Behav 4:405–420

Goy RW, McEwen BS (1980) Sexual differentiation of the brain. MIT Press, Cambridge

Grant LD, Bissette G, Nemeroff CB (1984) Distribution of peptides in the central nervous system. In: Nemeroff CB, Dunn AJ (eds) Peptides, hormones, and behavior. Spectrum, Jamaica, p 37

Greenough WT, Carter CS, Steerman C, DeVoogd TJ (1977) Sex differences in dendritic patterns in hamster preoptic area. Brain Res 126:63–72

Griffiths EC, Hooper KC, Jeffcoate SL, Holland DT (1975) The effects of gonadectomy and gonadal steroids on the activity of hypothalamic peptidases inactivating luteinizing hormone-releasing hormone (LH-RH). Brain Res 88:384–388

Harris GW, Michael RP (1964) The activation of sexual behaviour by hypothalamic implants of oestrogen. J Physiol (Lond) 17:275–301

Hart BL (1974) Medial preoptic-anterior hypothalamic area and the sociosexual behavior of male dogs: a comparative neuropsychological analysis. J Comp Physiol Psychol 86:328–349

Hart BL, Voith VL (1978) Changes in urine spraying, feeding, and sleep behavior of cats following medial preoptic-anterior hypothalamic lesions. Brain Res 145:406–409

Hayashi S (1976) Sterilization of female rats by neonatal placement of estradiol micropellets in anterior hypothalamus. Endocrinol J 23:55–60

Heimer L, Larsson K (1966/67) Impairment of mating behavior in male rats following lesions in the preoptic-anterior hypothalamic continuum. Brain Res 3:248–263

Hlinak Z, Madlafousek J, Mohapelova A (1979) Initiation of copulatory behavior in castrated male rats injected with critically adjusted doses of testosterone. Horm Behav 13:9–20

Kalra PS, McCann SM (1975) The stimulatory effect on gonadotropin release of implants of estradiol or progesterone in certain sites in the central nervous system. Neuroendocrinology 19: 289–302

Kelley DB, Pfaff DW (1978) Generalizations from comparative studies on neuroanatomical and endocrine mechanisms of sexual behaviour. In: Hutchison JB (ed) Biological determinants of sexual behaviour. Wiley, Chichester, p 225

King WJ, Green GL (1984) Monoclonal antibodies localize oestrogen receptor in the nuclei of target cells. Nature (Lond) 307:745–747

LaVelle A (1951) Nucleolar changes and development of Nissl substance in the cerebral cortex of fetal guinea pigs. J Comp Neurol 94:453–467

LaVelle A (1956) Nucleolar and Nissl substance development in nerve cells. J Comp Neurol 104: 175–201

Lieberburg I, McEwen BS (1977) Brain cell nuclear retention of testosterone metabolites, 5α-dihydrotestosterone and estradiol-17β, in adult male rats. Endocrinology 100:588–597

Lieberburg I, MacLusky N, McEwen BS (1980) Cytoplasmic and nuclear estradiol-17β binding in male and female rat brain: regional distribution, temporal aspects and metabolism. Brain Res 193:487–503

Lisk RD (1962) Diencephalic placement of estradiol and sexual receptivity in the female rat. Am J Physiol 203:493–496

Lisk RD (1967) Neural localization for androgen activation of copulatory behavior in the male rat. Endocrinology 80:754–761

Luine VN, McEwen BS (1983) Sex differences in cholinergic enzymes of diagonal band nuclei in the rat preoptic area. Neuroendocrinology 36:475–482

Luine VN, Rhodes JC (1983) Gonadal hormone regulation of MAO and other enzymes in hypothalamic areas. Neuroendocrinology 36:235–241

Luine VN, Khylchevskaya RI, McEwen BS (1974) Oestrogen effects on brain and pituitary enzyme activities. J Neurochem 23:925–934

Luine VN, McEwen BS, Black IB (1977) Effect of 17β-estradiol on hypothalamic tyrosine hydroxylase activity. Brain Res 120:188–192

Luttge WG (1979) Endocrine control of mammalian male sexual behavior: an analysis of the potential role of testosterone metabolites. In: Beyer C (ed) Endocrine control of sexual behavior. Raven, New York, p 341

MacLusky NJ, McEwen BS (1978) Oestrogen modulates progestin receptor concentrations in some brain regions and not others. Nature (Lond) 274:276–277

MacLusky NJ, McEwen BS (1980) Progestin receptors in rat brain: distribution and properties of cytoplasmic progestin binding sites. Endocrinology 106:192–202

MacLusky NJ, Naftolin F (1981) Sexual differentiation of the central nervous system. Science (Wash DC) 211:1294–1303

Madlafousek J, Hlinak Z, Beran J (1976) Decline of sexual behavior in castrated male rats: effects of female precopulatory behavior. Horm Behav 7:245–252

Marrone BL, Feder HH (1977) Characteristics of (^{3}H) estrogen and (^{3}H) progestin uptake and effects of progesterone on (^{3}H) estrogen uptake in brain, anterior pituitary and peripheral tissues of male and female guinea pigs. Biol Reprod 17:42–57

Martini L (1982) The 5α-reduction of testosterone in the neuroendocrine structures. Biochemical and physiological implications. Endocr Rev 3:1–15

Mathews D, Edwards DA (1977) Involvement of the ventromedial and anterior hypothalamic nuclei in the hormonal induction of receptivity in the female rat. Physiol Behav 19:319–326

Matsumoto A, Arai Y (1983) Sex difference in volume of the ventromedial nucleus of the hypothalamus in the rat. Endocrinol Jpn 30:277–280

Maurer RA, Woolley DE (1974) Demonstration of nuclear ³H-estradiol binding in hypothalamus and amygdala of female, androgenized-female and male rats. Neuroendocrinology 16:137–147

McEwen BS (1981) Neural gonadal steroid actions. Science (Wash DC) 211:1303–1311

Meisel RL, Ward IL (1981) Fetal female rats are masculinized by male littermates located caudally in the uterus. Science (Wash DC) 213:239–242

Moguilewsky M, Raynaud JP (1979a) Estrogen-sensitive progestin-binding sites in the female rat brain and pituitary. Brain Res 164:165–175

Moguilewsky M, Raynaud JP (1979b) The relevance of hypothalamic and hypophyseal progestin receptor regulation in the induction and inhibition of sexual behavior in the female rat. Endocrinology 105:516–522

Morrell JI, Pfaff DW (1982) Characterization of estrogen-concentrating hypothalamic neurons by their anoxal projections. Science (Wash DC) 217:1273–1276

Nance DM, Moger WH (1982) Ipsilateral hypothalamic deafferentiation blocks the increase in serum FSH following hemicastration. Brain Res Bull 8:299–302

Nance DM, Christensen LW, Shryne JE, Gorski RA (1977) Modifications in gonadotropin control and reproductive behavior in the female rat by hypothalamic and preoptic lesions. Brain Res Bull 2:307–312

Nance DM, White JP, Moger WH (1983) Neural regulation of the ovary: evidence for hypothalamic asymmetry in endocrine control. Brain Res Bull 10:353–355

Neill JD (1972) Sexual differences in the hypothalamic regulation of prolactin secretion. Endocrinology 90:1154–1159

Nordeen EJ, Yahr P (1982) Hemispheric asymmetries in the behavioral and hormonal effects of sexually differentiating mammalian brain. Science (Wash DC) 218:391–394

Nordeen EJ, Yahr P (1983) A regional analysis of estrogen binding to hypothalamic cell neclei in relation to masculinization and defeminization. J Neurosc 3:933–941

Nottebohm F (1980) Testosterone triggers growth of brain vocal control nuclei in adult female canaries. Brain Res 189:429–436

Nottebohm F (1981) A brain for all seasons: cyclical anatomical changes in song control nuclei of the canary brain. Science (Wash DC) 214:1368–1370

Nottebohm F, Arnold AP (1976) Sexual dimorphism in vocal control areas of the songbird brain. Science (Wash DC) 194:211–213

Numan M, Rosenblatt JS, Komisaruk BR (1977) Medial preoptic area and onset of maternal behavior in the rat. J Comp Physiol Psychol 91:146–164

Ogren L, Vertes M, Woolley D (1976) In vivo nuclear ³H-estradiol binding in brain areas of the rat: reduction by endogenous and exogenous androgens. Neuroendocrinology 21:350–365

Olsen KL (1979) Androgen-sensitive rats are defeminized by their testes. Nature (Lond) 279:238–239

Olsen KL, Whalen RE (1980) Sexual differentiation of the brain: effects on mating behavior and [³H]estradiol binding by hypothalamic chromatin in rats. Biol Reprod 22:1068–1072

Olsen KL, Whalen RE (1981) Hormonal control of the development of sexual behavior in androgen-insensitive (tfm) rats. Physiol Behav 27:883–886

Palay SL, Palade GE (1955) The fine structure of neurons. J Biochem Biophys Cytol 1:69–88

Palkovits M (1973) Isolated removal of hypothalamic or other brain nuclei of the rat. Brain Res 59:449–450

Pfaff DW (1970) Nature of sex hormone effects on rat sex behavior: specificity of effects and individual patterns of response. J Comp Physiol Psychol 73:349–358

Pfaff DW, Zigmond RE (1971) Neonatal androgen effects on sexual and non-sexual behavior of adult rats tested under various hormone regimes. Neuroendocrinology 7:129–145

Price EO (1975) Hormonal control of urine-marking in wild and domestic Norway rats. Horm Behav 6:393–397

Rainbow TC, Davis PG, McEwen BS (1980a) Anisomycin inhibits the activation of sexual behavior by estradiol and progesterone. Brain Res 194:548–555

Rainbow TC, Degroff V, Luine VN, McEwen BS (1980b) Estradiol 17β increases the number of muscarinic receptors in hypothalamic nuclei. Brain Res 198:239–243

Rainbow TC, Parsons B, McEwen BS (1982) Sex differences in rat brain oestrogen and progestin receptors. Nature (Lond) 300:648–649

Raisman G, Field PM (1971) Sexual dimorphism in the preoptic area of the rat. Science (Wash DC) 173:731–733

Raisman G, Field PM (1973) Sexual dimorphism in the neuropil of the preoptic area and its dependence on neonatal androgen. Brain Res 54:1–29

Rubin BS, Barfield RJ (1980) Priming of estrous responsiveness by implants of 17β-estradiol in the ventromedial hypothalamic nucleus of female rats. Endocrinology 106:504–509

Rubin BS, Barfield RJ (1983a) Progesterone in the ventromedial hypothalamus facilitates estrous behavior in ovariectomized, estrogen-primed rats. Endocrinology 113:797–804

Rubin BS, Barfield RJ (1983b) Induction of estrous behavior in ovariectomized rats by sequential replacement of estrogen and progesterone to the ventromedial hypothalamus. Neuroendocrinology 37:218–224

Sawchenko PE, Swanson LW (1982) Immunohistochemical identification of neurons in the paraventricular nucleus of the hypothalamus that project to the medulla or to the spinal cord in the rat. J Comp Neurol 205:260–272

Scouten CW, Burrell L, Palmer T, Cegavske CE (1980) Lateral projections of the medial preoptic area are necessary for androgenic influence on urine marking and copulation in rats. Physiol Behav 25:237–241

Stern JJ (1969) Neonatal castration, androstenedione, and the mating behavior of the male rat. J Comp Physiol Psychol 64:608–612

Swanson LW (1977) Immunohistochemical evidence for a neurophysin-containing autonomic pathway arising in the paraventricular nucleus of the hypothalamus. Brain Res 128:346–353

Swanson LW, Kuypers HGJM (1980) The paraventricular nucleus of the hypothalamus: cytoarchitectonic subdivisions and the organization of projections to the pituitary, dorsal vagal complex and spinal cord as demonstrated by retrograde fluorescence double-labelling methods. J Comp Neurol 194:555–570

Swanson LW, McKellar S (1979) The distribution of oxytocin- and neurophysin-stained fibers in the spinal cord of the rat and monkey. J Comp Neurol 188:87–106

Swanson LW, Sawchenko PE (1983) Hypothalamic integration: organization of the paraventricular and supraoptic nuclei. Annu Rev Neurosci 6:269–324

Wade GN, Zucker I (1970) Modulation of food intake and locomotor activity in female rats by diencephalic hormone implants. J Comp Physiol Psychol 72:328–336

Wallis CJ, Luttge WG (1980) Influence of estrogen and progesterone on glutamic acid decarboxylase activity in discrete regions of rat brain. J Neurochem 34:609–613

Welshons WV, Lieberman ME, Gorski J (1984) Nuclear localization of unoccuppied oestrogen receptors. Nature (Lond) 307:747–749

Whalen RE (1974) Sexual differentiation: models, methods, and mechanisms. In: Friedman RC, Richart RM, Vande Wiele RL (eds) Sex differences in behavior. Wiley, New York, p 467

Whalen RE, Massicci J (1975) Subcellular analysis of the accumulation of estrogen by the brain of male and female rats. Brain Res 89:255–264

Whalen RE, Olsen KL (1978) Chromatin binding of estradiol in the hypothalamus and cortex of male and female rats. Brain Res 152:121–131

Whalen RE, Luttge WG, Gorzalka BB (1971) Neonatal androgenization and the development of estrogen responsivity in male and female rats. Horm Behav 2:83–90

Wilson JD, George FW, Griffin JE (1981) The hormonal control of sexual development. Science (Wash DC) 211:1278–1284

Yahr P (1977) Central control of scent marking. In: Muller-Schwarze D, Mozell MM (eds) Chemical signals in vertebrates. Plenum, New York, p 547

Yahr P (1983) Hormonal influences on territorial marking behavior. In: Svare BB (ed) Hormones and aggressive behavior. Plenum, New York, p 145

Sexual Differentiation is a Biphasic Process in Mammals and Birds

M. SCHUMACHER[2] and J. BALTHAZART[1]

1 Introduction

In 1917, Lillie published his analysis of the development of the freemartin. Already in 1922 he raised the question as to whether homologous or heterologous gonadal hormones affect differentiation in embryonic life and questioned to what extent sex characters (including psyche) are reversible (Beach 1981).

However, the hypothesis that gonadal hormones determine in a permanent way during embryonic life the responses of the adult to hormones was rejected during the next decades (Smelser 1933; Beach 1945), and it was only in 1935 and 1936 that Pfeiffer furnished the evidence showing that in the rat the sex type of the hypophysis is not genetically determined but that its differentiation is dependent upon the gonad at birth.

Although several observations on the effect of perinatal endocrine manipulations on adult behaviour were made between 1937 and 1954 (Raynaud 1938; Dantchakoff 1938; Wilson et al. 1940; Beach and Holz 1946; Martins and Valle 1948; Barraclough and Leathem 1954) it is only in 1959 (37 years after Lillie) that Phoenix, Goy, Gerall, and Young established that the behavioural dimorphisms in the guinea pig are due to the action of androgens during pregnancy. They proposed that gonadal steroids have two different actions: activational and organizational. According to this concept, gonadal hormones activate their target tissues during adulthood in a reversible manner or organize ("differentiate") their target tissues during early development. They also suggested that the organizing actions of steroid hormones might occur only during special and limited periods of development, the so-called "critical periods of sexual differentiation".

2 The Progressive Differentiation in Rats

That steroid hormones influence brain differentiation only during critical periods of early development was suggested by many experiments in several species (for review, see MacLusky and Naftolin 1981; McEwen 1978; McEwen 1982). In rats, adult females

---

1 Laboratoire de Biochimie Générale et Comparée, Université de Liège, 17 place Delcour, 4020 Liège, Belgium
2 Laboratoire de Biochimie Générale et Comparée, Université de Liège, 17 place Delcour, 4020 Liège, Belgium

---

Neurobiology
(ed. by R. Gilles and J. Balthazart)
© Springer-Verlag Berlin Heidelberg 1985

show a cyclic pattern of LH secretion and oestradiol, in combination with progesterone, induces a release of an LH surge by the anterior pituitary gland (Castro-Vazquez and McCann 1975; Fink and Jamieson 1976). By contrast, male rats show a more tonic pattern of LH secretion and show no LH surge in response to oestradiol and progesterone (Brown-Grant 1974; Harlan and Gorski 1977). As a consequence, they fail to luteinize ovarian grafts (Gorski and Wagner 1965). This dimorphism is determined by the action of testicular androgens on the brain during a competent period extending until day 6 of life (Gorski 1968; Harris 1964).

In rats, neonatal androgens also suppress the capacity of the adult animal to show lordosis behaviour in response to E_2 and P (this process is called defeminization) and enhance the capacity of the adult to copulate in response to T (this process is called masculinization; Clemens et al. 1969; Beach et al. 1969).

Steroid hormones can only organize these dimorphic characteristics if administered during the first days of life in the rat (Harris 1964; Beach et al. 1969). During the critical period, a single exposure to steroid hormones organizes their target tissues in a permanent way. A hormonal stimulation lasting only a few hours is sufficient (Arai and Gorski 1968; Thomas et al. 1982; Thomas et al. 1983; Corbier et al. 1983).

That the critical period of sexual differentiation does not necessarily encompass the entire period during which gonadal hormones contribute to the organization of the brain was first suggested by the discovery of the delayed anovulatory syndrome (DAS). In females injected with low doses of androgen as neonates, ovulation occurs for a variable period after puberty before the appearance of the permanent anovulatory condition with persistent vaginal oestrus (Gorski 1968). This late appearance of the anovulatory condition is due to the action of postpubertal ovarian oestrogens and/or androgens as shown by Harlan and Gorski in 1978. They proposed that the exposure to a small dose of androgen during the critical period of sexual differentiation alters the sensitivity of the brain to subsequent irreversible effects of gonadal steroids (Harlan et al. 1979).

The hypothesis that a short perinatal exposure to steroids might sensitize hormone target tissues to the subsequent organizing effects of steroids was also suggested by Weisz and Ward (1980; see also Ward and Weisz 1980; Baum et al., this Vol. for studies in ferrets). In fact, during the perinatal period of rats, there is only a brief time during which circulating T concentrations are consistently higher in males than in females (Weisz and Ward 1980; Gogan et al. 1981; Corbier et al. 1978). According to Weisz and Ward, this short rise in plasma T sensitizes the tissues of the developing foetuses to the masculinizing actions of lower T levels at later stages of development.

Other studies in the rat also suggest that the organizing actions of ovarian hormones are not restricted to a critical period in perinatal life. Oestrogens given prior to weaning have permanent feminizing effects on adult open-field behaviour (Stewart and Cygan 1980) and Södersten (1976) presented evidence that ovarian secretions after the perinatal period determine the behavioural sensitivity of female rats to ovarian hormones. The androgen responsiveness of the liver is also determined by the action of gonadal secretions neonatally and after puberty (Gustafsson 1974). Oestrogens facilitate the development of synaptic structures in the sexually dimorphic arcuate nucleus of females during several weeks after birth (Arai and Matsumoto 1978).

3 The Process of Sexual Differentiation in Quail

The first attempt to permanently alter the behavioural sex in birds by steroid hormones was carried out by Domm (1939). He injected chicken eggs with oestrogens between the third and fifth day of incubation. As adults, males had a feminized plumage and rarely copulated. There was no behavioural effect in females. During the next decades, a lot of similar experiments were performed on chicken, quail, and pigeon (see Adkins 1978, for references). However, in all cases birds were observed as adults in the intact state and thus these experiments provided no evidence for a central organizing effect of embryonic hormone treatment.

The first demonstration of a permanent organizing effect of steroids in birds during a critical period in embryonic life was furnished by Wilson and Glick (1970). The treatment of chicken eggs with oestradiol benzoate (EB) or testosterone propionate (TP) suppressed mating behaviour in adult males treated with TP only if the egg treatment was given before day 13 of incubation (21-day incubation period). In 1975, Adkins showed that the injections of TP or EB into Japanese quail eggs on day 10 of incubation had permanent behavioural effects in males (17 days incubation period).

In this species males and females are sexually dimorphic (morphology and behaviour). In the presence of a female, males show the behaviour sequence: neck-grab, mount and cloacal contact movements whereas females never show male sexual behaviour. The cloacal gland (an epithelial foam-producing gland behind the cloaca) is big in males and rudimentary in females. The sternotracheal muscles (syringeal muscles) are heavy and large in males and small in females (Adkins 1975; Balthazart et al. 1983b; Schumacher and Balthazart 1983a). All these behavioural and morphological characteristics are androgen-dependent but the sexual dimorphism affecting them is not only due to the different endogenous hormones in both sexes. Even when injected with large amounts of TP or implanted with subcutaneous silastic implants of T producing physiological levels of circulating hormone similar in both sexes, photoregressed or ovariectomized female quail still do not copulate and grow smaller cloacal glands and sternotracheal muscles than males receiving the same treatment (Adkins 1975; Balthazart et al. 1983b).

Ovarian oestrogens are thought to cause this insensitivity of the females to the activating effects of T (demasculinization) by acting on their target tissues during a critical period in embryonic life ending on day 12 of egg incubation. This conclusion is based on the observation that oestrogens demasculinize male quail only if injected into male eggs before day 12 of egg incubation (Adkins 1979) and that injection of an anti-oestrogen (CI-628) on day 9 of incubation into female eggs prevents their demasculinization (Adkins 1976; for review, see Balthazart and Schumacher 1983; Balthazart 1983).

That E_2 is the hormone responsible for female demasculinization is also suggested by the observation that 5α-dihydrotestosterone, a non-aromatisable androgen, is ineffective in demasculinizing male embryos (Adkins et al. 1982). Testosterone has demasculinizing effects if injected in large amounts into male eggs probably because it is aromatized into E_2. In fact, the aromatization inhibitor ATD (1,4,6-androstatrien-3,17-dione) prevents TP but not EB from demasculinizing copulatory behaviour (Adkins et al. 1982).

4 The Progress of Sexual Differentiation in Quail

Hutchison (1978) was the first who showed that the permanent demasculinizing effects of ovarian secretions are not limited to a critical embryonic period in quail. When quail chicks were gonadectomized 6–12 h after hatching and treated with TP as adults, a significant proportion of the TP-treated females (57%) displayed male sexual behaviour when tested with a female. Her results also suggested that in the absence of ovarian hormones after hatching, female quail remain sensitive to the activating effects of T on behaviour until exposed to oestrogens. In one experiment, we confirmed the first of these results. A significant proportion of females ovariectomized as late as one week after hatching still showed male sexual behaviour patterns when treated with T as adults (Schumacher and Balthazart 1983b).

The next experiment was performed to analyze the exact time-course of postnatal demasculinization. Males and females were castrated at the age of 1 day or 1, 2, 4, and 6 weeks and treated as adults with T (Schumacher and Balthazart 1983c; Schumacher and Balthazart 1984). The age of castration had no effects on behaviour in males. However, a clear effect of the age of ovariectomy appeared in females. Although females of all groups were less sensitive to the activating effects of T than males, sexual behaviour was observed in a significantly higher proportion of females ovariectomized during the first 2 weeks after hatching than later in life (Fig. 1).

Similarly, postnatal testicular androgens had no permanent effects on morphological characteristics in male whereas postnatal ovarian secretions contributed to the full demasculinization of the cloacal gland and of the sternotracheal muscles in females

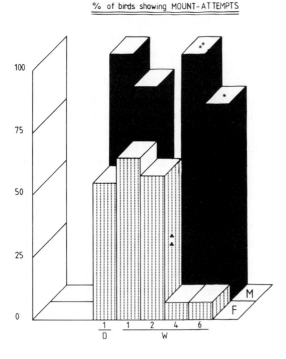

% of birds showing MOUNT-ATTEMPTS

Fig. 1. Percentage of males (*M posterior black columns*) and females (*F dotted anterior columns*) showing male sexual behaviour. Birds were gonadectomized 1 day (*D1*) or 1, 2, 4, or 6 weeks (*W1–6*) after hatching and treated as adults with T. **$2P < 0.01$; *$P < 0.05$ when compared to females. ▲▲ 2 $p < 0.01$ comparison between birds castrated before the age of 2 weeks or later in life. (Fisher's exact probability tests). (After Schumacher and Balthazart 1984)

(Fig. 2). Females glands tended to be smaller if ovariectomy had been performed later in life. Demasculinisation occured later in life for the sternotracheal muscles than for the cloacal gland. There was no sex difference in the weight of the syringeal muscles when castration has been performed before 2 weeks of age. The demasculinization of different reproductive characteristics is thus achieved in females at various times post-hatching.

A third experiment confirmed that postnatal ovarian in secretions contribute to full behavioural and morphological demasculinization (Schumacher and Balthazart 1984). Males and females were castrated at age 4 days or 4 weeks and treated as adults with T. As a control for the influence of stress on sexual differentiation, birds castrated 4 days after hatching were sham-operated at age 4 weeks and birds gonadectomized at age 4 weeks were sham-operated 4 days after birth. As in the previous experiment, the time of orchidectomy was without effect in males whereas females ovariectomized at age 4 weeks showed less copulatory behaviour and had smaller cloacal glands than females ovariectomized 4 days after hatching.

In another study, we determined the nature of the ovarian secretion responsible for the postnatal demasculinization of the females (Balthazart and Schumacher 1984a). As already mentioned, Adkins (1975, 1976, 1979) showed that E_2 is responsible for the demasculinization of male embryos and Hutchison (1978) suggested that E_2 is still capable of demasculinizing adult neonatally gonadectomized females but not males. It was interesting to investigate whether such a dimorphism in the sensitivity to the organizing effects of oestrogens is already present at hatching and if like in the embryo, E_2 is the differentiating hormone in postembryonic life.

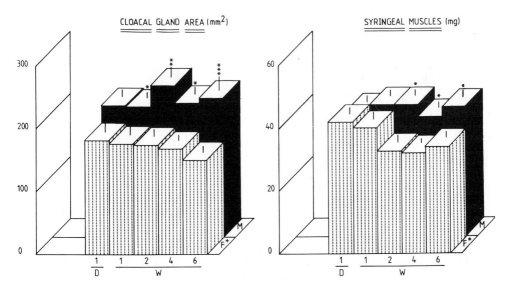

Fig. 2. Size of the cloacal gland (*left side*) and syringeal muscles (*right side*) of males (*M* posterior black columns) and females (*F* dotted anterior columns) gonadectomized 1 day (*D1*) or 1–6 weeks (*W1–6*) after hatching and treated as adults with T ($\bar{X}$ + SEM). ***2 $P < 0.001$; **2 $P < 0.01$; *2 $P < 0.05$; + 2 $P < 0.01$ when compared to females by 2-tailed t-tests or comparisons within a same sex by ANOVA if the asteriks is near the male or female sign. (After Schumacher and Balthazart 1984)

To answer these questions, males and females were gonadectomized at age 4 days and implanted for the first 4 weeks of life with empty or oestradiol-filled silastic capsules. After these 4 weeks, the capsules were removed and as adults, birds were implanted with T. As in the embryo, E_2 completed female demasculinization of copulatory behaviour and cloacal gland growth during the first weeks of life. By contrast, E_2 failed to demasculinize these characteristics in neonatally orchidectomized males (Fig. 3). Thus the postnatal reactivity to the organizing effects of E_2 is differentiated before hatching. Females are presensitized to the organizing actions of oestrogens and it is likely that embryonic E_2 is itself responsible for this effect.

It must, however, been pointed out that females are already partly demasculinized a few days after hatching. Their sexual behaviour is less vigourous than in males and is usually limited to mount attempts. Moreover, in contrast to males, neonatally ovariectomized females only show male sexual behaviour when tested in optimal conditions. Their sexual activity is weak in the test-arena usually used to test the behaviour in males and only becomes apparent when birds are tested in their home-cages. In the same manner, secondary sexual characteristics like the cloacal gland are already smaller in neonatally ovariectomized females than in males.

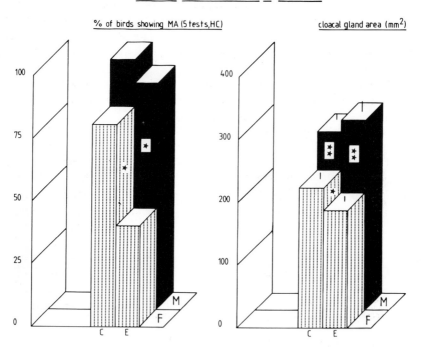

Fig. 3. Percentage of birds showing male sexual behaviour (*left side*) and cloacal gland development (*right side*, $\bar{X}$ + SEM). Males (*M* posterior black columns) and females (*F* dotted anterior columns) were gonadectomized at age 4 days and implanted for the first 4 weeks of life with empty silastic implants (*C*) or E_2-filled implants (*E*) and treated as adults with T. ⋆⋆ $2P < 0.01$; ⋆ $2P < 0.05$ when compared to the opposite experimental group of the same sex by Fisher's exact probability tests (behaviour) or by t-tests (cloacal gland). (After Balthazart and Schumacher 1984a)

Having shown that low amounts of E_2 can demasculinize females during the first weeks of life, we decided to see whether the same effect could be obtained in adult birds. For this reason, we removed the T implants of sexually active and neonatally castrated males and females from the previous experiment and implanted them with high amounts of E_2 for 50 days (Balthazart and Schumacher 1984a; see also Schumacher and Balthazart 1984). During this period of E_2 treatment, birds were tested for sexual behaviour. Whereas E_2 maintained full copulatory behaviour in nearly all males, it was ineffective in females. Thus the sensitivity to the activating effects of E_2 on behaviour is already differentiated at hatching. Although females are still sensitive to the activating effects of T on behaviour after hatching, they have already lost their sensitivity to the facilitating effects of oestrogens. After these 7 weeks of E_2 treatment, E_2 implants were removed and birds were implanted with T. In contrast to the pre-pubertal treatment, even large amounts of E_2 had been ineffective this time in further demasculinizing the adult neonatally ovariectomized females. This result is not necessarily in contradiction with that of Hutchison (1978), who suggested that even in adulthood E_2 might contribute to the full demasculinization of neonatally ovariectomized females. In fact, in contrast to her study, our females had sexual experience and had been exposed to the activating effects of T before the E_2 treatment. Testosterone treatment might end the sensitivity of females to the organizing effects of oestrogens.

The present results which show that female demasculinization in quail is a continuous process extending during the first weeks posthatching seem to be in contradiction with the data of Adkins (1979) which suggest that E_2 cannot demasculinize male quail embryos after day 11 of egg incubation. Several phenomena may account for these apparently different results. For example, the use of different strains of domestic quail may explain the observed differences. Our strain of quail is heavier than Adkins' strain and the process of sexual differentiation is perhaps slower in our birds. This possibility can now be discarded. In a recent experiment we replicated the results of Adkins for our strain of quail. We showed that 5 µg of EB injected into male eggs on day 9 of incubation were sufficient to produce full demasculinization of the males whereas an amount as large as 25 µg was ineffective on day 14 of incubation (Fig. 4). This confirms the presence of a "critical period" somehow related to sexual differentiation in our quail.

It is also possible that the injection of oestrogens into male eggs does not mimic the demasculinization of females by their ovarian oestrogens. As suggested by Hutchison (1978), embryonic hormonal treatments may act on the gonads rather than on brain mechanisms of sexual behaviour. In fact, during the "critical period", before day 12 of incubation, exogenous oestrogens can induce an ovarian cortex on the left testis (Haffen et al. 1975). The induced ovotestis would then secrete more oestrogens during the first weeks post-hatch and, like the ovary in females, progressively, demasculinize the young males. In this case, sexual differentiation in quail would simply be a continuous process and the critical period in embryonic life an artefact corresponding to a period during which steroids can affect the differentiation pattern of the gonads. On the basis of more recent data, this interpretation appears unlikely. In fact, 50-100 times less EB is required for the behavioural and morphological differentiation of male embryos on day 10 of egg incubation (Adkins 1979) than for the induction of an ovotestis (Haffen et al. 1975). Moreover, in a recent work Scheib and collaborators (1981) found that the induced ovotestis does not produce more oestrogens than a normal testis.

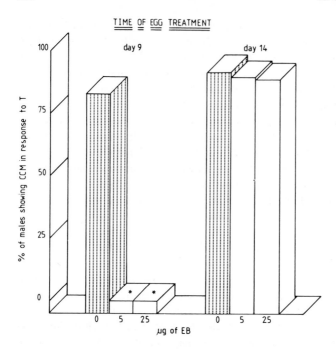

Fig. 4. Percentage of males performing cloacal contact movements (*CCM*). Male eggs were injected with 0.5 or 25 µg of EB dissolved in 50 µl of sesame oil on day 9 (*left side*) or day 14 (*right side*) of egg incubation. After hatching, birds were implanted with T and tested for sexual behaviour. * 2 *P* < 0.05 in comparison with oil injected males by Fisher's exact probability tests

Thus, we propose that, like in the rat, sexual differentiation might be a biphasic phenomenon in quail. A "critical period of sensitization" of the undifferentiated target tissues to the organizing actions of steroid hormones would be followed by a more "continuous period of organization" (differentiation) extending into adulthood or until the exposure to the activating effects of androgens (Schumacher and Balthazart 1984; Balthazart and Schumacher 1984b). As EB demasculinizes male embryos only if injected before day 12 of egg incubation, this stage of development would correspond to the end of the critical sensitization period.

In favour of this hypothesis is the observation that the left embryonic ovary but not the testis produces high amounts of E_2 only during a short time overlapping with this critical period (Guichard et al. 1977; Scheib et al. 1981). This rise in oestrogens would sensitize (like the rise of androgens in mammals) target tissues to the continuous differentiating effects of lower subsequent E_2 levels.

5 The Differentiation in Quail: Demasculinization or Masculinization?

Throughout the literature on sexual differentiation in quail and chicken, it has been accepted that sexual behaviour differentiates by a demasculinization of the females, the male phenotype being anhormonal (i.e. present without any hormonal influence). However, we do not believe that sufficient information is available to decide conclusively what the real process of sexual differentiation is in quail. As reported earlier (Balthazart and Schumacher 1984b), the identification of the differentiation process implies the knowledge of the "neutral" or "anhormonal" and of the "hormonally differentiated" sex. In this discussion we will consider the differentiation of the male phenotype only. Theoretically, adult male characteristics could be the result of three differentiation processes. These characteristics can be acquired following exposure to hormones (masculinization) or lost under the influence of steroids (demasculinization) or, finally, they can develop independent of the steroid milieu (be a "neutral" phenotype). These three mechanisms are by no means exclusive and can occur in the same animal at different times of its development or be observed following exposure to different levels of hormone. In rats, for example, Döhler et al. (1984) showed that sexual differentiation can operate by feminization and defeminization of sexual behaviour. During the critical period of differentiation, weak amounts of oestrogens are required for the maturation of the female phenotype whereas if high amounts of oestrogens are injected they lead to a loss of female characteristics. Another study also suggests that small amounts of oestrogens are required for the maturation of the neuropil (Toran-Allerand 1978; Toran-Allerand 1980), while most behavioural data point to a defeminizing effect of oestrogens in rats (McEwen 1982).

It is usually believed that the male is the "neutral" or "anhormonal" sex in quail and that the female phenotype results from a demasculinizing process (the loss of genetically determined male characteristics by the action of ovarian oestrogens). The only evidence for this asumption is based on the observation that the injection of an anti-oestrogen into female eggs prevents their demasculinization (Adkins 1976) and that injections of EB into male eggs cause an insensitivity of the adult to the activating effects of androgens (Adkins 1975). It is also established that ovarian oestrogens enhance this insensitivity by acting during the first weeks of life (Hutchison 1978; Balthazart and Schumacher 1984a).

However, these experiments do not exclude the possible contribution of a masculinizing action of testicular androgens in embryonic quail. We have recently shown that testicular secretions have differentiating effects on the regulation of LH and FSH during the first weeks after hatching (Schumacher and Balthazart 1984). Castrated T-implanted males have higher gonadotrophin levels than ovariectomized females treated with the same amount of hormone only if gonadectomy has been performed after 2 weeks of life (Fig. 5). Another possible contribution of masculinization in the sexual differentiation of quail is also suggested by the observation that injection of an anti-androgen (flutamide) into male eggs diminishes the sensitivity of the adult to T (Adkins, personal communication).

In fact, all results of the available experiments based on the injection of hormones or anti-hormones into eggs are compatible with a model of differentiation in quail based on a masculinization of male embryos rather than a demasculinization of females. To explain data in this way it is sufficient to postulate that oestrogens inhibit the organizing actions of androgens. Several experiments favour this hypothesis. First, we showed that E_2 inhibits androgen-induced crowing in chicks (Balthazart, Schumacher and Malacarne, unpublished data) and inhibits the androgen-activated development of the cloacal gland in adult males (Balthazart et al. 1984; Fig. 6). Oestradiol is also known to block the binding to the androgen receptor of both T and 5α-DHT (Bullock and Bardin 1974; Fox et al. 1978; Sheridan 1983).

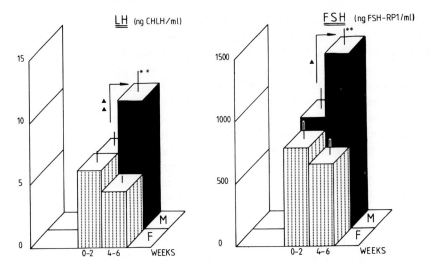

Fig. 5. Serum concentrations of *LH* (*left side*) and *FSH* (*right side*) of males (*M* posterior black columns) and females (*F* anterior dotted columns) castrated before 2 weeks (*0–2*) or after 2 weeks (*4–6*) of age and implanted as adults with T (X + SEM). ** 2 P < 0.01; * P < 0.05 when compared to females. ▲▲ 2 P < 0.01; ▲ P < 0.05 when compared to males castrated after the age of 2 weeks (ANOVA followed by Neuman-Keuls tests). (After Schumacher and Balthazart 1984)

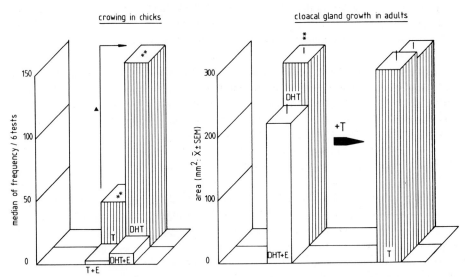

Fig. 6. Inhibitory effects of E_2 treatment (physiological amounts) on T and 5α-DHT induced crowing in male chicks (*left side*) and on 5α-DHT induced cloacal gland development (*right side*). The inhibitory effect of E_2 on cloacal gland growth was reversible: after removal of the E_2 and 5α-DHT implants, T implants induced full gland development in both experimental groups. ** 2 P < 0.01 comparison with the E_2-treated groups by two-tailed t-tests for cloacal gland development and by Mann-Whitney tests for crowing. T is less efficient than 5α-DHT in inducing crowing in male chicks (▲ P < 0.05 by Mann-Whitney test). (After Balthazart et al. 1983a)

If the hypothesis is true, the injections of anti-oestrogens into female eggs will prevent their oestrogens from inhibiting the masculinizing effects of their ovarian androgens. It is also interesting to note that anti-oestrogens like tamoxifen can change the embryonic ovary into a testis in chickens and quail (Scheib and Baulieu 1981; Salzgeber et al. 1981). Thus, anti-oestrogens injected into female eggs would not only inhibit the action of ovarian oestrogens but also enhance the production of masculining androgens by the affected gonad.

Similarily, injections of oestrogens into male eggs will inhibit the masculinizing action of testicular androgens. Moreover, injections of high amounts of E_2 into male eggs would correspond to a functional orchidectomy of the embryos (negative feedback effect or direct effect on the testis) and thus diminish the amount of available T. Indeed, oestrogens cause a regression of the testis in rats (Bendeck and Pomerantz 1984) and quail (Balander et al. 1980). There is, however, no reason to believe that exogenous oestrogens would inhibit the action of androgens only before day 12 of egg incubation in males. As EB affects male differentiation only if injected before day 12 of incubation, this period should correspond to a critical period for masculinization.

The observation that injections of TP into female eggs fail to masculinize female embryos and demasculinize male embryos might then be related to the pharmacological effects of the large amounts of TP (1–2 mg) used in these experiments. In fact, after the injection of 1–2 mg of TP into chicken eggs, plasma T-levels are 500 times higher than in control males (Gasc and Thibier 1979). Such large amounts of T may also induce a high aromatase activity producing amounts of E_2 sufficient to inhibit masculinization by the androgens. We showed that peripheral T treatment increases aromatase activity in quail chicks hypothalamus to levels seen in adult males (Schumacher and Hutchison, in preparation). In this respect it is worth remembering that the aromatization inhibitor ATD prevents TP from demasculinizing copulatory behaviour in quail (Adkins et al. 1982).

Unfortunately, nothing is known about the relative amounts of circulating androgens and oestrogens in male and female quail embryos. However, in chicken, where the differentiation process is probably similar to that observed in quail (Wilson and Glick 1970), female embryos have higher levels of circulating oestrogens than embryos of the opposite sex (Woods et al. 1975; Woods and Erton 1978; Woods and Brazzill 1981) whereas androgen levels seem to be similar in both sexes (Gasc and Thibier 1979). One study however reports higher T levels in male than in female embryos (Woods et al. 1975), but in both quail and chicken embryos, the in vitro production of androgens is similar for the ovaries and the testis whereas the left ovary produces more oestrogens than the testis during the critical period (Scheib et al. 1981; Guichard et al. 1977). According to our model, this higher amount of oestrogens in female embryos would protect them against the masculinizing actions of their own androgens.

All the experimental results available today support a differentiation process based on a demasculinization of the female embryos by their ovarian oestrogens as well as on a masculinization of the males by their endogenous T.

6 Postnatal Organizing Effects of Steroids in Quail

Whichever interpretation is retained, we must still explain why our female quail chicks, in contrast to adult females, are as sensitive to the activiting effects of T as male chicks for some characteristics. This is true for crowing, cloacal gland development, and the induction of aromatase activity but not for copulatory behaviour (Balthazart et al. 1983a; Schumacher and Hutchison, in preparation). This sensitivity is then progressively lost through the action of post-hatching ovarian oestrogens (Balthazart and Schumacher 1984b). Thus post-hatching ovarian E_2 contributes to the full insensitivity of the females to the activating effects of T. This could again result from a direct demasculinizing effect or from an inhibition of postnatal androgenic masculinization. In the latter case, females would be only partly protected against the masculinizing effects of their own androgens during embryonic development. Androgenic stimulation would be weak during the period of greatest sensitivity before day 12 of incubation due to the protecting oestrogens. As a consequence, the exposure to androgens would be required for a longer period extending after hatching. In contrast, androgen stimulation would be strong in males during the critical period and thus the process of masculinization would be completed during embryonic life so that males would not be sensitive to post-hatching oestrogens.

The observation that female chicks in contrast to males never copulate in response to T can be explained by the fact that T induces aromatase activity in the preoptic area (POA) of both male and female chicks (Schumacher and Hutchison, in preparation), a brain region important for the control of male sexual behaviour. This induction of intrahypothalamic E_2 would protect the POA against the further masculinization by the administered androgens. Thus T in chicks would masculinize structures with a low or no aromatase activity like the cloacal gland, the syrinx, and brain centres controlling vocal behaviour. Testosterone would also induce the aromatase in the POA, but then the produced E_2 would inhibit further masculinization of this structure and prevent the full maturation of the neuronal pathways involved in the expression of male sexual behaviour.

If quail are gonadectomized at different ages after hatching, T-treatment has the same activating effects in adult males irrespective of the age of castration. Their masculinization is probably completed during embryonic life because the androgenic stimulation is high. In females, by contrast, the suppression of post-hatching ovarian E_2 by removal of the left ovary will allow the androgens secreted by the adrenals and the rudimentary right ovary to complete the masculinization of these females. The adrenals of both male and female chickens are known to produce important amounts of androgens (Tanabe et al. 1979) and the remaining rudimentary right ovary also secretes some T (Guichard et al. 1980).

All the available experimental data which have always been interpreted within a conceptual framework refering to a differentiation by demasculinization of females can thus be reinterpreted and are compatible with a differentiation process by active masculinization by androgens of males which could be prevented by oestrogens.

7 Conclusions

The first experiment in which the behavioural sex in birds was altered permanently was performed in 1939 by Domm (see above). Forty-five years later the exact process of sexual differentiation in birds is still unknown. There is, in fact, no experimental evidence which permits the distinction between a differentiation in quail and chicken which would be based on a demasculinization of the females by their ovarian oestrogens or a masculinization of males by their testicular androgens. Thus it cannot be ascertained that the process of differentiation in quail is opposite to that observed in mammals

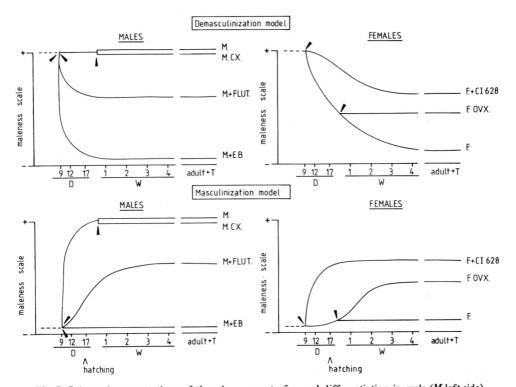

Fig. 7. Schematic presentations of the advancement of sexual differentiation in male (*M* left side) and female (*F* right side) quail according to the two differentiation models. The upper graphs show the hypothetical time-curves for male and female differentiation if the process is a demasculinization of the females by their ovarian oestrogens. The lower graphs present the hypothetical time-curves if the differentiation process is a progressive masculinization of the males by their testicular androgens. The Y-axis presents the "degree of maleness" (percentage of birds showing male sexual behaviour in response to testosterone as adults). The X-axis shows the age of the birds (*D* days of incubation; *W* weeks posthatch). The different curves correspond to different experimental groups receiving different treatments in embryonic and early life (*arrows* indicate the time of treatment). Birds were castrated (*CX*) after hatching or eggs were injected with oestradiol-benzoate (*EB*), flutamide (*FLUT.*, an anti-androgen) or nitromifene-citrate (*CI-628*, an anti-oestrogen). *M* and *F* represent the development of normal males and females. As adults, birds were tested after castration or after photoregression of the gonads followed by androgen-treatment for male sexual behaviour. For more details and references, see text

where oestrogens and/or androgens masculinize the young males. That the process of female demasculinization cannot be generalized to all avian species for all characteristics has already been shown by the work of Gurney and Konishi (1980) on zebra finches (Poephila guttata). In this species androgens and oestrogens masculinize the song system during early postnatal life.

On the basis of the experimental data actually available, we can propose 2 possible mechanisms for the sexual differentiation in quail and chicken:

1. The male is the anhormonal sex and females are demasculinized by their ovarian oestrogens.
2. The male phenotype results from a masculinizing action of testicular androgens. Females are protected against their own androgens by high levels of circulating oestrogens. Weak amounts of androgens and/or oestrogens derived from aromatization would be required for masculinization of males whereas higher oestrogen levels derived from aromatization of pharmacological levels of T injected into eggs or from ovarian secretions would have demasculinizing effects (Fig. 7).

Whatever the nature of the differentiation process (masculinization, demasculinization, feminization, defeminization), it appears that in both mammals and birds the permanent organizing effect of steroid hormones is not restricted to a critical period in early development and extends until and even after puberty. The process of sexual differentiation is probably biphasic: gonadal hormones determine during a short period of highest sensitivity the effects of steroid hormones. According to the mechanism of sexual differentiation, gonadal hormones by acting during the critical period of sexual differentiation will sensitize, desensitize, or maintain the sensitivity to the later continuous and permanent effects of steroid hormones.

Acknowledgements. We are indebted to Professor E. Schoffeniels for his continued interest in our research. This study was supported by a grant number 2.4158.80 from the Fonds de la Recherche Fondamentale Collective to Professor E. Schoffeniels and by a grant from the Belgian Fonds National de la Recherche Scientifique (FNRS; credit aux chercheurs) to J. Balthazart. M. Schumacher is "aspirant" du FNRS. We thank R.E. and J.B. Hutchison for stimulating and critical discussions which helped to develop some of the ideas presented in this chapter.

References

Adkins E (1975) Hormonal control of sexual differentiation in the Japanese quail. J Comp Physiol Psychol 89:61–71

Adkins EK (1976) Embryonic exposure to an antiestrogen masculinizes behavior of female quail. Physiol Behav 17:357–359

Adkins EK (1978) Sex steroids and the differentiation of avian reproductive behavior. Am Zool 18:501–509

Adkins EK (1979) Effect of embryonic treatment with estradiol or testosterone on sexual differentiation of the quail brain. Neuroendocrinology 29:178–185

Adkins-Regan EK, Pickett P, Koutnik D (1982) Sexual differentiation in quail: conversion of androgen to estrogen mediates testosterone-induced demasculinization of copulation but not other male characteristics. Horm Behav 16:259–278

Arai Y, Gorski RA (1968) Critical exposure time for androgenization of the developing hypothalamus in the female rat. Endocrinology 82:1010–1014

Arai Y, Matsumoto A (1978) Synapse formation in the hypothalamic arcuate nucleus during post-natal development in the female rat and its modification by neonatal estrogen treatment. Psycho-neuroendocrinology 3:35–45

Balander RJ, Van Krey HP, Siegel PB (1980) The effects of exogenous steroidal hormones on the testes of quail from selected high and low mating lines. Poultry Sci 59:1943–1946

Balthazart J (1983) Hormonal correlates of behavior. In: Farner DS, King JR, Parkes KC (eds) Avian Biology, vol 7. Academic, New York, pp 221–365

Balthazart J, Schumacher M (1983) Testosterone metabolism and sexual differentiation in quail. In: Balthazart J, Prove E, Gilles R (eds) Hormones and behaviour in higher vertebrates. Springer, Berlin Heidelberg New York, pp 237–260

Balthazart J, Schumacher M (1984a) Estradiol contributes to the postnatal demasculinization of female Japanese quail (Coturnix coturnix japonica). Horm Behav 18:287–297

Balthazart J, Schumacher M (1984b, in press) A two-step model for sexual differentiation. In: Komisaruk BR, Siegel HI (eds) Reproduction: a behavioural and neuroendocrine perspective. Ann NY Acad Sci

Balthazart J, Schumacher M, Malacarne G (1983a) Hormonal control of crowing in the Japanese quail (Coturnix coturnix japonica): inactivation of testosterone by the brain 5β-reducase. J Endocrinol 100:19–23

Balthazart J, Schumacher M, Ottinger MA (1983b) Sexual differences in the Japanese quail: behavior, morphology, and intracellular metabolism of testosterone. Gen Comp Endocrinol 51:191–207

Balthazart J, Schumacher M, Malacarne G (1984, in press) Interactions of androgens and estrogens in the control of sexual behavior in male Japanese quail. Physiol Behav

Barraclough CA, Leathem JH (1954) Infertility induced in mice by a single injection of testosterone propionate. Proc Soc Exp Biol Med 85:673–674

Beach FA (1945) Hormonal induction of mating responses in a rat with congenital absence of gonadal tissue. Anat Rec 92:289–292

Beach FA (1981) Historical origins of modern research on hormones and behavior. Horm Behav 15:325–376

Beach FA, Holz AM (1946) Mating behavior in male rats castated at various ages and injected with androgen. J Exp Zool 101:91–142

Beach FA, Noble RG, Orndoff RK (1969) Effects of perinatal androgen treatment on responses of male rats to gondal hormones in adulthood. J Comp Physiol Psychol 68:490–497

Bendeck MP, Pomerantz DK (1984) Developmental change in the ability of estradiol to suppress testosterone secretion by the testis of the rat. Biol Rep 30:816–823

Brown-Grant K (1974) Steroid hormone administration and gonadotrophin secretion in the gonad-ectomized rat. J Endocrinol 62:319–332

Bullock LP, Bardin CW (1974) Androgen receptors in mouse kidney: a study of male, female and androgen-insensitive (tfm/y) mice. Endocrinology 94:746–756

Castro-Vazquez A, McCann SM (1975) Cycle variations in the increased responsiveness of the pituitary to the luteinizing hormone-releasing hormone (LHRH) induced by LHRH. Endocrinology 97:13–19

Clemens LG, Hiroi M, Gorski RA (1969) Induction and facilitation of female mating behavior in rats treated neonatally with low doses of testosterone propionate. Endocrinology 84:1430–1438

Corbier P, Kerdelhue B, Picon R, Roffi J (1978) Changes in testicular weight and serum gonadotro-pin and testosterone levels before, during and after birth in the perinatal rat. Endocrinology 103:1985–1991

Corbier P, Roffi J, Rhoda J (1983) Female sexual behavior in male rats: effect of hour of castration at birth. Physiol Behav 30:613–616

Dantchakoff V (1983) Role des hormones dans la manifestation des instincts sexuels. CR Hebd Seances Acad Sci 206:945–947

Döhler KD, Hancke JL, Srivastava SS, Hofman C, Shryne JE, Gorski RA (1984) Participation of estrogens in female sexual differentiation of the brain: neuroanatomical, neuroendocrine and behavioral evidence. Prog Brain Res 61:99–117

Domm LV (1939) Intersexuality in adult brown leghorn males as a result of estrogenic treatment during early embryonic life. Proc Soc Exp Biol Med 42:310–312

Fink G, Jamieson MG (1976) Imunoreactive luteinizing hormone releasing factor in rat pituitary stalk blood: effects of electrical stimulation of the medial preoptic area. J Endocrinol 68:71–87

Fox TO, Vito CC, Wieland SJ (1978) Estrogen and androgen receptor proteins in embryonic and neonatal brain. Hypothesis for roles in sexual differentiation and behavior. Am Zool 18:525–537

Gasc JM, Thibier M (1979) Plasma testosterone concentration in control and testosterone-treated chick embryos. Experientia (Basel) 35:1411–1412

Gogan F, Slama A, Bizzini-Koutznetzova B, Dray F, Kordon C (1981) Importance of perinatal testosterone in sexual differentiation in the male rat. J Endocrinol 91:75–79

Gorski RA (1968) Influence of age on the response to paranatal administration of a low dose of androgen. Endocrinology 82:1001–1004

Gorski RA, Wagner JW (1965) Gonadal activity and sexual differentiation of the hypothalamus. Endocrinology 76:226–239

Guichard A, Cedard L, Mignot T-M, Scheib D, Haffen K (1977) Radioimmunoassay of steroids produced by cultured chick embryonic gonads: differences according to age, sex and side. Gen Comp Endocrinol 32:255–265

Guichard A, Scheib D, Haffen K, Mignot T-M, Cedard L (1980) Comparative study in steroidogenesis by quail and chick embryonic gonads in organ culture. J Steroid Biochem 12:83–87

Gurney ME, Konishi M (1980) Hormone-induced sexual differentiation of the brain and behavior in zebra finches. Science (Wash DC) 208:1380–1383

Gustafsson J-A (1974) Androgen responsiveness of the liver of developing rat. Biochem J 144:225–229

Haffen K, Scheib D, Guichard A, Cedard L (1975) Prolonged sexual bipotentiality of the embryonic quail testis and relation with sex steroid biosynthesis. Gen Comp Endocrinol 26:70–78

Harlan RE, Gorski RA (1977) Steroid regulation of luteinizing hormone secretion in normal and androgenized rats at different ages. Endocrinology 101:741–749

Harlan RE, Gorski RA (1978) Effects of postpubertal ovarian steroids on reproductive function and sexual differentiation of lightly androgenized rats. Endocrinology 102:1716–1724

Harlan RE, Gordon JH, Gorski RA (1979) Sexual differentiation of the brain: implications for neuroscience. In: Schneider DM (ed) Rev Neurosci, vol 4. Raven, New York, pp 31–71

Harris GW (1964) Sex hormones, brain development and brain function. Endocrinology 75:627–648

Hutchison RE (1978) Hormonal differentiation of sexual behavior in the Japanese quail. Horm Behav 11:363–387

Lillie FR (1917) The free-martin: a study of the action of sex hormones in the foetal life of cattle. J Exp Zool 23:371–392

MacLusky NJ, Naftolin F (1981) Sexual differentiation of the central nervous system. Science (Wash DC) 211:1294–1303

Martins T, Valle JR (1948) Hormonal regulation of the micturition behavior of dogs. J Comp Physiol Psychol 41:301–311

McEwen BS (1978) Sexual maturation and differentiation: the role of the gonadal steroids. Prog Brain Res 48:291–307

McEwen BS (1982) Sexual differentiation of the brain: gonadal hormone action and the current concepts of neuronal differentiation. In: Brown IR (ed) Molecular approaches to neurobiology. Academic, New York, pp 195–219

Pfeiffer CA (1935) Origin of functional differences between male and female hypophyses. Proc Soc Exp Biol Med 32:603–605

Pfeiffer CA (1936) Sexual differences of the hypophysis and their determination by the gonads. Am J Anat 58:195–226

Phoenix CH, Goy RW, Gerall AA, Young WC (1959) Organizing action of prenatally administered testosterone propionate on the tissues mediating mating behavior in the female guinea pig. Endocrinology 65:369–382

Raynaud A (1938) Comportement sexuel des souris femelles intersexuees. C R Soc Biol 1:993–995

Salzgeber B, Reyss-Brion M, Baulieu EE (1981) Modification des gonades femelles de l'embryon de poulet, apres action du tamoxifene. C R Acad Sci Paris 293:133–138

Scheib D, Baulieu EE (1981) Action antagoniste du tamoxifene sur la differenciation normale des gonades femelles de l'embryon de caille. C R Acad Sci Paris 293:513–514

Scheib D, Guichard A, Mignot T-M, Cedard L (1981) Steroidogenesis by gonads of normal and of diethylstilbestrol-treated quail embryos: radioimmunoassays on organ cultures. Gen Comp Endocrinol 43:519–526

Schumacher M, Balthazart J (1983a) The effects of testosterone and its metabolites on sexual behavior and morphology in male and female Japanese quail. Physiol Behav 30:335–339

Schumacher M, Balthazart J (1983b) The postnatal differentiation of sexual behavior in the Japanese quail (Coturnix coturnix japonica). Behav Processes 8:189–195

Schumacher M, Balthazart J (1983c) Effects of castration on postnatal differentiation in the Japanese quail (Coturnix coturnix japonica). IRCS Med Sci Libr Compend 11:102–103

Schumacher M, Balthazart J (1984) The postnatal demasculinization of sexual behavior in the Japanese quail (Coturnix coturnix japonica). Horm Behav 18:298–312

Sheridan PJ (1983) Androgen receptors in the brain: what are we measuring. Endocr Rev 4:171–178

Smelser GK (1933) The response of guinea pig mammary glands to sex hormones and ovarian grafts and its bearing on the problem of sex hormone antagonism. Physiol Zool 6:396–449

Södersten P (1976) Lordosis behaviour in male, female and androgenized female rats. J Endocrinol 70:409–420

Stewart J, Cygan D (1980) Ovarian hormones act early in development to feminize adult open-field behavior in the rat. Horm Behav 14:20–32

Tanabe Y, Nakamura T, Fujioka K, Doi O (1979) Production and secretion of sex steroid hormones by the testes, the ovary and the adrenal glands of embryonic and young chickens (Gallus domesticus). Gen Comp Endocrinol 39:26–33

Thomas DA, Barfield RJ, Etgen AM (1982) Influence of androgen on the development of sexual behavior in rats. Horm Behav 17:443–454

Thomas DA, Howard SB, Barfield RJ (1983) Influence of androgen on the development of sexual behavior in the rat. Horm Behav 17:308–315

Toran-Allerand CD (1978) Gonadal hormones and brain development: cellular aspects of sexual differentiation. Am Zool 18:553–565

Toran-Allerand CD (1980) Sex steroids and the development of the newborn mouse hypothalamus and preoptic area in vitro II. Morphological correlates and hormonal specificity. Brain Res 189:413–427

Ward IL, Weisz J (1980) Maternal stress alters plasma testosterone in fetal males. Science (Wash DC) 207:328–329

Weisz J, Ward IL (1980) Plasma testosterone and progesterone titers of pregnant rats, their male and female fetuses, and neonatal offspring. Endocrinology 106:306–316

Wilson JA, Glick B (1970) Ontogeny of mating behavior in the chicken. Am J Physiol 218:951–955

Wilson JG, Young WC, Hamilton JB (1940) A technique suppressing development of reproductive function and sensitivity to estrogen in the female rat. Yale J Biol Med 13:189–202

Woods JE, Brazzil DM (1981) Plasma 17β-estradiol levels in the chick embryo. Gen Comp Endocrinol 44:37–43

Woods JE, Erton LH (1978) The synthesis of estrogens in the gonads in the chick embryo. Gen Comp Endocrinol 36:360–370

Woods JE, Simpson RM, Moore PL (1975) Plasma testosterone levels in the chick embryo. Gen Comp Endocrinol 27:543–547

Woods JE, Congoran DD, Thomes RC (1982) Plasma estrone levels in the chick embryo. Poultry Sci 61:1729–1733

Sex Differences in the Anterior Pituitary Gland

M.O. DADA, J.F. RODRIGUEZ-SIERRA, and C.A. BLAKE [1]

1 Introduction

This chapter will review many of the sex differences we and other investigators have observed on the morphology and physiology of the anterior pituitary gland of the laboratory rat. Occasionally similarities and differences in other species are mentioned. When known, the age of onset and the underlying mechanisms of the sex differences are discussed.

2 Anterior Pituitary Gland (APG) Weight

When kept under highly controlled environmental conditions, male and female litter-mate rats increase in body weight similarly until about the sixth week after birth at which time males are heavier than females (Tables 1 and 2). Until this prepubertal growth spurt occurs in males, APG weights are similar in both sexes or tend to be a little higher in females. Even though the males continue to increase in body weight faster than do females, absolute APG weights tend to be higher in females. The APG weight/body weight ratio remains fairly constant in the female but decreases in the male with age. Whereas oestrogen but apparently not testosterone can cause an increase in APG weight in either sex under specific circumstances (Zondek 1936; Lisk 1969; Lloyd et al. 1973; Takahashi and Kawashima 1981), it is not clear whether or not oestrogen plays a physiological role in the sex difference in APG weight.

3 Morphology and Morphometry

3.1 Gonadotrophs

Light Microscopic Observations: A controversy exists as to whether all gonadotrophs in the rat contain luteinizing hormone (LH) and follicle-stimulating hormone (FSH) or whether some gonadotrophs contain both hormones while others contain only LH or FSH (see Girod 1984, for review). We recently obtained evidence strongly suggesting that in young adult (Dada et al. 1983) and prepubertal rats (Dada and Blake 1984,

---

1 Department of Anatomy, University of Nebraska Medical Center, Omaha, NE 68105, USA

Neurobiology
(ed. by R. Gilles and J. Balthazart)
© Springer-Verlag Berlin Heidelberg 1985

Table 1. Anterior pituitary gland (APG) and body wt. of male and female rats at different ages

Age (days)	Male			Female		
	Body wt. (g)	APG (mg)	APG (mg) 100 g^{-1} body wt.	Body wt. (g)	APG (mg)	APG (mg) 100 g^{-1} body wt.
7	16.4 ± 0.4[a] (18)	0.74 ± 0.02	4.61 ± 0.18	15.5 ± 0.6 (18)	0.71 ± 0.04	4.64 ± 0.26
15	26.4 ± 1.8 (13)	1.08 ± 0.06	4.23 ± 0.25	28.2 ± 1.6 (14)	1.32 ± 0.06[d]	4.81 ± 0.21
23	44.8 ± 4.6 (14)	1.68 ± 0.13	3.98 ± 0.25	44.8 ± 4.1 (12)	1.78 ± 0.08	4.50 ± 0.56
35	127 ± 3[d] (9)	4.27 ± 0.09	3.38 ± 0.06	110 ± 2 (9)	4.38 ± 0.24	3.97 ± 0.14[d]
40[b]	166 ± 4[d] (10)	5.0 ± 0.9	3.04 ± 0.07	133 ± 3 (9)	5.0 ± 0.1	3.77 ± 0.12[d]
80	389 ± 11[d] (16)	8.3 ± 0.3	2.15 ± 0.10	234 ± 4 (7)	9.2 ± 0.4	3.93 ± 0.18[d]
110	423 ± 17[d] (6)	8.6 ± 0.3	2.04 ± 0.12	246 ± 3 (7)	10.2 ± 0.5[c]	4.20 ± 0.24[d]

[a] Mean ± SE
[b] Vaginal opening and the first ovulation occured between 35 and 40 days of age
[c] $P < 0.05$
[d] $P < 0.01$ between the sexes (number of rats in each group is in parentheses)

Table 2. Anterior pituitary gland (APG) and body wt. of immature male and female rats

Age (days)	Male [b]			Female [b]		
	Body wt. (g)	APG (mg)	APG (mg) 100 g^{-1} body wt.	Body wt. (g)	APG (mg)	APG (mg) 100 g^{-1} body wt.
7	17.16 ± 0.23[a]	0.72 ± 0.02	4.19 ± 0.10	16.31 ± 0.37	0.77 ± 0.02	4.73 ± 0.11[d]
15	36.32 ± 0.49[c]	1.40 ± 0.04	3.87 ± 0.10	34.83 ± 0.55	1.51 ± 0.04	4.33 ± 0.09[d]
23	64.67 ± 1.27	2.25 ± 0.05	3.48 ± 0.08	60.77 ± 1.44	2.55 ± 0.07	4.21 ± 0.09[d]

[a] Mean ± SE
[b] Each group consists of 22–23 rats
[c] $P < 0.05$ and
[d] $P < 0.01$ between the sexes. These rats are different from those used in Table 1. The results are not identical, but the trends are similar

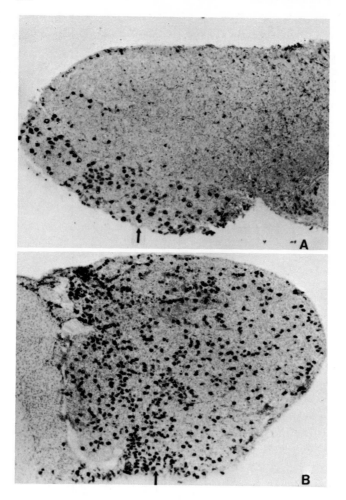

Fig. 1A,B. Photomicrographs of an entire half of the pars distalis in a section from a male rat (**A**) and a section from a female rat (**B**). Both sections were stained with anti-rat LH-S4. There are more cells in the anterior portion (*see arrow*) than the posterior portion in **A**, whereas the numbers of cells in both portions are roughly equal in **B** (× 65). Bar = 100 μm. (Dada et al. 1984a)

1985) of both sexes, virtually all FSH cells also contain LH, while the reverse is not true. The percentage of LH cells that also contained FSH was higher in adult male rats than in adult female rats (88.6 ± 3.3% vs 75.1 ± 1.7%), but such a sex difference was not observed in prepubertal rats (88.8 ± 2.0% for males vs. 84.8 ± 2.8% for females). The percentage of gonadotrophs that contain FSH may be controlled by the amount and pattern of LH releasing hormone (LHRH) released into the hypophyseal portal vessels. L.L. Garner in our laboratory has recently observed that SC administration of 1 μg LHRH twice daily for 7 days in adult male rats results in co-localisation of LH and FSH in virtually all gonadotrophs.

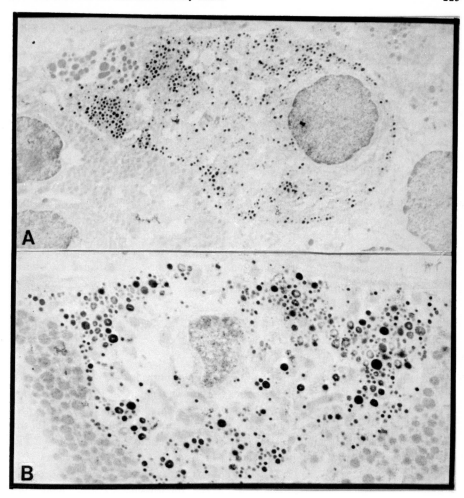

Fig. 2A,B. Electronmicrographs showing rat APG cells which stained immunocytochemically with anti-rat LHB. A Female LH cell (✕ 5,000). B Male LH cell (✕ 7,000)

The percentages of APG cells that contain LH and FSH cells are not different between young adult male and female rats (Dada et al. 1984a). The cells are usually polygonal or oval to polygonal in shape in both sexes (Blake 1980; Dada et al. 1983; Garner and Blake 1979, 1981), but the mean cross-sectional areas of gonadotrophs are bigger in adult male rats than in adult female rats ($104.2 \pm 5.9 \ \mu m^2$ vs. $81.2 \pm 3.2 \ \mu m^2$ for LH cells). The same is true for prepubertal rats ($101.8 \pm 4.8 \ \mu m^2$ vs $80.8 \pm 5.3 \ \mu m^2$ for LH cells).

There is also a sex difference in the distribution of gonadotrophs within the APG. In adult male rats (Dada et al. 1984a; Fig. 1) and in prepubertal male rats (M.O. Dada and C.A. Blake, unpublished observations), more gonadotrophs are located in the anterior portion of the APG than that which we observed in female rats of the same age. In the platyfish, the appearance of gonadotrophs in female rostral pars distalis antedates that in the male by about one year and in this position, the gonadotrophs are much more numerous in females than in males (Margolis-Kazan and Schreibman 1984).

Electron Microscopic Observations: It is possible to differentiate between male and female gonadotrophs at the ultrastructural level by marked differences in the populations of their secretion granules. In the female, almost all of the secretion granules are smaller than 200 nm in diameter (Garner and Blake 1981; Fig. 2). In contrast, the secretion granules in male gonadotrophs form two distinct populations, one which is similar to that seen in the female and a second population of larger granules which exceed 300 nm in diameter.

The large secretion granules may be testosterone dependent. Orchidectomy results within one day in a marked depletion of the large secretion granules. The presence of normal numbers of large secretion granules does not appear to be due to lack of negative feedback on gonadotrophin secretion per se. Maintenance of normal mean serum testosterone concentrations, by insertion of Silastic capsules containing testosterone, restores the population of large secretion granules in orchidectomized rats whereas oestrogen treatment does not. We are presently investigating whether or not testosterone capsules inserted into ovariectomized rats will stimulate the production of large secretion granules in female gonadotrophs.

3.2 Mammotrophs

A recent report suggests that a substantial number of individual APG cells can secrete both prolactin (PRL) and growth hormone (GH; Frawley and Neill 1983). Their observations were based on results found using reverse haemolytic plaque assays in vitro. However, it is unclear whether or not individual cells contain both PRL and GH in situ. Immunocytochemical staining of APG cells in tissue sections clearly shows that PRL and GH are stored in 2 morphologically distinct populations of cells (Nakane 1970; Dada et al. 1984b).

Using the classical ultrastructural criterion (i.e. the presence of large pleomorphic secretion granules), the percentages of PRL cells in the APG of female rats have been reported to be higher than those in male rats (Costoff 1973; Takahashi and Kawashima 1982). Nogami and Yoshimura (1982) showed with the use of alternate thick and thin sections that many cells in the APG of male rats that had small granules were immunoreactive with anti-PRL. The classical ultrastructural criterion, therefore, appears to be inadequate for the recognition of all PRL cells, at least in the male rat. Takahashi and Kawashima (1983) counted immunocytochemically (ICC) stained PRL cells from tissue sections directly and found lower percentages of PRL cells in male than in female rats. We found it impossible to count PRL cells directly using ICC-stained tissue and used an indirect method (Dada et al. 1984b). We calculated the percentages of PRL cells in the APG of adult male and female rats and found them to be similar. However, we observed the volume density of PRL cells in female rats to be significantly greater than that of PRL cells in male rats. This indicates that the PRL cells in female rats are bigger than those in male rats. No differences in the shape or distribution of PRL cells were observed between the sexes (Dada et al. 1984a).

Cyclic variation has been reported in the mitotic index of PRL cells of female rats, with the values in oestrus higher than those on other days of the oestrous cycle and those in male rats (Takahashi et al. 1984). There were no sex differences in mitotic index of PRL cells between male and female rats on other days of the oestrous cycle.

It is well known that old rats tend to develop spontaneous prolactinomas. The incidence is greater in female than in male rats (Trouillas et al. 1982) probably due to the tumorigenic activity of oestrogen (Clifton and Meyer 1956; Takahashi and Kawashima 1983).

3.3 Somatotrophs

In the rat and the mouse, immunocytochemically stained GH cells have been reported to be larger and more numerous in males than in females (Baker et al. 1969; Baker and Gross 1978; Gross 1980). However, these observations were not quantitative. In prepubertal rats (Dada et al. 1984c) and in adult rats (C.A. Blake, unpubl. observ.), we did not find any sex differences in the shape of GH cells, average cross-sectional area, volume density, or numerical density of GH cells, the percentage of APG cells which contain GH (Table 3), or the distribution of GH cells within the gland.

Table 3. Morphometric parameters observed in GH cells

	Prepubertal Rats[a]		Young Adult Rats[a]	
	Male, 40 days	Female, 35 days	Male, 85 days	Female, 85 days
Mean cross sectional area (μm^2)	65.6 ± 1.7	61.8 ± 1.6	54.1 ± 1.4[b]	52.7 ± 1.7
Volume density	26.8 ± 1.0	26.0 ± 1.5	22.6 ± 1.4	22.4 ± 1.1
Numerical density (no. of cells mm^{-3})	164.2 ± 7.7 × 10^3	174.6 ± 8.5 × 10^3	186.6 ± 14.4 × 10^3	173.7 ± 5.0 × 10^3
Percentage of GH cells in APG	26.9 ± 4.0	27.9 ± 3.6	22.7 ± 3.4	20.3 ± 1.7

[a] Each group consists of four rats
[b] Mean ± SE

No changes in any of the above parameters in GH cells were found 7 days after castration in either sex (C.A. Blake, unpubl. observ.). Five weeks after orchidectomy, Gross (1980) observed a reduction in the number and size of GH cells, and testosterone administration prevented this change. Five weeks after ovariectomy, he observed no consistent changes in the number and size of GH cells.

3.4 Thyrotrophs

The volume density of thyroid-stimulating hormone (TSH) cells and the percentage of APG cells that contain TSH are similar in adult male and female rats (Dada et al. 1984b). However, sex differences were observed in the percentages of APG cells which contain

TSH during post-natal development (Childs 1983; Childs et al. 1983). In both sexes, the percentages of TSH cells were higher in immature rats than in adults. In 15-day-old male rats, the percentage of TSH cells had decreased to adult levels (Childs 1983) but up to 22 days of age in female rats, the percentage of TSH cells remained twice the adult levels (Childs et al. 1983).

3.5 Corticotrophs

There appear to be no significant sexual differences in the size and numbers of adreno-corticotrophic hormones (ACTH) secreting cells in the APG of the rat (Dada et al. 1984b).

4 Physiology

4.1 Gonadotrophins

4.1.1 Pleomorphism in the Gonadotrophins

APG gonadotrophins are mixtures of various molecular species with different isoelectric points (Braselton and McShan 1970; Reichert 1971; Wakayabashi 1977). The various species of a particular hormone differ primarily in their carbohydrate moieties, particularly sialic acid (see Chappel et al. 1983, for review). Wakayabashi (1977) reported seven immunoreactive LH components in the rat APG. Differences existed in the relative amounts of some components between the sexes and between intact and castrated male rats. The biological activities of the components are directly proportional to the magnitude of their isoelectric points (Hattori et al. 1983). The female rat APG contained higher percentages of more bioactive LH components than did the APG of the intact male rat which in turn stored higher percentages of bioactive LH than the APG of the castrated male rat. It is therefore not surprising that the ratio of bioassay (BA; using testosterone production) values to radioimmunoassay (RIA) values for APG LH was in the following order: intact female rats > intact male rats > castrated male rats (Hattori et al. 1983).

In the rat, APG FSH is larger on gel chromatography in the male than in the female (Bogdanove et al. 1974b). APG FSH in orchidectomised rats is smaller and has a faster disappearance rate from the circulation compared to APG FSH in intact male rats. These changes were reversible by treatment with androgen (Bogdanove et al. 1974a,b). Blum and Gupta (1980) reported that the nature of pleomorphic forms of APG FSH as determined by gel chromatography was an age-dependent phenomenon in female but not in male rats. A "female type" of FSH observed on day 12 changed to a "male type" on day 17 and gradually reverted to the "female type" in the adult animal.

Using the human chorionic gonadotrophin BA for FSH (Steelman and Pohley 1953), Diebel et al. (1973) found the BA:RIA ratio of APG FSH to be higher in male than in female rats (a reverse of the situation for APG LH in the rat). It was also higher in testosterone-treated castrated male rats than in untreated male castrates. Interestingly, the ratio of radioreceptor assay (RRA; employing pregnant mare serum-treated immature rat ovaries) values to RIA values for serum FSH was reported to be greater in female than in male rats and was also greater in castrated male rats than in intact male rats (Minegishi et al. 1980). Since RRA is presumably closely related to BA, the results obtained from the pituitary FSH (Diebel et al. 1973) and the serum FSH (Minegishi et al. 1980) appear contradictory for reasons that are presently unclear. There is evidence, however, that there may be differences between the pituitary and serum forms of hormones at least in the rat (Campbell et al. 1978).

Sex differences in gonadotrophin pleomorphism also exist in primates. In the rhesus monkey, pituitary LH and FSH are larger on gel chromatography in the female than in the male (a reverse of the situation for FSH in rats; Peckam et al. 1973; Peckam and Knobil 1976a,b). In castrated monkeys of both sexes, the APG gonadotrophins are cleared less rapidly from the circulation compared to the APG gonadotrophins of intact animals (also a reverse of what occurs in rats). These castration-induced changes in female monkeys are reversible with oestrogen treatment (Peckam and Knobil 1976a).

The BA:RIA ratio for human serum LH is larger in men than in women and is higher in post-menopausal women and patients with Turner's syndrome than in cyclic women (Dufau et al. 1976). Similarly, the RRA:RIA ratio for human serum FSH is higher in men than in women, but it is lower in postmenopausal women than in cyclic women (Minegishi et al. 1982).

The sex differences in gonadotrophin pleomorphism thus have different patterns in different species, but in probably all species the gonadal steroid feedback plays an important role not only in the quantity, but also the quality of gonadotrophins synthesized and secreted by the APG (see Bogdanove et al. 1975, for review).

4.1.2 Gonadotrophin Content and Basal Release

In human foetuses, APG LH and FSH concentrations are higher in females than in males (Kaplan et al. 1976). In neonatal and juvenile rats, the APG concentrations and/or contents of LH and FSH are higher in female rats than in male rats; but in adult rats, these relationships are reversed (Lisk 1968; Dussault et al. 1977; Badger et al. 1982; Tables 4 and 5). In the period just before puberty, APG FSH concentrations are higher in male rats, but APG LH concentrations are similar in both sexes. In adult mice, APG contents of LH and FSH are higher in males (Cattanach et al. 1977) but in adult hamsters, APG LH concentrations are higher in males while APG FSH concentrations are similar in both sexes (Lamperti and Baldwin 1979; Lamperti and Blaha 1980).

The in vitro basal gonadotrophin release rates, especially those of FSH, tend to be higher in female rats than in male rats between 7 and 23 days after birth (Tables 4 and 5). Basal release is the release that is independent of the immediate presence of any hormones of non-APG origin (Elias and Blake 1981). Shortly prior to puberty and thereafter, the basal LH and FSH release rates are higher in male rats (Tables 4 and 5).

4.1.3 Serum Gonadotrophin Concentrations and Control of Gonadotrophin Secretion

Foetal Primates, Prepubertal Rats. In human and rhesus monkey foetuses serum gonadotrophin levels, particularly FSH levels, are higher in females (Kaplan et al. 1976; Ellinwood and Resko 1980). In female, but not in male rats, high levels of serum FSH are

Table 4. Anterior pituitary gland (APG) LH concentrations and contents and basal LH release rates in male and female rats of different ages

Age in days	APG LH: $(A; \mu g\ mg^{-1})$ and $(B; \mu g\ gland^{-1})$				Basal LH release rates: $(A; \mu g\ LH\ mg^{-1}\ 2\ h^{-1})$ and $(B; \mu g\ LH\ gland^{-1}\ 2\ h^{-1})$			
	Male		Female		Male		Female	
7 days	A	11.1 ± 2.3^{a}	A	26.7 ± 6.7	A	0.7 ± 0.1	A	1.2 ± 0.3
	B	8.5 ± 1.6	B	21.4 ± 6.3	B	0.5 ± 0.1	B	0.7 ± 0.2
		n = 6		n = 6		n = 6		n = 6
15 days	A	67.4 ± 21.0	A	117.7 ± 17.8^{c}	A	6.1 ± 0.9	A	8.8 ± 1.5
	B	71.5 ± 24.2	B	159.2 ± 27.2^{b}	B	6.4 ± 0.8	B	11.3 ± 1.7^{c}
		n = 5		n = 7		n = 13		n = 14
23 days	A	67.3 ± 15.5	A	152.0 ± 11.3^{c}	A	6.9 ± 1.4	A	9.4 ± 1.3
	B	93.9 ± 21.5	B	267.6 ± 19.4^{c}	B	11.6 ± 2.3	B	16.4 ± 2.3
		n = 7		n = 6		n = 14		n = 13
Prepubertal Male-40 days Female-35 days	A	30.6 ± 6.6	A	32.7 ± 3.3	A	8.5 ± 0.7^{c}	A	3.5 ± 0.9
	B	113.8 ± 21.6	B	101.5 ± 13.9	B	33.1 ± 4.2^{c}	B	10.4 ± 2.1
		n = 8		n = 8		n = 8		n = 8
Young adults 85 days	A	10.6 ± 0.9^{c}	A	5.2 ± 0.3	A	1.5 ± 0.1^{c}	A	0.9 ± 0.1
	B	79.1 ± 6.6^{c}	B	50.1 ± 3.2	B	12.3 ± 1.0^{c}	B	8.2 ± 0.8
		n = 16		n = 15		n = 16		n = 15

[a] Mean $\pm$ SE, [b] $P < 0.05$, and [c] $P < 0.01$ between the sexes, n = number of rats. Data from the young rats (7d, 15d, 23d), the peripubertal rats and the adult rats were obtained from 3 different radioimmunoassays and it would be invalid to make comparisons between data obtained from rats of different ages (i.e. vertical comparisons) except where such data were obtained from the same assay. The emphasis is on sex differences (i.e. horizontal comparisons)

observed during the second and third weeks of life. Serum LH levels are low throughout the postnatal period and are similar in both sexes (Ojeda and Ramirez 1972; Meijs-Roeloffs et al. 1975; Dussault et al. 1977; M.O. Dada, J.P. Metcalf, and C.A. Blake, unpublished observations). One reason that has been suggested for the sex differences in serum FSH levels in immature rats and foetal primates is that the FSH secretion in males is under the negative control of gonadal steroids at earlier ontogenetic stages compared to females (Ojeda and Ramirez 1972; Ellinwood and Resko 1980).

Shortly prior to puberty, serum LH levels are similar in rats of both sexes, but serum FSH levels are higher in male rats (M.O. Dada and C.A. Blake, unpubl. observ.).

Intact Adult Rats. Adult male rats release LH and FSH only in a tonic manner, but in adult female rats, both tonic and cyclic modes of release occur. In female rats, serum LH and FSH concentrations rise during the afternoon of proestrus and whereas serum LH concentrations fall during the evening of proestrus, serum FSH concentrations remain high until the morning of oestrus (see Blake 1983, for review). Serum LH levels in males are somewhat lower than non-surge LH levels in females, while serum FSH levels in males are higher than the non-surge FSH levels in females (Dada et al. 1983; D.R. Olson and C.A. Blake, unpubl. observ.).

Neonatally androgenized female rats are sterile as adults. They lack spontaneous cyclic preovulatory gonadotrophin surges and have persistent vaginal cornification.

Table 5. Anterior pituitary gland (APG) FSH concentrations and contents and basal FSH release rates in male and female rats of different ages

Age in days	APG FSH: $(A; \mu g\ mg^{-1})$ and $(B; \mu g\ gland^{-1})$		Basal FSH release rates: $(A; \mu g\ FSH\ mg^{-1}\ 2\ h^{-1})$ and $(B; \mu g\ FSH\ gland^{-1}\ 2\ h^{-1})$	
	Male	Female	Male	Female
7 days	A 5.3 ± 0.3 B 4.2 ± 0.5 n = 6	A 10.4 ± 1.4[c] B 8.0 ± 1.4[b] n = 6	A 0.9 ± 0.1 B 0.7 ± 0.2 n = 6	A 1.8 ± 0.3[c] B 1.1 ± 0.1 n = 6
15 days	A 14.7 ± 3.0 B 14.4 ± 3.5 n = 5	A 38.1 ± 3.5[c] B 51.5 ± 6.7[c] n = 6	A 5.6 ± 0.8 B 5.8 ± 0.8 n = 13	A 6.9 ± 0.9 B 8.9 ± 1.0[b] n = 14
23 days	A 15.7 ± 2.9 B 21.4 ± 3.7 n = 8	A 46.7 ± 6.6[c] B 79.7 ± 8.2[c] n = 6	A 4.8 ± 0.5 B 8.1 ± 1.2 n = 14	A 6.6 ± 0.9 B 11.4 ± 1.3 n = 12
Prepubertal Male-40 days Female-35 days	A 11.6 ± 0.8[c] B 44.9 ± 3.5[c] n = 8	A 3.9 ± 0.4 B 11.9 ± 0.9 n = 8	A 3.1 ± 0.4[c] B 12.9 ± 2.7[c] n = 8	A 1.0 ± 0.2 B 2.8 ± 0.5 n = 8
Young adults 85 days	A 10.3 ± 0.4[c] B 84.1 ± 3.2[c] n = 16	A 2.2 ± 0.1 B 21.4 ± 1.5 n = 15	A 1.2 ± 0.1[c] B 9.4 ± 0.5[c] n = 16	A 0.32 ± 0.03 B 3.1 ± 0.3 n = 15

[a] Mean ± SE, [b] P < 0.05, and [c] P < 0.01 between the sexes, n = number of rats. See legend to table 4 for further details

Conversely, male rats castrated during the neonatal period will exhibit cyclic patterns of gonadotrophin release as adults when grafted with ovarian tissue (see reviews by Gorski 1971; MacLusky and Naftolin 1981). Exposure of the brain to aromatisable androgens like testosterone in the early neonatal period appears to be a very important factor in the development of the male pattern of gonadotrophin release and in its absence the female pattern will develop. The results of several experiments (see Gorski 1971, for review) have suggested that the preoptic area (POA) of the rat regulates the cyclic gonadotrophin release while the arcuate region regulates the tonic release. There is evidence that the action of endogenous androgen in the male rat involves morphological alterations in the POA (see Gorski and Jacobson 1982, for review).

The LHRH neuronal system [the preoptico-suprachiasmatic-tuberoinfundibular system (PSTS)], functions as an integrated unit which synthesises, transports, stores, and ultimately releases LHRH (see Barraclough 1983, for review). The synthesis, transport, and storage of LHRH in the PSTS of androgen-sterilized female rats appears to be normal. Rather what appears to be lacking is the neural signal for the discharge of LHRH from the terminals in the median eminence (Lookingland et al. 1982). Considerable evidence suggests that the neural trigger for LHRH release in normal cyclic proestrous rats may be the discharge of norepinephrine into the vicinity of the LHRH system (see Barraclough 1983; Ramirez et al. 1984, for review).

Castrated Rats. After castration in adult rats, serum FSH levels rise rapidly in both sexes. Serum LH levels rise rapidly (within 8–12 h) in males, but do not rise in females until about 3 days and are not markedly elevated until about 3 weeks after ovariectomy (Savoy-Moore and Schwartz 1980; Garner and Blake 1981; Negro-Vilar et al. 1984; D.R. Olson and C.A. Blake, unpubl. observ.).

The reasons for the sex differences in the rate of the serum LH rise after castration are not clear. Genetic or developmental factors have been suggested (Gay and Hauger 1977) but neonatal androgenisation of female rats has been shown not to masculinize the post-castration LH response (Damassa et al. 1983). Another hypothesis is that "the last steroid seen by the hypothalamic-pituitary axis influences the LH response to castration" (Justo and Negro-Vilar 1979). In accordance with the latter hypothesis, some studies have shown that the nuclear retentions of oestradiol in the hypothalamus, the POA, and the APG are much more prolonged compared with testosterone retentions (reviewed in Negro-Vilar et al. 1984). This may account, at least in part, for the prolonged inhibition of LH release after ovariectomy.

Interestingly, the LH response to gonadectomy shifts from a masculine to a feminine type immediately after vaginal opening and the first ovulation (Lorenzen and Ramaley 1981). It is not clear whether the first oestradiol surge that precedes the first preovulatory LH surge is responsible for this shift. It is noteworthy that this sex difference in the rate of LH rise after castration is not seen in hamsters (Goldman and Porter 1970), a species in which oestrogen may not be absolutely necessary for inducing the proestrous gonadotrophin surge (Shander and Goldman 1978; Vomachka and Greenwald 1978).

Another sex difference in gonadotrophin secretion in castrated rats is the ability of oestradiol to induce LH surges in females (Caligaris et al. 1971; Neill 1972; Legan et al. 1975) but not in males (Neill 1972). Neonatally androgenized female rats have the male response while neonatally castrated male rats have the female response (Neill 1972). A retrochiasmatic cut in the hypothalamus prevents the oestrogen-induced LH surge in castrated female rats, suggesting that a site of oestrogenic action may be located rostrally in the hypothalamus. Unlike rodents, oestrogen-induced LH surges regularly occur in castrated male primates including men (seen Norman et al. 1983; Resko and Ellinwood 1984, for reviews). Also neonatally androgenized female rhesus monkeys ovulate, menstruate, and by deduction, have pre-ovulatory LH surges.

It is interesting to address the question "why is there no LH surge in the male". In primates the answer may be that the male does not have an ovary. In the rat, the answer appears to be largely in the exposure of the brain to androgens during the perinatal period.

4.1.4 LHRH and Pituitary Cyclic AMP Production

LHRH stimulates cyclic AMP (cAMP) production and LH release in hemi-APG's derived from adult male rats (Borgeat et al. 1972; Naor et al. 1975). In hemiglands derived from immature male rats or adult male rats that had been castrated for 10 days, LHRH induced LH release without a concomitant increase in pituitary cAMP levels. Testosterone administration to castrated male rats for 10 days restored the LHRH-induced pituitary cAMP increase (Naor et al. 1978, 1979). In hemi-APG's obtained from immature or proestrous female rats, LHRH was more effective in releasing LH compared to hemiglands derived from adult male rats, but without causing a parallel increase in gland cAMP levels (Naor et al. 1978). LHRH-induced cAMP production therefore appears to be androgen-dependent and therefore cAMP cannot be regarded as the second messenger for the LHRH action on LH release (see Naor 1982, for review).

4.1.5 5α-Reduction of Testosterone

It is well established that the APG like other androgen-sensitive tissues metabolizes testosterone into 5α-dihydrotestosterone (DHT) and subsequently into 3α-androstanediol (3α-DIOL). The 3β-isomer of androstanediol is formed in minute amounts. These conversions occur through an enzymatic complex that comprises a 5α-reductase and two (3α and 3β) hydroxysteroid dehydrogenases (see Martini 1982, for review).

At birth, there are no sex differences in the formation of DHT and 3α-DIOL by the rat APG. Between 10–15 days after birth, the formation of both metabolites is much higher in the APG of female rats than in those of male rats (Denef et al. 1974). APG's of adult male rats form 2.5 times more DHT and 1.5 times more 3α-DIOL than those of adult females (Denef et al. 1973). APG concentrations of DHT in adult male rats are 20% of those found in the adult prostate, and in contrast concentrations found in 10- to 15-day-old females exceed those found in the adult prostate (Denef et al. 1973, 1974). Castration at any age increased the DHT and 3α-DIOL formation in the APG of both sexes and also abolished sex differences (Denef et al. 1973, 1974). Neonatal androgenization did not affect the DHT formation in the APG of adult female rats (Denef et al. 1973). In the rat APG, DHT formation occurs primarily in gonadotrophs and the rate of 5α-reduction is proportional to the number and size of gonadotrophs (Denef 1979).

The results of several studies (reviewed in Denef 1983) suggest (1) that DHT and possibly 3α-DIOL are the active androgens which depress LH release in the gonadotroph and (2) DHT promotes the synthesis of FSH and at physiological LHRH concentrations, also its release. The latter suggestion may also explain why serum FSH levels in the 2nd and 3rd weeks after birth are higher in female rats than in male rats and why the reverse is observed in adult rats (Sect. 4.1.3).

4.1.6 Pituitary Cytosol Oestrogen Receptors

The affinity and concentrations of oestradiol-17β(E_2) receptors and the kinetics of interaction between E_2 and the receptors are similar in the APG of male and female rats (Korach and Muldoon 1972, 1974). Immature and gonadectomized adult rats of both sexes have values similar to those of intact adult rats (Korach and Muldoon 1974).

After the initial interaction between E_2 and its receptor, the hormone-receptor complex undergoes some transformation preparatory to its translocation to the nucleus. Cytosol receptors are depleted as a result of this nuclear translocation and are later replenished after several hours. The rate of cytosol receptor replenishment is always faster in the APG of adult male rats than that of adult female rats (Cidlowski and Muldoon 1976). This sex difference is not seen in immature rats and neonatally androgenized female rats have the male pattern of the receptor replenishment. Combined autoradiographic and immunocytochemical techniques have shown that all cell types in the APG of male and female rats show nuclear uptake of ^{3}H-oestradiol with the labelling density highest in gonadotrophs (Keefer 1981).

4.2 Prolactin

4.2.1 Pituitary Content and Basal Release

Rat APG concentration (K.A. Elias and C.A. Blake, unpubl. observ.) and content (Clayton and Bailey 1982) and mouse APG PRL content (Charlton et al. 1983) are higher in females than in males. This sex difference was not observed until puberty in mice (Charlton et al. 1983). There is evidence that oestrogens play an important role in this sex difference. Ovariectomy reduces the APG PRL content in mice and this reduction was prevented by sc implants of E_2. E_2 also increased the APG PRL content in normal male mice about 3.5-fold (Charlton et al. 1983). E_2 has been shown to increase ^{3}H-leucine incorporation into prolactin (Maurer and Gorski 1977) and to increase prolactin mRNA levels by increasing the transcription of the prolactin gene (Maurer 1982).

The in vitro basal PRL release rate/mg APG is higher in hemi-APG's derived from female rats than in those derived from male rats (K.A. Elias and C.A. Blake, unpubl. observ.).

4.2.2 Serum Prolactin Levels

In the adult male rat, PRL is released in a tonic acyclic fashion, while in the adult female rat, PRL is released in both a tonic and a cyclic manner. A prolactin surge occurs during the afternoon and evening of proestrus starting before the LH, FSH, and progesterone surges (Smith et al. 1975). Tonic levels of serum prolactin are similar in both sexes in the rat (Amenomori et al. 1970; Dohler and Wuttke 1975; Clayton and Bailey 1982) and in man (Frantz et al. 1972).

4.2.3 Regulation of Prolactin Secretion

Oestrogens. The stimulatory role of oestrogens in PRL secretion is well known. For example, the administration of antiserum to oestradiol to female rats on dioestrus day 2 blocks the PRL surge on proestrus (Neill et al. 1971). Oestrogen treatment of ovariectomized female rats for two days induces on the third day a serum PRL surge resembling the proestrous surge. Similar treatment of castrated male rats slightly increases the serum PRL levels, but does not induce a PRL surge (Neill 1972). Neonatally castrated male rats have PRL surges after oestrogen treatment and neonatally androgenized females do not have PRL surges, suggesting that androgenization of the hypothalamus is the basis of the sex difference. Furthermore, a retrochiasmatic hypothalamic cut prevents the oestrogen-induced PRL surges indicating that a site of oestrogen action may be in the rostral hypothalamus (Neill 1972).

Tranquilizing Agents and Pseudopregnancy. Brief treatment with reserpine (known to induce PRL secretion, Barraclough and Sawyer 1959) produces pseudopregnancy in female rats. Similar treatment of androgen-sterilized female rats or of castrated male rats bearing ovarian grafts (in which corpora lutea have been articially induced by human chorionic gonadotrophin) does not produce pseudopregnancy (corpus luteum function during an extended period; Zeilmaker 1963, 1964). This was interpreted to be due to a deficiency in prolactin secretion in the male rat because in castrated male rats bearing ovarian grafts, pituitary transplants under their kidney capsules will produce a pseudopregnancy (Zeilmaker 1963). The inability of the male rat to secrete enough prolactin to maintain a pseudopregnancy probably resides in the hypothalamus because male APG's transplanted under the median eminence of hypophysectomized females can support pseudopregnancy, pregnancy, and lactation (Harris and Jacobson 1952).

Dopamine and Hypothalamic Inhibitory Control. It is well established that in both sexes, the predominant hypothalamic influence on PRL secretion is inhibitory and that dopamine is a prolactin inhibitory factor (see Leong et al. 1983, for review). Female rats release more PRL in response to the removal of hypothalamic inhibition by median eminence lesions (Bishop et al. 1972) or to the blockade of dopaminergic receptors with pimozide than do male rats (Ojeda et al. 1977). These data suggest that the male APG is less responsive to dopamine compared to the female APG. Pituitary cells obtained from male rats are significantly less responsive to dopamine inhibition than those from pregnant and lactating female rats (Hoeffer et al. 1984) but unfortunately APG cells from non-pregnant, non-lactating female rats were not tested for dopamine inhibition in that study.

Neither neonatal androgenization nor neonatal orchidectomy affects the female or male response to pimozide (Ojeda et al. 1977). Injection of oestradiol benzoate (EB) to male rats increased PRL response to pimozide and ovariectomy reduced PRL response to pimozide. The sex difference in PRL response to blockade of dopaminergic receptors is not determined by neonatal androgenisation of the brain, but by the modulatory action of circulating oestrogen, probably at the pituitary level (Ojeda et al. 1977). Interestingly, the dopamine levels in hypophyseal stalk plasma are 2-6 times lower in male rats than in females (Ben-Jonathan et al. 1977), i.e., compared to the female rat, the male rat is less responsive to dopamine, and he is provided with less.

Thyrotrophin-Releasing Hormone (TRH). Prolactin response to injection of TRH is greater in women than in men (Frantz 1973) and in female rats than in male rats (Ojeda et al. 1977). Some investigators were in fact unable to demonstrate an increase in circulating PRL levels in male rats after injection of TRH (Valverde-R et al. 1972; Lu et al. 1972; C.A. Blake, unpubl. observ.).

Stress. PRL is one of the most responsive APG hormones to "stress". Human PRL response to the stress of major surgery and general anaesthesia is greater in women than in men (Noel et al. 1972).

Coitus. After sterile mating in rats, PRL is released daily in two large surges, a nocturnal surge and a diurnal surge. This goes on for 12-13 days and is characteristic of pseudopregnancy. This mating-induced PRL release is unique to female rats and does not even require male participation as vaginocervical stimulation with a glass rod will induce the PRL response (see Gunnet and Freeman 1983, for review). In humans, a significant rise in plasma PRL immediately after coitus has been noted in a limited number of women, all of whom experienced orgasm (Noel et al. 1972). Plasma PRL did not rise in their male partners. In women who did not experience orgasm, there was no change in plasma PRL. However, two women who had orgasm did not have any significant rise in plasma PRL.

Breast Stimulation. In normal menstruating women who are not lactating, breast stimulation produces a variable response. Some had little or no change in plasma PRL, others responded with a moderate rise of 2–3 times the basal levels, while a minority responded with a rise as high as that seen after suckling in lactating women (Noel et al. 1972; Frantz 1973). Breast stimulation in men regularly caused no change in plasma PRL levels.

Pup Presentation. Oestrogen-progesterone primed ovariectomized nulliparous female rats showed parental behaviour (after a latency of 2 days) when presented with pups that had just been suckled by a lactating rat. In addition, they showed prolactin surges that were comparable to those observed in lactating rats on pup presentation (Samuels and Bridges 1983). Similarly treated orchidectomized male rats showed parental behaviour (after a latency of 2 days) when presented with pups, but did not have an accompanying surge in PRL release. These data suggest a sex difference in the hormonal but not the behavioural responses to the young and may be indicative of sex differences in the hypothalamus-pituitary regulation of pup-induced PRL secretion (Samuels and Bridges 1983).

4.3 Growth Hormone

4.3.1 Pituitary Concentrations and Basal Release

APG GH concentrations and contents are higher in the adult male rat than in the adult female rat and this sex difference appears at puberty (Birge et al. 1967; C.A. Blake, unpubl. observ.). Similarly in prepubertal and young adult rats, the in vitro basal GH release rates are higher in male rats than in female rats (Dada et al. 1984c; Kaler et al. 1984; C.A. Blake, unpubl. observ.). Kaler et al. (1984) also observed that high potassium concentration in vitro caused a larger GH release from APG's derived from male rats than from APG's obtained from female rats, suggesting a larger releasable pool of GH in APG's of male rats.

Birge et al. (1967) reported oestrogen treatment of male rats to lower the APG GH concentration and testosterone treatment of female rats to increase the APG GH concentration. They also found castration of male rats to reduce the APG GH levels to those that were indistinguishable from pituitary GH levels of female rats. However, up to 35 days after castration, we did not observe any changes in the APG GH concentrations between castrated rats of either sex and the appropriate sham-castrated controls (C.A. Blake, unpubl. observ.).

4.3.2 Growth Hormone Release

The pulsatile release pattern of GH is sexually differentiated. In male rats, GH is released in regular pulses occurring at 3–4 h intervals, with low or undetectable levels between the peaks. In female rats, the peaks are lower and occur at shorter though more irregular intervals, but the levels between the peaks are higher compared to those in males (Saunders et al. 1976; Eden 1979; Millard et al. 1982). However, mean circulating GH levels are often similar between the sexes (Eden 1979; Mode et al. 1983).

Neonatal or prepubertal castration of male rats increases serum GH levels between the peaks and testosterone replacement therapy reverses this effect, indicating that a continuous presence of testosterone is important in maintaining low baseline serum GH levels in adult male rats (Millard et al. 1982; Jansson et al. 1984). Neonatal but not prepubertal castration decreased GH pulse height in male rats in adulthood, suggesting that neonatal androgenization of the brain is important in maintaining GH pulse amplitude in the adult male rat (Jansson et al. 1984). Neonatal castration does not, however, affect the 3-4 h periodicity of the GH pulses (Millard et al. 1982), suggesting that gonadal steroid environment during neonatal development or adulthood is not the sole determinant of GH release pattern in the male rat.

In female rats, neonatal androgenization has no effect on the pattern of the GH release (Millard et al. 1982). Neonatal gonadectomy of female rats, however, increases the GH pulse amplitude and decreases baseline GH levels, but the mean plasma levels are increased (Jansson et al. 1984). There is no information yet on the periodicity of the pulses after neonatal ovariectomy. Also, the effects of prepubertal ovariectomy and oestrogen replacement after neonatal ovariectomy on GH release pattern have not been reported.

Willoughby and Martin (1978) lesioned the medial preoptic area (MPOA; the source of somatostatin in the median eminence) in male rats and observed that the period between the GH pulses reduced from 3.63 ± 0.40 h to 2.11 ± 0.74 h ($P < 0.001$). It is not clear whether sex differences in the early MPOA maturation contributes to the sex differences that occur in the periodicity of GH pulses.

Female rat liver normally has higher concentrations of PRL receptors (Kelly et al. 1974), higher 5α-reductase activity and lower mixed-function oxidase activity (see Colby 1980, for review) than the male rat liver. Mode et al. (1982) have provided evidence to indicate that the sexually differentiated pattern of GH secretion may be responsible for the sex differences that exist in the hepatic steroid metabolism and the hepatic concentration of PRL receptors. Also, high pulses and lower baseline levels of plasma GH stimulate body growth more effectively than a constant level of the hormone (Jansson et al. 1982). This suggests that sex differences in the pattern of GH may also explain in part why male rats are bigger than female rats after puberty.

Recently, we castrated or sham-castrated male and female rats and decapitated them at different periods up to 35 days after surgery. Immediately after surgery the mean serum GH levels were depressed in castrated and sham-castrated rats of both sexes, presumably due to "stress". Whereas normal mean serum GH levels were later observed in sham-castrated rats of both sexes and in castrated male rats, castrated female rats continued to maintain low mean serum GH levels. Interestingly, APG GH concentrations and the in vitro basal GH release rates did not change throughout the study in either sex. This suggests that the gonads are important in maintaining normal mean circulating GH levels in female rats, but not in male rats (C.A. Blake, unpubl. observ.). However, we point out that the normal serum levels in castrated male rats do not necessarily imply that the pulsatile release patterns are unchanged after castration.

4.4 Thyroid-Stimulating Hormone

Plasma TSH concentrations in male rats are approximately twice as much as those in female rats (Rapp and Pyun 1974; Fukuda et al. 1975; Tonooka and Kobayashi 1980). This sex difference was not observed until after one month after birth (Fukuda et al. 1975). Circulating thyroxine (T_4) concentrations are also slightly but significantly higher in male rats than in female rats (Rapp and Pyun 1974; Fukuda et al. 1975), and in men more than in women (Kelstrup 1973). However, plasma triiodothyronine levels are higher in female rats than in male rats (Fukuda et al. 1975). Interestingly, Rapp and Pyun (1974) showed that there was no correlation between plasma TSH and T_4 levels in the rat.

Plasma corticosterone levels are higher in female rats than in male rats (Fukuda et al. 1975) and this may partly explain the sex differences observed in circulating TSH levels, because glucocorticoids have been shown to suppress pituitary TSH secretion presumably by inhibiting the release of the thyrotrophin releasing hormone (TRH; Wilber and Utiger 1969). Arguing against this explanation was the observation that adrenalectomy did not induce any significant changes in plasma TSH levels in female rats (Fukuda et al. 1975).

Women show a greater TSH response to TRH than men and this sex difference may be oestrogen-related since oestrogen administration to men enhances TSH response to TRH (see Scanlon et al. 1980, for review).

4.5 ACTH

We do not know of any studies that have addressed sex differences in circulating ACTH levels. In rats, plasma corticosterone levels are higher in females than in males (Fukuda et al. 1975). Also on subjection to stressful conditions, plasma corticosterone levels rose more rapidly in females than in males (Kant et al. 1983). In humans, there are no sex differences in circulating corticosteroid levels (Krieger et al. 1971). It is not clear whether these data indicate sex differences in ACTH levels in rats, but not in humans.

4.6 Substance P

The APG of adult male rats have higher concentrations of substance P-like immuno-reactivity (SP-LI) than those of adult female rats (DePalatis et al. 1982; Yoshikawa and Hong 1983b). Sex differences in APG levels of SP-LI were not observed in 15-day-old rats and castration of adult rats of either sex did not induce any changes in the APG SP-LI when compared to those of sham-castrated controls (DePalatis et al. 1982a). Similarly, treatment of female rats with DHT or male rats with oestradiol cypionate did not affect the APG levels of SP-LI (Yoshikawa and Hong 1983b). Neonatal gonadectomy (on day 1) resulted in a marked decrease of the SP-LI levels in adult males and this decrease was restored by neonatal testosterone replacement (days 2, 4, and 6) but not by androgen replacement in adulthood. Testosterone injection of neonatal female rats (days 2, 4, and 6) caused a significant increase in APG SP-LI concentrations after puberty (Yoshikawa and Hong 1983b). These results taken together indicate that the sex difference in APG SP-LI levels is not attributable to circulating gonadal hormones in adulthood but rather to neonatal exposure to testosterone.

Very recent evidence indicates that the SP-LI levels in the APG of adult male rats depend on their thyroid status. Thyroidectomy increases the gland SP-LI concentrations while the administration of T_4 reduces the SP-LI levels (Aronin et al. 1984). It is not clear at present how this relates to the sex difference in pituitary SP-LI levels. As mentioned in Sect. 4.4 plasma T_4 levels tend to be lower in female rats than in male rats, but plasma T_3 levels are higher in female rats (Fukuda et al. 1975; Tonooka and Kobayashi 1980).

In the rat, SP-LI has been localized immunocytochemically on gonadotrophs and lactotrophs (Morel et al. 1982) but in the guinea pig, SP-LI was localized almost exclusively on thyrotrophs (DePalatis et al. 1982b).

4.7 Endogenous Opioid-Peptides

4.7.1 β-Endorphin

Higher concentrations of APG β-endorphin-like immunoreactivity (βE-LI) have been reported in male rats than in female rats as determined by RIA (Hong et al. 1981). The antiserum used in that study also recognized β-lipotrophin and pro-opiomelanocortin, both of which are present in the APG. Sex differences in the APG βE concentrations were not evident in the study of Baizman and Cox (1978) who used RRA to measure βE levels. However, they reported that in both sexes the βE concentrations in the APG increased markedly at the onset of sexual maturity. βE has been localized in the ACTH cells of the APG (Li et al. 1979; Tramu and Beauvillain 1980; Dacheux 1981). If sex differences really do exist in the βE-LI levels in the rat APG our observations that the numbers and size of the ACTH cells are similar in both sexes (Dada et al. 1984b) would suggest that on the average individual ACTH cells in the male rat store more radioimmunoassayable βE compared to ACTH cells in female rats. The resting levels and stress-induced increase in serum βE concentrations are higher in male than in female rats and both are depressed by treating male rats with oestradiol benzoate (Mueller 1980).

4.7.2 The Enkephalins

Both methionine-enkephalin-like immunoreactivity (ME-LI) and leucine-enkephalin-like immunoreativitiy (LE-LI) levels are higher in the APG's of male rats than in those of female rats as determined by RIA (Hong et al. 1982a,b). The sex difference in the APG levels of ME-Li appeared shortly before puberty (day 35).

These sex differences may be due to a stimulatory action of androgen and an inhibitory action of oestrogen. Implantation of oestradiol-containing Silastic capsules into male rats for 3 weeks markedly reduced the ME-LI (by 81%) and LE-LI (by 67%) levels in the APG (Hong et al. 1982a). Similar treatment of female rats with dihydrotestosterone (DHT) increased the APG levels of ME-LI (Yoshikawa and Hong 1983a). Orchidectomy decreased APG levels of both ME-LI and LE-LI and these decreases were partially reversed by the administration of DHT. Ovariectomy induced increases in the APG levels of ME-LI and LE-LI and these elevations were completely prevented by oestradiol treatment (Yoshikawa and Hong 1983a).

Both ME-LI and LE-LI have been observed immunocytochemically in the APG of the guinea pig and the rat (Tramu and Leonardelli 1979). In both species immunoreactivity was found in the intermediate lobe, ACTH cells, and TSH cells. In the guinea pig, but not the rat, gonadotrophs were also immunoreactive with antisera to both enkephalins. Sex differences do not exist in the concentrations of ME-LI and LE-LI in the neuro-intermediate lobe (NIL) of the rat and castration or treatment with gonadal steroids has no effect on the levels of both enkephalins in the rat NIL (Hong et al. 1982a; Yoshikawa and Hong 1983a).

4.7.3 Dynorphin

There is a suggestion of sex differences in the concentration of dynorphin in the rat APG from the study of Goldstein and Ghazarossian (1980). The APG concentration of male rats (n = 5) was 42.4 ± 5.4 pmol g^{-1} (mean $\pm$ SE), while the concentration in pooled tissues from 6 female rats was 13.5 pmol g^{-1}.

5 Concluding Remarks

Although this review is by no means exhaustive, a wide variety of sex differences in the APG of the rat have been cited. The mechanisms responsible for some of the sex differences are yet unknown. Some sex differences (e.g. cyclic gonadotrophin release, oestrogen-induced PRL surges, APG levels of Substance P) are to a large extent due to whether or not steroids act on the brain very early in life. Other sex differences (e.g. large secretion granules in gonadotrophin, and APG enkephalin concentrations) appear to be modulated by circulating gonadal steroids in adult life.

Acknowledgements. Experiments conducted in the authors' laboratories were supported by grants from the NIH (HD 11011 and 13219) and the College of Medicine, University of Lagos, Lagos, Nigeria.

References

Amenomori Y, Chen CL, Meites J (1970) Serum prolactin levels in rats during different reproductive states. Endocrinology 86:506–510

Aronin N, Morency K, Leeman SE, Braverman LE, Coslovsky R (1984) Regulation by thyroid hormone of the concentration of substance P in the rat anterior pituitary. Endocrinology 114: 2138–2142

Badger TM, Millard WJ, Martin JB, Rosenblum PM, Levenson SE (1982) Hypothalamic-pituitary function in adult rats treated neonatally with monosodium glutamate. Endocrinology 111: 2031–2038

Baizman ER, Cox BM (1978) Endorphin in rat pituitary glands: its distribution within the gland and age related changes in gland content in male and female rats. Life Sci 22:519–526

Baker BL, Gross DS (1978) Cytology and distribution of secretory cell types in the mouse hypophysis as demonstrated with immunocytochemistry. Am J Anat 153:193–216

Baker BL, Midgley AR Jr, Gerstein BE, Yu YY (1969) Differentiation of growth hormone- and prolactin-containing acidophils with peroxidase-labeled antibody. Anat Rec 164:163–172

Barraclough CA (1983) The role of catecholamines in the regulation of gonadotropin secretion. Acta Morphol Acad Sci Hung 31:101–116

Barraclough CA, Sawyer CH (1959) Induction of pseudopregnancy in the rat by reserpine and chlorpromazine. Endocrinology 65:563–571

Ben-Jonathan M, Oliver C, Weiner HJ, Mical RS, Porter JC (1977) Dopamine in hypophysial portal plasma of the rat during the estrous cycle and throughout pregnancy. Endocrinology 101:452–458

Birge CA, Peake GT, Mariz IK, Daughaday WH (1967) Radioimmunoassayable growth hormone in the rat pituitary gland: effects of age, sex and hormonal state. Endocrinology 81:195–204

Bishop W, Fawcett CP, Krulich L, McCann SM (1972) Acute and chronic effects of hypothalamic lesions on the release of FSH, LH, and prolactin in intact and castrated rats. Endocrinology 91: 643–656

Blake CA (1980) Correlative study of changes in the morphology of the LH gonadotroph and anterior pituitary gland LH secretion during the 4-day rat estrous cycle. Biol Reprod 23:1097–1108

Blake CA (1983) Anterior pituitary gland FSH secretion during the rat estrous cycle: control mechanisms which result in parallelism and nonparallelism in serum FSH and LH concentrations. In: Bhatnagar AS (ed) The anterior pituitary gland. Raven, New York, pp 227–237

Blum W, Gupta D (1980) Age and sex-dependent nature of polymorphic forms of rat pituitary FSH: the role of glycosylation. Neuroendocrinol Lett 2:357–365

Bogdanove EM, Campbell GT, Blair ED, Mula ME, Miller AE, Grossman GH (1974a) Gonad-pituitary feedback involves qualitative change: androgens alter the type of FSH secreted by the rat pituitary. Endocrinology 95:219–228

Bogdanove EM, Campbell GT, Peckam WD (1974b) FSH pleomorphism in the rat – regulation by gonadal steroids. Endocr Res Commun 1:87–99

Bogdanove EM, Nolin JM, Campbell GT (1975) Qualitative and quantitative gonad-pituitary feedback. Recent Prog Horm Res 31:567–619

Borgeat P, Chavancy G, Dupont A, Labrie F, Arimura A, Schally AV (1972) Stimulation of adenosine 3′:5′-cyclic monophosphate accumulation in anterior pituitary gland in vitro by synthetic luteinizing hormone-releasing hormone. Proc Natl Acad Sci USA 69:2677–2681

Braselton WE, McShan WH (1970) Purification and properties of follicle-stimulating and luteinizing hormones from horse pituitary glands. Arch Biochem Biophys 139:45–88

Caligaris L, Astrada JJ, Taleisnik S (1971) Release of luteinizing hormone induced by oestrogen injection into ovariectomized rats. Endocrinology 88:810–815

Campbell GT, Blair ED, Grossman GH, Miller AE, Small ME, Bogdanove EM (1978) Distribution and disappearance of radioimmunoassayable circulating luteinizing hormone in the rat: an apparent difference between stored and released forms of the hormone. Endocrinology 103: 674–682

Cattanach BM, Iddon CA, Charlton HM, Chappa SA, Fink G (1977) Gonadotrophin-releasing hormone deficiency in a mutant mouse with hypogonadism. Nature (Lond) 269:338–340

Chappel SC, Ulloa-Aguirre A, Coutifaris C (1983) Biosynthesis and secretion of follicle-stimulating hormone. Endocr Rev 4:179–211

Charlton HM, Speight A, Halpin DMG, Bramwell A, Sheward WJ, Fink G (1983) Prolactin measurements in normal and hypogonadal (hpg) mice: developmental and experimental studies. Endocrinology 113:545–548

Childs GV (1983) Neonatal development of the thyrotrope in the male rat pituitary. Endocrinology 112:1647–1652

Childs GV, Hyde C, Naor Z (1983) Morphometric analysis of thyrotropes in developing and cycling female rats: studies of intact pituitaries and cell fractions separated by centrifugal elutriation. Endocrinology 113:1601–1607

Cidlowski JA, Muldoon TG (1976) Sex-related differences in the regulation of cytoplasmic estrogen receptor levels in responsive tissues of the rat. Endocrinology 98:833–841

Clayton RN, Bailey LC (1982) Hyperprolactinaemia attenuates the gonadotrophin releasing hormone receptor response to gonadectomy in rats. J Endocrinol 95:267–274

Clifton KH, Meyer RK (1956) Mechanism of anterior pituitary tumor induction by estrogen. Acta Anat 125:65–81

Colby HD (1980) Regulation of hepatic drug and steroid metabolism by androgens and estrogens. In: Thomas JA, Singhal RL (eds) Advances in sex hormone research, vol 4. Urban and Schwarzenberg, Baltimore, pp 27–73

Costoff A (1973) Ultrastructure of rat adenohypophyses: correlation with function. Academic, New York, pp 130–146

Dacheux F (1981) Ultrastructural localization of corticotropin, β-lipotropin, and α- and β-endorphin in the porcine pituitary. Cell Tissue Res 215:87–101

Dada MO, Blake CA (1984) Administration of monosodium glutamate to neonatal male rats: alterations in the gonadotrophs and in gonadotrophin secretion. Neuroendocrinology 38:490–497

Dada MO, Blake CA (1985) Monosodium L-glutamate administration: effects on gonadotrophin secretion, gonadotrophs and mammotrophs in prepubertal female rats. J Endocrinol 104:185–192

Dada MO, Campbell GT, Blake CA (1983) A quantitative immunocytochemical study of the luteinizing hormone and follicle-stimulating hormone cells in the adenohypophysis of adult male rats and adult female rats throughout the estrous cycle. Endocrinology 113:970–984

Dada MO, Campbell GT, Blake CA (1984a) The localization of gonadotrophs in normal adult male and female rats. Endocrinology 114:397–406

Dada MO, Campbell GT, Blake CA (1984b) Pars distalis cell quantification in normal adult male and female rats. J Endocrinol 101:87–94

Dada MO, Campbell GT, Blake CA (1984c) Effects of neonatal administration of monosodium glutamate on somatotrophs and growth hormone secretion in prepubertal male and female rats. Endocrinology 115:996–1003

Damassa DA, Rabii J, Sawyer CH (1983) Responses of serum LH and FSH to the removal of steroid feedback inhibition: effects of neonatal androgen sterilization and of anterior hypothalamic deafferentiation. Neuroendocrinology 37:122–130

Denef C (1979) Evidence that pituitary 5α-dihydrotestosterone formation is regulated through changes in the proportional number and size of gonadotrophic cells. Neuroendocrinology 29:132–139

Denef C (1983) 5α-dihydrotestosterone formation and its functional significance in rat anterior pituitary, subpopulations of gonadotrophs and cell cultures. J Steroid Biochem 19:235–239

Denef C, Magnus C, McEwen BS (1973) Sex differences and hormonal control of testosterone metabolism in rat pituitary and brain. J Endocrinol 59:605–621

Denef C, Magnus C, McEwen BS (1974) Sex-dependent changes in pituitary 5α-dihydrotestosterone and 3α-androstanediol formation during postnatal development and puberty in the rat. Endocrinology 94:1265–1274

DePalatis LR, Negro-Vilar A, McCann SM (1982a) Age and sex related changes of substance P-like immunoreactivity in the anterior pituitary gland of the rat. Fed Proc 41:1353 (abstract)

DePalatis LR, Fiorindo RP, Ho RH (1982b) Substance P immunoreactivity in the anterior pituitary gland of the guinea pig. Endocrinology 110:282–284

Diebel ND, Yamamoto M, Bogdanove EM (1973) Discrepancies between radioimmunoassays and bioassays for rat FSH: evidence that androgen treatment and withdrawal can alter bioassay-immunoassay ratios. Endocrinology 92:1065–1078

Dohler KD, Wuttke W (1975) Changes with age in levels of serum gonadotropins, prolactin and gonadal steroids in prepubertal male and female rats. Endocrinology 97:898–907

Dufau ML, Rock P, Neubauer A, Catt KJ (1976) In vitro bioassay of LH in human serum: the rat interstitial cell testosterone (RICT) assay. J Clin Endocrinol Metab 42:958–969

Dussault JH, Walker P, Dubois JD, Labrie F (1977) The development of the hypothalamo-pituitary axis in the neonatal rat: sexual maturation in male and female rats as assessed by hypothalamic LHRH and pituitary and serum LH and FSH concentrations. Can J Physiol Pharmacol 55:1091–1097

Eden S (1979) Age- and sex-related differences in episodic growth hormone secretion in the rat. Endocrinology 105:555–560

Elias KA, Blake CA (1981) A detailed in vitro characterization of the basal follicle-stimulating hormone and luteinizing hormone secretion rates during the rat four-day estrous cycle. Endocrinology 109:708–713

Ellinwood WE, Resko JA (1980) Sex differences in biologically active and immunoreactive gonadotropins in the fetal circulation of rhesus monkeys. Endocrinology 107:902–907

Frantz AG (1973) The regulation of prolactin secretion in humans. In: Ganong WF, Martini L (eds) Frontiers in neuroendocrinology. Oxford University Press, London, pp 337–374

Frantz AG, Kleinberg DL, Noel GL (1972) Studies on prolactin in man. In: Pincus G (ed) Recent progress in hormone research, vol 28. Academic, New York, pp 527–573

Frawley LS, Neill JD (1983) Identification of a pituitary cell type that secretes both growth hormone and prolactin: detection by reverse hemolytic plaque assays. Program of the Endocrine Society, 65th annual meeting, abstract No 918

Fukuda H, Greer MA, Roberts L, Allen CF, Critchlow V, Wilson M (1975) Nyctohemeral and sex-related variations in plasma thyrotropin, thyroxine and triiodothyronine. Endocrinology 97: 1424–1431

Garner LL, Blake CA (1979) Morphological correlates for LHRH self-priming and anterior pituitary gland refractoriness to LHRH in proestrous rats: an immunocytochemical study. Biol Reprod 20:1055–1066

Garner LL, Blake CA (1981) Ultrastructural, immunocytochemical study of the LH secreting cell of the rat anterior pituitary gland: changes occurring after ovariectomy. Biol Reprod 24:461–474

Gay VL, Hauger RL (1977) A sex-related pattern of gonadotropin secretion in the castrated rat: effects of changing the inhibitory steroid on pituitary LH content. Biol Reprod 16:527–535

Girod C (1984) Fine structure of the pituitary pars distalis. In: Motta PM (ed) Ultrastructure of endocrine cells and tissues. Martinus Nijhoff, Boston, pp 12–28

Goldman BD, Porter JC (1970) Serum LH levels in intact and castrated golden hamsters. Endocrinology 87:676–679

Goldstein A, Ghazarossian VE (1980) Immunoreactive dynorphin in pituitary and brain. Proc Natl Acad Sci USA 77:6207–6210

Gorski RA (1971) Gonadal hormones and the perinatal development of neuroendocrine function. In: Martini L, Ganong WF (eds) Frontiers in neuroendocrinology. Oxford University Press, London, pp 237–290

Gorski RA, Jacobson CD (1982) Sexual differentiation of the brain. Front Horm Res 10:1–14

Gross DS (1980) Role of somatostatin in the modulation of hypophysial growth hormone production by gonadal steroids. Am J Anat 158:507–519

Gunnet JW, Freeman ME (1983) The mating-induced release of prolactin: a unique neuroendocrine response. Endocr Rev 4:44–61

Harris GW, Jacobson D (1952) Functional grafts of the anterior pituitary gland. Proc R Soc Lond Biol Sci 139:263–276

Hattori M, Sakamoto K, Wakayabashi K (1983) The presence of LH components having different ratios of bioactivity to immunoreactivity in the rat pituitary glands. Endocrinol Jpn 30:289–296

Hoeffer MT, Herman ML, Ben-Jonathan N (1984) Prolactin secretion by cultured anterior pituitary cells: influence of culture conditions and endocrine status of the pituitary donor. Mol Cell Endocr 35:229–235

Hong JS, Lowe C, Squibb RE, Lamartinere CA (1981) Monosodium glutamate exposure in the neonate alters hypothalamic and pituitary neuropeptide levels in the adult. Regul Pept 2:347–352

Hong JS, Yoshikawa K, Hudson PM, Uphouse LL (1982a) Regulation of pituitary and brain enkephalin systems by estrogen. Life Sci 31:2181–2184

Hong JS, Yoshikawa K, Lamartiniere CA (1982b) Sex-related difference in the rat pituitary (Met5)-enkephalin level-altered by gonadectomy. Brain Res 251:380–383

Jansson J-O, Albertson-Wikland K, Eden S, Thorngren K-G, Isaksson G (1982) Circumstantial evidence for a role of the secretory pattern of growth hormone in control of body growth. Acta Endocrinol 99:24–30

Jansson J-O, Ekberg S, Isaksson OGP, Eden S (1984) Influence of gonadal steroids of age- and sex-related secretory patterns of growth hormone in the rat. Endocrinology 114:1287–1294

Justo SN, Negro-Vilar A (1979) A female-like rise in luteinizing hormone and follicle-stimulating hormone after gonadectomy in male rats induced by oestradiol pretreatment. J Endocrinol 80: 111–116

Kaler LW, Dyke A, Critchlow V (1984) Release of somatostatin (SRIF) and growth hormone (GH) during perifusion of the preoptic-hypothalamus (PO-HTH) and anterior pituitary (AP) in male and female rats. Anat Rec 208:86A (abstract)

Kant GJ, Lenox RH, Bunnell BN, Mougey EH, Pennington LL, Meyerhoff JL (1983) Comparison of stress response in male and female rats: pituitary cyclic AMP and plasma prolactin, growth hormone and corticosterone. Psychoneuroendocrinology 8:421–428

Kaplan SL, Grumbach MM, Aubert ML (1976) The ontogenesis of pituitary hormones, hypothalamic factors in the human fetus: maturation of central nervous system regulation of anterior pituitary function. Recent Prog Horm Res 32:161–243

Keefer DA (1981) Induction by progesterone of a sexual dimorphism of estrogen uptake by anterior pituitary cells in situ. Cell Tissue Res 215:75–86

Kelly PA, Posner BI, Tsushima T, Friesen HG (1974) Studies of insulin, growth hormone and prolactin binding: ontogenesis, effects of sex and pregnancy. Endocrinology 95:532–539

Kelstrup J (1973) Free and total thyroxine in serum: ranges and sex differences for selected normals, patients with thyroid disease, and pregnant women. Scand J Clin Lab Invest 32:227–231

Korach KS, Muldoon TG (1972) Comparison of specific 17β-estradiol-receptor interactions in the anterior pituitary of male and female rats. Endocrinology 92:322–326

Korach KS, Muldoon TG (1974) Characterization of the interaction between 17β-estradiol and its cytoplasmic receptor in the rat anterior pituitary gland. Biochemistry 13:1932–1938

Krieger DT, Allen W, Rizzo F, Krieger HP (1971) Characterization of the normal temporal plasma corticosteroid levels. J Clin Endocrinol Metab 32:266–284

Lamperti A, Baldwin DA (1979) The effects of gonadal steroids on gonadotropin secretion in hamsters with a lesion of the arcuate nucleus of the hypothalamus. Endocrinology 104:1041–1045

Lamperti A, Blaha G (1980) Further observations on effects of neonatally administered monosodium glutamate on the reproductive axis of hamsters. Biol Reprod 22:687–693

Legan SJ, Coon GA, Karsch FJ (1975) Role of estrogen as initiator of daily LH surges in the ovariectomized rat. Endocrinology 96:50–56

Leong DA, Frawley LS, Neill JD (1983) Neuroendocrine control of prolactin secretion. Annu Rev Physiol 45:109–127

Li JY, Dubois MP, Dubois PM (1979) Ultrastructural localization of immunoreactive corticotropin, β-lipotropin, α- and β-endorphin in cells of human fetal anterior pituitary. Cell Tissue Res 204:37–51

Lisk RD (1968) Luteinizing hormone in the pituitary gland of the albino rat: concentration and content as a function of sex and age. Neuroendocrinology 3:18–24

Lisk RD (1969) Estrogen: direct effects on hypothalamus or pituitary in relation to pituitary weight changes. Neuroendocrinology 4:368–373

Lloyd HM, Meares JD, Jacobi J (1973) Early effects of stilboestrol on growth hormone and prolactin secretion and on pituitary mitotic activity in the male rat. J Endocrinol 58:227–231

Lookingland KJ, Wise PM, Barraclough CA (1982) Failure of the hypothalamic noradrenergic system to function in adult androgen-sterilized rats. Biol Reprod 3:18–24

Lorenzen JR, Ramaley JA (1981) Ontogeny of sex differences in LH and FSH levels 48 h after castration in the rat. Am J Physiol 241:E460–E464

Lu K-H, Shaar CJ, Kortright KH, Meites J (1972) Effects of synthetic TRH on in vitro and in vivo prolactin release in rat. Endocrinology 91:1540–1545

MacLusky NJ, Naftolin F (1981) Sexual differentiation of the central nervous system. Science (Wash DC) 211:1294–1303

Margolis-Kazan H, Schreibman MP (1984) Sexually dimorphic age-related changes in pituitary gonadotrope distribution. Mech Ageing Dev 24:325–333

Martini L (1982) The 5α-reduction of testosterone in the neuroendocrine structures. Biochemical and physiological implications. Endocr Rev 3:1–25

Maurer RA (1982) Estradiol regulates the transcription of the prolactin gene. J Biol Chem 257:2133–2136

Maurer RA, Gorski J (1977) Effects of estradiol-17β and pimozide on prolactin synthesis in male and female rats. Endocrinology 101:76–84

Meijs-Roelofs HMA, DeGreef WJ, Uilenbroek JThJ (1975) Plasma progesterone and its relationship to serum gonadotrophins in immature female rats. J Endocrinol 64:329–336

Millard WJ, Martin JB, Fox TO (1982) Analysis of sexually dimorphic patterns of growth hormone secretion in rats: effects of gonadal steroids during the neonatal period. Program of the endocrine society, 64th annual meeting, abstract No 982

Minegishi T, Igarashi M, Wakayabashi K (1980) Measurement of rat serum FSH by radioreceptor assay and comparison with radioimmunoassay. Endocrinol Jpn 27:717−725

Minegishi T, Igarashi M, Wakayabashi K (1982) Measurement of human FSH by radioreceptor assay. Endocrinol Jpn 29:233−240

Mode A, Gustafsson J-A, Jansson J-O, Eden S, Isaksson O (1982) Association between plasma level of growth hormone and sex differentiation of hepatic steroid metabolism in the rat. Endocrinology 111:1692−1697

Mode A, Norstedt G, Eneroth P, Gustafsson J-A (1983) Purification of liver feminizing factor from rat pituitaries and demonstration of its identity with growth hormone. Endocrinology 113:1250−1260

Morel G, Chayvialle JA, Kerdelhue B, Dubois PM (1982) Ultrastructural evidence for endogenous substance-P-like immunoreactivity in the rat pituitary gland. Neuroendocrinology 35:86−92

Mueller GP (1980) Attenuated pituitary β-endorphin release in estrogen-treated rats. Proc Soc Exp Biol Med 165:75−81

Nakane PK (1970) Classification of anterior pituitary cell types with immunoenzyme histochemistry. J Histochem Cytochem 18:9−20

Naor Z (1982) Cyclic nucleotide production and hormonal control of anterior pituitary cells. INSERM 110:395−418

Naor Z, Koch Y, Chobsieng P, Zor U (1975) Pituitary cyclic AMP production and mechanism of luteinizing hormone release. FEBS Lett 58:318−321

Naor Z, Zor U, Meidan R, Koch Y (1978) Sex difference in pituitary cyclic AMP response to gonadotropin-releasing hormone. Am J Physiol 235:E37−E41

Naor Z, Fawcett CP, McCann SM (1979) Differential effects of castration and testosterone replacement on basal and LHRH-stimulated cAMP and cGMP accumulation and on gonadotropin release from the pituitary of the male rat. Mol Cell Endocr 14:191−198

Negro-Vilar A, Tesone M, Johnston CA, DePaolo L, Justo SN (1984) Sex differences in regulation on gonadotropin secretion: involvement of central monoaminergic and peptidergic systems and brain steroid receptors. In: Serio M, Motto M, Zanisi M, Martini L (eds) Sexual differentiation: basic and clinical aspects. Raven, New York, pp 107−118

Neill JD (1972) Sexual differences in the hypothalamic regulation of prolactin secretion. Endocrinology 90:1154−1159

Neill JD, Freeman ME, Tillson SA (1971) Control of proestrus surge of prolactin and luteinizing hormone secretions by estrogens in the rat. Endocrinology 89:1448−1453

Noel GL, Suh HK, Stone JG, Frantz AG (1972) Human prolactin and growth hormone release during surgery and other conditions of stress. J Clin Endocrinol Metab 35:840−851

Nogami H, Yoshimura F (1982) Fine structural criteria of prolactin cells identified immunohistochemically in the male rat. Anat Rec 202:261−274

Norman RL, Levine JE, Spies HG (1983) Control of gonadotropin secretion in primates: observations in stalk-sectioned rhesus macaques. In: Norman RL (ed) Neuroendocrine aspects of reproduction. Academic, New York, pp 263−284

Ojeda SR, Ramirez VD (1972) Plasma level of LH and FSH in maturing rats: response to gonadectomy. Endocrinology 90:466−472

Ojeda SR, Castro-Vazquez A, Jameson HE (1977) Prolactin release in response to blockade of dopaminergic receptors and to TRH injection in developing and adult rats: role of estrogen in determining sex difference. Endocrinology 100:427−439

Peckam WD, Knobil E (1976a) The effects of ovariectomy, estrogen replacement and neuraminidase treatment on the properties of the adenohypophysial glycoprotein hormones of the rhesus monkey. Endocrinology 98:1054−1060

Peckam WD, Knobil E (1976b) Qualitative changes in the pituitary gonadotropins of the male rhesus monkey following castration. Endocrinology 98:1061−1064

Peckam WD, Yamaji T, Dierschke DJ, Knobil E (1973) Gonadal function and the biological and physiochemical properties of follicle-stimulating hormone. Endocrinology 92:1660−1666

Ramirez VD, Feder HH, Sawyer CH (1984) The role of brain catecholamines in the regulation of the LH secretion: a critical inquiry. In: Martini L, Ganong WF (eds) Frontiers in neuroendocrinology, vol 8, pp 27–84

Rapp JP, Pyun LL (1974) A sex difference in plasma thyroxine and thyroid stimulating hormone in rats. Proc Soc Exp Biol Med 146:1021–1023

Reichert LE Jr (1971) Electrophoretic properties of pituitary gonadotrophs as studied by electrofocusing. Endocrinology 88:1029–1044

Resko JA, Ellinwood WE (1984) Sexual differentiation of the brain of primates. In: Serio M, Motta M, Zanisi M, Martini L (eds) Sexual differentiation: basic and clinical aspects. Raven, New York, pp 169–181

Samuels MH, Bridges RS (1983) Plasma prolactin concentrations in parental male and female rats: effects of exposure to rat young. Endocrinology 113:1647–1654

Saunders A, Terry LC, Audet J, Brazeau P, Martin JB (1976) Dynamic studies of growth hormone and prolactin secretion in the female rat. Neuroendocrinology 21:193–203

Savoy-Moore RT, Schwartz NB (1980) Differential control of FSH and LH secretion. In: Greep RO (ed) Reproductive physiology III. International review of physiology, vol 22. University Park Press, Baltimore, pp 203–248

Scanlon MF, Lewis M, Weightman DR, Chan V, Hall R (1980) The neuroregulation of human thyrotropin secretion. In: Martini L, Ganong WF (eds) Frontiers in neuroendocrinology, vol 6. Raven, New York, pp 333–380

Shander D, Goldman B (1978) Ovarian steroid modulation of gonadotropin secretion and pituitary responsiveness to luteinizing hormone-releasing hormone in the female hamster. Endocrinology 103:1383–1393

Smith MS, Freeman ME, Neill JD (1975) The control of progesterone secretion during the estrous cycle and early pseudopregnancy in the rat: prolactin, gonadotropin and steroid levels associated with rescue of the corpus luteum of pseudopregnancy. Endocrinology 96:219–226

Steelman SL, Pohley FM (1953) Assay of the follicle stimulating hormone based on the augmentation with human chorionic gonadotrophin. Endocrinology 53:604–616

Takahashi S, Kawashima S (1981) Responsiveness to estrogen of pituitary glands and prolactin cells in gonadectomized male and female rats. Annot Zool Jpn 54:73–84

Takahashi S, Kawashima S (1982) Age-related changes in prolactin cell percentage and serum prolactin levels in intact and neonatally gonadectomized male and female rats. Acta Anat 113:211–217

Takahashi S, Kawashima S (1983) Age-related changes in prolactin cells in male and female rats of the Wistar/TW strain. J Sci Hiroshima Univ Ser B 31:185–191

Takahashi S, Okazaki K, Kawashima S (1984) Mitotic activity of prolactin cells in the pituitary glands of male and female rats of different ages. Cell Tissue Res 235:497–502

Tonooka N, Kobayashi S (1980) Effect of propylthiouracil on nycthemeral and sex related variation on plasma TSH in rats. Endocrinol Jpn 27:27–32

Tramu G, Beauvillain JC (1980) Pituitary polypeptide-secreting cells: immunocytochemical identification of ACTH, MSH and peptides related to LPH. In: Justisz M, McKerne KW (eds) Synthesis and release of adenohypophyseal hormones. Plenum, New York, pp 39–66

Tramu G, Leonardelli J (1979) Immunohistochemical localization of enkephalins in median eminence and adenohypophysis. Brain Res 168:457–471

Trouillas J, Girod C, Claustrat B, Cure M, Dubois MP (1982) Spontaneous pituitary tumors in the Wistar/Furth/ICo rat strain. Am J Pathol 109:57–70

Valverde-R C, Chieffo V, Reichlin S (1972) Prolactin-releasing factor in porcine and rat hypothalamic tissue. Endocrinology 91:982–993

Vomachka AJ, Greenwald GS (1978) Acute negative feedback effects of ovarian steroid removal and replacement in cyclic female hamster. Biol Reprod 19:1040–1045

Wakayabashi K (1977) Heterogeneity of rat luteinizing hormone revealed by radioimmunoassay and electrofocusing studies. Endocrinol Jpn 24:473–485

Wilber JF, Utiger RD (1969) The effect of glucocorticoids on thyrotropin secretion. J Clin Invest 48:2096–2103

Willoughby JO, Martin JB (1978) Pulsatile growth hormone secretion: inhibitory role of medial preoptic area. Brain Res 148:240–244

Yoshikawa K, Hong JS (1983a) The enkephalin system in the rat anterior pituitary: regulation by gonadal steroids, hormones and psychotropic drugs. Endocrinology 113:1218–1227

Yoshikawa K, Hong JS (1983b) Sex related difference in substance P level in rat anterior pituitary: a mode of neonatal imprinting by testosterone. Brain Res 273:362–365

Zeilmaker GH (1963) Experimental studies on the regulation of corpus luteum in castrated male rats bearing a transplanted ovary. Acta Endocrinol 43:246–254

Zeilmaker GH (1964) Aspects of regulation of corpus luteum function in androgen-sterilized female rats. Acta Endocrinol 46:571–579

Zondek B (1936) Tumor of the pituitary induced with follicular hormone. Lancet 230:776–778

Symposium IV

Comparative Aspects of Aminergic Neurons

Organizers I. ORCHARD and R. H. G. DOWNER

Estimation of Biogenic Amines in Biological Tissues

R.G.H. DOWNER, B.A. BAILEY, and R.J. MARTIN[1]

1 Introduction

The availability of appropriate analytical procedures is of fundamental importance in achieving a holistic understanding of the biochemistry and physiology of biogenic amines in animals. Ideally, the analytical procedure should provide sensitive quantitation of specific compounds and should permit routine processing of relatively large numbers of samples without the need for expensive instrumentation. A variety of techniques have been used to analyze biogenic amines and these are discussed below with particular emphasis placed on the estimation of catecholamines, indoleamines, and monohydroxy-phenolamines in a single sample. The use of high performance liquid chromatography with electrochemical detection is discussed in some detail and procedures for sample preparation and extraction of monoamines are also described.

2 Methods Available for Estimation of Monoamines

2.1 Radioenzymology

The radioenzymatic method provides sensitive estimation of individual monoamines and has been applied to the determination of a variety of such compounds (Saavedra 1984). In discussing the technique it is convenient to consider its application to the estimation of a specific compound and, in the present account, discussion will be limited to the determination of octopamine. The procedure is based on specific conversion of octopamine to radiolabelled synephrine in the presence of radiolabelled methyl-S-adenosyl-L-methionine and the enzyme, phenylethanolamine N-methyl transferase (PNMT). Norepinephrine also serves as substrate for PNMT and must be degraded by alkaline conditions and heat in order to prevent interference with the estimation of octopamine (Harmar and Horn 1976; Buck et al. 1977; Talamo 1979). In addition, β-hydroxylated amines including normetanephrine, synephrine, and phenylethanolamine are methylated by PNMT; therefore, the methylated products of these compounds must be separated by chromatographic and/or crystallization procedures in order to ensure the specificity of the assay (Harmar and Horn 1976; Buck et al. 1977; Kobayashi

---

1 Department of Biology, University of Waterloo, Waterloo, Ontario, Canada N2L 3G1

Neurobiology
(ed. by R. Gilles and J. Balthazart)
© Springer-Verlag Berlin Heidelberg 1985

et al. 1980;Candy 1981). A further constraint associated with the radioenzymatic assay results from the use of liquid-liquid solvent extraction methods that are typically employed to recover the radioactive reaction products from the aqueous buffer. The extraction efficiency of monoamines into organic solvents is often low due to the amphoteric nature of these compounds and this decreases the sensitivity of the analytical procedure. In spite of these difficulties, the radioenzymatic method provides estimation of octopamine levels as low as 25 pg (Axelrod et al. 1976; Buck et al. 1977; Danielson et al. 1977; Dymond and Evans 1979;Kobayashi et al. 1980); however, the somewhat laborious nature of the procedure together with the fact that only a single compound is determined at any one time renders the procedure limited in application.

2.2 Chromatography with Mass Fragmentographic Detection

Thin layer chromatography and gas chromatography may be combined with mass spectroscopy to provide greater specificity than the radioenzymatic method (Williams and Couch 1978; Karoum et al. 1979; Edwards et al. 1979) especially when high resolution instrumentation is employed (Davis and Durden 1982; Durden et al. 1980; Durden and Boulton 1982; Boulton and Juorio 1982). In addition, a metabolic profile of several amines can be obtained during a single analysis although, more frequently, selected ion monitoring (SIM) of one compound is used to provide greater sensitivity (Williams and Couch 1978; Edwards et al. 1979; Karoum et al. 1979; Davis and Durden 1982; Durden and Boulton 1982). SIM increases the time available to monitor each ion and, therefore, results in a greater signal to noise ratio at the detector. Indeed, a sensitive negative ion chemical ionisation assay enables the detection of femtogram quantities of octopamine and tyramine (Duffield et al. 1983) and, thus, affords the greatest sensitivity of available analytical techniques. A major constraint associated with mass spectrometric methods is the complex sample-processing procedure that involves solvent extraction, derivatization and chromatographic separation in order to reduce the background signal. The accuracy and reliability of mass spectroscopic methods commend the use of these techniques, which are particularly valuable as a confirmational tool, however, the complexity and high cost of instrumentation render the methods impracticable for most laboratories.

2.3 Gas Chromatography with Electron Capture

Gas chromatography with electron capture detection combines high sensitivity with the convenience of enabling several compounds to be separated and detected in a single sample (Edwards and Blau 1972; Martin and Baker 1976; Legatt et al. 1981; Baker et al. 1981, 1982; Coutts and Baker 1982). The electron capture detector requires that the amines are first derivatized to compounds containing electron affinitive moieties. Such derivatives as N-dinitrophenol-0-trimethylsilyl ethers have been used successfully (Edwards and Blau 1972) but, more recently, derivatization with fluorinated and chlorinated acylating reagents have been preferred because of the increased sensitivity that they offer and the fewer reaction steps required for derivatization (Baker et al. 1981, 1982). N-acetylation of the amines with acetic anhydride prior to solvent extraction increases the efficiency of extracting the amines from aqueous homogenates (Baker et al. 1980). The N-acetylated amines are then derivatized for analysis by hydrolyzing the acetyl group with ammonium hydroxide and reacting the amine with trifluoroacetic anhydride (Baker et al. 1980, 1981, 1982; LeGatt et al. 1981). The advent of high resolution capillary columns enhances further the utility of the method (Hampson et al. 1984); however, the complexity of preparing halogenated derivatives together with the non-selectivity of electron capture detection has dissuaded wide scale adoption of the technique.

2.4 High Performance Liquid Chromatography (HPLC)

HPLC is widely accepted as a convenient technique for the separation of catecholamines and indoleamines in a single biological sample (Christensen and Blank 1979; Mefford 1981; Kissenger et al. 1981; Allenmark 1982; Warsh et al. 1982). The use of reversed-phase columns in HPLC systems enhances the ability to separate compounds of varying polarity through such strategies as adjustment of buffer pH to control the extent of ionization of the compounds, addition of organic modifiers to the mobile phase to reduce surface tension between the sorbent and the mobile phase and the formation of ion pairs to reduce the polarity of the compounds. Furthermore, the small-diameter spherical particles that are now available in HPLC columns provide a large surface area for rapid mass transfer of substances between the mobile and stationary phases, thereby reducing band broadening and increasing resolution.

Two detection methods are commonly employed to estimate the eluted amines; these are fluorescence and electrochemical. Electrochemical detection [ElCD] is the more favoured procedure because no derivatization is required for the hydroxylated amines and some degree of specificity is provided as a result of the oxidation characteristics of the different compounds. However, such amines as 2-phenylethylamine and 2-phenyl-ethanolamine, which do not contain ring hydroxyl moieties, are not electroactive at the potentials normally employed for detection and, therefore, must be converted to an electrochemically active derivative for ElCD.

By contrast with the wide application of HPLC for estimation of catecholamines and indoleamines, the technique has not been used extensively with monohydroxy-phenolamines. HPLC with fluorescence detection was used to analyze urinary tyramine levels (Davis et al. 1978, 1979) and octopamine levels in *Aplysia california* (Mell and Carpenter 1980), whereas HPLC/ElCD has been applied to the analysis of tyramine, octopamine, and synephrine in plant products (Kenyhercz and Kissenger 1978a,b) and octopamine in insects (Nassel and Laxmyr 1983; Bailey et al. 1984a; Martin et al. 1984).

3 Electrochemical Oxidation of Monoamines

Monoamines undergo oxidation at ring hydroxyl groups to produce orthoquinnone derivatives with the relase of electrons (Fig. 1). Electrochemical detectors exploit this oxidation by providing the required electropotential between two electrodes to effect oxidation and then amplifying and monitoring the current produced as a result of electron transfer to the electrode. The amount of current generated by the oxidation is

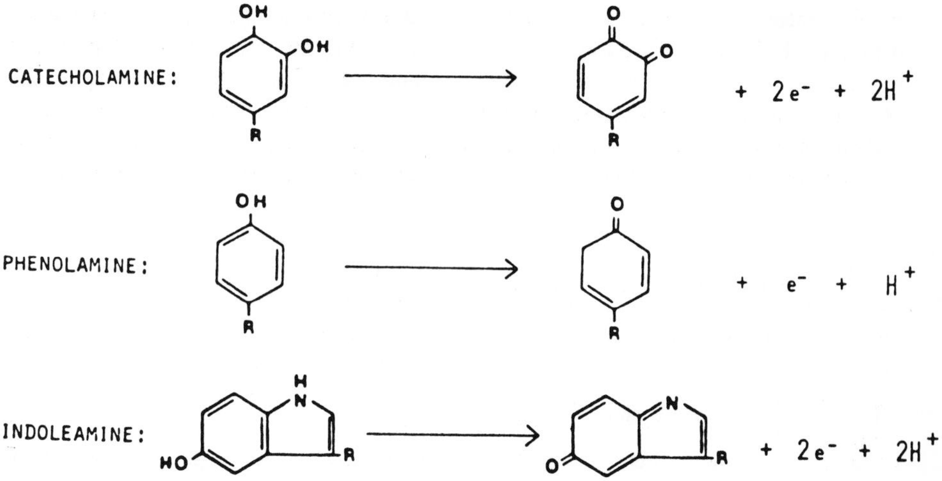

CATECHOLAMINE: (structure) $\longrightarrow$ (structure) $+ \ 2e^- \ + \ 2H^+$

PHENOLAMINE: (structure) $\longrightarrow$ (structure) $+ \ e^- \ + \ H^+$

INDOLEAMINE: (structure) $\longrightarrow$ (structure) $+ \ 2e^- \ + \ 2H^+$

Fig. 1. Oxidation of catecholamines, phenolamines and indoleamines. (After Marsden 1983)

directly proportional to the number of molecules oxidized; thus quantitative detection is achieved.

Electrochemical detectors oxidize any oxidizable material present in the eluant, however, the relatively low oxidation potentials required to effect oxidation of catecholamines and indoleamines ensure a high degree of selectivity for the compounds. By contrast, the monohydroxyphenolamines, tyramine and octopamine, require higher oxidation potentials in order to undergo electrooxidation. This is illustrated in Fig. 2 which demonstrates the relationship between the voltage applied to produce oxidation

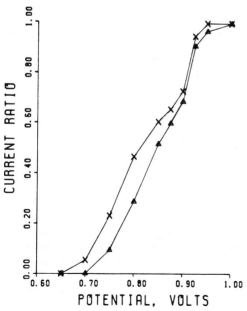

Fig. 2. Hydrodynamic voltammograms of tyramine (x) and octopamine (▲). Detection by thin-layer amperometric detector. (Bailey et al. 1982)

and the current generated as a result of the oxidation reaction (hydrodynamic voltam-mogram). It is evident from Fig. 2 that an oxidation potential of close to 1 V is needed to bring about adequate oxidation of tyramine and octopamine whereas hydrodynamic voltammograms for catecholamines obtained under identical conditions indicate that maximal oxidation current is generated at applied potentials of less than 0.70 V. The need to use high potentials for oxidation of tyramine and octopamine results in loss of the selectivity that was identified above as an advantage of ElCD for the estimation of catecholamines and indoleamines; furthermore, the application of high potentials to column eluants produces a variety of oxidized products which foul the relatively small surface area of the tubular electrodes or thin layer cells that are employed in amper-ometric electrochemical detectors.

3.1 Amperometric Detection of Biogenic Amines

In spite of the constraints identified above, HPLC with amperometric electrochemical detection has been used for simultaneous estimation of catecholamines and phenol-amines (Bailey et al. 1982; Nassel and Laxmyr 1983; Laxmyr 1984; Fuzeau-Braesch and Papin 1983). The method employs a reversed-phase C-18 column and permits estimation of amines at concentrations below 100 pg/injection with a signal to noise ratio $\geqslant 4$ (Bailey et al. 1982). A typical chromatogram of standard compounds is il-lustrated in Fig. 3 and the chromatographic conditions are described in the legend.

3.2 Coulometric Detection of Biogenic Amines

Many of the problems inherent in the use of a single amperometric detector for simul-taneous estimation of catecholamines, indoleamines, and monohydroxyphenolamines may be overcome by use of a dual electrode coulometric detector (Martin et al. 1983).

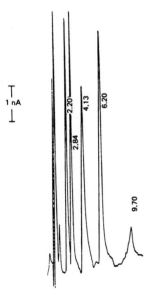

Fig. 3. Chromatogram of standard solution containing 5 ng nor-epinephrine (RT:2.20), octopamine (RT:2.84), dopamine (RT: 4.13), tyramine (RT:6.20). Chromatography on Ultrasphere RP-18 column with mobile phase comprising acetic acid-am-monium hydroxide buffer (pH 6.0), EDTA, sodium octane sul-phonic acid and methanol; flow rate was 2.0 ml min^{-1}. (Bailey et al. 1982)

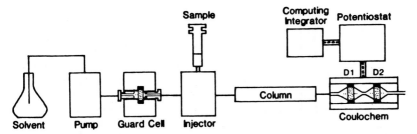

Fig. 4. Chromatographic system for separation and estimation of catecholamines, phenolamines, and indoleamines by HPLC/EICD. (Downer et al. 1984)

The larger surface area of coulometric detector electrodes is less susceptible to fouling by oxidation products and provides greater redox efficiency, effecting 100% oxidation of the oxidizable eluant. Furthermore, the use of dual electrodes enables differential screening of compounds that oxidize at low potentials from those that require higher potentials for oxidation. Thus, the first detector may be set at a relatively low potential to monitor and completely oxidize catecholamines and indoleamines while phenolamines are detected at the second detector which is set at a higher potential. The complete chromatographic system is illustrated in Fig. 4. An important feature of the system is the inclusion of a guard cell between the solvent reservoir and the injector. By operating the guard cell at a high potential, oxidizable contaminants present with the mobile phase are oxidized before they elute from the column and this, therefore, reduces extraneous signals from the mobile phase at the analytical detector.

Typical chromatograms obtained with standard compounds and with insect nervous tissue are illustrated in Fig. 5. The first detector, which is set at 0.5 V, oxidizes norepinephrine, epinephrine, 3,4-dihydroxybenzylamine (internal standard), dopamine, 5-hydroxytryptamine, and tryptophan. Tyramine, octopamine, 5-hydroxytryptamine, and tryptophan are oxidized at the second detector which is set at 0.75 V (note that a lower oxidation potential is required than with amperometric detection; see Martin et al. 1983 for discussion). The advantages of the dual electrodes are evidenced by reference to the detection of 3,4-dihydroxybenzylamine and p-octopamine which have similar retention times (6.40 min and 6.19 min respectively) but are detected at different oxidizing potentials and, therefore, are completely resolved by the detector. The detection of 5-hydroxytryptamine and tryptophan at both detectors results from these molecules undergoing oxidation reactions at both detectors; thus the first oxidation of 5-hydroxytryptamine occurs at the 5-OH group of the indole while the second reaction involves oxidation of ring nitrogen to N^+ (Svendsen and Greibrokk 1981).

A profile of some of the standard compounds that have been separated and detected with the system is presented in Table 1. These data demonstrate that most amino acids and acid metabolites are eluted before elution of the first amine, norepinephrine. Only tryptophan, a fairly lipophilic amino acid is retained for longer than most amines. The polar N-acetyl metabolites of dopamine and 5-hydroxytryptamine also elute with the early fractions and do not interfere with the resolution of amines. The metanephrines, normethanephrine and metanephrine, elute in regions where no major amine fractions appear and, therefore, do not interfere with the estimation of such compounds. Table 1

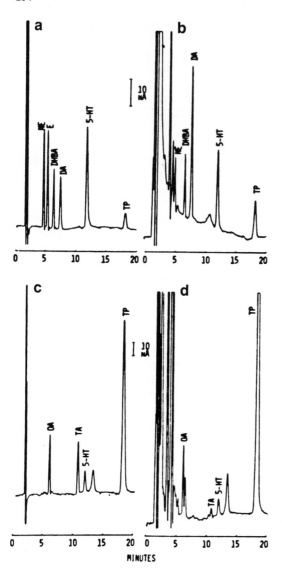

Fig. 5a–d. Typical chromatograms obtained by HPLC/EICD using dual coulometric detectors with detector 1 set at 0.5 V (**a, b**) and detector 2 set at 0.75 V (**c, d**). **a** Standard: 500 pg norepinephrine, epinephrine, dopamine, 5-hydroxytryptamine; 250 pg dihydroxybenzylamine; 1,000 pg tryptophan. **c** Standard: 500 pg octopamine, tyramine, 5-hydroxytryptamine; 1,000 pg tryptophan. **b** and **d** Supernatant from whole brain of *Periplaneta americana* (1/5 brain equivalent).

Chromatography on Ultrasphere IPC-18 column with mobile phase comprising sodium phosphate buffer (pH 3.2). EDTA, sodium dodecyl sulphate, TCA, acetonitrile, and methanol; flow rate was 0.8 ml min^{-1}. (Martin et al. 1984)

indicates also the ability of the chromatographic system to separate the para, meta, and ortho isomers of octopamine and synephrine. Finally, it should be noted that phenylethylamine, phenylethanolamine, and their amino acid precursor, phenylalanine, lack the structural characteristics necessary for oxidation under the conditions employed in this study and consequently were not detected. However, precolumn derivatives of these compounds have been formed and detected electrochemically (Joseph and Davies 1983; Shimada et al. 1983; Leroy et al. 1983; Allison et al. 1984). The amino acid tryptamine should undergo oxidation and be detected at a high oxidation potential (Richards 1979; Svendsen and Greibrokk 1981), however, the lipophilic nature of this amine suggests that it may be retained on the column beyond the 30-min run time used in the current study.

Table 1. Retention of amines, amino acid precursors, and amine metabolites on a reversed-phase HPLC column

	Retention time (min)	Detector response 0.5 V	0.75 V
Amino acid precursors			
Phenylalanine	–	–	–
Tyrosine	3.84	slight	+
3,4-Dihydroxyphenylalanine	3.08	+	slight
Tryptophan	17.58	+	+
5-Hydroxytryptophan	4.62	+	+
Amines			
Norepinephrine	4.81	+	–
Epinephrine	5.48	+	–
p-Octopamine	6.19	–	+
3,4-Dihydroxybenzylamine	6.40	+	–
p-Synephrine	7.20	–	+
Dopamine	7.48	+	–
m-Octopamine	9.48	–	+
m-Synephrine	11.00	–	+
p-Tyramine	11.10	–	+
5-Hydroxytryptamine	11.78	+	+
o-Octopamine	15.55	–	+
o-Synephrine	17.75	–	+
Tryptamine	–	–	–
Phenylethylamine	–	–	–
Phenylethanolamine	–	–	–
Metabolites			
Homovanillic acid	2.73	+	–
p-Hydroxymandelic acid	1.82	+	+
p-Hydroxyphenylacetic acid	2.57	+	+
5-Hydroxyindoleacetic acid	2.37	+	+
N-Acetyldopamine	2.18	+	–
N-Acetyl,5-Hydroxytryptamine	6.80	+	+
Normetanephrine	6.80	+	–
Metanephrine	8.00	+	–

The dual electrode coulometric detector offers several advantages over the amperometric detector including the lower applied potential required to oxidize the amines (e.g. 0.75 V compared with 0.95 V for octopamine) and the ability to screen compounds that oxidize at high potentials from those that are more electroactive.

The technique has been used to estimate biogenic amine levels in a variety of tissues from several species and some of these results are presented in Table 2. The values indicated in Table 2 are consistent with those reported previously for rat brain (Wenk and Greenland 1980; Doshi and Edwards 1981; Hegstrand and Eichelman 1981; Lyness 1982; Wagner et al. 1982; Todoriki et al. 1983), mouse brain (Sasa and Blank 1977; Christensen and Blank 1979), rat heart (Yui et al. 1980, Shoup et al. 1981; Eriksson and Persson 1982), cockroach nerve cord (Evans 1978) and cockroach haemolymph (Davenport and Evans 1984) and thus provide excellent vindication for the validity and widespread applicability of the technique.

Table 2. Estimations of amine concentrations in various biological tissues using HPLC/EICD

	Amine concentration (ng g^{-1})			
	NE	DA	OA	5-HT
Rat heart	752 ± 123 (10)	23 ± 2 (2)	12 ± 9 (6)	253 ± 74 (10)
Rat brain	376 ± 28 (12)	906 ± 70 (12)	5 ± 2 (6)	341 ± 47 (12)
Mouse brain	473 ± 24 (16)	1,424 ± 115 (16)	ND	587 ± 55 (16)
Cockroach nerve cord	ND	311 ± 65 (8)	888 ± 128 (8)	336 ± 77 (8)

NE, norepinephrine; DA, dopamine; OA, octopamine; 5-HT, 5-hydroxytryptamine

4 Tissue Preparation and Extraction of Monoamines

4.1 Direct Injection of Supernatant Following Homogenization

Preparation of samples for analysis of tissue amine levels typically involves precipitation of proteins with dilute perchloric acid followed by centrifugation and extraction (Boulton et al. 1976; Martin and Baker 1976; Wagner et al. 1982; Eriksson and Persson 1982). Several reports have indicated that, with certain tissues, the extraction step may be eliminated and the perchloric acid supernatant injected directly onto the HPLC column (Yui et al. 1980; Anderson et al. 1980; Roston et al. 1982; Pleece et al. 1982; Nielson and Johnston 1982; Mayer and Shoup 1983; Taylor et al. 1983). This procedure effects considerable time-saving, although the more rapidly eluting fractions such as norepinephrine may not be resolved from contaminants eluting with the solvent front (Anderson et al. 1980; Pleece et al. 1982; Morier and Rips 1982; Nielson and Johnston 1982).

Macromolecular polyanions such as heparin and dextran sulphate form insoluble complexes with lipoproteins (Burnstein et al. 1970) and the addition of either substance to the tissue sample prior to the precipitation step yields an increased amount of precipitate and a cleaner chromatogram when the supernatant is injected directly onto the column (Martin et al. 1983; Sloley and Downer 1984). Furthermore, the recovery of tissue amines is not affected by the addition of heparin. Figure 6 illustrates chromatograms obtained by direct injection of supernatant derived from rat brain homogenized in perchloric acid and heparin. The chromatograms may be further improved by increasing the amount of perchloric acid in which the tissues are homogenized (Fig. 6c, d).

4.2 Extraction of Octopamine and Tyramine

The amphoteric nature of octopamine and tyramine renders them difficult to extract from aqueous homogenates (Harmar and Horn 1976; Baker et al. 1980). Catecholamines are also amphoteric but selective extraction methods, based on the ability of the 3,4-dihydroxyphenyl moiety to form cyclic complexes with boric acid or alumina, are available (Allenmark 1982). The monohydroxy equivalents are not readily extracted by these techniques and, consequently, less selective procedures have been employed

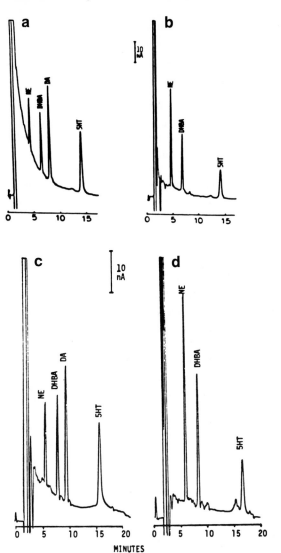

Fig. 6a–d. Chromatograms of supernatant from homogenates of rat brain (a, c) and rat heart (b, d) when low (a, b) and increased (c, d) amounts of perchloric acid are included in the homogenisation medium. Chromatography on Ultrasphere IP, C18 column with mobile phase comprising sodium phosphate buffer (pH 3.2). EDTA, sodium dodecyl sulphate, TCA, acetonitrile, and methanol; flow rate was 0.8 ml min^{-1}

to extract these compounds from biological tissues. These include liquid-liquid solvent extraction (Molinoff et al. 1969; Edwards and Blau 1972; Harmar and Horn 1976; Danielson et al. 1977; Buck et al. 1977; Kenyhercz and Kissenger 1978a,b), acetylation in aqueous medium prior to solvent extraction (Baker et al. 1980, 1981; LeGatt et al. 1981), ion exchange (Boulton et al. 1976; Martin and Baker 1976; Slingsby and Boulton 1976; Nassel and Laxmyr 1983) and ion exchange followed by Sephadex G-10 chromatography (Kamata et al. 1982). Another possible extraction technique is provided by the recent availability of disposable C-18 reversed-phase extraction columns. Octopamine and tyramine are ionized at acidic pH and, therefore, are poorly retained on C-18 silica packing. However, the retention can be increased either by adjusting the pH towards the relatively high pK values of these compounds (Mack and Bonisch 1979) or by ion-pair formation between an alkylsulfate and the monoamine.

4.2.1 Extraction from Reversed-Phase Columns by pH Adjustment

The effect of pH on the retention of some catecholamines and monohydroxyphenol-amines on C-18 reversed-phase columns is illustrated in Fig. 7. The recovery of catechol-amines is less than that of monohydroxyphenolamines especially at more alkaline pH, thus the procedure is particularly useful for selective extraction of monohydroxyphenol-amines. Elution of amines from the extraction column is achieved with acidic methanol (Bailey et al. 1984b). The recovery of octopamine and tyramine is linear when up to 150 ng of amine is applied to the disposable columns used in this study. The availability of disposable columns also accommodates the criticism that the use of high pH to in-crease the retention of monoamines on reversed-phase columns reduces the life of columns by increasing the solubility of the silica-based column particles (Majors 1980). The technique has been employed in this laboratory to extract octopamine from insect haemolymph and nerve cord and from rat brain and heart (Bailey et al. 1984b) and by other workers to extract metanephrines from urine (Canfeil et al. 1982) and indolic tryptophan metabolites from urine (Tonelli et al. 1982). In each case the column could be used for up to fifty times without loss of performance.

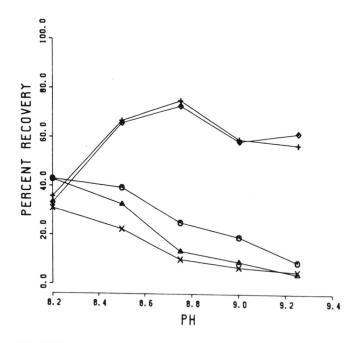

Fig. 7. Effect of pH on the recovery of norepinephrine (o), epinephrine (△), octopamine (+), dop-amine (x), and tyramine (◊) from reversed-phase extraction columns without ion-pairing

4.2.2 Extraction from Reversed-Phase Columns by Ion-Pair Formation

Sodium dodecyl sulphate (SDS) forms an ion-pair complex with catecholamines, mono-hydroxyphenolamines, and indoleamines at acidic pH. The amine-SDS ion-pair complex is a relatively large, lipophilic complex and is not eluted from the reversed-phase column matrix with water. Indeed an aqueous solution containing 20% methanol may be used to wash the column and elute potential contaminants with only minimal loss of recovery. Amines may then be eluted from the column using 100% methanol. Complete recovery of 1 ng amounts of individual amines was obtained when concentrations of SDS greater than 3 mM were applied to the extraction column. Furthermore, the recoveries of norepinephrine, octopamine, dopamine, and tyramine remain linear when up to 500 ng are applied to the column (Fig. 8).

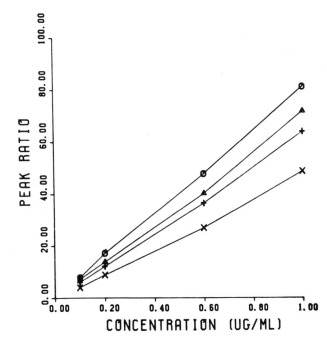

Fig. 8. Recovery of varying concentrations of norepine-phrine (o), octopamine (△), dopamine (+), and tyramine (x) from reversed-phase extraction columns

The extraction efficiency of these reversed-phase extraction columns, when used in combination with ion-pairing techniques, surpasses that of other extraction methods for monohydroxyphenolamines. However, at present, the method lacks absolute specificity. For example, magnesium ions from brain homogenates are absorbed onto the column with SDS in a manner similar to that described for the association of octane sulphate and various cationic metals (Johansson 1981). Attempts to chelate the metal prior to extraction were unsuccessful and it is necessary to alter the composition of the mobile phase in order to shift the metal peak to a region of the chromatograph that does not interfere with major amines.

5 Future Trends

The foregoing account indicates the potential of HPLC/ElCD for analysis of mono-amines, their metabolites and, by extrapolation, the activity of enzymes involved in their metabolism in samples of biological tissues. It is reasonable to predict that advances in column technology and increased sophistication of detector design, including the use of multiple detector systems will result in increased resolution and sensitivity in the future. Electrochemical principles may also be applied to continuous monitoring of these substances in vivo and it is within this context that the most significant advances are likely to occur. Detection in vivo requires miniaturization of the electrode system and implantation into the tissue under investigation. The major problem to be over-come in this regard is that of selectivity in order that the oxidation currents that are measured reflect the oxidation of specific compounds. The use of highly selective electrodes together with differential pulse voltammetry offers encouragement that the problems of selectivity will be overcome (Marsden 1983; Hutson and Curzon 1983). Thus it is with confidence that we predict increasing application of electrochemical principles to the analysis and monitoring of monoamines in the nervous system.

References

Allenmark S (1982) Analysis of catecholamines by HPLC. J Liq Chromatogr 5 Suppl 1:1–41

Allison LA, Mayer GS, Shoup RE (1984) opthalaldehyde derivatives of amines for high-speed li-quid chromatography/electrochemistry. Anal Chem 56:1089–1096

Anderson GM, Batter DK, Young JA, Shaywitz BA, Cohen DJ (1980) Simplified liquid chromato-graphic-electrochemical determination of norepinephrine and dopamine in rat brain. J Chroma-togr 181:453–455

Axelrod J, Saavedra J, Usdin E (1976) Trace amines in the brain. In: Usdin E, Sandler M (eds) Trace amines and the brain. Dekker, New York, p 1

Bailey BA, Martin RJ, Downer RGH (1982) Simultaneous determination of dopamine, norepine-phrine, tyramine and octopamine by reverse-phase liquid chromatography with electrochemical detection. J Liq Chromatogr 5:2435–2452

Bailey BA, Martin RJ, Downer RGH (1984a) Haemolymph octopamine levels during and following flight in the American cockroach, *Periplaneta americana* L. Can J Zool 62:19–22

Bailey BA, Martin RJ, Downer RGH (1984b) A rapid and specific technique for the extraction of tyramine and octopamine from biological tissues for HPLC analysis. In: Boulton AA, Baker GB, Dewhurst WG, Sandler M (eds) Neurobiology of the trace amines. Humana, Clifton, NJ, pp 85–90

Baker GB, Coutts RT, LeGatt DF (1980) A procedure for extraction and separation of phenylethyl-amine, tyramine and octopamine. Biochem Soc Trans 8:622–623

Baker GB, Coutts RT, Martin IL (1981) Analysis of amines in the central nervous system by gas chromatography with electroncapture detection. Prog Neurobiol (NY) 17:1–24

Baker GB, Coutts RT, LeGatt DF (1982) Gas chromatographic analysis of amines in biological systems. In: Baker GB, Coutts RT (eds) Analysis of biogenic amines, techniques and instrumenta-tion in analytical chemistry, vol 4. Elsevier, Amsterdam, pp 109–128

Boulton AA, Juorio AV (1982) Brain trace amines. In: Lajtha A (ed) Handbook of neurochemistry, 2nd ed, vol 1. Plenum, New York, p 189

Buck SH, Murphy RC, Mollinoff PB (1977) The normal occurrence of octopamine in the central nervous system of the rat. Brain Res 122:281–297

Burstein M, Scholnick HR, Morfin R (1970) Rapid method for the isolation of lipoproteins from human serum by precipitation with polyanions. J Lipid Res 11:583–595

Candy DJ (1981) Hormonal regulation of substrate transport and metabolism. In: Downer RGH (ed) Energy metabolism in insects. Plenum, New York, pp 19–52

Canfeil C, Bindr SR, Khayam-Bashi H (1982) Quantitation of urinary normetanephrine and metanephrine by reversed-phase extraction and mass-fragmentographic analysis. Clin Chem 28:25–28

Christensen HD, Blank CL (1979) The determination of neurochemicals in tissue samples at subpicomole levels. In: Hawk GL (ed) Biological/biomedical applications of liquid chromatography. Part II. Dekker, New York, pp 133–164

Coutts RT, Baker GB (1982) Gas chromatography. In: Lajtha A (ed) Handbook of neurochemistry, 2nd edn, vol 2. Plenum, New York, pp 429–448

Danielson TJ, Boulton AA, Robertson HA (1977) m-octopamine, p-octopamine and phenylethanolamine in rat brain: a sensitive, specific assay and the effects of some drugs. J Neurochem 29: 1131–1135

Davenport, Evans PD (1984) Stress induced changes in the octopamine levels of insect haemolymph. Insect Biochem 14:135–141

Davis BA, Durden DA (1982) Quantitative high resolution mass spectrometry of biogenic amines. In: Baker GB, Coutts RT (eds) Analysis of biogenic amines, techniques and instrumentation in analytical chemistry, vol 4. Elsevier, Amsterdam, pp 129–150

Davis TP, Gehrke CW, Gehrke CW Jr, Cunningham TD, Kuo KC, Gerhardt KO, Johnson HD, Williams GH (1978) High-performance liquid-chromatographic separation and fluorescence measurement of biogenic amines in plasma, urine and tissue. Clin Chem 24:1317–1324

Davis TP, Gehrke CW, Gehrke CW Jr, Cunningham TD, Kuo KC, Gerhardt KO, Johnson HD, Williams CH (1979) High-performance liquid chromatographic analysis of biogenic amines in biological materials as opthalaldehyde derivatives. J Chromatogr 162:293–310

Doshi PS, Edwards DJ (1981) Effects of L-dopa on dopamine and norepinephrine concentrations in rat brain assessed by gas chromatography. J Chromatogr 210:505–511

Downer RGH, Bailey BA, Martin RJ (1984) Estimation of biogenic amines by HPLC and the electrochemical detector. SP Chromatographic Review 11:5–7

Duffield PH, Dougan DFH, Wade DN, Low GKC, Duffield AM (1983) A negative ion chemical ionization GCMS assay for octopamine, tyramine and their α-methylated analogs in regions of rat brain after administration of amphetamine. Spectros Int J 2:311–317

Durden DA, Boulton AA (1982) Mass spectrometric analysis of some neurotransmitters and their precursors and metabolites. In: Lajtha A (ed) Handbook of neurochemistry, 2nd ed, vol 2. Plenum, New York, pp 397–428

Durden DA, Juorio AV, Davies BA (1980) Thin-layer chromatographic and high resolution mass spectrometric determination of β-hydroxyphenylethylamines in tissues as dansyl-acetyl derivatives. Anal Chem 52:1815–1820

Dymond GR, Evans PD (1979) Biogenic amines in the nervous system of the cockroach, *Periplaneta americana* association of octopamine with mushroom bodies and dorsal unpaired median (DUM) neurones. Insect Biochem 9:535–545

Edwards DJ, Blau K (1972) Analysis of phenylethylamines in biological tissues by gas-liquid chromatography with electron-capture detection. Anal Biochem 45:387–402

Eriksson B-M, Persson B-A (1982) Determination of catecholamines in rat heart tissue and plasma samples by liquid chromatography with electrochemical detection. J Chromatogr 228:143–154

Evans PD (1978) Octopamine distribution in the insect nervous system. J Neurochem 30:1009–1013

Fuzeau-Braesch S, Papin C (1983) Dosage de l'octopamine par chromatographie liquide à haute performance (HPLC) et détection électrochemique (ED): essais sur le cerveau du criquet *Locusta migratoria cinerascens*. Agressologie 24:377–399

Hampson DR, Baker GB, Coutts RT (1984) A rapid and sensitive gas chromatographic method for quantitation of 2-phenylethylamine in brain tissue and urine. Res Commun Chem Pathol Pharmacol 43:169–172

Harmar AJ, Horn AS (1976) Octopamine in mammalian brain: rapid post mortem increase and effects of drugs. J Neurochem 26:987–993

Hegstrand LR, Eichelman B (1981) Determination of rat brain catecholamines using liquid chromatography with electrochemical detection. J Chromatogr 222:107–111

Hutson PH, Curzon G (1983) Monitoring in vivo of transmitter metabolism by electrochemical methods. Biochem J 211:1–12

Johansson M (1981) Retention in reversed-phase ion-pair chromatography of amines on alkyl-bonded phases. J Liq Chromatogr 4:1435–1457

Kamata S, Imura K, Okada A, Kawashima Y, Yamatodani A, Watanabe T, Wade H (1982) Simultaneous analyses of phenylethylamine, phenylethanolamine, tyramine and octopamine in rat brain using fluorescamine. J Chromatogr 231:291–299

Karoum F, Nasrallah H, Potkin S, Chuang L, Moyer-Schwing J, Phillips I, Wyatt RJ (1979) Mass fragmentography of phenylethylamine, m- and p-tyramine and related amines in plasma, cerebrospinal fluid, urine and brain. J Neurochem 33:201–212

Kenyhercz TM, Kissinger PT (1978a) Identification and quantification of tryptophan and tyrosine metabolites in the banana by liquid chromatography with electrochemical detection. J Food Sci 43:1354–1356

Kenyhercz TM, Kissinger PT (1978b) Determination of selected acidic, neutral and basic natural products in cocao bean and processed cocoa. Liquid chromatography with electrochemical detection. Lloydia (Cinci) 41:130–139

Kissinger PT, Bruntlett CS, Shoup RE (1981) Neurochemical applications of liquid chromatography with electrochemical detection. Life Sci 28:455–465

Kobayashi K, Foti A, Dequattro V, Kolloch R, Miano L (1980) A radioenzymatic assay for free and conjugated normetanephrine and octopamine excretion in man. Clin Chim Acta 107:163–173

Laxmyr L (1984) Biogenic amines and DOPA in the central nervous system of decapod crustaceans. Comp Biochem Physiol 77C:139–143

LeGatt DF, Baker GB, Coutts RT (1981) Simultaneous extraction and separation of trace amines of biological interest. J Chromatogr 225:301–308

Leroy P, Nicolas A, Moreau A (1983) Electrochemical detection of sympatomimetric drugs following pre-column o-pthalaldehyde derivatization and reversed-phase high performance liquid chromatography. J Chromatogr 282:561–559

Lyness WH (1982) Simultaneous measurement of dopamine and its metabolites, 5-hydroxytryptamine, 5-hydroxyindoleacetic acid and tryptophan in brain tissue using liquid chromatography and electrochemical detection. Life Sci 31:1435–2443

Mack F, Bonisch H (1979) Dissociation constants and lipophilicity of catecholamines and related compounds. Arch Pharmacol (Weinheim) 310:1–9

Majors RE (1980) Practical operation of bonded-phase columns in high-performance liquid chromatography. In: Horvath C (ed) High-performance liquid chromatography: advances and perspectives, vol 1. Academic, New York, pp 75–111

Marsden CA (1983) Application of electrochemical detection to neuropharmacology. Trends Biochem Sci 1983:148–152

Martin IL, Baker GB (1976) Procedural difficulties in the gas liquid chromatographic assay of the arylalkylamines. J Chromatogr 123:45–50

Martin RJ, Bailey BA, Downer RGH (1983) Rapid estimation of catecholamines, octopamine and 5-hydroxytryptamine from biological tissues using high performance liquid chromatography with coulometric detection. J Chromatogr 278:265–274

Martin RJ, Bailey BA, Downer RGH (1984) Analysis of octopamine, dopamine, 5-hydroxytryptamine and tryptophan in the brain and nerve cord of the American cockroach. In: Boulton AA, Baker GB, Dewhurst WG, Sandler M (eds) Neurobiology of the trace amines. Humana, New York, pp 91–96

Mayer GS, Shoup RE (1983) Simultaneous multiple electrode liquid chromatographic-electrochemical assay for catecholamines, indoleamines and metabolites in brain tissue. J Chromatogr 255:533–544

Mefford JN (1981) Application of high performance liquid chromatography with electrochemical detection to neurochemical analysis: measurement of catecholamines, serotonin and metabolites in rat brain. J Neurosci Methods 3:207–224

Mell LD, Carpenter DD (1980) Fluorometric determination of octopamine in tissue homogenates by high performance liquid chromatography. Neurochem Res 5:1089–1096

Molinoff PB, Landsberg L, Axelrod J (1969) An enzymatic assay for octopamine and other c-hydroxylated phenylethylamines. J Pharmacol Exp Ther 170:253–261

Morier E, Rips R (1982) A new technique for simultaneous assay of biogenic amines and their metabolites in unpurified mouse brain. J Liq Chromatogr 5:151–164

Nassel DR, Laxmyr L (1983) Quantitative determination of biogenic amines and dopa in the CNS of adult and larval blowflies, *Calliphora erythrocephala*. Comp Biochem Physiol 75C:259–265

Nielson JA, Johnston CA (1982) Rapid, concurrent analysis of dopamine, 5-hydroxytryptamine, their precursors and metabolites utilizing high performance liquid chromatography with electrochemical detection: analysis of brain tissue and cerebrospinal fluid. Life Sci 31:2847–2856

Pleece SA, Redfern PN, Riley CM, Tomlinson E (1982) Biogenic amine resolution in tissue extracts of rat brain using ion-pair high-performance liquid chromatography with electrochemical detection. Analyst 107:755–760

Richard DA (1979) Electrochemical detection of tryptophan metabolites following high-performance liquid chromatography. J Chromatogr 175:293–299

Roston DA, Shoup RE, Kissinger PT (1982) Liquid chromatography/electrochemistry: thin-layer multiple electrode detection. Anal Chem 54:1417–1434

Saavedra JM (1984) The use of enzymatic radioisotopic microassays for the quantification of β-phenylethylamine, phenylethanolamine, tyramine and octopamine. In: Boulton AA, Baker GB, Dewhurst WG, Sandler M (eds) Neurobiology of the trace amines. Humana, Clifton, NJ, pp 41–55

Sasa S, Blank L (1977) Determination of serotonin and dopamine in mouse brain tissue by high performance liquid chromatography with electrochemical detection. Anal Chem 49:354–359

Shimada K, Tanaka M, Nambara T (1983) New derivatization of amines for high performance liquid chromatography with electrochemical detection. J Chromatogr 280:271–277

Shoup RE, Bruntlett CS, Jacons WA, Kissinger PT (1981) LCEC: a powerful tool for biomedical problem solving. Am Lab (Fairfield Conn) 151:144–153

Slingsby JM, Boulton AA (1976) Separation and quantitation of some urinary arylalkylamines. J Chromatogr 123:51–56

Sloley BD, Downer RGH (1984, in press) Distribution of 5-hydroxytryptamine and indolealkylamine metabolites in the american cockroach, *Periplaneta americana* L. Comp Biochem Physiol

Svendsen H, Greibrokk T (1981) High-performance liquid chromatographic determination of biogenic amines. Comparisons of detection methods. J Chromatogr 213:429–437

Talamo BR (1979) Function of octopamine in the nervous system. In: Mosnaim AD, Wolf ME (eds) Noncatecholic phenylethylamine. Part II. Phenylethanolamine, tyramine and octopamine. Dekker, New York, pp 261–292

Taylor RB, Reid R, Kendle KE, Geddes C, Curle PF (1983) Assay procedures for the determination of biogenic amines and their metabolites in rat hypothalamus using ion-pairing reversed-phase high performance liquid chromatography. J Chromatogr 277:101–114

Todoriki H, Hayashi T, Naruse H, Hirakawa AY (1983) Sensitive high-performance liquid chromatographic determination of catecholamines in rat brain using a laser fluorimetric detection system. J Chromatogr 276:45–54

Tonelli D, Gattavecchia E, Gandolfi M (1982) Thin-layer chromatographic determination of indolic tryptophan metabolites in human urine using Sep-Pak C-18 extraction. J Chromatogr 231:283–289

Wagner J, Vitali P, Palfreyman MG, Zraika M, Huot S (1982) Simultaneous determination of 3,4-dihydroxyphenylalanine, 5-hydroxytryptophan, dopamine, 4-hydroxy-3-methoxyphenylamine, norepinephrine, 3,4-dihydroxyphenylacetic acid, homovanollic acid, serotonin, and 5-hydroxyindoleacetic acid in rat cerebrospinal fluid and brain by high-performance liquid chromatography with electrochemical detection. J Neurochem 38:1241–1254

Warsh JJ, Chiu AS, Godse DD (1982) Determination of biogenic amines and their metabolites by high-performance liquid chromatography. In: Baker GB, Coutts RT (eds) Analysis of biogenic amines, techniques and instrumentation in analytical chemistry, vol 4. Elsevier, Amsterdam, pp 203–236

Wenk G, Greenland R (1980) Investigation of the performance of a high-performance liquid chromatography system with an electrochemical detector. J Chromatogr 183:261–267

Williams CM, Couch MW, Midgeley JM (1984) Natural occurrence and metabolism of the isometric octopamines and synephrines. In: Boulton AA, Baker GB, Dewhurst WG, Sandler M (eds) Neurobiology of the trace amines. Humana, New York, pp 97–103

Yui Y, Itokawa Y, Kawai C (1980) A rapid and highly sensitive method for determination of picogram levels of norepinephrine and epinephrine in tissues by high-performance liquid chromatography. Anal Biochem 108:11–15

Neurotransmitters, Neuromodulators, and Neurohormones

G. HOYLE [1]

1 Introduction

The above broad title was selected for me by the organizers of this symposium, and while I should love to expound on the comparative aspects, physiological and biochemical, such an undertaking would of itself fill the entire volume. Therefore, most of my remarks will be restricted to my current interests and experience, which means that one substance will have centre stage, namely octopamine, and insects will be the primary experimental subject. Nevertheless, my overall perspective will be truly comparative.

2 Definitions

The three classes are all household names, but there is no agreement as to what each should refer to: the topic of their designations occupied a lead article by Dismuskes in *Behavioral and Brain Sciences* with numerous commentaries (Dismukes 1979), several by persons who produced alternative definitions, including myself. Some authors prefer to include all neuroactive substances under the single rubric neurotransmitters. For them, neuromodulators are a type of transmitter, and neurohormones a type of neuromodulator. I doubt if there will ever be general agreement about definitions, especially since the term neurotransmitter has, historically, been used very loosely indeed. This was inevitable when both the biophysical/biochemical events of chemical action on neural tissue were unknown, and before the ultrastructural details were worked out. In light of current overall knowledge we can, if we wish, ignore historical precedents without undue risk, and produce simple, rational definitions from scratch. I shall start by giving you my own abbreviated definitions: an expanded version can be found in my commentary to the Dismukes article. It is unlikely that a set of definitions proposed by a clinically-oriented investigator, will seem satisfactory from the perspective of a truly comparative physiologist, so these definitions could prove useful. At least they will aid the reader of this article.

---

1 Institute of Neuroscience, University of Oregon, Eugene, OR 97403, USA

Neurobiology
(ed. by R. Gilles and J. Balthazart)
© Springer-Verlag Berlin Heidelberg 1985

2.1 Natural Neuroactive Substance (NAS)

A chemical agent synthesized by a neuron which affects the properties of other neurons and/or muscle cells.

2.2 Neurotransmitter (NT)

A NAS which is released at a synapse and alters the ion permeability of the postsynaptic membrane.

2.3 Neuromodulator (NM)

A NAS which is released in the general vicinity of a group of synapses and affects synaptic transmission by either pre- or postsynaptic action, or both.

2.4 Neurohormone (NH)

A NAS which is released into blood and acts at distant as well as proximal target sites. It may act on any neuronal property, on muscle cell properties or (unfortunately from the point of view of simple definitions) growth, reproductive system maturation, pigment synthesis, diuresis, tanning etc. Fortunately, there is another term which we can use to cover some of these non-neural actions, namely neuroendocrine activity. Likewise agents transported in both directions within neurons which are used for long-term reciprocal influences on other neurons, and/or muscle cells which are innervated.

In interpreting the above definitions it should be realized that the *functions* of the substances overlap freely, especially of NM's and NH's. Also, NM's, and NH's may, or may not, combine with specific receptors located on the outside of membranes, which in turn may, or may not, be linked to adjustable ion channels. The alternative is that they exert their actions after passing into the target cells. Furthermore, it is increasingly apparent that at any given synapse more than one substance may be released together, at the same, or different, rates. Only one of these may be a transmitter, the other a modulator either of the same synapse or of distant ones, even having a neurohormonal action. Possibly synapses will be found at which a NM, or even a NH, is released which does not have any action on the synapse at which it is released, but only on other, distant ones. Such an anomaly could have easily occurred in association with an evolutionary shift in function. For example, in distant related grasshoppers and stenopelmatide the original hind-leg slow extensor tibiae has become the fast, and vice versa (Wilson and Hoyle 1978; Hoyle and Field 1983b). The definition covers these options by referring only to the types of action involved.

3 Common NAS

According to the above definitions there are only three transmitters which are truly widespread, two excitory and one inhibitory. The excitors are acetylcholine and l.glutamate and the inhibitor is gamma amino butyric acid (GABA). The use of acetylcholine as an inhibitor by vertebrate hearts is a rare exception. In principle any NAS could produce any kind of physiological action provided it interacts with a receptor attached to an openable ion channel. There is nothing special about any NAS as such, or even its receptors, only the consequences of their interaction. It is only the channel properties which truly matter.

The number of substances known to be used as modulators is already relatively large, and can be expected to continue to grow as new ones are discovered. The list includes simple and complex amines, and several peptides, currently about 40 total, of which several are truly widespread. These are in four distinct groups by chemical structure: the catecholamines epinephrine, norepinephrine, and dopamine, and the phenolamine octopamine in one group, the imidazole 5-hydroxytryptamine, the indolamine histamine, and the pentapeptide proctolin forming the other three. No one will be surprised to find these substances turning up and having functions in any animal species. The four chemical structures are so different that a steric key-in-the-lock resemblance seems unlikely, nor are they all serving as simple surface-acting channel openers. Some of their actions depend on entering a cell, either pre- or post-synaptically, and there promoting the release of a second messenger, commonly either calcium or cAMP. The messenger sets in motion a chain of events, different in detail for a particular cell, but principally of two kinds. One affects the internal calcium concentration by actions on calmodulin/calsequestrin calcium-pumping mechanisms. The other promotes protein phosphorylation, giving rise to molecules which enter, and alter properties of membrane. The former affects mobilization and release of transmitter directly, the latter indirectly, by altering the membrane time constant. A variety of post-synaptic events are also affected by both.

There are currently about 30 well-characterized neurohormones, but the eventual list seems likely to be extremely long and will almost certainly exceed that of modulators. Most are complex molecules such as steroids, or large peptides, and they are generally highly species-specific. The latter constraint, in many instances, may be due to characteristic proteins attached to the fundamental moiety. NAS of the vertebrate pituitary are all neurohormones, and while they influence a variety of events in invertebrates, and many instances of invertebrate CNS neurons showing immunoreactivity to labelled antibodies to them, none has been conclusively shown to be produced by invertebrates. The long vertebrate list also includes gonadotrophin, vasopressin, vasotocin, oxytocin, neurophysins, ACTH, dynorphin, calcitonin, TRF, STH, insulin, glucagon, gastrin, cholecystokinin, secretin, enkephalins, endorphins, substance P, and somatostatin.

Medical text-books cover the vertebrate literature on all of these. There has been a fair amount of work on specific NH of vertebrates in invertebrates, but very little that is truly satisfactory and none which is conclusive: none of these substances is yet known with confidence to be produced and utilized by an invertebrate. Immunoreactivity to cholecystokinin, which is a peptide having central as well as peripheral actions in vertebrates, has been found in the entire *Aplysia* nervous system and in crustacean brains. There is reactivity to insulin and gastrin in the silkworm, the tobacco hornworm, and *Aplysia*. There has unfortunately been very little in the way of study of the functions any vertebrate NH might have in any invertebrate even by those who assume that some are indeed produced and utilized by the latter. Reciprocally, the known invertebrate NH, egg-laying hormone and FMRamide in molluscs, bursicon, eclosion hormone, adipokinetic hormone, and proctolin in insects, are peculiar to the class and are not known to have effects on vertebrates. All of these are peptides, but with a wide range of mol. wt. Proctolin is only a pentapeptide, eclosion hormone at least ten times as large. They have probably evolved as disposable bits of RNA which happen to be taken up by specific cells in which they initiate otherwise dormant replications. Specific surface receptors may be needed to "recognize" them and help them cross the membrane, but an earlier notion that for every NAS there had to be a specific receptor is currently open to question. This is unquestionably true only for the few NT's.

4 Functional Roles of NT's

NT's have long been the intensive target for investigation by an host of comparative, as well as "general" physiologists, so need not concern us. A NT diffuses across the short gap between the pre-synaptic terminal membrane and the post-synaptic membrane and combines briefly with specific receptors linked to specific openable ion channels. The direct physiological actions of NT's are confined to the membrane potential effects which follow the changes in ion conductance which they promote.

5 Functional Roles of NM's

NM's, by contrast, play multiple roles which are only now beginning to be understood, and only in a few systems have intensive investigations been carried out. It is already apparent that there will be a great variety of actions.

The first to be well worked out is 5 H-T, which is synthesized by several small neurons of the right half of the Aplysia abdominal ganglion (Eisenstadt et al. 1973) and for which there is immunoreactivity in several cells of leech ganglia (Zipser and McKay 1981): the giant Retzius cells of the leech are 5 H-Tergic (Bianchi 1967). In the leech 5 H-T relaxes longitudinal muscles via hyperpolarization caused by increased gCl. This peripheral action is the functional role played by the Retzius cells; it facilitates swimming, which is evoked at the same time, either if the blood concentration is sufficiently great (Willard 1981) or more probably because 5 H-T is released at specific sites in the neuropile from small interneurons. The duration of an evoked swim is proportional to the blood 5 H-T concentration. Activity in a single identified neuron known as 204 can initiate swimming, and also maintain it, as well as modulate it by changing phase characteristics (Weeks and Kristan 1978). It is significant that the same substance has both peripheral and central actions which work together in promoting and modulating the single behaviour. Probably all the physiological actions are effected via direct and indirect local release of 5 H-T, which then alters properties of neurons of the motor program generator (MPG) neural circuit for swimming.

As will probably turn out to be the case with many other animals, the same NM is used in more than one behaviour. In the leech 5 H-T is used not only in swimming, but also in feeding (Lent and Dickinson 1984), and quite likely in the circadian rhythm, and in aspects of sexual behaviour also.

In *Aplysia*, 5 H-T exerts a general arousing action whose cellular basis has been worked out (Kandel and Schwartz 1982). It promotes phosphorylation of several proteins, one of which is a membrane protein in presynaptic neurons. The action is either after entering or by interacting with a receptor which somehow triggers the chain of events, which certainly involves cAMP activation. An end result is decreased gK, associated with increased input resistance, so that the depolarization caused by an incoming impulse lasts longer, releasing more transmitter, transmission being potentiated.

This is an important example, of one of many possible forms of modulator action. Comparable research is needed on other systems, both on 5 H-T action, and also that of other modulators.

In insects the principal modulator is not 5 H-T but the phenolamine equivalent of norepinephrine, octopamine (OCT). Octopamine is the NM synthesized and released by dorsal unpaired median (DUM) neurons (Hoyle 1975; Hoyle and Barker 1975; Evans and O'Shea 1978). Many varied modulatory actions and behavioural effects of OCT in insects are now known and many more can be expected. The first to be discovered were all peripheral: inhibition of intrinsic rhythmic muscular contractions (Hoyle 1975, 1978) at concentrations as low as 10^{-10} M, then potentiation of slow extensor tibiae neuromuscular EJP's (O'Shea and Evans 1979). The latter action is due partly to enhanced transmitter release, partly to an effect on the post-synaptic membrane (Evans 1981). Therefore, there are at least three different peripheral locales for OCT action, possibly indicating the existence of as many different receptors. Each has a different time-course in regard to: delay in onset, time to peak effect, rates of rise and decay of effect, and overall duration. The local action on muscle cell membrane potential can be either nil, depolarizing, or hyperpolarizing (Hoyle 1978) suggesting involvement of altered gCl, but no details are known.

The presynaptic action of OCT on neuromuscular junctions is best seen in the nocturnal primitive New Zealand stenopelmatid orthopteran insects known by their Maori name "wetas" (night devils). A quiescent daytime preparation shows potentiation of the overall mechanical response to SETi (slow extensor tibiae) by 10^{-8} M dl OCT which exceeds sevenfold for a steady tetanus and is essentially infinite for twitches, which are non-existent without the OCT. Excitatory junctional potentials (EJP's) are enhanced up to fivefold, the larger ones eliciting graded electrogenic responses (Hoyle 1984). Full potentiation is reached about 8 min from onset. At about this length of time a second effect is apparent, drastic slowing of relaxation. After a brief burst in SETi there is almost no relaxation, the muscle having gone into a catch-like tension (C-T) condition. American relatives of the weta, the Jerusalem cricket, show the same condition (Fig. 1). The C-T relaxes very slowly over a period of about 8–30 min, unless a single inhibitory junctional potential (IJP) comes along. One is sufficient to restore the C-T to zero in less than 1 s.

The catch-condition is a post-synaptic action which locks the membrane potential in the synaptic regions in the depolarized state after a burst of SETi impulses (Fig. 2). This condition, and also presynaptic potentiation, are also set up by natural release of OCT from the neurons which innervates the extensor muscle (dorsal unpaired median neuron innervating the extensor tibiae; DUMETi), in a fraction of the time, about 60 s,

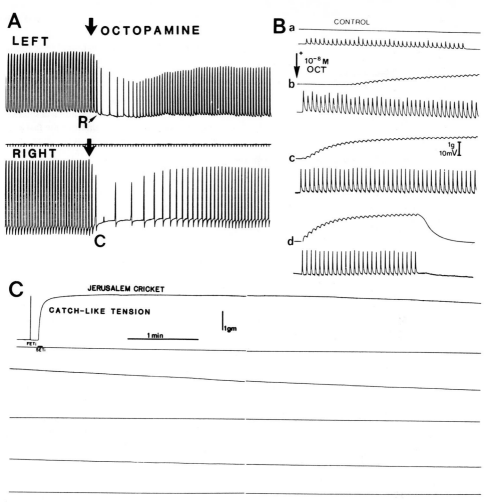

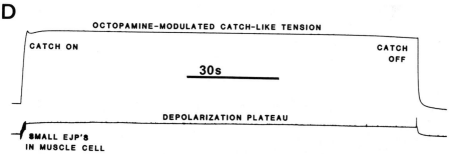

Fig. 1 A–D. Multiple modulatory actions of octopamine (*OCT*) on insect nerve-muscle. **A** Inhibition of intrinsic rhythmicity, in locust (*S.gregaria*) extensor tibiae, by a brief injected pulse of 10^{-7} M OCT, at *arrows*. On one side basic tonus was relaxed (*R*), on the other side increased (*C*). Isometric tension records from *left* and *right* sides simultaneously. Time in seconds. (Hoyle 1975) **B** Potentiation of junctional potentials and tension responses, of *Hemideina femorata* (N.Z. weta) metathoracic SETi (slow extensor tibiae) by 10^{-8} M OCT. (Hoyle 1984) **C** Switching SETi response to catch-like tension. Fast extensor tibiae FETi twitch, followed by brief SETi burst, in metathoracic leg of a Jerusalem cricket, after infusion of saline containing 10^{-6} M dl^{-1} octopamine into the leg. SETi evokes catch-like tension (C-T) which decays extremely slowly. (Hoyle, unpubl.) **D** Intracellular recorded depolarization plateau in muscle cell of *Hemideina* in response to SETi in the presence of 10^{-6} M OCT, accompanying isometric C-T, which was relaxed by a single, late EJP. (Hoyle 1984)

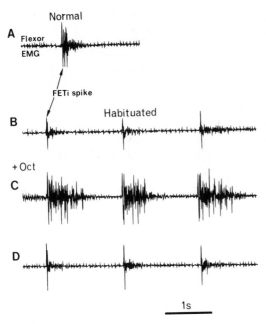

Fig. 2A–D. Dishabituation of the partially habituated proprioceptive inputs of the resistance reflex to fast extension, by a single slug of octopamine iontophoresed into the region of synaptic inputs by a current pulse. Fast extension was elicited by applying single stimuli to the fast excitatory motor neuron innervating the extensor tibiae muscle (*FETi*), and the response was recorded electromyographically from the flexor tibia muscle. **D** was recorded 1 min following the cessation of the iontophoretic current pulse. (Sombati and Hoyle 1984b)

that can be achieved by bath-applied OCT. This C-T phenomenon is not an artifact of physiology but a natural behavioural event, a weta or a Jerusalem cricket utilizes it to produce a long-lasting posture, especially threat posture (Hoyle and Field 1983a). The insect's control of C-T is so accurate, and so adjustable, that it uses it successfully, in operant-conditioning tests, to hold a joint angle coupled to negative reinforcement to within 5° arc (Hoyle and Field 1983b). To achieve this, they must first release OCT, then fire a SETi burst with a precise mean frequency and duration.

The DUM neurons have central as well as peripheral dendrites, some of which are outgoing, within integrating regions of neuropile. Nevertheless, no behavioural events are discernible when OCT is injected into locust/grasshopper haemolymph. Such injections wake up sleepy wetas and in crayfish and lobsters they cause abdominal extension (Livingstone et al. 1980; Glanzman and Krasne 1983). But the weta effect is peripheral only: the CNS of insects, unlike that of crustaceans, is surrounded by a barrier. If OCT has actions in the insect neuropile they will be discernible only with injection into neuropile. The DUM neurons each have different, dendritic morphologies, suggesting that their influences in the neuropile are local not global.

Accordingly, Sombati and Hoyle (1984a) iontophoresed OCT from micropipettes with about 0.2 μm diameter into regions of neuropile known to have input synapses to motor neurons. Several significant effects were obtained, but only when the tip of the pipette was precisely located. Movement of the tip away from a region at which an effect was obtained, of as little as 5 μm in any direction, resulted in total loss of the effect. Therefore the limit of the radius of effectiveness of iontophoresed OCT was not more than about 3 μm. Bath-applied OCT was completely ineffective unless major nerve trunks were cut close to the ganglion. Even then, effects took about 40 min to develop. The following effects were obtained:

1. Dishabituation. Habituated synaptic inputs to identified motor neurons are dishabituated by OCT release in a dose-dependent manner. At a sensitive site an effect is apparent within 2 s of the onset of iontophoretic current. The duration of dishabituation is indefinite with continuous pulsing of OCT, and outlasts termination by at least 1.5 min for a fairly strong dose (30 nA × 30 s).

2. Sensitization. Excitatory synaptic inputs and motor responses generated by standardized stimuli in reflex actions are routinely enhanced by local iontophoretic release of OCT into sites of synaptic input to motor neurons, or bath-applied after cutting major nerve trunks close to the ganglion (Fig. 3). The amount and duration of effectiveness using iontophoresis are dose-dependent.

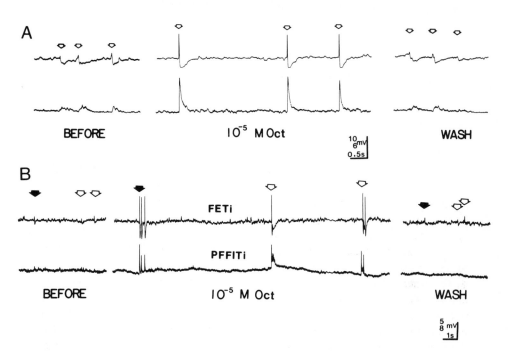

Fig. 3A, B. Sensitization of reflexes by bath-applied octopamine in locust (*S. americana*) metathoracic ganglion. The responses were recorded intracellularly from identified motor neurons FETi (*top traces*) and its antagonist, the (posterior fast flexor fibiae motor neuron; PFFITi) simultaneously, with two electrodes. After placing the electrodes and identifying the neurons all nerve trunks except the abdominal connectives and the auditory nerves were cut close to the ganglion, to permit OCT to enter the neuropile. The stimuli used were: touch of the ipsilateral knee with a fine brush in **A** (*at arrows*); standardized air puffs (*open arrows*) or loud handclaps (*solid arrows*) in **B**. (Sombati and Hoyle 1984b)

3. Potentiation. Many direct responses to specific inputs are enhanced up to several-fold by iontophoresed OCT. The dishabituated response to any type of input after habituation has steadied is not just restored to normal by OCT, but enhanced to supranormal provided the OCT dose is sufficiently great (Fig. 4). Proprioceptive sensory

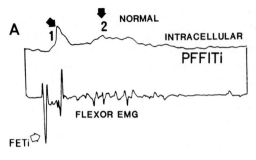

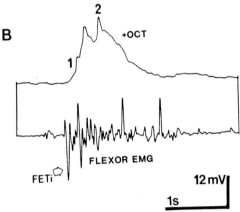

Fig. 4A,B. Potentiation of postsynaptic responses in identified motor neuron PFFITi to a single action potential in FETi by OCT iontophoresed into neuropile at the region indicated in the inset. The earlier response (1) was due to direct synaptic inputs, the earliest of which is monosynaptic. The later response (2) was due to proprioceptive input of the resistance reflex to extension.
A Normal. B Following iontophoretic injection of OCT into the region of synaptic inputs to flexors from collaterals of FETi. (Sombati and Hoyle 1984b)

inputs to motor neurons are potentiated to a much greater extent than direct inputs from other motor neurons. Sensory inputs to motor neurons are cholinergic (Harrow et al. 1982); inputs to motor neurons appear to be glutamatergic (Sombati and Hoyle 1984c).

4. Direct Excitation. Since there are continuous incoming inputs from various sources in intact ganglia it was not possible to distinguish between potentiating some excitatory ones and directly depolarizing the neuronal membrane. Potentiation of background inputs certainly does occur, and the membrane potential recorded at either the soma or the neuropile also fall, when OCT is iontophoresed at a sensitive site. Some otherwise silent motor neurons were caused to discharge long trains of impulses in response to OCT released at a sensitive site (Fig. 5).

5. Generation of Bouts of Specific Behaviour. One site, indicated in Fig. 6, was located in neuropile, at which iontophoretic release of OCT evoked a bout of rhythmic flex/ extend movements of the metathoracic tibia of the injected side. If the entire leg was free to move the movements resembled stepping and occurred at a steady frequency of 2.2 s^{-1}, equivalent to fast walking (Fig. 6). A shift of the pipette no more than 3μm away from the optimal site resulted in loss of the response. Placing the electrode in precisely the equivalent location on the contralateral side, followed by similar OCT iontophoresis, caused the contralateral leg to step similarly.

In exploring the effects of similar iontophoretic releases at other neuropilar sites, two were found, along with contralateral homologues, four in all, at which OCT release

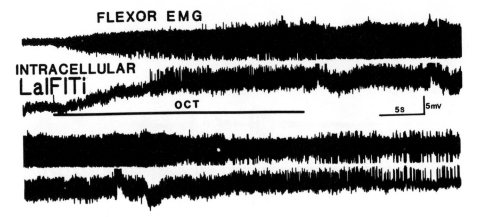

Fig. 5. Direct depolarization and excitation of flexor motor neurons by OCT iontophoresed at a site near that used in the experiment of Fig. 4. *Above* is the flexor EMG, below the intracellular response of the lateral intermediate flexor tibiae motor neuron (LaIFITi) – continuous record. (Sombati and Hoyle 1984b)

was followed by a bout of fictive flight. This involved movements of both sides of the insect equally, i.e. the whole flight motor was turned on (Fig. 7). The duration of the bout, but not either the frequency or the amplitude, of the movements, was dose-dependent. The longest sequence obtained lasted 25 min, for an injection time of 1.5 min.

It begins to look as though there may have been a phylogenetic split, with annelids and molluscs exploiting 5 H-T as a potentiating modulator, whereas arthropods have concentrated on OCT, or have utilized both substances. In one molluscan preparation potentiation of biphasic synaptic transmission by activity in a neuron considered to be 5 H-Tergic, is exactly mimicked by either 5 H-T or OCT (Shimahara and Tauc 1978). Thus not only can their effects be similar, they may be two different keys each capable of opening the same lock.

6 Functions of NH

One well-characterized invertebrate neurohormone whose actions have been extensively studied at the cellular level is the bag-cell or egg-laying hormone (ELH) of marine molluscs, a polypeptide which has been sequenced (Mahon and Scheller 1983). ELH causes a long-lasting stereotyped behaviour in which other activities are suppressed, a suitable substrate for the egg string is located, and then the eggs are carefully laid. The neural mechanism has not been worked out, but long-lasting effects on neuronal properties, excitation of some neurons, inhibition of others, are known, and the whole process can, in principle at least, be worked out. It is possible, though it seems unlikely, that all the various effects are directly brought about by the peptide. More likely is that the neurohormone does some things by direct actions on membrane properties and others

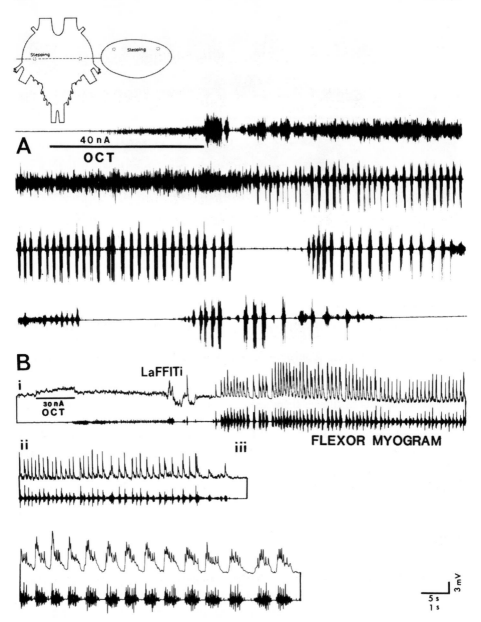

Fig. 6 A, B. Bouts of stepping evoked by OCT iontophoresed into the restricted specific site in the neuropile indicated in the inset. **A** Strong, prolonged flexion, followed by rhythmical flex/extend movements. Extracellular myogram from the flexor tibiae. **B** Weak flexion which was soon followed by a nice bout of stepping movements. Intracellular recording from identified neuron LaFFlTi accompanies EMG. An excerpt at higher speed shows the depolarizing potentials and bursts of spikes in the motor neuron. (Sombati and Hoyle 1984a)

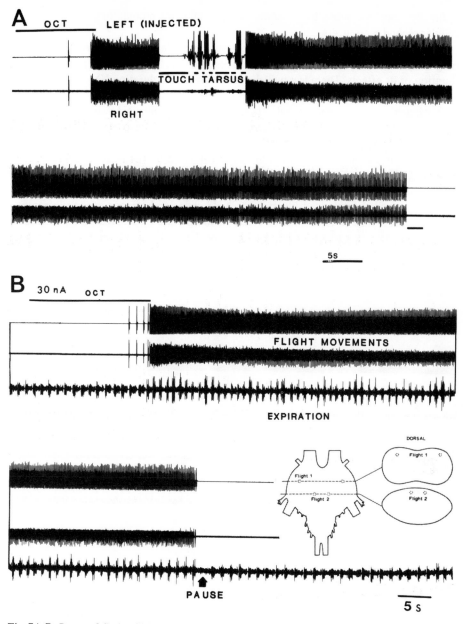

Fig. 7A,B. Bouts of fictive flight evoked by OCT iontophoresed in one of the four region shown in the inset. The movements and their frequency are identical regardless of site, except that tarsal inhibition is less complete on the ipsilateral site. The duration of a bout is dose-dependent. A coupled stepwise increase in the intensity and frequency of respiratory movements precisely accompanies the bout. (Sombati and Hoyle 1984a)

indirectly, some via activation of other neurons releasing modulators, others via intracellular second messengers.

A major difference between the actions of a modulator and a neurohormone is a long delay before any action is apparent as a result of the latter, and the extremely long duration of its effects. There is a twilight zone where long-duration NM actions overlap with the shorter-duration NH actions and indeed there are some NAS which serve in both capacities in the same animal. There is no reason why a NAS should not be able to serve as all three, NT, NM, and NH, in one animal, and possibly some amines do this, for it depends only on the nature of the release site and the target. In vertebrates norepinephrine is a likely candidate for the triple role. In arthropods, acetylcholine, octopamine (OCT), proctolin (PRN) have each been shown to serve at least dual roles, ACh as NT and NM, OCT and PRN as NM and NH.

Another well-characterized invertebrate NH is eclosion hormone of the silk moth, a large peptide which is released into blood in the mature pupa. After a 20-min delay following release, a species-specific pre-eclosion behaviour starts, and lasts for about 1.5 h (Fig. 8A). The abdomen rotates and undulates vigorously for 20–30 min, then continues the same movements, but weakly, for 30 min, followed by a final 1/2 h of vigorous movement. This behaviour serves to loosen the stiff pupal cuticle. True eclosion

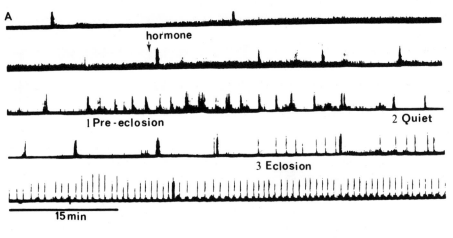

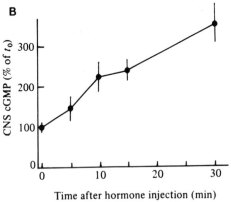

Fig. 8A,B. Example of the elicitation of a long-lasting behaviour sequence by a neurohormone: pre-eclosion behaviour, followed by eclosion, of the abdomen of the silk moth *Hyalophora cecropia* in response to addition of eclosion NH to bathing fluid. A Monitored as extracellular electrical activity in motor axons from an isolated CNS preparation. (From Truman 1978) B Rise in cGMP in nervous system following addition of eclosion NH. (Truman et al. 1980)

then commences. There is a rise in cAMP which occurs early, and which initiates other relevant events, before falling. The most significant following action appears to be a slow steady rise of cGMP in some of the neurons of the pre-eclosion MPG (Fig. 8B). The involvement of cGMP explains the initial delay, since its concentration rises only slowly, to reach the threshold level for turning on the behaviour either by clutching, intensification, or turning on, of the MPG.

There are two ways in which the need for a second, or third, messenger might be linked to the slow progression of such a behaviour. Different regions of the MPG may have progressively higher thresholds, or the rise in concentration of the intermediary may be different in different regions.

7 Discussion

If we are ever fully to understand the generation of behaviour there is no doubt that we must have a much better understanding than we currently do of the chemical diversity, overall functions, and specific physiological actions, of NM and NH in diverse organisms. It no longer seems likely that any major circuit functions solely by virtue of the intrinsic properties of its component neurons and their synaptic connections. The problem with recognizing that modular functions are of such importance is that it is already apparent that their more existence makes it less likely that we shall ever be able to comprehend MPG. In a recent article Selverston (1980) presciently drew attention to the impending difficulties. He works with the smallest organized functionally cohesive set of neurons known, except for arthropod cardiac ganglia, namely the lobster stomatogastric ganglion. There are only 30 neurons, divided into two independent groups of 14 and 16, each set having different functions. One set controls three teeth which rhythmically grind up food in the cardiac (anterior) stomach, the other simply controls opening and closing of the pyloric sphincter. Yet in spite of their simple functions, it is now apparent that the neuronal circuits, for all the subtlety of their connections and intrinsic properties, could not operate alone. They must be triggered, by ACh which is then serving as a modulator (Nagy and Dickinson 1983), or alternatively/complementarily by dopamine (Kushner 1979). In addition though, 5 H-T is involved as an adjustor of timing, and possibly also histamine and one or more peptides (Marder and Eisen 1984).

The prospect must be faced that natural functioning includes modulation of modulations. All this is doubtless nice from the organism's point of view, since fine-tuning has homeostatic and therefore adaptive value. Even a lobster must function better if it is not suffering from indigestion! But from the investigator's point of view, particularly if a global, analytical, perspective is desired rather than a mere descriptive catalogue, the realization is at once exhilarating intellectually and demoralizing in practice. A technically-talented international team, with some 30-plus participants, has been constantly at work unravelling the secrets of the lobster cardiac ganglion food-chewing MPG for the past 15 years and is still finding out new facts! What, then, are the prospects for understanding MPG's in more complex parts of a nervous system, especially for arhythmic behaviour sequences of evolutionarily more advanced animals? We already

posses the technical ability to collect the needed data, short of discovering new phenomena. What is needed now is a realistic understanding of the magnitude, as well as
the nature, of the task, and the will, patience and above all very long-term financial
support, necessary to sustain the research.

References

Bianchi S (1967) On the different types of fluorescent neurons in the leech *(Hirudo medicinalis)*.
    Atti Soc Peloritana Sci Fis Mat Nat 13:39–47
Dismukes RK (1979) New concepts of molecular communication among neurons. Behav Brain Sci
    2:427–429
Eisenstadt M, Goldman JE, Kandel ER, Koike H, Koester J, Schwartz JH (1973) Intrasomatic in-
    jection of radioactive precursors for studying transmitter synthesis in identified neurons of
    Aplysia californica. Proc Natl Acad Sci 70:3371–3375
Evans PD (1981) Multiple receptor types for octopamine in the locust. J Physiol (Lond) 318:99–
    122
Evans PD, O'Shea M (1978) The identification of an octopaminergic neurone and the modulation
    of a myogenic rhythm in the locust. J Exp Biol 73:235–260
Glanzman DC, Krasne FB (1983) Serotonin and octopamine have opposite modulatory effects on
    the crayfish's lateral giant escape reaction. J Neurosci 3:2263–2269
Harrow ID, David JA, Satelle DB (1982) Acetylcholine receptors of identified insect neurons. In:
    Neuropharmacology of insects. CIBA Symp 88:12–31
Hoyle G (1975) Evidence that insect dorsal unpaired median (DUM) neurons are octopaminergic. J
    Exp Zool 193:425–431
Hoyle G (1978) The dorsal, unpaired, median neurons of the locust metathoracic ganglion. J Neuro-
    biol 9:43–57
Hoyle G (1984) Neuromuscular transmission in a primitive insect: modulation by octopamine, and
    catch-like tension. Comp Biochem Physiol 77C:219–232
Hoyle G, Barker DL (1975) Synthesis of octopamine by DUM neurons. J Exp Zool 193:433–439
Hoyle G, Field LH (1983a) Defense posture and leg-position learning in a primitive insect utilize
    catchlike tension. J Neurobiol 14:285–298
Hoyle G, Field LH (1983b) Elicitation and abrupt termination of behaviorally significant catchlike
    tension in a primitive insect. J Neurobiol 14:299–312
Kandel ER, Schwartz JH (1982) Molecular biology of learning: modulation of transmitter release.
    Science (Wash DC) 218:433–443
Kushner PD (1979) The presence and function of dopamine in the lobster stomatogastric nervous
    system: the generation and regulation of motor rhythms. Ph.D. Dissertation, Univ Oregon
Lent CM, Dickinson MH (1984) Serotonin integrates the feeding behavior of the medicinal leech.
    J Comp Physiol A Sens Neural Behav Physiol 154:457–471
Livingstone MS, Harris-Warrick RM, Kravitz EA (1980) Serotonin and octopamine produce opposite
    postures in lobsters. Science (Wash DC) 208:76–79
Mahon AC, Scheller RH (1983) The molecular basis of a neuroendocrine fixed action pattern: egg
    laying in *Aplysia*. In: Molecular neurobiology. Cold Spring Harbor Symp Quant Biol 68:405–
    412
Marder E, Eisen E (1984) Electrically coupled pacemaker neurons respond differently to the same
    physiological inputs and neurotransmitters. J Neurophysiol (Bethesda) 51:1362–1374
Nagy F, Dickinson PS (1983) Control of a central pattern generator by an identified modulatory
    interneurone in crustacea. J Exp Biol 105:33–58
O'Shea M, Evans PD (1979) Potentiation of neuromuscular transmission by an octopaminergic
    neurons in the locust. J Exp Biol 79:169–190
Selverston AI (1980) Are central pattern generators understandable? Behav Brain Sci 3:535–571

Shimahara T, Tauc L (1978) The role of cyclic AMP in the modulation of synaptic efficacy. J Physiol (Lond) 74:515–519

Sombati S, Hoyle G (1984a) Central nervous sensitization and dishabituation of reflex action in an insect by neuromodulator octopamine. J Neurobiol 15:455–480

Sombati S, Hoyle G (1984b) Generation of specific behaviors in a locust by local release into neuropil of the natural neuromodulator octopamine. J Neurobiol 15:481–506

Sombati S, Hoyle G (1984c) Glutamatergic central nervous transmission in insects. J Neurobiol 15: 507–516

Truman JW (1978) Hormonal release of stereoytped motor programmes from the isolated nervous system of the Cecropia silkmoth. J Exp Biol 74:151–173

Truman JW, Mumby SM, Welch SK (1980) Involvement of cyclic GMP in the release of stereotyped behavior patterns in moths by a peptide hormone. J Exp Biol 84:201–212

Weeks JC, Kristan WB (1978) Initiation, maintenance and modulation of swimming in the medicinal leech by the activity of a single neuron. J Exp Biol 77:71–88

Willard AL (1981) Effects of serotonin on the generation of the motor program for swimming by the medicinal leech. J Neurosci 1:936–944

Wilson JA, Hoyle G (1978) Serially homologous neurones as concomitants of functional specialization. Nature (Lond) 274:377–379

Zipser B, McKay R (1981) Monoclonal antibodies distinguish identifiable neurones in the leech. Nature (Lond) 289:549–554

The Distribution of Biogenic Monoamines in Invertebrates

N. KLEMM [1]

This Chapter presents a short overview about our knowledge of the presence and localization of biogenic monoamines (bMA) in invertebrates. Biogenic MA are known as neuroactive substances and their occurence in the nervous system will be of main concern in this article. Their distribution was studied in several invertebrate phyla by numerous authors and it has not been possible to list all the citations in the reference list. The limited number of neurons, the location of the cell bodies at the surface of the ganglia, and their large size in some species has made the invertebrate neurons accessible to experimental approach. As an example the most compelling evidence that serotonin act as a transmitter and as a modulatory substance was achieved by studying the metacerebral giant 5-HT-containing cell in *Aplysia* (see Pentreath et al. 1982).

Although histamine (HA) and tryptamine are also biogenic monoamines (bMA) our attention here will be focussed on catecholamines (CA), octopamine (OCT), and serotonin (5-HT). Several histochemical methods are available to selectively demonstrate bMA-containing neurons but this article will focus on information obtained by the most specific histochemical methods as the formaldehyde-induced fluorescence method (Falck-Hillarp method, such FIF method) and its glyoxylic acid derivates for the intracellular demonstration of "fluorogenic" bMA as the CA dopamine (DA), noradrenaline (NA), adrenaline (A), and the indolylalkylamine (IA) 5-HT. Using routine filtre setting CA emit green and IA yellow light.

Unfortunately these methods do not differentiate between the amines and their precursor amino acids L-DOPA or 5-HTP and information about the presence of DOPA and 5-HTP and about their concentrations is important before the fluorophore can be interpreted as being of CA or IA-type. The aldehyde method is not very sensitive to 5-HT thus the reports on the presence of 5-HT achieved by the FIF method may in many cases be fragmentary. The recently introduced specific antibody to 5-HT helps to solve some of the pitfalls of the FIF methods provided that appropriate specificity tests are made. The specificity of the present histochemical methods for the cellular localization of other bMA such as OA, HA, and tryptamine remains to be demonstrated.

---

1 Department of Zoology, University of Lund, Lund, Sweden

Neurobiology
(ed. by R. Gilles and J. Balthazart)
© Springer-Verlag Berlin Heidelberg 1985

1 Protozoa

There are only few fragmentary reports on the presence of bMA in Protozoa. CA and 5-HT seem to occur in ciliates (see Welsh and Moorehead 1960; Welsh 1972).

2 Metazoa

2.1 Coelenterata

The Coelenterata which include hydra, jelly fish and sea anemones represent the lowest phylum of the phylogenetic tree of animals which have a nervous system. Biogenic MA were detected in many species. Its content varies from species to species and differs even in closely related forms. DA and NA was found in many but not all forms investigated. 5-HT so far has been found only in a scyphozoan. No A was found. In the hydrozoan *Hydra attenuata* DA (0.3 μg gww^{-1}), NA (0.003 μg gww^{-1}), and L-DOPA (0.0015 μg gww^{-1}) were detected. In *Tubularia indivisa* these data were 0.8 μg gww^{-1}, 0.3 μg gww^{-1}, and 0.07 μg gww^{-1} respectively as given by Carlberg and Rosengren (1985) using HPLC/EC analyses. They could not find A or 5-HT. No histochemical reaction were seen in Hydrozoa after aldehyde treatment by Dahl et al. (1963) or by Plotnikova and Govyrin (1966). 5-HT and HA are likely to be a part of the toxin of the scyphozoan sea wasp *Chironex fleckeri* and in the sea nettle *Chrysaora quinquecirrha* (see Burnett and Calton 1977). Green fluorescent neurons which may be sensory or sensorymotoric were found in the ectoderm of Anthozoa. These cell bodies have one process to the surface, while the others proceed proximally and contribute fibres to the green fluorescent basiepithelial nervous network, close to the basal membrane. Plotnikova and Govyrin (1966) reported similar distribution of fluorescence in *Actinia equina* and *Burodactis stella*, which may be due to L-DOPA as no fluorogenic MA could be detected in actinians. Instead several μg gww^{-1} L-DOPA were estimated. The polype of the octocorallian *Kophobelemnon stroemi*, however, contains DA, NA, and L-DOPA but no A or 5-HT (Carlberg and Rosengren 1985). In the ctenoporan *Beroe* sp. the presence of DA, NA, and L-DOPA were reported by Carlberg and Rosengren (1985).

2.2 Plathelminthes

2.2.1 Turbellaria

In whole aminal extracts of the free living flatworm *Dugesia tigrina* the presence of 5-HT (1.5-3.5 μg gww^{-1}) (Welsh and Moorehead 1960), DA (1.3 μg gww^{-1}), and NA (0.2 μg gww^{-1}) was established (Welsh 1972). The distribution of fluorogenic MA was studied in *Euplanaria* sp. (Dahl et al. 1963), in *Dendrocoeleums lacteum* (Plotnikova and Kuzmina 1968), in *Phagocata oregonensis, Proctotyla fluviatilis,* and *Dugesia tigrina* (Welsh and Williams 1970), in *Polycelis nigra* (Lurje 1975), and in *Microstomum lineata* (Reuter et al. 1980) by means of the Falck-Hillarp method. In *Microstomum* only green fluorescent neurons were found but green and yellow neurons were detected in all other species studied. Both types of fluorophores were found in cell bodies and fibres in the paired cerebral ganglia and in the cerebral commisure connecting both ganglia. Along the paired nerve cord green and yellow fluorescent cell bodies are distributed at intervals without obvious clustering into ganglia. In *Protoctyla* and *Dugesia* cell bodies with an indole-type of fluorophore are situated at the base of each commisure between both nerve cords. One of their processes follows the commisure to the contralateral nerve cord, while the other processes run to the periphery. In *M. lineata, D. lacteum,* and *P. nigra* only green fibres were reported to leave the CNS to supply the peripheral muscles. These fibres form a subepithelial plexus together with monopolar and multipolar green fluorescent cell bodies.

In *Turbellaria* a system of neurons is separated from the CNS and innervates the intestine ("autonomic" nervous system). Its apical part, the stomatogastric nervous system, closely surrounds the pharynx. It contains many scattered green fluorescent fibres and cell bodies whose fibres are continuous with the CNS. Fibres from the stomatogastric nervous system innervate the pharyngeal muscles (Plotnikova and Kuzmina 1968; Welsh and Williams 1970; Lurje 1975; Reuter et al. 1980). Welsh and Williams (1970) and Reuter et al. (1980) found many green fluorescent multipolar neurons just beneath the outer muscle layer of the pharynx and yellow fluorescent cells were found in deeper muscle layers (Welsh and Williams 1970). Single green fluorescent fibres were also found to supply the midgut (Reuter et al. 1980).

2.2.2 Trematoda

In the parasitic trematode *Schistosoma mansoni* Chou et al. (1972) analysed 5-HT (2.0–3.5 μg gww^{-1}) and NA (0.2–0.4 μg gww^{-1}) but did not find DA. In *Sch. haematobium* they found only 5-HT and no CA, while in *Sch. japonicum* DA, NA, and 5-HT were found. Bennet and Bueding (1973) could not find any evidence that *Sch. mansoni* can synthesize 5-HT from tryptophan. They found, however, that 5HT and 5-HTP can be taken up from the medium into the CNS of the worms against a concentration gradient by an active uptake process. In the CNS 5-HTP is converted into 5-HT. They concluded that 5-HT and/or 5-HTP had to be supplied from the host. Although 5-HT is the dominant bMA in schistosomides it was not found in the liver fluke *Fasciola hepatica* were only DA (0.3–0.7 μg gww^{-1}) was detected (Chou et al. 1972).

The location of bMA was studied in *Sch. mansoni* by Bennet and Bueding (1971) and by Machado et al. (1972). Green and yellow fluorescent cell bodies were found in the cerebral region and in regular intervals along the nerve trunks. Fibres of both cell types emerge from the paired central nerve trunks and run to the periphery to end below the integument. No fluorescent cell bodies were seen in the integument (Bennet and Bueding 1971). Other fibres proceed centrally and are distributed throughout the parenchyma between the nerve trunks.

2.2.3 Cestoda

Chemical analyses of whole tapeworms of the species *Mesocestoides corti* (Hariri 1974) and *Hymenolepis diminuates* (Chou et al. 1972) revealed the presence of 5-HT but no CA was detected. Shield (1971) studied bMA in *Dipylidium caninum* and found aldehyde induced fluorescence in the CNS of the scolex and in the longitudinal nerve cords in the proglotids, in the musculature of the body wall, in the suckers, in the rostellar pad and rostellar gland of the scolex, in the cirrus pouch and in the wall of the copulation canal in the genital apparatus. The fluorophore was not further characterized. The more primitive tapeworm *Diphyllobotrium dendriticum* was studied by Gustafsson and Wikren (1981) and they found only neurons with yellow fluorescence. The cell bodies were located in the cerebral ganglia and in the nerve cord. From the cerebral ganglia fluorescent fibres (probably sensory) run to the tip of the bothridia. Yellow fluorescent monopolar and bipolar cell bodies are situated peripherally along the nerve cords at frequent intervals. One of their processes extends peripherally into the parenchyma. A network of fluorescent fibres was reported in the longitudinal muscle layer with fibres interspaced between the subtegumental cells.

2.3 Nemertini

5-HT was quantified in extracts of the ribbon worm *Lineus ruber* and *Cerebratulus lacteus* by Welsh and Moorhead (1960). In both species the highest concentration was found in the head, 0.43 μg gww^{-1} in the former species and 2.9 μg gww^{-1} in the latter species. Green fluorescent cell bodies were seen in the cerebral ganglion of *Lineus sanguineus* by Reutter (1969). Green fibres extend from the cerebral ganglion to the head region where they form a green subepithelial fibre plexus. Green fluorescent, presumably sensory fibres, extend to the frontal organs. The ribbon worms have a retractable proboscis dorsally to the mouth and the forgut. In *Lineus* nerve fibres with green fluorescence were found to supply the muscle layer on the proboscis, mouth, and foregut. No cell bodies were detected in this region. The retractor muscle of the proboscis receives CA fibres. The nerve fibres in the proboscis and in the mouth and foregut region were supposed to be sensoric and motoric (Reutter 1969).

2.4 Nematoda

In the wild type of *Caenorhabditis elegans* DA (145 ng gww^{-1}) and DOPA (16 ng gww^{-1}) has been assayed by Sulston et al. (1975). Plotnikova et al. (1969) reported green fluorescent fibres in the four nerve trunks of the CNS in the parasite *Ascaris suum*. Green fibres, probably of central origin, project along the papillary nerve to the rostral papillae. Several green fluorescent cells were also found in the CNS of the tail regions. In young larva of *Ascaris lumbricoides* (Sulston et al. 1975) and in adults of *Phocanema decipiens* (Goh and Davey 1976) four cephalic neurons were seen, each sends a process forward to the rostral papillae and one presumed efferent process rearward into the nerve ring. The arrangement of green fluorescent neurons is remarkably similar in the tiny (1 mm) free living nematode *C. elegans* and the much larger (40 cm) parasitic *A. lumbricoides*. In *C. elegans* different mutations are known that do not synthesize DA (Sulston et al. 1975).

2.5 Annelida

2.5.1 Polychaeta

The concentration of DA, NA, and 5-HT was assayed in the cerebral ganglia and in the ventral cord of *Glycera convulata* by Manaranche and LéHermite (1973) who measured

5-HT (17.7 μg gww^{-1}; 21.9 μg gww^{-1}), DA (2.48 and 0.48 μg gww^{-1}), NA (3.25 and 1.64 μg gww^{-1}). They also claimed to have detected A (7.0 and 9.1 μg gww^{-1} respectively, see also Welsh and Moorhead (1960).

Detailed histochemical studies were performed on *Nephtys* sp. by Clarke (1966) and on *Nereis virens* by White and Marsden (1978). In both species green fluorescent neurons were found to dominate in the cerebral ganglion and yellow fluorescence dominate in the ventral cord were they form a repetitive pattern in successive segments. No fluorescence was found in the giant fibres (Clarke 1966). Green processes from small CA-containing cells in the dorsal tegumental epidermis project from the prostomial epidermis via the n. tegmentalis into the CNS in *Nephtys* (Clarke 1966). Contrary to the findings in *Nephtys* no fluorescence was found in the tegumental nerve in *N. virens* (White and Marsden 1978). In *Nephtys* yellow fluorescent fibres of central origin were reported to project to the periphery. In *N. virens*, however, White and Marsden (1978) could not detect any 5-HT fibre outside the CNS. In no species fluorogenic MA were seen in the palpal nerves, nuchal nerves, or optic nerves. In *Nephtys* (Clarke 1966) yellow fluorescent fibres from the circumoesophageal connective invade the pharynx. Small yellow fluorescent cell bodies were found in the epithelium of the gut.

2.5.2 Oligochaeta

Biogenic MA were quantified in the CNS of the earthworm *Lumbricus terrestris*. The concentration of 5-HT in the nerve cord was 10.4 μg gww^{-1} (Welsh and Moorhead 1960) and that of DA, NA, and OCT 1.8 μg gww^{-1}, 0.8 μg gww^{-1}, and 3.6 μg gww^{-1} respectively (Robertson and Osborne 1979).

Rude (1966) and Myhrberg (1967) contributed the most detailed studies on the location of bMA in the earthworm. In the cortex of the cerebral ganglia approximately equal numbers of numerous green and yellow fluorescent cells were seen distributed among the non-fluorescent cells of the cortex; they did not seem to be concentrated into clusters. Their processes run into the fluorescent neuropil. The ventral cord contains 150–170 ganglia each with approx. 1,000 neurons. Each ganglion contains about 50 yellow or green fluorescent cells after aldehyde treatment. One pair of green fluorescent fibre tracts proceeds uninterruptedly on the dorsal part of the neuropil of both halves of the whole nerve cord and has many green fluorescent cross-connections between both sides (Rude 1966). Some yellow fluorescent fibres leave the CNS while green fibres originate from green fluorescent bipolar cells in the body wall (Rude 1966; Myhrberg 1967). In these cells DA was analyzed by microspectrofluorometry (Ehinger and Myhrberg 1971). Their proximal processes branch into the green fluorescent network beneath the epidermis (basiepithelial network) from which fibres proceed further along the segmental nerve into the CNS (Myhrberg 1967).

Myhrberg (1967) found bipolar and tripolar green fluorescent nerve cells in the pharyngeal wall of the earthworm. One of their processes seems to supply the musculature of the pharynx. Other processes join the basiepithelial network of the pharynx. Another type of cell lies subepithelialy and has a process directed towards the epithelial surface. No CA or 5-HT were seen in the alimentary canal posterior to the pharynx.

2.5.3 Hirudinea

Only 5-HT (3.7 μg gww^{-1} – Ehinger et al. 1968; Marsden and Kerkut 1969) but almost no CA (Marsden and Kerkut 1969) was quantified in the CNS of the leech *Hirudo medicinalis*.

The distribution of fluorogenic amine-containing neurons was studied in *Hirudo medicinalis* by several authors (see Lent 1977). A total of 129–138 yellow cells and 25–29 green cells were counted in the 34 ganglia of *Hirudo* (Rude 1969). Principally each unfused segmental ganglion contains seven cell bodies containing 5-HT two of which are the large (diameter: 80–90 μm) Retzius cells. This pattern of cellular distribution can be followed in every segmental ganglion. In some ganglia a pair of green fluorescent cell bodies were seen. Each root ganglion contains a pair of DA-containing cell bodies each with a process that proceeds into the CNS. The brain consists of two ganglia and has only two pairs of green fluorescent cell bodies (Rude 1969). Yellow fluorescent longitudinal fibre tracts extend along the whole length of the CNS. The majority of the neurons seems to be interneurons. Only the Retzius cell axons were seen to leave the CNS where they supply the muscles of the body wall (Mason and Leake 1978).

Contrary to the other annelides no fluorescent cell bodies or CA-containing fibres were found in the peripheral tissue (Ehinger et al. 1968; Marsden and Kerkut 1969; Rude 1969).

Rude (1969) reported the presence of green fluorescent fibres in the stomatogastric nerve ring, but according to Marsden and Kerkut (1969) only yellow fibres supply the muscles of the pharynx.

2.6 Mollusca

2.6.1 Gastropoda

Biogenic MA have been measured in the CNS of several species of molluscs, e.g. *Helix pomatia* (Guthrie et al. 1976) and *Aplysia californica* (Carpenter et al. 1971) (see also Welsh and Moorhead 1960; Welsh 1972). DA, OA, and 5-HT were found in all species investigated. NA was present in *Helix* (Guthrie et al. 1976) but no detectable amounts were seen in *Aplysia* (Carpenter et al. 1971). Adrenaline has not yet been found in any mollusc. Some 5-HTP was reported in *H. pomatia* but L-DOPA was undetectable (Dolezalova et al. 1973). Hiripi and Salanki (1973) reported seasonal variation of the 5-HT concentration in the CNS in *H. pomatia*; 5-HT content was highest in the autumn and the lowest in spring.

Histochemical studies revealed green and yellow fluorescent cell bodies which may occur together in the same ganglion (cerebral ganglion) or alone, as in the right parietal ganglion and visceral ganglia of *P. corneus* where only 5-HT cells were found (Marsden and Kerkut 1970). In the cerebral ganglion of *A. californica*, Tritt et al. (1983) found 8–10 CA and 10–25 5-HT-containing neurons using the glyoxylic acid technique. Almost all cell bodies in the CNS of *Aplysia*, including the bag cells (Tritt et al. 1983), are surrounded by 5-HT (Tritt et al. 1983) or 5-HT-immunoreactive (5-HTi) (Goldstein et al. 1984; Ono and McCaman 1984) fibres which may make axo-somatic contacts (Tritt et al. 1983; Goldstein et al. 1984; Ono and McCaman 1984). The majority of the 5-HT-containing cell processes do not leave the CNS.

Some molluscan MA-containing cells are very large, especially the giant serotonin-containing cell (GSC) of the cerebral ganglion that is found in many species (Pentreath et al. 1982). In the giant Brasilian land snail *Strochocheilus oblongus* the cell body diameter reaches 500 μm (Jaeger et al. 1971). Its axons project into the neuropil of other ganglia and contact several cell bodies. Some of its axons leave the CNS and supply the muscles involved in feeding (Pentreath et al. 1982). Another giant DA-containing cell body (GDC) (about 200 μm in diameter) lies in the left pedal ganglion i.e. in *P. corneus* (Marsden and Kerkut 1970). Its processes course into several central ganglia and some of them project inwards the periphery (Pentreath and Berry 1975).

The heart of *H. pomatia* receives CA and 5-HT fibres from the visceral nerve (Cardot 1971; Jaeger et al. 1971). According to Cardot (1971) the concentration of 5-HT in the heart varies and is highest in June and lowest in February, at the end of the hibernation period similar as in the CNS.

In the slug *Limax maximus* CA fibres reach several somatic muscles, including the retractors of the head, tentacles, and pharynx, and some glands, including the pedal mucus glands (Osborne and Cottrell 1971). The muscles of the gill in *Aplysia* are innervated by CA and 5-HT fibres (Peretz and Estes 1974). Fibres with 5-HT innervate the visceral musculature of the fore gut in *P. corneus* (Marsden and Kerkut 1970) and *A. californica* (Goldstein et al. 1984). The musculature of the pharynx receives 5-HT fibres and small green cells were found in the wall of the oesophagus (Marsden and Kerkut 1970).

CA-containing fibres were found to be scattered throughout the integument of *L. maximus*. They concentrate in the tentacles, the facial grooves and near the mouth (Osborne and Cottrell 1971). Monopolar and bipolar cells containing DA are scattered in the gill of *A. californica* (Peretz and Ester 1974). Presumed sensory cells containing CA were seen in the statocyst (Tritt et al. 1983) and the tentacle, mantle, and siphon epithelium of *Aplysia* (Luborsdky-Moore and Jacklet 1976).

Presumed neurosecretory neurons containing 5-HT are present in the neuronal sheath of the CNS of the marine species *Philine aperta* (Barber 1982) and *A. californica* (Goldstein et al. 1984). These fibres originate in the CNS and their varicosities in this regions are exposed directly to the blood (Barber 1982).

2.6.2 Bivalvia

In the bivalve CNS, 5-HT (Welsh and Moorhead 1960) and DA, but no NA or A (Myers and Sweeney 1972) were detected. In *Mytilus edulis* the concentration of 5-HT in the CNS was found to vary seasonaly being highest ($57.3\ \mu g\ gww^{-1}$) in August and lowest ($25.1\ \mu g\ gww^{-1}$) in January (Stefano and Catapane 1977).

A detailed histochemical study using the Falck-Hillarp method was performed by Sweeney (1968) on the 5-mm-long species *Spaerium sulcatum*. A total number of aprox. 2,000 cell bodies were found to be fluorescent. In each half of the cerebral ganglion about 120 yellow and 50 green fluorescent cells were seen. The pedal ganglion contains about 250 yellow fluorescent cell bodies but no green ones and the visceral ganglion about 125 green fluorescent cells but no yellow ones. In the very reduced buccal ganglion only green cells were detected. All ganglia contain green and yellow fluorescent fibres. In the visceral ganglion of *M. edulis*, some 5-HT cells occur in addition to CA-containing cell bodies (Stefano and Aiello 1975). The green cells in the buccal ganglion contribute to fibres which form a nervous plexus around the oesophagus.

The branchial nerve innervates the gills of *M. edulis* with yellow and green fluorescent fibres of central origin (Stefano and Aiello 1975). No innervation of the heart of *S. sulcatum* by fluorogenic MA could be detected (Sweeney 1968).

Sweeney (1968) reported three green cells in the wall of the statocyst in *S. sulcatum*. Presumed sensory cells containing CA were seen also in the edge of the mantle, in the foot, in the posterior pallial region and in the siphons.

In *M. edulis* Stefano and Aiello showed some bMA fibres of neurosecretory type around the sheath of the CNS.

2.6.3 Cephalopoda

Dopamine, NA, OA, and 5-HT were detected in all parts of the CNS of cephalopods. Generally the concentration of bMA is higher in *Octopoda* than in *Decapoda*. For quantitative data see Robertson and Juorio (1976).

Aldehyde induced fluorescence of CA and 5-HT was seen in many regions of the CNS. Cell bodies and fluorescent fibres were found in the superior buccal lobe, in the posterior buccal and lateral frontal lobes. Strong fluorescence which was not further specified appears in the median inferior frontal lobes which receives "taste fibres" from the labial lobe, in subfrontal lobes, superior frontal lobes, vertical lobes, subvertical lobes, and the peduncle and basal lobes. Some CA and 5-HT fibres were seen in some of the plexiform layers of the optic lobe but not in the photoreceptor cells or optic nerve (Matus 1973).

The posterior salivary gland in *Octopus* is rich in bMA (Robertson and Juorio 1976). For example in *Octopus vulgaris* the salivary gland contents of OCT, DA, NA, and 5-HT are respectively 1,300 μg gww^{-1}, 3,100 μg gww^{-1}, 5,800 μg gww^{-1}, and 460 μg gww^{-1}. In the cuttle fish *Sepia officinalis* the salivary gland concentrations of bMA are much lower: respectively 0.09 μg gww^{-1}, 0.89 μg gww^{-1}, 1.5 μg gww^{-1}, and less than 0.070 μg gww^{-1} (Robertson and Juorio 1976). There is evidence that some of these amines originate in the CNS and reach the gland via the posterior salivary nerve (Martin and Barlow 1972; Arluison and Ducrois 1977).

Fluorescent fibres originating in the inferior buccal ganglion were found to innervate the crop and the oesophagus in several octopod species, while the rest of the alimentary canal receives non-fluorescent fibres from the gastric ganglion. No fluorescence was detected in the systemic or branchial heart, which is contrary to the findings in gastropods (Juorio and Killick 1973).

2.7 Arthropoda

In arthropod nervous tissue DA, NA, OCT, and 5-HT but no A have been found (Klemm 1976; Evans 1980). Biogenic MA occur also in the haemolymph (Evans 1980; Beltz and Kravitz 1983) and in arthropods DA is further involved in wound healing and in the sclerotinization and melanization of newly formed exoskeleton (Brunet 1980). The neuronal and non-neuronal CA pools seem to be separated by the initial step of synthesis from tyrosine to L-DOPA. In the nervous system this step involves tyrosine hydroxylase, as in mammals (Maxwell et al. 1978; Laxmyr, in press), while in the cuticle tyrosinases convert tyrosine to L-DOPA and its further o-quinone products (Brunet 1980; Laxmyr, in press). The following description focuses on bMA in the nervous system of some crustacea and insects that have been intensively studied.

2.7.1 Crustacea

The concentration of DA, NA, OCT, and 5-HT was studied in the CNS of several species of decapod crustacea (Laxmyr 1984). For example in the cerebral ganglion (brain) of the crayfish *Pacifastacus leniusculus* the concentration of DA is 0.30 μg gww^{-1}, NA 0.19 μg gww^{-1}, OA 0.88 μg gww^{-1}, and 5-HT 0.20 μg gww^{-1}. Quantitative data of other authors are summarized by Laxmyr (1984). Besides CA considerable amounts of L-DOPA (0.20 μg gww^{-1}) were found. After stress (i.e. prolonged handling) the L-DOPA concentration reached values of 2.0 μg gww^{-1} whereas the concentration of bMA remained unaltered (Elofsson et al. 1982).

The distribution of bMA was studied mainly with the Falck-Hillarp method. Recently data obtained with immunocytological methods for the detection of 5-HT are added. In the brain of the crayfish green cell bodies were found in two of the six cell agglomerizations (Elofsson et al. 1966) and 5-HTi cells occur in five of the six (Elofsson 1983). Green fluorescent fibres and 5-HT-immunoreactive (5-HTi) fibres pervade large parts of the neuropil and accumulate in many regions (central body, protocerebral bridge, olfactory glomeruli in the deutocerebrum etc.). In the crab *Carcinus maenas* green fluorescent cells occur in five of the six cell clusters (Goldstone and Cook 1971). In neither crayfish nor crab, was fluorescence found to be associated with the neurosecretory X-organ and sinus gland. The brains of several non-malacostracan and malacostracan species were studied by Aramant and Elofsson (1976). In all species green fluorescent interneurons were always found in the central body but their presence in other structures varied in different species. A comparative interpretation of the data is difficult because of the lack of comparative neuroanatomical information about the crustacean brain.

In *Malacostraca* the optic lobe contains four regions of structured neuropil: the outermost lamina ganglionaris, followed by the medulla externa, m. interna and m. terminalis. The m. interna is lacking in non-malacostraca. In a few species green fibres were detected in the l. ganglionaris (e.g. *Asselus aquaticus, Pandalus montagui,* - but not in *P. borealis,* and occasionally in *Astacus astacus*). In the m. externa and m. interna the green and 5-HTi fibres form several perpendicular strata. In the crayfish the m. externa contains three layers with green and 5-HTi fibres. The m. interna has five green layers and two of them additionally contain 5-HTi neurons (Elofsson and Klemm 1972; Elofsson 1983).

The connective (circumoesophageal) ganglion of *Crustacea* contains green cell bodies (Plotnikova and Govyrin 1966; Goldstone and Cook 1971; Kushner and Maynard 1977) and one 5-HTi cell (Beltz and Kravitz 1983). According the Goldstone and Cook (1971) a cell of the connective ganglion supplies CA to the pericardial organ of crabs.

Beltz and Kravitz (1983) have counted about 100 5-HTi cells in the ventral cord of *Homarus americanus*. There is at least one pair in each ganglion. In some ganglia their processes cross to the contra-lateral side while in others they project ipsi-laterally. They always project into the preceeding ganglion or ganglia where they arborize and supply the longitudinal tracts of the ventral nerve cord. Some 5-HTi fibres leave in the segmental nerves of the thoracic ganglia.

In the stomatogastric ganglion of *Homarus vulgaris* green fluorescent cells were seen by Osborne and Dando (1970). Dopamine-containing fibres in the stomatogastric ganglion of *Panulirus interruptus* originate in the connective ganglion (Kushner and Maynard 1977). No 5-HTi cell bodies but immunoreactive fibres of presumed central origin were reported in the oesophageal, stomatogastric, and cardiac ganglion by Beltz and Kravitz (1983). In the cardiac ganglion of the American lobster all the five motorneurons which innervate the heart were reported to contain NA (Ocorr and Berlind 1983).

Green fluorescent fibres were seen to supply the hindgut of *Astacus* (Elofsson et al. 1966) and some other species (see Aramant and Elofsson 1976).

Neurohaemal organs containing bMA have been reported in *Crustacea*. Cells with OA are located in the second segmental nerve of the thoracic ganglia in *H. americanus* and release OCT into the haemolymph (Livingstone et al. 1981). The second thoracic segmental nerve is covered by a dense 5-HTi fibre plexus of yet unknown origin, which is exposed to the body fluid (Beltz and Kravitz 1983). The pericardial organ, which is composed of several anastomosing segmental nerves from the thoracic ganglia, contains fibres carrying peptides, CA (Goldstone and Cook 1971) and 5-HT (Goldstone and Cook 1971; Beltz and Kravitz 1983) originating in the CNS (Goldstone and Cook 1971).

2.7.2 Insecta

Biogenic MA in insects were found in nervous and non-nervous tissues. The involvement of DA in tanning of the cuticle was already mentioned. DA, NA, A, and 5-HT were reported as constituents of the venom in wasps, hornets, and honey bees (see Owen 1978).

In the brain of the desert locust *Schistocerca gregaria* OCT (2.43 μg gww^{-1}) is reported to be the quantitatively dominating bMA, while the values for 5-HT were between 0.79 and 1.50 μg gww^{-1}, for DA between 0.8 and 0.9 μg gww^{-1}, and for NA 0.11 μg gww^{-1} (Klemm 1976; Robertson 1976). No A was found. Nässel and Laxmyr (1983) detected considerable amounts of L-DOPA (4.7 μg gww^{-1}) in the larval CNS of the blowfly *Calliphora erythrocephala*, a concentration which is 10-20 times higher than that of any other bMA. In adults the content of L-DOPA was half that of amines. In *Periplaneta americana* L-DOPA is low (less than 0.1 μg gww^{-1}; Murdock and Klemm, unpublished observation). A low concentration of 5-HTP (0.02 nmol mg^{-1} prot) was reported in the CNS of locusts by Clarke and Donnellan (1982). For further quantitative data on insects see Evans (1980), Nässel and Laxmyr (1983), Mercer et al. (1983).

The distribution of bMA in the CNS was studied by aldehyde-fluorescence methods (Klemm 1976) and recently by using antibodies directed against 5-HT (Klemm 1983; Klemm and Sundler 1983; Bishop and O'Shea 1983; Mercer et al. 1983; Klemm et al. 1984; Schurmann and Klemm 1984). The cell bodies appear either singly or in clusters in different part of the brain. They occur regularly in the posterior brain but vary in their distribution in other regions. In the cockroach *Blaberus craniifer* 190-240 green fluorescent and 220-280 5-HTi cell bodies were counted (Klemm 1983; Klemm et al. 1984). Thus approximately 0.2% of the cell bodies of the brain (without the optic lobes) contain CA and 5-HTi. The number of CA and 5-HT-containing cell bodies appear to be higher in locusts, though quantitative counts were not given (Klemm and Falck 1978). In the bee *Apis mellifera* only 40-60 cell bodies were found to be 5-HTi (Schurmann and Klemm 1984) and 70-90 are green fluorescent (Klemm, unpublished observation). Thus in bees approx. only 0.03% of the cerebral cells (without the optic lobes) contain fluorogenic amines. In adult blowflies approx. 0.05% of the cerebral and optic cells are 5-HT-immunoreactive (Klemm and Nässel, to be published). Catecholamine and 5-HT-containing processes are distributed all over the brain. Some of them concentrate in tracts and supply several distinct neuropilar regions. Some regions receive CA-containing fibres (e.g. the ellipsoid body of the central body complex (Klemm 1976, 1983); others receive 5-HTi terminals (e.g. the pons of locusts, crickets, and cockroaches and the calyx of the mushroom body in locusts and flies (Klemm 1976; Klemm et al. 1984; Klemm and Nässel, to be published), and some regions are innervated by both types of fibres (e.g. the fan-shaped body of the central body complex; the alpha and beta lobes of all insects studied; the calyx and peduncle in cockroaches, the peduncle in honey bees; the pons of flies (Klemm 1976; Klemm and Sundler 1983; Klemm et al. 1984; Schurmann and Klemm 1984). The pons of honey bees, however, lacks CA or 5-HTi fibres (Klemm 1976; Schurmann and Klemm 1984).

Biogenic MA's seem to be involved in antennal sensoric transmission. Fibres with CA and 5-HT supply the olfactory glomeruli in cockroach (Klemm 1983; Klemm et al. 1984) and honey bee (Klemm 1976; Mercer et al. 1983; Schurmann and Klemm 1984), whereas in olfactory glomeruli of locusts (Klemm and Sundler 1983) and blowfly (Klemm and Nässel, to be published) only 5-HTi neurons could be detected. In cockroach, bee, and fly the antenno-sensory system is highly developed, thus there is no obvious correlation between function and the occurence of bMA in their olfactory lobe (Klemm 1976).

The distribution of bMA in the optic lobe varies in different insects. They never occur in photoreceptor cells. The dragonfly *(Odonata)*, and the honey bee *(Hymenoptera)* for example both have highly developed eyes but they show a different pattern of innervation of the optic neuropils. In *Odonata* all three neuropil regions are richly supplied by CA and 5-HT fibres of local and cerebral origin. In the lamina the fibres are often oriented retinotopically, but in the medulla and lobula they form several perpendicularly oriented strata (Elofsson and Klemm 1972). In the optic lobe of the bee no CA could be detected (Elofsson and Klemm 1972; Mercer et al. 1983) but 5-HT fibres form one stratum in each of the three neuropil region (Mercer et al. 1983; Schurmann and Klemm 1984).

Cell bodies with DA were demonstrated in the ventral nerve cord of caddisflies (Klemm 1971); 5-HTi cell were seen in *Periplaneta* (Bishop and O'Shea 1983) and blowfly (Nässel and Cantera, in press). These cells send fibres into the neuropil of the ventral cord. Longitudinal fibre tracts with fluorogenic MA connect all ganglia of the ventral cord to the brain. Some fibres of the tract originate in the brain (Klemm 1971, 1983; Klemm et al. 1984). Commisural 5-HTi fibres connect both sides of the nerve cord (Nässel and Cantera, in press). The CA-containing and 5-HTi fibres do not leave the ventral cord by the segmental nerves. In the ventral ganglia of several insects dorsal unpaired median (DUM) cells containing OCT were reported. Their processes, leave the ganglia and supply peripheral organs like the DUMeti cells in the thoracic ganglion in locusts which supply the extensor tibiae (Hoyle et al. 1974) or the four DUM-cells in the terminal ganglion of the larval firefly *Photurus versicolor* which innervates the light organ (Christensen and Carlson 1982).

The stomatogastric nervous system contains CA and 5-HT. The frontal ganglion of the silver fish Lepisma contains two pairs of CA cells. In other species the frontal ganglion contains two (caddisflies) to 50–70 (dragonflies) yellow fluorescent cell bodies. No green fluorescent cell bodies have been observed in their frontal ganglion. The yellow fibres contribute to the fibre tracts with travel the whole length of the stomatogastric nervous system. The majority of the CA fibres seem to originate in the brain, while at least many of the 5-HT fibres have cell bodies in the stomatogastric nervous system. In locusts both CA and 5-HTi cell bodies occur in the occipital ganglion and ingluvial ganglion. Fibres of both types, partly originating in these two ganglia, innervate the muscles of the foregut. In the stomatogastric nervous system of crickets only 5-HTi cell bodies were detected. They lie in the frontal ganglion. The visceral muscles of crickets receive 5-HTi fibres but no supply of CA fibres (Klemm 1979; Klemm and Hustert 1984). Lafon-Cazal and Arluison (1976) found OA in the occipital ganglion of the locust.

The salivary gland in several insects e.g. locusts and cockroaches is innervated by DA-containing fibres (Klemm 1972; see Evans 1980).

Biogenic MA were found to be secreted into the haemolymph (Evans 1980; Orchard 1982). The site of their release is still unknown but principally three sites of release can be considered: (a) The storage lobe of the corpora cardiaca (an analog of the pituitary of vertebrates) which in some insects, i.e. locusts (Klemm and Falck 1978) and cockroaches (Gersch et al. 1974) contain CA and 5-HT of cerebral origin. The corpora allata were never found to contain fluorogenic MA. (b) The medial nerve of the ventral cord is surrounded by neurosecretory fibres which in locusts and cockroaches were reported to contain DA, NA, and OCT (Evans 1980). (c) In the flies *Calliphora* and *Drosophila* many 5-HTi fibres of central origin form a dense plexus in the neuronal sheath of central ganglia and peripheral nerves and thus closely appose to the body fluid (Nässel and Elekes, in press, to be published). In *Odonata* green fluorescent fibres penetrate the neuronal sheath of the cerebral ganglion (Klemm, unpublished observation).

2.8 Echinodermata

Dopamine was found to be present already in the preneuronal phase of embryonic starfish and sea urchin. Its content rises drastically with the development of the nervous system in the bipinnaria and pluteus larvae (Toneby 1980). Ryberg (1974) reported CA fluorescence in neuron-like systems and 5-HT fluorescence in the endodermal wall of the pluteus of *Psammechinus miliaris*. In the planktonic larva of the starfish *Pisaster ochraceus* green fluorescence was found to be associated with the ciliary bond, which is a principal locomotory and feeding organ of the larvae (Burke 1983). In the nervous system of adult echimoderms DA and NA were found. CA fluorescence was seen in the nervous system associated with presumed interneurons in the ectoneural tissue.

Some of their fibres supply the side walls of the podia in the starfish *Asterias rubens*. The stomach of *A. rubens* is innervated by CA-containing neurons. No fluorescence was found in the motoric hyponeural nervous system (Cottrell and Pentreath 1970).

3 Concluding Comments

Our understanding of the distribution of bMA's in invertebrates is fragmentary. Nevertheless some conclusions can already be drawn: primary CA and 5-HT occur in the nervous system in almost all animals. Its presence, content, and distribution varies not only in species of different phyla but can also vary in closely related species. The presence of A remains to be established. 5-HT is the quantitative dominant bMA in the CNS of flatworms, annelids, and molluscs, whereas OCT seems to dominate in arthropods. The concentration of bMA's can vary circadianly, seasonally, or with stress. With the exception of nematods and probably leeches, there is no worm, mollusc, crustacea, or insect which can be taken as a typical representative of its phylum concerning the distribution of bMA. Biogenic MA are always involved with interneurons. Many of their cell bodies are arranged in clusters. Their processes form widespread networks which supply many different targets within the brain and the ventral nerve cord. Several targets are shared by CA and 5-HT neurons, others have only one of them. The innervation of the targets by bMA's varies in different species. Thus these CA and 5-HT-containing neurons in the CNS of invertebrates seem to represent an analog of the amine-containing diffuse ascending and descending reticular modulating system of vertebrates. Catecholamines or 5-HT or both are present in the stomatogastric nervous system in all phyla investigated and supply the visceral muscles of the foregut. Only in few cases 5-HT or CA fibres were found to supply some somatic muscles. Sensory cells with CA were found in almost all phyla investigated, but seem never to occur in arthropods. Involvement of 5-HT in neurosecretion seems to be shared by all invertebrates.

References

Aramant R, Elofsson R (1976) Monoaminergic neurons in the nervous system of crustaceans. Cell Tissue Res 170:231–351

Arluison M, Ducrois C (1977) Localization of monoamine nerve fibers by formaldehyde fluorescence histochemistry in the posterior salivary duct and gland of Octopus vulgaris. Tissue Cell 8:61–72

Barber A (1982) Monoamine-containing varicosities in the neural sheath of a gastropod mollusc demonstrated by glyoxylic acid histofluorescence. Cell Tissue Res 226:267–273

Barlow J, Juorio AV, Martin R (1974) Monoamine transport in the octopus posterior salivary gland nerves. J Comp Physiol 89:105–122

Beltz BS, Kravitz EA (1983) Mapping of serotonin-like immunoreactivity in the lobster nervous system. J Neurosci 3:585–602

Bennett J, Bueding E (1971) Localization of biogenic amines in Schistosoma mansoni. Comp Biochem Physiol 39:857–867

Bennett JL, Bueding E (1973) Uptake of 5-hydroxytryptamine by Schistosoma masoni. Mol Pharmacol 9:311–319

Bishop CA, O'Shea M (1983) Serotonin immunoreactive neurons in the central nervous system of an insect (Periplaneta americana). J Neurobiol 14:251–269

Brunet PCJ (1980) The metabolism of the aromatic amino acids concerned in the cross-linking of insect cuticle. Insect Biochem 10:467–500

Burke DR (1983) The structure of the larval nervous system of Pisaster ochrauceus (Echinodermata: Asteroidea). J Morphol 178:23–35

Burnett JW, Calton GJ (1977) The chemistry and toxicology of some venomous pelagic coelenterates. Toxicon 15:177–196

Cardot J (1971) Variations saisonnieres de la 5-hydroxytryptamine dans les tissus nerveux et cardiaque chez le Mollusque Helix pomatia. CR Soc Biol 165:338–341

Carlberg M, Rosengreen E (1985) Biochemical basis for adrenergic neurotransmission in coelenterates. J Comp Physiol 155:251–255

Carpenter D, Breese G, Schanberg S, Kopin I (1971) Serotonin and dopamine: distribution and accumulation in Aplysia nervous and non-nervous tissues. Int Neurosci 2:49–56

Chou TCT, Bennett J, Bueding E (1972) Occurrence and concentration of biogenic amines in trematodes. J Parasitol 58:1098–1102

Christensen TA, Carlson AD (1982) The neurophysiology of larval firefly luminescence: direct activation through four bifurcating (DUM) neurons. J Comp Physiol 148:503–514

Clarke BS, Donnellan JF (1982) Concentrations of some putative neurotransmitters in the CNS of quick-frozen insects. Insect Biochem 12:623–638

Clarke ME (1966) Histochemical localization of monoamines in the nervous system of the polychaete Nephtys. Proc Soc Lond B Biol Sci 165:308–325

Cottrell GA, Pentreath VW (1970) Localization of catecholamines in the nervous system of a starfish, Asterias rubens, and of a brittlestar, Ophiothrix fragilis. Comp Gen Pharmacol 1:73–81

Dahl E, Falck B, von Mecklenburg C, Myhrberg H (1963) An adrenergic nervous system in sea anemones. Q J Microsc Sci 104:531–534

Dolesalova H, Giacobini E, Stipita-Klauco M (1973) An attempt to identify putative neurotransmitter molecules in the central nervous system of the snail. Int J Neurosci 5:53–59

Ehinger B, Myhrberg H (1971) Neuronal localization of dopamine, noradrenaline and 5-hydroxytryptamine in the central and peripheral nervous system of Lumbricus terrestris (L.). Histochemie 28:265–275

Ehinger B, Falck B, Myhrberg H (1968) Biogenic monoamines in Hirudo medicinalis. Histochemie 15:140–149

Elofsson R (1983) 5-HT-like immunoreactivity in the central nervous system of the crayfish, Pacifastacus leniusculus. Cell Tissue Res 232:221–236

Elofsson R, Klemm N (1972) Monoamine-containing neurons in the optic ganglia of crustaceans and insects. Z Zellforsch Mikrosk Anat 133:475–499

Elofsson R, Kauri T, Nielson S-O, Stömberg J-A (1966) Localization of monoaminergic neurons in the central nervous system of Astacus astacus L. (Crustacea). Z Zellforsch Mikrosk Anat 74: 464–473

Elofsson R, Kauri T, Nielson S-O, Strömberg J-O (1968) Catecholamine-containing nerve fibers in the hind-gut of the crayfish Astacus astacus (Crustacea, Decapoda). Experientia (Basel) 24: 1159–1160

Elofsson R, Laxmyr L, Rosengren E, Hansson C (1982) Identification and quantitative measurements of biogenic amines and DOPA in the central nervous system and haemolymph of the crayfish, Pacifastacus leniusculus (Crustacea). Comp Biochem Physiol 71C:195–201

Evans PD (1980) Biogenic amines in the insect nervous system. Adv Insect Physiol 15:317–473

Gersch M, Hentschel E, Ude J (1974) Aminerge Substanzen im lateralen Herznerven und im stomatogastrischen Nervensystem der Schabe Blaberus craniifer Burm. Zool Jahrb Abt Allg Zool Physiol Tiere 78:1–15

Goh SL, Davey KG (1976) Localization and distribution of catecholaminergic structures in the nervous system of Phocanema decipiens (Nematoda). Int J Parasitol 6:403–411

Goldstein R, Kistler HB, Steinbusch HWM, Schwartz JH (1984) Distribution of serotonin-immunoreactivity in juvenile Aplysia. Neuroscience 11:535–547

Goldstone MW, Cooke IM (1971) Histochemical localization of monoamines in the crab central nervous system. Z Zellforsch Mikrosk Anat 116:7–19

Goosey MW, Candy DJ (1980) The d-octopamine content of the haemolymph of the locust, Schistocerce americana gregaria, and its elevation during flight. Insect Biochem 10:3934–397

Gustafsson MKS, Wikgren MC (1981) Peptidergic and aminergic neurons in adult Diphyllobothri-um dendriticum Nitzsch. 1824 (Cestoda, Pseudophyllidae). Z Parasitenkd 64:121–134

Guthrie PB, Neuhoff V, Osborne NN (1976) Dopamine, noradrenaline, octopamine and tyrosine-hydroxylase in the gastropod Helix pomatia. Comp Biochem Physiol 52C:109–111

Hariri M (1974) Occurrence and concentration of biogenic amines in Mesocestodes corti (Cestoda). J Parasitol 60:737–743

Hiripi L, Salanki J (1973) Seasonal and activity-dependent changes of the serotonin level in the CNS and heart of the snail (Helix pomatia L.). Comp Gen Pharmacol 4:285–292

Hoyle G (1975) Evidence that insect dorsal unpaired median (DUM) neurones are octopaminergic. J Exp Zool 193:425–431

Hoyle G, Dagan D, Mohorly B, Colquhoun W (1974) Dorsal unpaired median insect neurons make neurosecretory endings in sceletal muscle. J C Zool 187:109–165

Jaeger CP, Jaeger EC, Welsh JH (1971) Localization of monoamine-containing neurons in the nervous system of Strophocheilus oblongus Gastropoda. Z Zellforsch Mikrosk Anat 112:54–68

Juorio AV, Killick SW (1973) The distribution of monamines and some of their acid metabolites in the posterior salivary glands and viscera of some cephalopods. Comp Biochem Physiol 44A: 1059–1067

Klemm N (1971) Monoaminhaltige Strukturen im Zentralnervensystem der Trichoptera (Insecta). Teil II. Z Zellforsch Mikrosk Anat 117:537–558

Klemm N (1972) Monoamine-containing nervous fibres in foregut and salivary gland of the desert locust. Schistocerca gregaria Forskal (Orthoptera, Acrididae). Comp Biochem Physiol 43A: 207–211

Klemm N (1976) Histochemistry of putative transmitter substances in the insect brain. Prog Neur-biol (NY) 7:99–169

Klemm N (1979) Biogenic monoamines in the stomatogastric nervous system of members of several insect orders. Entomol Gen 5:113–121

Klemm N (1983) Monoamine-containing neurons and their projections in the brain (supraoesopha-geal ganglion) of cockroaches. An aldehyde fluorescence study. Cell Tissue Res 229:379–402

Klemm N, Falck B (1978) Monoamines in the pars intercerebralis-corpus cardiacum complex of locusts. Gen Comp Endocrinol 34:180–192

Klemm N, Hustert R (1984) The distribution of 5-HT and catecholamines in the stomatogastric nervous system of orthopteroid insects. In: Vizi ES, Magyar K (eds) Regulation of transmitter function. Budapest, pp 537–540

Klemm N, Sundler F (1983) Organization of catecholamine and serotonin-immunoreactive neurons in the corpora pedunculata of the desert locust, Schistocerca gregaria Forsk. Neurosci Lett 36: 13–17

Klemm N, Steinbusch HWM, Sundler F (1984) Distribution of serotonin-containing neurons and their pathways in the supraoesophageal ganglion of the cockroach Periplaneta americana (L.) as revealed by immunocytochemistry. J Comp Neurol 225:387–395

Kushner PD, Maynard EA (1977) Localization of monoamine fluorescence in the stomatogastric nervous system of lobsters. Brain Res 129:13–28

Lafon-Cazal M, Arluison M (1976) Localization of monoamines in the corpora cardiaca and the hypocerebral ganglion of locusts. Cell Tissue Res 172:517–527

Laxmyr L (1984) Biogenic amines and DOPA in the central nervous system of decapod crustaceans. Comp Biochem Physiol 77C:139–143

Laxmyr L (1984, in press) Tyrosine hydroxylase in the central nervous system of the crayfish, Pacifastacus leniusculus (Crustacea, Decapoda)

Lent CM (1977) The Retzius cell within the central nervous system of leeches. Prog Neurobiol (NY) 8:81–117

Livingstone MS, Schaeffer SF, Kravitz EA (1981) Biochemistry and ultrastructure of serotoninergic nerve endings in lobster: serotonin and octopamine are contained in different nervous endings. J Neurobiol 12:27–54

Luborsky-Moore JL, Jacklet JW (1976) Localization of catecholamines in the eyes and other tissues of Aplysia. J Histochem Cytochem 24:1150–1158

Lurje BL (1975) Monoamine-containing neurons in planaria Polycellis nigra (Turb). Vestn Mosk Univ 2:3–13 (in Russian)

Machado CRS, Machado ABM, Pellegrino S (1972) Catecholamine-containing neurons in Schistosoma mansoni. Z Zellforsch Mikrosk Anat 124:230–237

Manaranche R, L'Hermite P (1973) Etudes des amines biogenes de Glycera convulata K. (Annelide, Polychete). Z Zellforsch Mikrosk Anat 137:21–36

Marsden CA, Kerkut GA (1969) Fluorescent microscopy of the 5-HT- and catecholamine-containing cells in the central nervous system of the leech Hirudo medicinalis. Comp Biochem Physiol 31:851–862

Marsden CA, Kerkut GA (1970) The occurrence of monoamines in Planorbis corneus: a fluorescence microscopic and microspectrometric study. Comp Gen Pharmacol 1:101–116

Martin R, Barlow J (1972) Localization of monoamines in nerves of the posterior salivary gland and salivary center in the brain of octopus. Z Zellforsch Mikrosk Anat 125:16–30

Mason A, Leake LD (1978) Morphology of leech Retzius cells demonstrated by intracellular injection of horse radish peroxidase. Comp Biochem Physiol 61A:213–216

Matus AI (1973) Histochemical localization of biogenic monoamines in the cephalic ganglia of Octopus vulgaris. Tissue Cell 5:591–601

Maxwell GD, Tait JF, Hildebrand JG (1978) Regional synthesis of neurotransmitter candidates in the CNS of the moth Manduca sexta. Comp Biochem Physiol 61C:109–119

Mercer AR, Mobbs PG, Davenport AP, Evans PD (1983) Biogenic amines in the brain of the honeybee, Apis mellifera. Cell Tissue Res 234:655–677

Myers PR, Sweeney DC (1972) The determination of catcholamines and their metabolites in the pedal ganglia of Quadratula pustulosa (Mollusca, Pelecypoda). Comp Gen Pharmacol 3:277–282

Myhrberg H (1967) Monoaminergic mechanisms in the nervous system of Lumbricus terrestris (L.). Z Zellforsch Mikrosk Anat 81:311–343

Nässel DR, Cantera R (1984, in press) Mapping of serotonin-immunoreactive neurons in the larval nervous system of the flies Calliphora erythrocephala and Sarcophaga bullata. Cell Tissue Res 239:423–434

Nässel DR, Elekes K (1984) Ultrastructural demonstration of serotoninimmunoreactivity in the nervous system of an insect (Calliphora erythrocephala). Neurosci Lett 48:203–210

Nässel DR, Laxmyr L (1983) Quantitative determination of biogenic amines and DOPA in the CNS of adult and larval blowflies, Calliphora erythrocephala. Comp Biochem Physiol 75C:259–265

Ocorr KA, Berlind A (1983) The identification and localization of a catecholamine in the motor neurons of the lobster cardiac ganglion. J Neurobiol 14:51–59

Ono JK, McCaman RE (1984) Immunocytochemical localization and direct assay of serotonin-containing neurons in Aplysia. Neuroscience 11:549–560

Orchard I (1982) Octopamine in insects: neurotransmitter, neurohormone, and neuromodulator. Can J Zool 60:659–669

Osborne NN, Cottrell GA (1971) Distribution of biogenic amines in the slug, Limax maximus. Z Zellforsch Mikrosk Anat 112:15–30

Osborne NN, Dando MR (1970) Monoamines in the stomatogastric ganglion of the lobster Homarus vulgaris. Comp Biochem Physiol 32:327–331

Owen MD (1978) Venom replenishment, as indicated by histamine, in honey bee (Apis mellifera) venom. J Insect Physiol 24:433–437

Owen MD, Bridges AR (1982) Catecholamines in the honey bee (Apis melliferra L.) and various vespid (Hymenoptera) venoms. Toxicon 20:1075–1084

Pentreath VW, Berry MS (1975) Ultrastructure of the terminals of an identified dopamine-containing neurone marked by intracellular injection of radioactive dopamine. J Neurocytol 4:249–260

Pentreath VW, Berry MS, Osborne NN (1982) The serotonergic cerebral cells in gastropods. In: Osborne NN (ed) The biology of serotonergic transmission. Wiley, Chichester, pp 457–514

Peretz B, Estes J (1974) Histology and histochemistry of the peripheral neural plexus in the Aplysia gill. J Neurobiol 5:3–19

Plotnikova SI, Govyrin VA (1966) The distribution of catecholamine-containing nerve elements in coelenterates and protostomes. Arch Anat Gist Embryol 50:79–87 (in Russian)

Plotnikova SI, Kuzmina LV (1968) Distribution of monoamine-containing nervous elements in Planaria Dendrocoeleum lacteum (Turbellaria). Sh Evol Biochem Fisiol Suppl 23–29 (in Russian)

Plotnikova SI, Shishov BA, Kuzmina LV (1969) On the study of biogenic monoamines in the nervous system of Ascaris suum. Tr Gelmintol Lab 20:103–108 (in Russian)

Pree J, Rutschke E (1983) Zur circadianen Rhythmik des Dopamingehaltes im Gehirn von Periplaneta americana L. Zool Jahrb Abt Allg Zool Physiol Tiere 87:455–460

Reuter M, Wikgren M, Palmberg I (1980) The nervous system of Microstomum lineare (Turbellaria,
Macrostomida). Cell Tissue Res 211:31–40

Reutter K (1969) Biogene Amine im Nervensystem von Lineus sanguineus Rathke (Nemertini). Z
Zellforsch Mikrosk Anat 94:391–406

Robertson HA (1976) Octopamine, dopamine and noradrenaline content of the brain of the locust,
Schistocerca gregaria. Experientia (Basel) 32:552–553

Robertson HA, Juorio AV (1976) Octopamine and some related noncatecholic amines in invertebrate nervous systems. Int Rev Neurobiol 19:173–224

Robertson HA, Osborne NN (1979) Putative neurotransmitters in the annelid central nervous system: presence of 5-hydroxytryptamine and octopamine-stimulate adenylate cyclases. Comp
Biochem Physiol 64C:7–14

Rude S (1966) Monoamine-containing neurons in the nerve cord and body wall of Lumbricus terrestris. J Comp Neurol 128:397–412

Rude S (1969) Monoamine-containing neurons in the central nervous system and peripheral nerves
of the leech, Hirudo medicinalis. J Comp Neurol 136:349–372

Ryberg E (1974) The localization of biogenic amines in the echinopluteus. Acta Zool (Stockh) 55:
179–189

Schurmann FW, Klemm N (1984) Serotonin-immunoreactive nerves in the brain of the honey bee.
J Comp Neurol

Shield JM (1971) Histochemical localization of monoamines in the nervous system of Dipylidium
canium (Cestoda) by the formaldehyde fluorescence technique. Int J Parasitol 1:135–138

Stefano GB, Aiello E (1975) Histofluorescent localization of serotonin and dopamine in the nervous
system and gill of Mytilus edulis (Bivalvia). Biol Bull 148:141–156

Stefano GB, Catapane EJ (1977) Seasonal monoamine changes in the central nervous system of
Mytilus edulis (Bivalvia). Experientia (Basel) 33:1341–1342

Sulston J, Dew M, Brenner S (1975) Dopaminergic neurons in the nematode Caenorhabditis elegans.
J Comp Neurol 163:215–226

Sweeney DC (1968) The anatomical distribution of monoamines in a freshwater bivalve mollusc,
Sphaerium sulcatum (L.). Comp Biochem Physiol 25:601–613

Toneby M (1980) Dopamine in developing larvae of the sea urchin Psammechinus miliaris Gmelin.
Comp Biochem Physiol 65C:139–142

Tritt SH, Lowe IP, Byrne JH (1983) A modification of the glyoxylic acid induced histofluorescence
technique for demonstration of catecholamines and serotonin in tissue of Aplysia californica.
Brain Res 259:159–162

Welsh JH (1972) Catecholamine in invertebrates. In: Blaschko H, Muscholl E (eds) Handbuch der
experimentellen Pharmakologie, vol 33. Springer, Berlin Heidelberg New York, pp 79–109

Welsh JH, Moorhead M (1960) The quantitative distribution of 5-hydroxytryptamine in the invertebrates, especially in their nervous system. J Neurochem 6:146–169

Welsh JH, Williams LD (1970) Monoamine-containing neurons in Planaria. J Comp Neurol 138:
103–116

White D, Marsden JR (1978) Microspectrofluorimetric measurements on cells containing biogenic
amines in the cerebral ganglion of the polychaete Nereis virens (Sars). Biol Bull 155:395–409

Amine-Sensitive Adenylate Cyclases and Their Role in Neuronal Function

R.P. BODNARYK[1]

1 Introduction

Recognition that nervous tissue contains especially high specific activities of the enzymes needed to synthesize and degrade cyclic AMP and high concentrations of proteins such as calmodulin that can regulate the activities of these enzymes has lead to the belief that cAMP is involved in synaptic transmission. The further recognition that in neural membranes receptors for biogenic amines are functionally coupled, via a guanine nucleotide-binding regulatory protein, to adenylate cyclase gave great incentive to research aimed at establishing a nervous function for cAMP and defining in molecular terms its action in synaptic transmission (Drummond 1983). The hypothesis that the effects of cAMP in various tissues (Kuo and Greengard 1969) including the central nervous system (Greengard 1976, 1978; Greengard and DeCamilli 1982) are mediated through a family of enzymes called protein kinases recently has been strengthened by the exciting discovery of synapsin 1, a nerve terminal-specific phosphoprotein associated with synaptic vesicles (DeCamilli et al. 1983a, b; Huttner et al. 1983). Undoubtedly, phosphorylation-dephosphorylation reactions form the molecular basis for cAMP-mediated effects on synaptic transmission, perhaps through regulation of vesicle function and transmitter release. Yet, in spite of many years of intensive and biochemically productive research in these areas, only in a few cases has the action of biogenic amines in the nervous system been linked to an identified cAMP-dependent biological response. It is perhaps not surprising, given the reductionist tendencies of the scientific process, that the clearest examples of how cAMP is involved in physiological and behavioural processes have been sought and found in lower animals whose nervous systems are simpler both in terms of fewer and larger cells. Some of these neurons are readily identifiable, enabling the experimenter to return with precision to the same neurone, to impale it with electrodes for electrophysiological measurement, to inject it with drugs or biologically-active macromolecules, to extract it for biochemical determination of active substances and to correlate results with a biological response. It is the intent of this review to examine some of the physiological and behavioural systems in lower animals that have contributed significantly to our understanding of the role of amine-sensitive adenylate cyclase in neuronal function. In particular, an account is given of recent advances in the neural function of octopamine-sensitive and serotonin-sensitive adenylate cyclases. Octopamine-sensitive adenylate cyclase, widely distributed in in-

---

1 Agriculture Canada Research Station, 195 Dafoe Road, Winnipeg, Manitoba, R3T 2M9, Canada

Neurobiology
(ed. by R. Gilles and J. Balthazart)
© Springer-Verlag Berlin Heidelberg 1985

vertebrates (Bodnaryk 1983b) but apparently absent in vertebrates (Harmar and Horn 1977), is often excluded from general reviews of cyclic nucleotides in the nervous system (Drummond 1983). Yet, octopamine likely has the same functional importance in invertebrates as noradrenalin and adrenalin have in the vertebrates (revs by Evans 1980; Bodnaryk 1982a, 1983b; Orchard 1982; Klem 1984, this chap.; Robertson 1984, this chap.). Serotonin, serotonin-sensitive adenylate cyclase and cAMP-mediated protein phosphorylation of neural membrane components, as studied in large identified neurons of lower animals such as the mollusc *Aplysia*, are at the centre of recent neurochemical discoveries that have importance for understanding learning and memory functions at the molecular level (Kandel and Schwartz 1982).

2 Role of Octopamine-Sensitive Adenylate Cyclase in Neural Function

2.1 Pharmacology and Toxicology of Octopamine Receptors Coupled to Adenylate Cyclase

2.1.1 Pharmacology

In their paper reporting the discovery of an octopamine-sensitive adenylate cyclase in the thoracic ganglia of the cockroach, *Periplaneta americana*, Nathanson and Greengard (1973) found that the α-adrenergic antagonist phentolamine strongly inhibited the activation of adenylate cyclase by octopamine, whereas the β-adrenergic antagonist propranolol had little effect. Their observation has been repeated many times with octopamine-sensitive adenylate cyclase from diverse invertebrates (Bodnaryk 1982a, 1983b). In particular, detailed pharmacological studies of the effects of agonists and antagonists on the isolated spontaneously beating ventricle of the venus clam, *Tapes watlingi* (Dougan and Wade 1978a,b) and on the extensor tibiae neuromuscular preparation from the hind leg of the locust, *Schistocerca americana gregaria* (Evans 1981) have shown that octopamine receptors have many similarities with vertebrate α-adreno-receptors. However, the parallel between vertebrate α-adrenoreceptors and octopamine receptors does not appear to extend to their respective modes of action (Evans 1981). Octopamine receptors are positively coupled to adenylate cyclase and octopamine receptor activation leads to pronounced increases in cAMP formation (Bodnaryk 1982a, 1983b). The exact association of α-adrenergic receptors and adenylate cyclase in vertebrates remains unsettled (Drummond 1983). In some systems, α-adrenergic receptor activation *inhibits* cAMP formation (McCarthy and de Vellis 1978; Kahn et al. 1982). Other studies indicate that α-adrenergic mechanisms activate adenylate cyclase indirectly by facilitating β-adrenergic, histaminergic or adenosine receptors (Daly et al. 1980a,b).

2.1.2 Stereospecificity

Erspamer (1952), who first described octopamine in the posterior salivary gland of the ocotpus, *Octopus vulgaris*, showed that the naturally occurring octopamine was pharmacologically more potent than an equimolar concentration of racemic DL-octopamine but was unable to specify which was the natural isomer. Using an enzymic technique, Goosey and Candy (1980) showed that D-octopamine occurs in the blood of the locust *S. americana gregaria*. Proof that D-octopamine is the natural isomer in the CNS of diverse invertebrates (a moth, beetle, snail, and crayfish) was obtained by separating derivatized radioactive octopamine enantiomers from CNS preparations by HPLC (Starratt and Bodnaryk 1981).

Although it is invariably found that D-octopamine is more potent than L-octopamine, the relative potency ratios of the two stereoisomers can vary considerably from one experimental preparation to the next.

For octopamine-stimulated adenylate cyclase in cockroach *(P. americana)* brain homogenates, D-octopamine is 200 times more potent than L-octopamine (Harmar and Horn 1977). For intracellular recordings of polarization in isolated ganglia of the horseshoe cray, *Limulus polyphemus*, the potency ratio is 100, but for recordings in isolated abdominal ganglia of the cockroach, *P. americana*, it is only 2.5 (Roberts and Walker 1981). For the isolated spontaneously beating ventricle of the venus clam, *T. watlini*, the ratio is 20 (Dougan and Wade 1978a,b) and for different octopamine receptors in locust hind leg neuromuscular preparation the potency ratio various from 2 to 10 (Evans 1981). Wide variations exist in the potency ratio among various tissues in the same animal. For example, in elevating cAMP levels in circulating hematocytes of the lobster, *Homarus americanus*, D-octopamine is only twice as potent as L-octopamine, but in increasing tension in the claw opener muscle D-octopamine is 50 times more potent (Battelle and Kravitz 1978). Variability of octopamine receptor stereoselectivity in these various systems remains unexplained.

2.1.3 Multiple Receptor Subtypes

An octopamine receptor classification scheme based on the effects of agonists and antagonists on the locust hind leg extensor-tibiae neuromuscular preparation has been proposed by Evans (1981):

Octopamine$_1$ receptors mediate the slowing of the myogenic rhythm of contraction and relaxation and are located post-synaptically on the muscle fibers of the proximally located myogenic bundle. Antagonists: chlorpromazine ($>$ yohimbine) $\gg$ metoclopramide. Agonists: clonidine $\gg$ naphazoline.

Octopamine$_2$ receptors mediate the increase in twitch-tension amplitude of the slow motoneurone to the extensor-tibiae (called SETi) and may be located presynaptically on SETi nerve terminals. Antagonists: metoclopramide $\gg$ chlorpromazine ($>$ yohimbine). Agonists: naphazoline $\gg$ tolazoline and naphazoline $\gg$ tolazoline.

Octopamine$_{2B}$ receptors mediate the increase in relaxation rate of twitch tension induced by firing either the fast (FETi) or slow (SETi) motoneurones and are located post-synaptically on muscle fibers. Antagonists: metoclopramide $\gg$ chlorpromazine ($>$ yohimbine). Agonists: naphazoline $\gg$ clonidine and tolazoline $\gg$ clonidine.

Octopamine$_{2A}$ receptors are blocked by low concentrations of cyproheptadine, mianserin, and metoclopramide and are thus further distinguished from octopamine$_{2B}$ receptors which are at least ten times less sensitive to these drugs.

Although this classification system of multiple octopamine receptor subtypes is undoubtedly useful for precise definition of the effects of octopamine on the locust hind leg neuromuscular preparation, it has yet to be shown to have general applicability either in peripheral or central systems.

2.1.4 Toxicology

Formamidines are a relatively new class of insect and acarine pest control agents (Hollingworth 1976) whose mode of action appears to be the disruption of octopamin-ergic systems. Behavioural, biochemical, pharmacological, and toxicological studies have all indicated that these compounds interact with octopamine receptors coupled to adenylate cyclase at peripheral and central neural sites (Hollingworth and Murdock 1980; Murdock and Hollingworth 1980; Evans and Gee 1980; Nathanson and Hunnicutt 1981; Bodnaryk 1982b; Gole et al. 1983) and at non-neural sites (Orchard et al. 1982).

The interaction of the formamidines, chlordimeform, and N-demethylchlordime-form (Fig. 1), with octopamine-sensitive adenylate cyclase has been studied in detail in two well-defined preparations: the firefly light organ (Nathanson and Hunnicutt 1981) and the cockroach nerve cord (Gole et al. 1983). In the intact nerve cord, chlordime-form, and N-demethylchlordimeform mimic the action of octopamine in elevating cAMP. In nerve cord homogenates, N-demethylchlordimeform also mimics the action of octopamine but chlordimeform has no demonstrable effect, suggesting that chlor-dimeform may be active in vivo as a result of its conversion to N-demethylchlordime-form (Gole et al. 1983), a suggestion supported by the slow-acting, weak in vivo action of chlordimeform on the intact firefly lantern (Hollingworth and Murdock 1980) and locust hind leg neuromuscular junction (Evans and Gee 1980).

Biochemical and pharmacological studies of the highly active octopamine-sensitive adenylate cyclase in washed membranes from the firefly light organ (Nathanson and Hunnicutt 1981) and crude homogenate of cockroach nerve cord (Gole et al. 1983) have established that N-demethylchlordimeform is a potent *partial agonist* of the octo-pamine receptor, whereas chlordimeform at high concentrations is an antagonist. Activation of octopamine-sensitive adenylate cyclase by N-demethylchlordimeform is competitively inhibited by the receptor antagonists cyproheptadine, clozapine, flu-

HO—⬡—COH-CH₂-NH₂

OCTOPAMINE

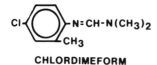

CHLORDIMEFORM

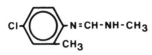

N-DEMETHYLCHLORDIMEFORM

Fig. 1. Structure of octopamine, chlordimeform, and N-de-methylchlordimeform

phenzine, and phentolamine. Propranolol is relatively ineffective. The inhibitory constants of the various drugs correlate well with those for inhibiting octopamine stimulation.

Dopamine-sensitive adenylate cyclase in the rat caudate nucleus and isoproterenol-sensitive adenylate cyclase in rat heart and liver are little effected by N-demethylchlordimeform, indicating that its agonist activity is specific to octopamine-sensitive adenylate cyclase (Nathanson and Hunnicutt 1981).

Activation of octopamine-sensitive adenylate cyclase in insects and ticks by formamidine treatment has deleterious behavioural and physiological consequences that are likely the product of a cascade of neuroendocrinological responses mediated by release of peptide neurohormones (whose second messenger is cAMP) from neurosecretory cells (Orchard et al. 1982, 1983; Singh and Barker 1983). Such interactions will likely continue to provide a rich and productive field of study for physiologist and toxicologist alike. Of special interest to comparative biochemistry and physiology are exact comparisons of toxicological effects of formamidines in vertebrates which may have octopamine receptors that are not coupled to adenylate cyclase and in invertebrates whose octopamine receptors are positively coupled to adenylate cyclase (see following Section).

Synergism. A several-fold increase in the level of cAMP, but not cGMP, occurs in the adult moth of *Mamestra configurata* treated with chlordimeform (Bodnaryk 1982b). When treatment with chlordimeform is combined with permethrin, a synthetic pyrethroid insecticide which causes levels of cGMP but not cAMP to rise, levels of both cyclic nucleotides are increased and a synergistic effect on mortality (termed AG synergism) is obtained (Bodnaryk 1982b,c). AG synergism may of practical value for insect pest control (Plapp 1976; Bodnaryk 1982).

2.2 Are all Octopamine Receptors Coupled to Adenylate Cyclase?

Although it is now clear that receptors for biogenic amines are individual proteins distinct from adenylate cyclase (Ross and Gilman 1980), it is by no means certain that all receptors or receptor subtypes for biogenic amines are positively coupled to adenylate cyclase (Cooper 1983), or that all or the effects of a given biogenic amine are mediated through cAMP. For example, there are two subtypes of dopamine receptor in the rat striatum: D-1 receptors whose effects involve activation of adenylate cyclase and D-2 receptors not linked to the stimulation of adenylate cyclase (Kebabian and Calne 1979; Huff and Molinoff 1982). The situation is less clear with respect to octopamine receptors. Recent research has given definition to some of the problems encountered when dealing with octopamine receptor binding and adenylate cyclase activity.

2.2.1 High-Affinity Octopamine-Binding Sites and Adenylate Cyclase

The pharmacological properties of high-affinity $[^3H]$ octopamine-binding sites in head homogenates of *Drosophila* (Dudai 1982; Dudai and Zvi 1984) are *not* identical with those of octopamine-sensitive adenylate cyclase present in head homogeneates (Uzzan and Dudai 1982). The rank order of potency of aminergic ligands in blocking the stimulation of adenylate cyclase by octopamine in the head homogenates was: phentolamine > dihydroergotamine > metergoline > chlorpromazine > clonidine > D,L-propranolol > phenylephrine whereas the rank order in displacing [³H] octopamine from its binding sites was: dihydroergotamine > phentolamine > clonidine > metergoline > chlorpromazine > phenylephrine > D,L-propranolol. The concentration of drugs such as phentolamine, dihydroergotamine, and clonidine needed for half-maximal blocking of the stimulation of saturating concentrations of adenylate cyclase in head homogenates is $10-100\ \mu M$, but the half-maximal concentration needed to displace [³H] octopamine from its binding sites is many times lower (Dudai and Zvi 1984). The concentration of octopamine needed for half-maximal stimulation of adenylate cyclase in *Drosophila* head homogenates (Uzzan and Dudai 1982) as well as in neural tissues of other insects (Bodnaryk 1983b) is in the low μM range, whereas the apparent Kd of octopamine for the [³H] octopamine binding site in *Drosophila* is at the nM range (Dudai 1982; Dudai and Zvi 1984). The threshold concentrations at which octopamine is active in physiological preparations, such as the locust neuromuscular junction (Evans 1981) is also at the nM range. The discrepancy between these observations may be more apparent than real. For instance, changes may occur in vitro during homogenization that convert the drug-binding site into a high-affinity state, or convert the adenylate cyclase-coupled receptor into a low affinity state. Dudai and Zvi (1984) consider the latter more likely since they observed that even a low concentration of guanyl-nucleotide reduced the total number of high-affinity [³H] octopamine-binding sites. Since adenylate cyclase is routinely assayed in the presence of GTP, it is conceivable that no high affinity binding sites would be detected under such conditions. On the other hand, it is possible that [³H] octopamine-binding sites detected in *Drosophila* head homogenates are octopamine receptors which do not mediate their physiological effect via adenylate cyclase and cAMP. Alternatively, the high-affinity [³H] octopamine-binding sites may be coupled to adenylate cyclase, but may comprise only a small part of the total population of octopamine receptors coupled to adenylate cyclase (Dudai and Zvi 1984). It is further possible that receptors that do not activate adenylate cyclase in vivo may do so in broken cell preparations (Rodbell 1980) or that there may be differences between receptor-mediated activation of adenylate cyclase in membrane preparations and intact cells (Porzig 1982). Unfortunately, it is not possible to distinguish among these possibilities with current biochemical techniques.

2.2.2 The "Spare-Receptor" Hypothesis

The concentration of octopamine needed for threshold physiological effects (10^{-8} to 10^{-9} M) on neuromuscular transmission and muscle tension in the locust hind leg extensior tibiae muscle preparation causes only the slightest increase in the level of cAMP in the preparation. Maximal increases in cAMP occur at octopamine concentrations of 10^{-3} to 10^{-4} M (Evans 1984a,b). The concept of "spare receptors" (Levitzki 1976) for octopamine has been evoked by Evans (1984a) to explain the apparent discrepancy. The hypothesis has two elements: (1) at low hormone concentrations, a physiological system responds efficiently to the hormone because the probability of a hormone occupying a receptor is proportional to the number of available receptors; (2) at high hormone concentrations, the occupancy of many receptors results in a redundant production of cAMP that is not accompanied by any further increase in physiological response. The latter might occur when the concentration of cAMP ex-

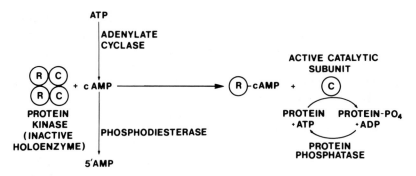

Fig. 2. Protein phosphorylation catalyzed by cAMP-dependent protein kinase. cAMP-dependent protein kinase is a tetramer composed of two dissimilar subunits, called regulatory (*R*) and catalytic (*C*). Binding of cAMP to the regulatory subunit of the inactive holoenzyme releases the catalytic subunit which is an active protein phosphotransferase. (Glass and Krebs 1980)

ceeds that of cAMP-dependent protein kinase to the extent that all of the available regulatory subunits of the protein kinase have interacted with cAMP (Fig. 2). Under these circumstances the availability of regulatory subunits of protein kinase would therefore limit the magnitude of the response or its duration and, as such, might constitute a useful mechanism for specifying an "upper control limit" for a physiological response such as muscle contraction.

Since cAMP that is bound to the regulatory subunit of cAMP-dependent protein kinase represents the amount of active catalytic subunits (Fig. 2), measurement of bound cAMP may provide more meaningful physiological information on octopamine-mediated events in the locust extensor tibia muscle preparation than measurement of total cAMP (see Bodnaryk 1981).

2.3 Regulation by Ca^{2+} and Calmodulin

The regulation of neuronal adenylate cyclase by Ca^{2+} and calmodulin from vertebrates (Drummond 1983) and invertebrates has many common features. Thus, adenylate cyclase activity in washed membranes prepared from the brain of the moth, *M. configurata*, is stimulated in the presence of calmodulin by low concentrations of free Ca^{2+} (0.08 μM) and strongly inhibited by higher concentrations (Fig. 3; Bodnaryk 1983a). It seems significant that neuronal adenylate cyclase responds to a range of concentrations of free Ca^{2+} thought to be present intracellularly (Kretsinger 1979). The activity of octopamine-sensitive adenylate cyclase in the washed membranes from the brain of *M. configurata* is also modified by Ca^{2+} and calmodulin. The maximal reaction velocity in the presence of 0.08 μM free Ca^{2+} was increased 1.4-fold by calmodulin but the Ka for octopamine (1.6 μM) remained unchanged (Bodnaryk 1983a). The increase in maximal reaction velocity of octopamine-sensitive adenylate cyclase from moth brain caused by Ca^{2+}-calmodulin is relatively small (1.4-fold). It is possible that Ca^{2+}-calmodulin-stimulated adenylate cyclase activity represents only a proportion of the total adenylate cyclase present in the moth brain membranes. Bovine brain adenylate cyclase solubilized by detergent can be resolved into two fractions using cal-

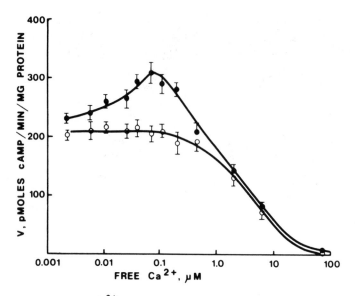

Fig. 3. Effect of Ca^{2+} on the activity of adenylate cyclase in washed membranes from the brain of a moth, *Mamestra configurata. Open circles* in the absence of calmodulin; *closed circles* in the presence of 0.17 μM calmodulin. (Bodnaryk 1983a)

modulin-Sepharose affinity chromatography. The major fraction, representing 80% of the total, was *not* calmodulin-sensitive and did not bind to the affinity column. The remainder, which was calmodulin-sensitive, could be eluted from the column with the calcium chelator, EGTA (Westcott et al. 1979).

2.4 Functions of Octopamine-Sensitive Adenylate Cyclase in the CNS and in Peripheral Systems

2.4.1 Function in the CNS

In spite of many biochemical and pharmacological studies of octopamine-sensitive adenylate cyclase in the CNS of diverse invertebrates (Bodnaryk 1982a, 1983b), a role for octopamine in invertebrate CNS function has yet to be established. One experimental difficulty in defining a role for octopamine is the lack of specific octopamine agonists and antagonists (Harmar and Horn 1977). Another is the lack of a well-defined, intact cellular system to which modern methods of neurophysiology, pharmacology, and biochemistry can be used in conjunction with broken cell studies. The firefly light organ may provide a useful peripheral system for establishing a neural function for octopamine.

2.4.2 Neural Control of Firefly Flashing

The control of flashing in the firefly, *Photuris*, is via neuronal afferents running to the light organ or "lantern". Electrical stimulation of afferent nerves or the lantern itself causes light emission and control of flashing is abolished after denervation. Application of octopamine or its N-methyl derivative, synephrine (Carlson 1968a,b, 1972) or the octopamine agonists chlordimeform and its N-demethylated derivatives (Hollingworth and Murdock 1980) (but not acetylcholine, serotonin or GABA) is effective in eliciting light production in intact or decentralized light organs. It is currently thought that neuronal activity in the form of a volley of afferent nerve impulses causes the release of an amine neurotransmitter, likely octopamine (Robertson and Carlson 1976), that mediates control of light emission.

The lantern of adult (Nathanson 1979; Copeland and Robertson 1982) and larval *Photuris* (Nathanson and Hunnicutt 1979) contains an adenylate cyclase that is activated by as much as 25-fold by low concentrations of octopamine. The relative potency of octopamine and various other amines in stimulating adenylate cyclase, and the effects of antagonists in blocking activation by octopamine, correlate well with the effects of these agents in affecting light production (Nathanson 1979). Thus cAMP might be an intracellular mediator of light activation in the firefly lantern. Several features of the lantern, and especially the larval lantern, offer advantages for studying the neural function of octopamine in an intact cellular system that is amenable to biochemical, pharmacological, and neurophysiological analyses.

2.4.3 Effects at the Neuromuscular Junction

Post-Synaptic Effects. A single, octopamine-containing neurone, called DUMETi (Hoyle et al. 1974; Hoyle 1975), affects neuromuscular transmission and various forms of muscle tension in the extensor tibiae muscle of the hind leg of the locust, *S. americana gregaria*. The neurone can be easily identified physiologically and selectively stimulated. The neurone does not form discrete synaptic junctions with the muscle fibers but ends as blind neurosecretory terminals in the outer layers of the sarcolemmal complex of fibers (Hoyle et al. 1980). According to Evans (1981), octopamine released from these terminals acts as a neuromodulator or local hormone, modulating the effectiveness of neuromuscular transmission.

Stimulation of the octopaminergic neurone to the extensor tibiae muscle increases the level of cAMP (but not cGMP) in locust extensor tibiae neuromuscular preparations, as does the application of octopamine. The post-synaptic effect of octopamine was calcium sensitive, potentiated by the phosphodiesterase inhibitor 3-isobutyl-1-methyl-xanthine (IBMX) and mimiced by the cAMP analog 8-(4-chlorophenylthio)adenosine cyclic $3':5'$-monophosphate (CPT cAMP) and the diterpene adenylate cyclase activator forskolin (Evans 1984a,b). Pharmacological analyses with agonists and antagonists indicated that the octopamine-mediated increases in cAMP in the preparation are mediated by octopamine$_2$ class receptors which modulate neuromuscular transmission and muscle tension (Evans 1981).

At present, little, if anything is known about mechanisms that link increased levels of cAMP to a physiological response of the muscle. Octopamine induced increases in cAMP might also be related in part to the regulation of carbohydrate metabolism in the extensor tibiae muscle, as suggested for locust flight muscle (Candy 1978; Worm 1980).

Presynaptic Effects. Treatment of the locust hind leg neuromuscular preparation with IBMX, CPT cAMP or forskolin also mimics the *presynaptic* effect of octopamine on spontaneous release of transmitter from the slow motoneurone (called SETi) to the extensor tibiae muscles as measured by the frequency of SETi spontaneous miniature endplate potentials (m.e.p.p.s.). Presynaptic octopamine$_2$ receptors on the terminals of the slow motoneurone are involved in transmitter release (Evans 1981, 1984b). Evans (1984b) hypothesizes that the elevation of presynaptic cAMP levels by octopamine is likely to affect transmitter release by altering the levels of free Ca^{2+} in the nerve terminals, possibly by the action of a specific protein kinase. The hypothesis is consistent with the observed calcium sensitivity of the effects of octopamine on the locust neuromuscular preparation (Evans 1984b) but lacks further biochemical detail.

Low levels (10^{-10} to 10^{-7} M) of octopamine cause enhanced post-synaptic potentials in the opener muscle in the claw of the freshwater crayfish, *Procambarus clarkii* (Breen and Atwood 1983). The authors attribute this to a presynaptic effect of octopamine which increases quantal release of transmitter. Most significantly, the effect is more pronounced and longer lasting when octopamine is applied to active neuromuscular preparations, suggesting a mechanism for strengthening pathways used during specific activities. It will be of interest to determine whether the effect also occurs in the central nervous system and whether regulation of K^+ channels via membrane protein phosphorylation is involved.

3 Role of Serotonin-Sensitive Adenylate Cyclase in Neuronal Function

3.1 Regulation of Potassium Channels

The *exit* of K^+ from cells is mediated by trans-membrane K^+ channels. Unlike Na^+ channels, which appear to exist as a single type, there are several kinds of K^+ channels that occur in different ratios in different neurons giving rise to neuronal diversity (Meech 1978; Reichardt and Kelly 1983; Petersen and Maryama 1984). In the nervous system these channels are important in regulating electrical activity, and in particular, in regulating changes in synaptic efficiency that lead to altered behaviour and memory function. At least some of these channels appear to be regulated by neurotransmitters and cAMP-dependent protein kinases.

3.2 Pre-Synaptic Regulation of K^+ Channels

3.2.1 Learning in *Aplysia*

Habituation and sensitization are elementary forms of non-associative learning, habituation being broadly defined as the decrease in a behavioural response on repeated presentation of the same stimulus and sensitization as an increase in an animal's responsiveness after a strong or novel stimulus. Kandel and colleagues have established a molecular basis for sensitization of the gill-withdrawal reflex in the marine mollusc *Aplysia californica*, the essence of which is cAMP-mediated protein phosphorylation leading to the closure of a specific K^+ channel, with consequent increases in the duration of the action potential, Ca^{2+} influx and transmitter release at monosynaptic connections between sensory neurons and motor cells (Kandel 1981; Siegelbaum et al. 1982; Kandel and Schwartz 1982) (Fig. 4).

The ingenious technique of intracellular protein kinase injection, made possible by the enormous size of the cell body of sensory neurons in *Aplysia*, has been used by Castellucci et al. (1980) to establish that cAMP-mediated protein phosphorylation is an essential component of behavioural sensitization of the gill-withdrawal reflex. They injected the purified catalytic subunit of a cAMP-dependent protein kinase (Fig. 2) into cell bodies of individual sensory neurons and simultaneously assayed transmitter release postsynaptically either in an interneuron or in a motor neuron of the gill-withdrawal reflex. Injection of active catalytic subunit mimiced the action of serotonin and cAMP by simulating the physiological changes that accompany presynaptic facilitation, i.e., by broadening the action potential and accompanying increase in Ca^{2+} current by decreasing the input conductance of the cell as a result of a decrease in the K^+ current and by increasing the amount of transmitter released by terminals of the sensory cell onto follower neurons. The results are consistent with the hypothesis (Castellucci et al. 1980) that the protein that is phosphorylated by the catalytic subunit of cAMP-dependent protein kinase is either a component of the K^+ channel itself or a modulator protein that acts on the channel (Fig. 4).

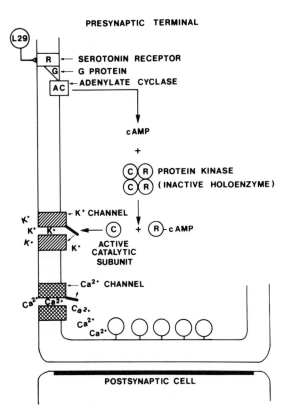

Fig. 4. A molecular model of presynaptic facilitation and sensitization. (After Klein and Kandel 1980)

3.2.2 Learning in *Hermissenda*

Additional support for the idea that protein phosphorylation is an essential event in some forms of learning has been obtained from studies of the nudibranch *Hermissenda crassicornis* by Neary et al. (1981). The authors report that there is an increased level of incorporation of ^{32}P in a M_r 20,000 phosphoprotein in the eye of *Hermissenda* after training with paired light and rotation but not after control procedures. The possible role of protein phosphorylation in regulating two voltage dependent K^+ currents (I_A and I_B) in type B photoreceptors in the eye has been investigated by protein kinase injection by Alkon et al. (1983). Injection of the catalytic subunit of a cAMP-dependent protein kinase preferentially reduced I_B more than I_A, whereas injection of Ca^{2+}-calmodulin-dependent protein kinase reduced I_A more than I_B. Since the early voltage-dependent K^+ current I_A was reduced and inactivated more rapidly in trained than in control type B cells (Alkon et al. 1982), it seems possible that increased phosphorylation of the M_r 20,000 protein in the eye of associatively-trained *Hermissenda* could result from increased Ca^{2+}-calmodulin-dependent protein kinase activity (Alkon et al. 1983).

3.2.3 Learning in *Drosophila*

Mutants of *Drosophila melanogaster* having impared learning and memory ability and altered cAMP metabolism have been used to seek the molecular basis of these functions (Quinn and Greenspan 1984).

The *dunce* mutants of *Drosophila* do not learn to avoid an ordorant associated with an electric shock or quinine powder, even though both of these punishments are effective reinforces of avoidance behaviour in normal flies. The *dunce* mutant is capable of sensing the odorant as shown in separate experiments and has the same morphology and general vigour as normal flies. The *dunce* mutant, however, lacks form 11 cAMP phosphodiesterase and has elevated body levels of cAMP (Davis and Kiger 1978; Byers et al. 1981; Solti et al. 1983), indicating at least that the *dunce* gene and one isozyme of cAMP phosphodiesterase are closely related (Byers et al. 1981). It has not yet been established that *dunce* is the structural gene of form 11 phosphodiesterase or that the normal product of the *dunce* gene forms an integral part of a molecular apparatus of learning at the cyclic nucleotide level.

In the memory mutant *rutabaga* of *Drosophila*, the activity of a membrane-bound adenylate cyclase present in homogenates of body regions of adult flies is lower than in corresponding homogenates from normal flies (Dudai et al. 1983). Washing the membranes does not abolish the difference between mutant and normal flies, indicating that a soluble cytosolic factor is not involved. Adenylate cyclase activity of washed membranes from *rutabaga* displays a lower V_{max}, a higher K_m and an abnormal response to Mg^{2+} ions compared to normal flies, an effect especially pronounced in washed membranes from the abdomen. Although low adenylate cyclase activity is consistent with abnormal short-term memory as seen in the preceding section, proof establishing a link between the lesion in adenylate cyclase and memory deficit in *rutabaga* is not yet at hand. It will be of interest to study protein phosphorylation in genetic mutants of *Drosophila* that have impaired learning and memory function.

3.3 Post-Synaptic Regulation of K^+ Channels

The identified neuron R15 in *Aplysia* exhibits a regular pattern of endogenous "bursting" activity which consists of alternating depolarizing and hyperpolarizing membrane oscillations. Neurophysiological, pharmacological, and biochemical evidence indicates that the hyperpolarizing phase in R15 is due to a serotonin-induced *increase* in K^+ conductance that is mediated by cAMP. Thus, addition of inhibitors of phosphodiesterase, such as theophylline or IBMX to the bathing medium increased the concentration of cAMP in the abdominal ganglion and augmented the hyperpolarizing phases, as did intraneural injection of cAMP analogues or an inhibitor of adenylate cyclase, guanylylimidodiphosphate (Treistman and Levitan 1976a,b; Levitan et al. 1979; Levitan and Norman 1980). Voltage clamp analysis indicated that serotonin and cAMP analogues both cause an increase in membrane slope conductance in R15 in a manner consistent with increased K^+ conductance. The effect of saturating concentrations of serotonin and cAMP analogues on K^+ conductance were not additive, consistent with the idea that cAMP mediates the effect of serotonin. In unclamped neuron R15, low concentrations of serotonin (0.1 μM) are potentiated by the phosphodiesterase inhibitor Ro20-1724 and high concentrations of serotonin (10 μM) can inhibit bursting completely (Drummond et al. 1980a).

Pharmacological analysis supports the idea that the serotonin receptor that mediates hyperpolarization in R15 (Drummond et al. 1980a) is similar to the serotonin receptor that is coupled to adenylate cyclase (Levitan 1978; Drummond et al. 1980b,c). In particular, the rank order of potency of a series of pharmacological agents that alter the electrical activity of R15 is generally similar to the EC50 (K_i) of these agents acting on serotonin-sensitive adenylate cyclase in the abdominal ganglion (Drummond et al. 1980a).

The serotonin-induced increase in K^+ conductance that is mediated by cAMP in R15 suggests that protein phosphorylation by a protein kinase might be important in regulating the K^+ channel. To investigate this possibility, Adams and Levitan (1982) injected a specific inhibitor of cAMP-dependent protein kinase intracellularly into neuron R15. The injection blocked the serotonin-induced increase in K^+ conductance completely. Full recovery of the serotonin response occurred spontaneously 5–13 h after the injection, presumably as a result of intracellular proteolysis of the protein kinase inhibitor. The effect of the inhibitor was specific because the response of the neuron to dopamine was not inhibited and because injection of other proteins (alpha-bungarotoxin; bovine serum albumin) did not affect the serotonin response. These results provide convincing evidence that protein phosphorylation is a necessary step in the process that leads to activation of K^+ channels by serotonin in neuron R15 (Adams and Levitan 1982).

In an attempt to identify the phosphorylated substrates involved in the activation of K^+ channels by serotonin in neuron R15, Lemos et al. (1982) injected [γ^{32}P]ATP into R15. Intracellular injection offers the precision of localizing radioactivity to the soma and neuropile processes of an identified living neuron. At least 15 phosphoproteins of M_r 22,000–230,000 were labelled in R15 during 50 min following the injection. When serotonin was added to the incubation, there was a change in the pattern of labelling of the phosphoproteins. Several high mol. wt. proteins (M_r 230,000; 205,000; 135,000) and one low mol. wt. protein (M_r 26,000) showed significant increases in phosphorylation and one protein (M_r 43,000) showed a significant decrease in phosphorylation (Lemos et al. 1982). At least some of the proteins phosphorylated in vivo were also found in in vitro experiments, making it possible to use an in vitro system to study physiologically relevant phosphorylation (Novak-Hofer and Levitan 1983). No doubt future research will focus on the possible role of these phosphoproteins in the regulation of the K^+ channel in R15 and elsewhere.

3.4 Regulation of Ca^{2+}-Activated K^+ Channels

In the nervous system, Ca^{2+}-activated K^+ channels, of which there appear to be three distinctive types, play a major role in regulating electrical activity (Meech 1978; Schwarz and Passow 1983; Peterson and Maruyama 1984). Evidence that Ca^{2+}-activated K^+ conductance in non-identified neurons in the snail, *Helix roseneri*, is enhanced by protein phosphorylation has been provided by DePeyer et al. (1982). Addition of physiological concentrations of the catalytic subunit of cAMP-dependent protein kinase to the internal perfusing medium enhanced the outward current produced by depolarizing voltage clamp steps with no apparent effect on the inward current. Internal perfusion with catalytic subunit inactivated by 5,5'-dithiobis (2-nitrobenzoic acid), a reaction that causes only minor modification of the structure of the protein but completely abolishes its enzymatic activity, was without effect on the outward current. The result provides convincing evidence that the enhancement of outward current produced by active catalytic subunit is due to protein phosphorylation and not due to some non-specific effect. Decreasing the external Ca^{2+} concentration from 10 mM to 1 mM eliminated the effect of the catalytic subunit, as did internal perfusion with the Ca^{2+} chelator EGTA, showing the Ca^{2+} ions play an important role in enhanced outward current. These results indicate that cAMP-dependent protein phosphorylation regulates the Ca^{2+}-activated K^+ conductance in the *Helix* neuron, possibly by phosphorylation of a regulatory component of the K^+ channel such as to increase its affinity for Ca^{2+} (DePeyer et al. 1982).

References

Adams WB, Levitan IB (1982) Intracellular injection of protein kinase inhibitor blocks the serotonin-induced increase in K^+ conductance in *Aplysia* neuron R15. Proc Natl Acad Sci USA 79: 3877–3880

Alkon DL, Lederhendler I, Shoukimas JJ (1982) Primary changes of membrane current during retention of associative learning. Science (Wash DC) 215:693–695

Alkon DL, Acosta-Urquidi J, Olds J, Kuzma G, Neary JT (1982) Protein kinase injection reduces voltage-dependent potassium currents. Science (Wash DC) 219:303–306

Alkon DL, Acosta-Urquidi J, Olds J, Kuzma G, Neary JT (1983) Protein kinase injection reduces voltage-dependent potassium currents. Science (Wash DC) 219:303–306

Battelle BA, Kravitz EA (1978) Targets of octopamine action in the lobster: cyclic nucleotide changes and physiological effects in hemolymph, heart and exoskeletal muscle. J Pharmacol Exp Ther 205:438–448

Bodnaryk RP (1979a) Identification of specific dopamine- and octopamine-sensitive adenylate cyclases in the brain of *Mamestra configurata* Wlk. Insect Biochem 9:155–162

Bodnaryk RP (1979b) Characterization of an octopamine-sensitive adenylate cyclase from insect brain (*Mamestra configurata* Wlk.). Can J Biochem 57:226–232

Bodnaryk RP (1979c) Basal, dopamine- and octopamine-stimulated adenylate cyclase activity in the brain of the moth, *Mamestra configurata*, during its metamorphosis. J Neurochem 33:275–282

Bodnaryk RP (1981) Free and bound cyclic AMP in the brain of the moth *Mamestra configurata* Wlk during pupal-adult metamorphosis. Can J Zool 59:1629–1634

Bodnaryk RP (1982a) Biogenic amine-sensitive adenylate cyclases in insects. Insect Biochem 12:1–6

Bodnaryk RP (1982b) The effect of single and combined doses of chlordimeform and permethrin on cAMP and cGMP levels in the moth, *Mamestra configurata* Wlk. Pestic Biochem Physiol 18:334–340

Bodnaryk RP (1982c) The effects of pesticides and related compounds on cyclic nucleotide metabolism. Insect Biochem 12:589–597

Bodnaryk RP (1983a) Regulation by Ca^{2+} and calmodulin of brain adenylate cyclase from the moth, *Mamestra configurata* Wlk. Insect Biochem 13:111–114

Bodnaryk RP (1983b) Cyclic nucleotides. In: Downer RGH, Laufer H (eds) Endocrinology of insects, vol 1. Liss, New York, pp 567–614

Breen CA, Atwood HL (1983) Octopamine – a neurohormone with presynaptic activity-dependent effects at crayfish neuromuscular junctions. Nature (Lond) 303:716–718

Byers D, David RL, Kiger JA (1981) Defect in cyclic AMP phosphodiesterase due to the *dunce* mutation of learning in *Drosophila melanogaster*. Nature (Lond) 289:79–81

Candy DJ (1978) The regulation of locust flight muscle metabolism by ocotpamine and other compounds. Insect Biochem 8:177–181

Carlson AD (1968a) Effect of adrenergic drugs on the lantern of the larval Photuris firefly. J Exp Biol 48:381–387

Carlson AD (1968b) Effect of drugs on luminescence in larval fireflies. J Exp Biol 49:195–199

Carlson AD (1972) A comparison of transmitter and synephrine on luminescence induction in the firefly larva. J Exp Biol 57:737–743

Castellucci VF, Kandel ER, Schwartz JH, Wilson FD (1980) Intra-cellular injection of the catalytic subunit of cyclic AMP-dependent protein kinase simulates facilitation of transmitter release underlying behavioral sensitization in *Aplysia*. Proc Natl Acad Sci USA 77:7492–7496

Cooper DMF (1983) Receptor-mediated stimulation and inhibition of adenylate cyclase. Curr Top Membr Transp 18:67–84

Copeland J, Robertson HA (1982) Octopamine as the transmitter at the firefly lantern: presence of an octopamine-sensitive and a dopamine-sensitive adenylate cyclase. Comp Biochem Physiol 72c:125–127

Daly JW, McNeal E, Partington C, Neuwirth M, Creveling CR (1980a) Accumulations of cAMP in adenine-labelled cell-free preparations from guinea pig cerebral cortex: role of alpha-adrenergic and H_1-histaminergic receptors. J Neurochem 35:326–337

Daly JW, Padgett W, Nimitkitpaisan Y, Creveling CR, Cantacuzene D, Kirk KL (1980b) Fluoro-norepinephrines: specific agonists for the activation of *alpha* and *beta* adrenergic-sensitive cyclic AMP-generating systems in brain slices. J Pharmacol Exp Ther 212:382–389

Davis RL, Kiger JA (1978) Genetic manipulation of cyclic AMP levels in *Drosophila melanogaster*. Biochem Biophys Res Commun 81:1180–1186

DeCamilli P, Cameron R, Greengard P (1983a) Synapsin I (Protein I), a nerve terminal-specific phosphoprotein I. Its general distribution in synapses of the central and peripheral nervous system demonstrated by immunofluorescence in frozen and plastic sections. J Cell Biol 96:1337–1354

DeCamilli P, Harris SM, Huttner WB, Greengard P (1983b) Synapsin I (Protein I), a nerve terminal-specific phosphoprotein II. Its specific association with synaptic vesicles demonstrated by immunocytochemistry in agarose-embedded synaptosomes. J Cell Biol 96:1355–1373

DePeyer JE, Cachelin AB, Levitan IB, Reuter H (1982) Ca^{2+}-activated K^+ conductance in internally perfused snail neurons is enhanced by protein phosphorylation. Proc Natl Acad Sci USA 79:4207–4211

Dougan DFH, Wade DN (1978a) Action of octopamine agonists and stereo isomers at a specific octopamine receptor. Clin Exp Pharmacol Physiol 5:333–339

Dougan DFH, Wade DN (1978b) Differential blockade of octopamine and dopamine receptors by analogues of clozapine and metoclopramide. Clin Exp Pharmacol Physiol 5:341–349

Drummond GI (1983) Cycle nucleotides in the nervous system. Adv Cyclic Nucleotide Res 15: 373–496

Drummond AH, Benson JA, Levitan IB (1980a) Serotonin-induced hyperpolarization of an identified *Aplysia* neuron is mediated by cyclic AMP. Proc Natl Acad Sci USA 77:5013–5017

Drummond AH, Bucher F, Levitan IB (1980b) d-[³H] Lysergic acid diethylamide binding to serotonin receptors in the molluscan nervous system. J Biol Chem 255:6679–6686

Drummond AH, Bucher F, Levitan IB (1980c) Distribution of serotonin and dopamine receptors in Aplysia tissues: analysis by [³H]LSD binding and adenylate cyclase stimulation. Brain Res 184:163–177

Dudai Y (1982) High-affinity octopamine receptors revealed in *Drosophila* by binding of [³H] octopamine. Neurosc. Lett 28:163–167

Dudai Y, Zvi S (1984) High-affinity [³H] octopamine-binding sites in *Drosophila melanogaster*: interaction with ligands and relationships to octopamine receptors. Comp Biochem Physiol 77c: 145–151

Dudai Y, Uzzan A, Zvi S (1983) Abnormal activity of adenylate cyclase in the *Drosophila* memory mutant rutabaga. Neurosci Lett 42:207–212

Erspamer V (1952) Identification of octopamine as 1-p-hydroxyphenylethanolamine. Nature (Lond) 169:375–376

Evans PD (1980) Biogenic amines in the insect nervous system. Adv Insect Physiol 15:317–473

Evans PD (1981) Multiple receptor types for octopamine in the locust. J Physiol (Lond) 318:99–122

Evans PD (1984a) A modulatory octopaminergic neurone increases cyclic nucleotide levels in locust skeletal muscle. J Physiol (Lond) 348:307–324

Evans PD (1984b) The role of cyclic nucleotides and calcium in the mediation of the modulatory effects of octopamine on locust skeletal muscle. J Physiol (Lond) 384:325–340

Evans PD, Gee JD (1980) Action of formamidine pesticides on octopamine receptors. Nature (Lond) 287:60–62

Glass DB, Krebs EG (1980) Protein phosphorylation catalyzed by cyclic AMP-dependent and cyclic GMP-dependent protein kinases. Annu Rev Pharmacol Toxicol 20:363–388

Gole JWD, Orr GL, Downer RGH (1983) Interaction of formamidines with octopamine-sensitive adenylate cyclase receptor in the nerve cord of *Periplaneta americana* L. Life Sci 32:2939–2947

Goosey MW, Candy DJ (1980) The D-octopamine content of the haemolymph of the locust, *Schistocerca americana gregaria* and its elevation during flight. Insect Biochem 10:393–397

Greengard P (1976) Possible role for cyclic nucleotides and phosphorylated membrane proteins in postsynaptic actions of neurotransmitters. Nature (Lond) 260:101–108

Greengard P (1978) Phosphorylated proteins as physiological effectors. Science (Wash DC) 199: 146–152

Greengard P, DeCamilli P (1982) Protein phosphorylation in neurons. In: Schotland DL (ed) Disorders of the motor unit. Wiley, New York, pp 441–460

Harmar AJ, Horn AS (1977) Octopamine-sensitive adenylate cyclase in cockroach brain: effects of agonists, antagonists and guanylyl nucleotides. Mol Pharmacol 13:512–520

Hollingworth RM (1976) Chemistry, biological activity, and uses of formamidine pesticides. Environ Health Perspect 14:57–69

Hollingworth RM, Murdock LL (1980) Formamidine pesticides: octopamine-like actions in a firefly. Science (Wash DC) 208:74–76

Hoyle G (1975) Evidence that insect dorsal unpaired median (DUM) neurons are octopaminergic. J Exp Zool 193:425–431

Hoyle G, Dagon D, Moberly B, Colquhoun W (1974) Dorsal unpaired median insect neurons make neurosecretory endings on skeletal muscle. J Exp Zool 187:159–165

Huff RM, Molinoff PB (1982) Quantitative determination of dopamine receptor subtypes not linked to activation of adenylate cyclase in rat striatum. Proc Natl Acad Sci USA 79:7561–7565

Huttner WB, Schiebkler W, Greengard P, DeCamilli P (1983) Synapsin I (Protein I), a nerve terminal-specific phosphoprotein III. Its association with synaptic vesicles studied in a highly purified synaptic vesicle preparation. J Cell Biol 96:1374–1388

Kahn DJ, Mitrius JC, U'Prichard DC (1982) Alpha$_2$-adrenergic receptors in neuroblastoma × glioma hybrid cells. Characterization with agonist and antagonist radioligands and relationship to adenylate cyclase. Mol Pharmacol 21:17−26

Kandel ER (1981) Calcium and the control of synaptic strength by learning. Nature (Lond) 293: 697−700

Kandel ER, Schwartz JH (1982) Molecular biology of learning: modulation of transmitter release. Science (Wash DC) 218:433−443

Kebabian JW, Calne DB (1979) Multiple receptors for dopamine. Nature (Lond) 277:93−96

Klein M, Camardo J, Kandel ER (1982) Serotonin modulates a specific potassium current in the sensory neurons that show presynaptic facilitation in *Aplysia*. Proc Natl Acad Sc USA 79: 5713−5717

Kretsinger RH (1979) The informational role of calcium in the cytosol. Adv Cyclic Nucleotide Res 11:1−26

Kuo JF, Greengard P (1969) Cyclic nucleotide-dependent protein kinases IV. Widespread occurrence of adenosine 3',5'-monophosphate dependent protein kinase in various tissues and phyla of the animal kingdom. Proc Natl Acad Sci USA 64:1349−1355

Lemos JR, Novak-Hofere I, Levitan IB (1982) Serotonin alters the phosphorylation of specific proteins inside a single living nerve cell. Nature (Lond) 298:64−65

Levitan IB (1978) Adenylate cyclase in isolated Helix and Aplysia neuronal cell bodies: stimulation by serotonin and peptide-containing extract. Brain Res 154:404−408

Levitan IB, Norman J (1980) Different effects of cAMP and cGMP derivatives on the activity of an identified neuron: biochemical and electrophysiological analysis. Brain Res 187:415−429

Levitan IB, Harmar AJ, Adams WB (1979) Synaptic and hormonal modulation of a neuronal oscillator: a search for molecular mechanisms. J Exp Biol 81:131−151

Levitzki A (1976) Catecholamine receptors. In: Cuatrecasas P, Greaves MF (eds) Receptors and recognition, ser A, vol 2. Chapman and Hall, London, pp 199−229

McCarthy KD, deVellis J (1978) Alpha-adrenergic receptor modulation of beta-adrenergic, adenosine and prostaglandin E$_1$ increased adenosine 3':5'-cyclic monophosphate levels in primary cultures of glia. J Cyclic Nucleotide Res 4:15−26

Meech RW (1978) Calcium-dependent potassium activation in nervous tissues. Annu Rev Biophys Bioeng 7:1−18

Murdock LL, Hollingworth RM (1980) Octopamine-like actions of formamidines in the firefly light organ. Insect neurobiology and pesticide action. Soc Chem Indust, London, pp 415−422

Nathanson JA (1976) Octopamine-sensitive adenylate cyclase and its possible relationship to the octopamine receptor. In: Usdin E, Sandler M (eds) Trace amines and the brain. Dekker, New York, pp 161−190

Nathanson JA (1979) Octopamine receptors, adenosine 3',5'-monophosphate, and neural control of firefly flashing. Science (Wash DC) 203:65−68

Nathanson JA, Greengard P (1973) Octopamine-sensitive adenylate cyclase: evidence for a biological role of octopamine in nervous tissue. Science (Wash DC) 180:308−310

Nathanson JA, Hunnicutt EJ (1979) Neural control of light emission in Photuris larvae: identification of octopamine-sensitive adenylate cyclase. J Exp Zool 208:255−262

Nathanson JA, Hunnicutt EJ (1981) N-demethylchlordimeform. A potent partial agonist of octopamine-sensitive adenylate cyclase. Mol Pharmacol 20:68−75

Neary JT, Crow T, Alkon DL (1981) Changes in a specific phosphoprotein band following associative learning in *Hermissenda*. Nature (Lond) 293:658−660

Novak-Hofer I, Levitan IB (1983) Ca^{++}/Calmodulin-regulated protein phosphorylation in the *Aplysia* nervous system. J Neuroci 3:473−481

Orchard I (1982) Octopamine in insects: neurotransmitter, neurohormone, and neuromodulator. Can J 2001 60:659−669

Orchard IG, Singh GJP, Loughton BG (1982) Action of formamidine pesticides on octopamine receptors on locust fat body. Comp Biochem Physiol 73C:331−334

Orchard I, Gole JWD, Downer RGH (1983) Pharmacology of aminergic receptors mediating an elevation in cyclic AMP and release of hormone from locust neurosecretory cells. Brain Res 288: 349−353

Petersen OH, Maruyama Y (1984) Calcium-activated potassium channels and their role in secretion. Nature (Lond) 307:693–696

Plapp FW (1976) Chlordimeform as a synergist for insecticides against the tobacco budworm. J Econ Entomol 69:91–92

Porzig H (1982) Are there differences in the beta-receptor-adenylate cyclase systems of fragmented membranes and living cells? Trends Pharmacol Sci 3:75–78

Quinn WG, Greenspan RJ (1984) Learning and courtship in *Drosophila*: two stories with mutants. Annu Rev Neurosci 7:67–93

Reichardt LF, Kelly RB (1983) A molecular description of nerve terminal function. Annu Rev Biochem 52:871–926

Roberts CJ, Walker RJ (1981) Octopamine receptors on *Limulus* and *Periplaneta* central neurons. Comp Biochem Physiol 69C:301–306

Robertson HA, Carlson AD (1976) Octopamine: presence in firefly lantern suggests transmitter role. J Exp Zool 195:159–164

Robertson HA, Osborne NN (1979) Putative neurotransmitters in the annelid central nervous system: presence of 5-hydroxytryptamine and octopamine-stimulated adenylate cyclases. Comp Biochem Physiol 64C:7–14

Rodbell M (1980) The role of hormone receptors and GTP-regulatory proteins in membrane transduction. Nature (Lond) 284:17–22

Schwarz W, Passow H (1983) Ca^{2+}-activated K^+ channels in erythrocytes and excitable cells. Annu Rev Physiol 45:359–374

Siegelbaum SA, Camardo JS, Kandel ER (1982) Serotonin and cyclic AMP close single K^+ channels in *Aplysia* sensory neurones. Nature (Lond) 299:413–417

Singh GJP, Barker JF (1983) Ultrastructural studies on formamidine-induced release of neurosecretion in *Locusta migratoria* (Orthoptera:Locustidae). Can Entomol 115:1147–1153

Solti M, Devay P, Kiss I, Londesborough J, Friedrich P (1983) Cyclic nucleotide phosphodiesterases in larval brain of wild type and *dunce* mutant strains of *Drosophila melanogaster*: isoenzyme pattern and activation by Ca^{2+}/calmodulin. Biochem Biophys Res Commun 111:652–658

Starratt AN, Bodnaryk RP (1981) Stereoisomeric identity of octopamine in the central nervous system of invertebrates. Insect Biochem 11:645–648

Treistman SN, Levitan IB (1976a) Alteration of electrical activity in molluscan neurones by cyclic nucleotides and peptide factors. Nature (Lond) 261:62–64

Treistman SN, Levitan IB (1976b) Intraneuronal guanylyl-imidodiphosphate injection mimics long-term synaptic hyperpolarization in *Aplysia*. Proc Natl Acad Sci USA 73:4689–4692

Uzzan A, Dudai Y (1982) Aminergic receptors in *Drosophila melanogaster*: responsiveness of adenylate cyclase to putative neurotransmitters. J Neurochem 38:1542–1550

Westcott KR, LaPorte DC, Storm DR (1979) Resolution of adenylate cyclase sensitive and insensitive to Ca^{2+} and calcium-dependent regulatory protein (CDR) by CDR-Sepharose affinity chromatography. Proc Natl Acad Sci USA 76:204–208

Worm RAA (1980) Involvement of cyclic nucleotides in locust flight muscle metabolism. Comp Biochem Physiol 67C:23–27

Biogenic Amines and the Regulation of Peptidergic Neurosecretory Cells

I. ORCHARD [1]

1 Introduction

Neurosecretory cells, defined as neurons which release chemical messengers (neurohormones) into the circulatory system for transport to their target sites, are found extensively throughout vertebrates and invertebrates (see Gabe 1966; Finlayson and Osborne 1975). Within these animal groups, there is a striking similarity in the anatomical arrangement of the neurosecretory systems, a similarity which was appreciated early in the development of neurosecretion (e.g. Scharrer and Scharrer 1944; Hanström 1953). Neurosecretory cells are usually found grouped in specific areas of the central nervous system connected, via axonal tracts, to a neurohaemal organ. This neurohaemal organ is usually a bulbous structure, swollen by virtue of the immense number of branched endings which increase the surface area for release (Fig. 1). Intrinsic cells may or may not be associated with this neurohaemal organ. Cell bodies and axons containing peptidergic hormones are often found interspersed with others containing biogenic amines (Cooke and Goldstone 1970; Baumgarten et al. 1972; Bjorklund 1968; Klemm and Axelsson 1973; Oksche 1976).

In addition to this similarity in structure, it also appears that the basic physiological and biochemical properties of neurosecretory cells are also similar (see Finlayson and Osborne 1975; Yagi and Iwasaki 1977; Cooke and Sullivan 1982; Orchard 1983). Functionally, these systems release neurohormones which control both metabolic and developmental processes.

While the morphological, physiological, and biochemical properties of the neurosecretory cells per se are similar, it has also been postulated that the mechanisms of integration may also possess some common features (Scharrer and Scharrer 1944; Orchard 1984). In particular, attention has focussed on the close anatomical relationship between aminergic and peptidergic neurons, and the presence of aminergic axons within neurohaemal organs. Physiologically, there may be two reasons for such a close association. The first is simply that amines may be neurohormones, and a neurohaemal organ would be a logical site from which to release these amines into the circulatory system. Secondly, amines may regulate the activities of peptidergic neurosecretory cells by acting as neurotransmitters or neuromodulators (Fig. 2). As we shall see there is evidence for both of these possibilities in vertebrates and invertebrates. In particular, there is now an enormous body of information on the hypothalamo-pituitary complex

---

1 Department of Zoology, University of Toronto, Toronto, Ontario, Canada M5S 1A1

Neurobiology
(ed. by R. Gilles and J. Balthazart)
© Springer-Verlag Berlin Heidelberg 1985

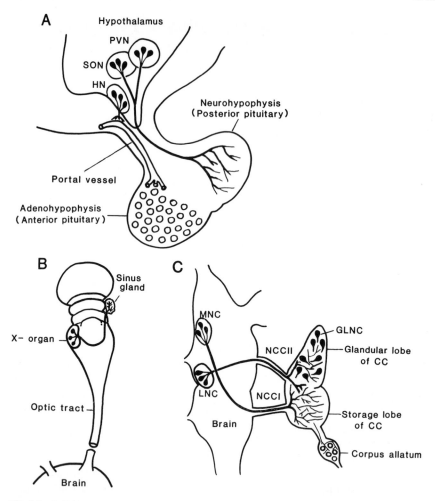

Fig. 1A–C. Diagram to illustrate the structural similarities between **A** hypothalamo-pituitary complex of mammals; **B** brain-X-organ-sinus gland of decapod crustacea; and **C** brain-corpus cardiacum complex of insects, as represented by the locust. *CC* corpus cardiacum; *GLNC* glandular lobe neurosecretory cells; *HN* hypothalamic nuclei; *LNC* lateral neurosecretory cells; *MNC* medial neurosecretory cells; *NCCI* and *NCCII* nervi corporis cardiaci I and II; *PVN* paraventricular nucleus; *SON* supraoptic nucleus. Neurosecretory cells *shaded*; gland cells *clear*. (After Andrew 1983; Orchard 1984)

of vertebrates concerning the regulation of release of peptidergic hormones by biogenic amines (see below). That this topic has attracted wide attention is illustrated by the referencing of 509 papers in an early review (Weiner and Ganong 1978). Attention has also focussed on this means of integration within invertebrates, and information is now available illustrating just such as relationship.

This review is aimed at collecting the evidence for aminergic regulation of peptidergic neurosecretory cells in vertebrates and invertebrates. Two invertebrate groups are examined, insects and crustacea, because more is known about their endocrinology than for other invertebrates.

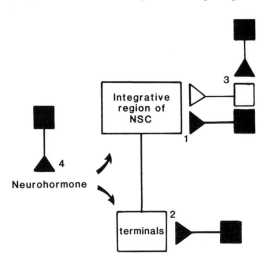

Fig. 2. Possible sites at which aminergic neurons (*solid figures*) could act to affect secretion from peptidergic neurosecretory cells (*NSC*). Aminergic neurons could synapse with the integrative region of *NSC* (*1*) or terminals (*2*) of the *NSC*. They could act via one (*clear figure*) or many neurons in pathway converging onto *NSC* (*3*) or they could release amine close to the terminal or into the haemolymph which may influence terminal in a neurohormonal fashion (*4*). (After Orchard 1984)

2 Vertebrates

The vertebrate literature (largely mammalian) on this topic is vast and has been reviewed extensively (see Weiner and Ganong 1978; Krulich 1979; Ajika 1980; McCann 1980; Buonomo et al. 1981). It goes beyond the scope of the present review to detail all of the work which has led to the current understanding in this field, and so a general synthesis will be presented which will lay the foundation for the rest of the review.

In vertebrates, it is now well established that biogenic amines regulate the release of peptidergic hormones from the hypothalamo-pituitary complex (eg. Arita and Porter 1984; Fehrer et al. 1983; Meyer et al. 1984; Clemens et al. 1978; Dufy et al. 1979; see also McCann et al. 1972; Krulich 1979; Weiner and Ganong 1978; McCann 1980). Included among these peptidergic hormones are oxytocin released from the posterior pituitary, and hypothalamic-hypophysiotropic hormones (releasing factors) released from the hypothalamus. These releasing factors enter the hypophyseal-portal blood vessels and regulate the release of the six established anterior pituitary hormones. There are at least seven releasing factors: corticotropin-releasing hormone (CRH) which increases the secretion of adrenocorticotropic hormone (ACTH); growth hormone-releasing hormone (GHRH) and somatostatin which increase and decrease respectively the secretion of growth hormone (GH); thyrotropin-releasing hormone (TRH) which stimulates the secretion of thyroid-stimulating hormone (TSH); luteinizing hormone-releasing hormone (LHRH) which stimulates the secretion of luteinizing hormone (LH) and follicle-stimulating hormone (FSH); prolactin-releasing hormone (PRH) and prolactin-inhibiting hormone (PIH) which stimulate and inhibit respectively the secretion of prolactin. Except for PIH these releasing factors are believed to be peptides (see Weiner and Ganong 1978).

The hypothalamus is innervated by aminergic neurons which have been shown to contain dopamine, norepinephrine, epinephrine, histamine, and serotonin (5-hydroxytryptamine, 5-HT) (see Nakai et al. 1983; Ajika 1980). Some of the dopaminergic neurons secrete dopamine into the hypophyseal portal blood where it is transported to, and acts directly upon, the anterior pituitary to inhibit tonic prolactin secretion (ie. dopamine itself acts as a neurohormone and is the PIH) (see McCann et al. 1984). Evidence for this comes from the demonstration that dopamine inhibits prolactin release from pituitary glands in vitro, high concentrations of dopamine occur in hypophyseal portal vessels, and dopaminergic receptors occur in the anterior pituitary. Similar experiments have also shown dopamine to inhibit TSH release (Foord et al. 1983). Amines also appear to function as neurotransmitters involved in controlling the hypothalamic hormone-secreting neurons which secrete releasing factors, and there is evidence to show that aminergic neurons make synaptic contact with these neurons (McNeill and Sladek 1977; Ajika 1979, 1980). While it may be argued that the systems are not fully characterized, there is sufficient information to make some generalised comments and provide some examples. Norepinephrine may act in an inhibitory manner upon CRH-secreting neurons (Jones et al. 1976) thereby inhibiting ACTH release. This effect is mediated by α-adrenergic receptors which probably lie on the dendrites or cell bodies of the CRH-secreting neurons in the medial basal hypothalamus, since norepinephrine has no effect upon the median eminence. Norepinephrine also has no effect upon ACTH secretion when incubated with anterior pituitary in vitro. In a similar manner, norepinephrine appears to stimulate TSH secretion by stimulating TRH-secreting neurons (e.g. Krulich et al. 1977) and GH secretion by stimulating GHRH-secreting neurons (Jones et al. 1976; Kakucoka and Makara 1983). Dopamine and norepinephrine influence the activities of LHRH-secreting neurons but the effect is dependent upon gonadal steroids and may be excitatory or inhibitory (Schneider and McCann 1970; Negro-Vilar et al. 1979; Adler et al. 1983). Conflicting results have been published concerning the effect of dopamine on GH release (see Kakucoka and Makara 1983). In some studies dopamine inhibits GH release, in others it stimulates GH release. As mentioned earlier tonic prolactin secretion is under the direct inhibitory control of PIH which appears to be dopamine. During times of rapid increase in prolactin secretion i.e. during suckling or estrogen-induced surges, 5-HT containing neurons appear to be stimulatory on prolactin secretion. 5-HT does not act directly upon the pituitary and its effect seems to be on the hypothalamus. At the present time it is not altogether clear if this stimulatory effect is a result of increased secretion of PRH or decreased secretion of PIH, although there is certainly evidence for stimulated secretion of PRH (Clemens et al. 1978).

The peptidergic hormones released from the posterior pituitary may also be under aminergic control. A central aminergic component has been implicated in the release of oxytocin during the milk-ejection reflex of rats (Tribollet et al. 1978). Norepinephrine terminals synapse with neurosecretory cells (Carlsson et al. 1962) and norepinephrine, dopamine, and 5-HT influence the firing rate of identified neurosecretory cells when applied iontophorectically (Barker et al. 1971).

3 Invertebrates

In comparison to the enormous body of information on the hypothalamo-pituitary complex of vertebrates, relatively little is known about the control of neurosecretory cells in invertebrates (in particular the involvement of amines). While the association of biogenic amines with the peptidergic neurosecretory systems of invertebrates has been stressed by several authors (see Evans 1980; Cooke and Goldstone 1970) experiments on a functional relationship have been rare. This of course has been due to a lack of basic information on the identity of neurohormones, the functions they control and the specific neuronal pathways through which they are activated. However, there have been recent advances in these fields and evidence is now forthcoming for a physiological relationship between aminergic and peptidergic neurons in invertebrates and there is sufficient knowledge to make some comparisons with vertebrates.

3.1 Insects

The distribution of amines in the insect neurosecretory system and the role of amines in peptide-release has recently been reviewed (Orchard 1984). Fluorescence histochemistry has revealed the presence of aminergic cell bodies located among the neurosecretory cells of the anterior pars intercerebralis of several insect species (Klemm and Falck 1978; Klemm 1983). In locusts, there are several hundred green-fluorescent cell bodies, containing dopamine and possibly norepinephrine, and one yellow fluorescent cell body containing an unidentified indolalkylamine (Klemm and Falck 1978). Double staining of sections for amines and peptidergic material indicates that the two cell types are distinct.

Dopamine, an unidentified yellow fluorescent indolalkylamine, and an unidentified fluorophore have also been demonstrated in the corpus cardiacum (a neurohaemal organ) of locusts and cockroaches (Klemm and Falck 1978; Lafon-Cazal 1981; Lafon-Cazal and Arluison 1976; Gersch et al. 1974). Radioenzymatic assays have demonstrated the presence of dopamine, norepinephrine and octopamine in the corpus cardiacum of the same insects (Dymond and Evans 1979; Evans 1978; Lafon-Cazal 1981; Orchard and Loughton 1981a; David and Lafon-Cazal 1979). The presence of 5-HT has also been noted by Gersch et al. (1961) and Migliori-Natalizi et al. (1970). The tract which connects the cells of the anterior pars intercerebralis to the corpus cardiacum (NCC1) is highly fluorescent, while the tract which connects the lateral neurosecretory cells of the brain to the corpus cardiacum (NCCII) is not (Klemm and Falck 1978).

In the locust, the corpus cardiacum is separated into the storage lobe (consisting largely of terminals of neurosecretory cells located within the pars intercerebralis of the brain) and glandular lobe (consisting of intrinsic neurosecretory cells interspersed with extrinsic axons from the brain). Fluorescence histochemistry reveals that the fluorescent amines are restricted to the storage lobe, with only a few fibers passing to the glandular lobe (Klemm and Falck 1978; Lafon-Cazal 1981). The glandular lobe itself is apparently devoid of fluorescent amines. Octopamine, however, a non-fluorogenic amine, is present in both glandular and storage lobe (David and Lafon-Cazal 1979; Orchard and Loughton 1981; Lafon-Cazal 1981; Goosey and Candy 1982).

Octopamine is a neurohormone in insects, released into the haemolymph during flight or following various forms of stress (Orchard et al. 1981; Goosey and Candy 1980; Bailey et al. 1983; Davenport and Evans 1984). Functions for octopamine as a neurohormone include its ability to stimulate release of lipid or trehalose from fat body. Octopamine also increases the activity of glycogen phosphorylase, stimulates glycogenolysis in ventral nerve cord and increases the rate of glucose oxidation in flight muscles (see Orchard 1982). Octopamine appears to be the mediator of a generalized response to excitation, the analogy with epinephrine and norepinephrine and the "fight or flight" response of vertebrates having been pointed out previously (Hoyle 1975; Gole and Downer 1979; Downer 1980). A neurohormonal function for other amines has yet to be demonstrated in insects.

Recent studies have now established a role for biogenic amines in the regulation of peptidergic cells in insects. In locusts, the glandular lobe of the corpus cardiacum is the source of two adipokinetic hormones, AKHI (Stone et al. 1976) and AKHII (Carlsen et al. 1979). The neurosecretory cells containing these hormones are activated during flight (Rademakers and Beenakkers 1977) and are thereby stimulated to release both hormones (Orchard and Lange 1983a,b). The release of AKH's is under the synaptic control of axons in NCCII (Rademakers 1977a,b) and electrical stimulation of NCCII results in the release of both hormones (Orchard and Loughton 1981a,b; Orchard and Lange 1983a). Synaptic contact with the neurosecretory cells is made from axons containing both large electron-dense granules (100 nm diameter) as well as smaller clear vesicles (20 nm diameter). The characteristics of these electron-dense granules are similar to those of identified octopaminergic neurons (Livingstone et al. 1981; Hoyle et al. 1980) in that the density of the granules varies and a substructure of rod-like tubular subunits is visible in the less dense granules (Krogh and Normann 1977; Rademakers and Beenakkers 1977). Physiological evidence indicates that these synapses are aminergic and in fact, octopaminergic (see Orchard 1984). Electrical stimulation of NCCII results in the release of AKH's (Orchard and Loughton 1981a,b; Orchard and Lange 1983a,b) and is accompanied by an elevation in cyclic AMP in the neurosecretory cells (Orchard et al. 1983a,c). Both of these effects are prevented following in vivo exposure to reserpine, and both effects are antagonized by α-aminergic receptor antagonists. Octopamine is present in the glandular lobe (Orchard and Loughton 1981a) and in NCCII (Martin and Orchard, unpublished observation). The most potent naturally occuring amine capable of mimicking both of the synaptically activated events is the monophenolic amine octopamine (Orchard et al. 1983a), and the effect of octopamine is antagonized by α-aminergic receptor antagonists. The control of release of AKH's therefore appears to be via synaptic activation of the neurosecretory cells from octopaminergic neurons. The cell bodies of these neurons lie within the brain and project to the neurosecretory cells via NCCII (Rademakers 1977b).

An interesting facet of the octopaminergic control of release of AKH's is that flight induces a short term elevation in haemolymph octopamine levels (Goosey and Candy 1980). Octopamine can act as a neurohormone (see earlier, also Orchard 1982) and in the locust acts upon the fat body to cause the release of lipid (Orchard et al. 1981, 1982). An intriguing possibility is that the haemolymph octopamine levels may reach a sufficient magnitude to potentiate the neurally evoked (octopamine-mediated) release of AKH's. Thus there may be dual control of the neurosecretory cells of the glandular lobe; synaptic input utilizing octopamine as the transmitter and hormonal input from circulating octopamine.

Similar evidence for an involvement of octopamine in regulating hormone release has recently been obtained in cockroaches (Downer et al. 1984), where a hyperglycaemic hormone is released from the corpus cardiacum. Electrical stimulation of NCCII results in the release of hyperglycaemic hormone (Gersch 1972) via an adrenergic system

(Gersch et al. 1974). Electrical stimulation also induces an elevation in cyclic AMP within the corpus cardiacum (Downer et al. 1984). Octopamine, applied to corpora cardiaca in vitro mimics both of these neurally evoked events, and the action of antagonists is consistent with there being α-aminergic receptors involved with the control of release of hyperglycaemic hormone. It was originally believed that hyperglycaemic hormone was manufactured in cell bodies in the brain and transported to the corpus cardiacum for release. The effect of octopamine was therefore believed to be on the terminals. Recent work has cast some doubt on this. O'Shea et al. (1984) have recently isolated two myoactive peptides from cockroach corpus cardiacum (MI and MII), which are synthesised in the corpus cardiacum and released from it into the haemolymph. MI appears to be the same hormone as neurohormone D of Baumann and Gersch (1982) which also appears to be the hyperglycaemic hormone. It thus appears that hyperglycaemic hormone may well be synthesised within the corpus cardiacum. If this is the case then one would anticipate that the cell bodies of the hyperglycaemic hormone-containing cells must lie within the corpus cardiacum. The system would thus be identical to that of the AKH system in locusts, with both metabolic hormones synthesised and released from the corpus cardiacum and both under neural control of octopaminergic axons in NCCII.

Recent experiments have provided evidence for aminergic regulation of certain medial neurosecretory cells of adult females of the blood sucking assassin bug (Orchard et al. 1983b; Orchard 1984) and, just as in vertebrates where the effects of dopamine and norepinephrine on LHRH release are dependent upon gonadal steroids, so too is the effects of dopamine in this bug. The timing and rate of oviposition in mature females is governed by a myotropic peptidergic ovulation hormone derived from ten large neurosecretory cells in the brain (Kriger 1981). In mated females, the electrical activity of these median neurosecretory cells and their axons, and the associated release of ovulation hormone, are stimulated by the appearance of ecdysteroid in the haemolymph (Ruegg et al. 1981, 1982). It is believed that the presence of the ovaries are required for ecdysteroid to appear in the haemolymph. Thus in ovariectomized, mated females, the peak of ecdysteroid is absent and so too is the characteristic pattern of electrical activity in the corpus cardiacum. However, injection of 20-hydroxyecdysone into ovariectomized mated females restores both the patterning of electrical activity and the resultant release of ovulation hormone (Ruegg et al. 1981, 1982). The enhancement of electrical activity of the neurosecretory cells in the brain and corpus cardiacum induced by 20-hydroxyecdysone has been used as a means of examining the possible role of aminergic neurons in this reflex (Orchard et al. 1983b). The response of the brain and corpus cardiacum, from mated ovariectomized females, to 20-hydroxyecdysone is blocked by the α-adrenergic receptor antagonists phentolamine and phenoxybenzamine, but not by the β-adrenergic receptor antagonist propranolol. Treatment of insects with reserpine is also effective at abolishing the response to 20-hydroxyecdysone, and dopamine is capable of mimicking the action of 20-hydroxyecdysone in mated ovariectomized females as well as in reserpine-treated ovariectomized females. The action of 20-hydroxyecdysone on the neurosecretory cells does not therefore appear to be direct, but involves aminergic interneurons located within the brain. The simplest interpretation would have aminergic neurons sensitive to the ecdysteroid, and synaptically linked to the neurosecretory cells. However these experiments cannot distinguish the number of pathways involved within this reflex.

Schooneveld (1974) described synaptic contacts between neurosecretory axons, and axons containing dense-core vesicles of a size to be expected in aminergic cells. This provides some ultrastructural evidence that median neurosecretory cells of Colorado potato beetle may be controlled synaptically by aminergic neurons.

Other evidence for a relationship between aminergic and peptidergic cells has been obtained from histological and ultrastructural studies. Flour beetles fed with a 1% reserpine diet demonstrate conspicuous changes in the median neurosecretory cells, with an accumulation of paraldehyde fuchsin material in the cell bodies and axons (Masner et al. 1970). These results indicate a reduction in the release of neurohormone, suggestive of an inhibitory aminergic control over neurosecretory activity. More recent studies examined the ultrastructure of neurosecretory cells following administration of norepinephrine (Warton and Dutkowski 1978), reserpine (Warton and Dutkowski 1977), or disulfiram, an inhibitor of norepinephrine synthesis (Warton 1981). Treatment of the wax moth with these agents produces ultrastructural changes in neurosecretory cells in the brain consistent with the hypothesis that aminergic neurons exert inhibitory control over these cells.

3.2 Crustacea

There are three major neurosecretory centres in decapod crustacea (see Andrew 1983; Cooke and Sullivan 1982). The neurosecretory cells which constitute the X-organ possess a neurohaemal organ called the sinus gland. These structures lie on an extension of the brain within the eyestalk. The X-organ/sinus gland complex produces a number of hormones, some of which have been purified and sequenced e.g. erythrophore-concentrating hormone (Fernlund and Josefsson 1972); light-adapting hormone (Fernlund 1976); and hyperglycaemic hormone (Kleinholz 1976). The pericardial organs are neurohaemal organs that lie in the venous cavity surrounding the crustacean heart. The pericardial organs are located distally in the second thoracic root of the lobster and in the homologous distal thoracic segmental nerves of crabs. They are believed to release two cardioexcitatory peptides (see Berlind and Cooke 1970; Sullivan 1979). Cell bodies (root cells) and neurosecretory terminals are also located more proximally on these roots. Distinct from the pericardial organs are the post-commisural organs, small neurohaemal organs attached to the tritocerebral commissure which are believed to secrete hormones affecting pigment movement in certain chromatophores (Fingerman 1966).

Fluorescence histochemistry (Elofsson et al. 1966; Goldstone and Cooke 1971) demonstrates positive staining for aminergic cell tracts and neuropile processes in the brain and eyestalk ganglia, however, there is little information concerning the association of biogenic amines with the X-organ/sinus gland complex, or the postcommissural organs. Andrew et al. (1978) reported the presence of several hundred small diameter cell bodies ($< 20 \mu m$) interspersed among the larger neurosecretory cells of the X-organ in crayfish. Ultrastructurally these cell bodies possess dense-cored vesicles (90 nm diameter) suggestive of amine-containing neurons. Furthermore, the Falck-Hillarp fluorescence technique for amines reveals the presence of one cell body exhibiting green fluorescence. No dense-cored vesicles, or fluorescence, are observed in the sinus gland indicating that the small diameter cell bodies do not project to this structure. Presumably if these several hundred cell bodies are aminergic, then they contain a non-fluorogenic amine (octopamine?).

Fluorescence histochemistry has revealed the presence of 5-HT and dopamine-containing terminals in the pericardial organs (Cooke and Goldstone 1970; Goldstone and Cooke 1971), and radioenzymatic assay has demonstrated the presence of octopamine (Evans et al. 1976a,b). All of these amines have been shown to by synthesized and released from the pericardial organs (review by Cooke and Sullivan 1982), as too have octopamine and 5-HT from areas more proximal, near the root cells (see Kravitz et al. 1980).

Berlind et al. (1970) examined the possible involvement of dopamine and 5-HT in release of the cardio-excitor from pericardial organs and concluded that there was no evidence for a role of these amines in the acute control of peptide hormone release. Since it is now known that octopamine is also present within the pericardial organs it would be of interest to repeat their experiments with this amine. However, their results with reserpine would argue against a role of any amine in the release of this hormone. It is clear that 5-HT, dopamine, and octopamine appear to be neurohormones released from these structures. Physiological effects of these neurohormones include decreased blood clotting time and modulation of neuromuscular transmission and muscle contraction (see Kravitz et al. 1980; Cooke and Sullivan 1982).

Fingerman and Rao (1970) found that injection of 5-HT into whole fiddler crabs or crayfish, induced dispersion of erythrophore pigments, while dopamine induced concentration of these pigments (Rao and Brannan 1978). Dispersion and aggregation of the pigment in the erythrophore are regulated by a red pigment-dispersing hormone, and a red pigment-concentrating hormone. Since neither 5-HT nor dopamine affected the erythrophores in isolated legs, these authors attributed the actions of the amines to a stimulation of release of the two peptide hormones. The receptors mediating these effects were further characterised by injecting agonists and antagonists of these amines into whole animals (Fingerman et al. 1981a). In a similar series of experiments, Fingerman et al. (1981b) associated norepinephrine with the control of melanin-dispersing hormone in the fiddler crab, and considered that histamine inhibited the release of this hormone (Hanumante and Fingerman 1982). It is unfortunate that all of the above experiments were carried out on whole animals, and as a result the site of action of these amines is not known. If, as suggested by the authors, the amines mimic the action of the natural transmitter used in the pathway of peptide-hormone release, then it should be feasable to incubate the neurosecretory system in these amines and stimulate or inhibit release of bioassayable hormone in vitro. At the present time we do not know at what position in the neural pathway these amines act, or indeed whether they are acting directly upon the neurosecretory terminals.

4 Conclusion

In both vertebrates and invertebrates there is a close anatomical association between aminergic cells and peptidergic neurosecretory cells. Neurosecretory cells and aminergic cells are grouped together within the central nervous system, and neurohaemal organs contain axons belonging to both classes of cells. Octopamine, dopamine, norepinephrine, 5-HT, and histamine have been identified within neurohaemal organs using radioenzymatic assays and fluorescence histochemistry.

The evidence in this review indicates that the close physiological relationship which is known to exist between aminergic and peptidergic neurosecretory cells in vertebrates is also found within invertebrates. It seems likely that multiple aminergic neuronal systems are involved in the control of secretion of a number of neurohormones. Octopamine acts as an excitatory transmitter stimulating the release of AKH's in locusts (Orchard and Loughton 1981a; Orchard 1982) and hyperglycaemic hormone in cockroaches (Downer et al. 1984). Octopamine also has a neurohormonal role in these insects. The action of ecdysteroid in stimulating the median neurosecretory cells in an assassin bug is mediated via aminergic interneurons with dopamine being capable of mimicking the effect of 20-hydroxyecdysone (Orchard et al. 1983b). Aminergic cells appear to make synaptic contact with peptidergic neurosecretory cells in beetles (Schooneveld 1974) and norepinephrine may be an inhibitory transmitter on some of the neurosecretory cells in the wax moth. In crustacea, the release of red pigment-dispersing hormone and red pigment-concentrating hormone appear to be under the excitatory control of 5-HT and dopamine respectively (Fingerman and Rao 1970; Rao and Brannon 1978). Norepinephrine apparently stimulates release of melanin-dispersing hormone, while histamine inhibits the release of this hormone (Fingerman et al. 1981b; Hanumante and Fingerman 1982). Octopamine, 5-HT, and dopamine all act as neurohormones within crustacea.

Acknowledgement. I am most grateful to Angela B. Lange for helpful suggestions and for the preparation of the manuscript.

References

Adler BA, Johnson MD, Lynch CO, Crowley WR (1983) Evidence that norepinephrine and epinephrine systems mediate the stimulatory effects of ovarian hormones on luteinizing hormone and luteinizing hormone-releasing hormone. Endocrinology 113:1431–1438

Ajika K (1979) Simultaneous localization of LHRH and catecholamines in rat hypothalamus. J Anat 128:331–347

Ajika K (1980) Relationship between catecholaminergic neurons and hypothalamic hormone-containing neurons in the hypothalamus. In: Martini L, Ganong F (eds) Frontiers in neuroendocrinology, vol 6. Raven, New York, pp 1–32

Andrew RD (1983) Neurosecretory pathways supplying the neurohemal organs in crustacea. In: Gupta AP (ed) Neurohemal organs of arthropods. Thomas, Springfield, pp 90–117

Andrew RD, Orchard I, Saleuddin ASM (1978) Structural re-evaluation of the neurosecretory system in the crayfish eyestalk. Cell Tissue Res 190:235–246

Arita J, Porter JC (1984) Relationship between dopamine release into hypophysial portal blood and prolactin release after morphine treatment in rats. Neuroendocrinology 38:62–67

Bailey BA, Martin RJ, Downer RGH (1983) Haemolymph octopamine levels during and following flight in the American cockroach, *Periplaneta americana* L. Can J Zool 62:19–22

Barker JL, Crayton JW, Nicoll RA (1971) Noradrenaline and acetylcholine responses of supraoptic neurosecretory cells. J Physiol (Lond) 218:19–32

Baumann E, Gersch M (1982) Purification and identification of neurohormone D, a heart accelerating peptide from the corpora cardiaca of the cockroach *Periplaneta americana*. Insect Biochem 12:7–14

Baumgarten HG, Bjorklund A, Holstein AF, Nobin A (1972) Organization and ultra-structural identification of catecholamine nerve terminals in the neuronal lobe and pars intermedia of the rat pituitary. Z Zellforsch Mikrosk Anat 126:483–517

Berlind A, Cooke IM (1970) Release of a neurosecretory hormone as peptide by electrical stimulation of crab pericardial organs. J Exp Biol 53:679–686

Berlind A, Cooke IM, Goldstone MW (1970) Do the monoamines in crab pericardial organs play a role in peptide neurosecretion? J Exp Biol 53:669–677

Bjorklund A (1968) Monoamine-containing fibres in the pituitary neuro-intermediate lobe of the pig and rat. Z Zellforsch Mikrosk Anat 89:573–589

Buonomo FC, Rabii J, Scanes CG (1981) Aminergic involvement in the control of luteinizing hormone secretion in domestic fowl. Gen Comp Endocrinol 45:162–166

Carlsen J, Herman WS, Christensen M, Josefsson L (1979) Characterisation of a second peptide with adipokinetic and red pigment-concentrating activity from the locust corpora cardiaca. Insect Biochem 9:497–501

Carlsson A, Falck B, Hillarp NA (1962) Cellular localization of brain monoamines. Acta Physiol Scand 56:1–28

Clemens JA, Roush ME, Fuller RW (1978) Evidence that serotonin neurons stimulate secretion of prolactin releasing factor. Life Sci 22:2209–2214

Cooke IM, Goldstone MW (1970) Fluorescence localization of monoamines in crab neurosecretory structures. J Exp Biol 53:651–668

Cooke IM, Sullivan RE (1982) Hormones and neurosecretion. In: Atwood HL, Sanderman DC (eds) The biology of crustacea, vol 3. Academic, New York, pp 205–290

Davenport AP, Evans PD (1984) Stress-induced changes in the octopamine levels of insect haemolymph. Insect Biochem 14:135–143

David J-C, Lafon-Cazal M (1979) Octopamine distribution in the *Locusta migratoria* nervous and nonnervous systems. Comp Biochem Physiol 64C:161–164

Downer RGH (1980) Short term trehalosemia by excitation in *Periplaneta americana*. J Insect Physiol 25:59–63

Downer RGH, Orr GL, Gole JWD, Orchard I (1984) The role of octopamine and cyclic AMP in regulating hormone release from corpora cardiaca of the american cockroach. J Insect Physiol 30:457–462

Dufy B, Vincent J-D, Fleury H, Du Pasquier P, Gourdji D, Tixier-Vidal A (1979) Dopamine inhibition of action potentials in a prolactin secreting cell line is modulated by oestrogen. Nature (Lond) 282:855–857

Dymond GR, Evans PD (1979) Biogenic amines in the nervous system of the cockroach, *Periplaneta americana*: association of octopamine with mushroom bodies and dorsal unpaired median (DUM) neurones. Insect Biochem 9:535–545

Elofsson R, Kauri T, Nielsen S-O, Stromberg J-O (1966) Localization of monoaminergic neurons in the central nervous system of *Astacus astacus* Linne (Crustacea). Z Zellforsch Mikrosk Anat 74:464–473

Evans PD (1978) Octopamine distribution in the insect nervous system. J Neurochem 30:1009–1013

Evans PD (1980) Biogenic amines in the insect nervous system. Adv Insect Physiol 15:317–474

Evans PD, Kravitz EA, Talamo BR (1976a) Octopamine release at two points along lobster nerve trunks. J Physiol (Lond) 262:71–89

Evans PD, Kravitz EA, Talamo BR, Wallace BG (1976b) The association of octopamine with specific neurones along lobster nerve trunks. J Physiol (Lond) 262:51–70

Fehrer SC, Silsby JL, El Halawani ME (1983) Serotonergic stimulation of prolactin release in the young turkey *(Meleagris gallopavo)*. Gen Comp Endocrinol 52:400–408

Fernlund P (1976) Structure of a light-adapting hormone from the shrimp, *Pandalus borealis*. Biochim Biophys Acta 439:17–25

Fernlund P, Josefsson L (1972) Crustacean color-change hormone: amino acid sequence and chemical synthesis. Science (Wash DC) 177:173–175

Fingerman M (1966) Neurosecretory control of pigmentary effectors in crustaceans. Am Zool 6:169–179

Fingerman M, Rao KR (1970) Action of biogenic amines on crustacean chromatophores III. Antagonism by lysergic acid diethylamide on the effect of serotonin and colour changes in the fiddler crab, *Uca pugilator*. Comp Gen Pharmacol 1:341–348

Fingerman M, Hanumante MM, Fingerman SW (1981a) The effects of biogenic amines on color changes of the fiddler crab, *Uca pugilator*: further evidence for roles of 5-hydroxytryptamine and dopamine as neurotransmitters triggering release of erythrophorotropic hormones. Comp Biochem Physiol 68C:205–211

Fingerman M, Hanumante MM, Fingerman SW, Reinschmidt DC (1981b) Effects of norepinephrine and norepinephrine agonists and antagonists on the melanophores of the fiddler crab *Uca pugilator*. J Crustacean Biol 1:16–27

Finlayson LH, Osborne MP (1975) Secretory activity of neurons and related electrical activity. Adv Comp Physiol Biochem 6:165–258

Foord SM, Peters JR, Dieguez C, Scanlon MF, Hall R (1983) Dopamine receptors on intact anterior pituitary cells in culture: functional association with the inhibition of prolactin and thyrotropin. Endocrinology 112:1567–1577

Gabe M (1966) "Neurosecretion". Int Ser Monog Biol, vol 28. Pergamon, New York

Gersch M (1972) Experimentelle Untersuchungen zum Freisetzungsmechanismus von Neurohormonen nach elektrischer Reizung der Corpora cardiaca von *Periplaneta americana* in vitro. J Insect Physiol 18:2425–2439

Gersch M, Fischer F, Unger H, Kabitza W (1961) Vorkommen von Seratonin im Nervensystem von *Periplaneta americana* L. (Insecta). Z Naturforsch Mikrosk Anat 16B:351–352

Gersch M, Hentschel E, Ude J (1974) Aminergic Substanzen in lateralen Herznerven und im stomatogastrischen Nervensystem der Schabe *Blaberus craniifer* burm. Zool Jahrb Abt Allg Zool Physiol Tiere 78:1–15

Goldstone M, Cooke I (1971) Histochemical localization of monoamines in the crab central nervous system. Z Zellforsch Mikrosk Anat 116:7–19

Gole JWD, Downer RGH (1979) Elevation of adenosine 3′,5′-monophosphate by octopamine in fat body of the American cockroach *Periplaneta americana* L. Comp Biochem Physiol 64C: 223–226

Goosey MW, Candy DJ (1980) The D-octopamine content of the haemolymph of the locust, *Schistocerca americana gregaria* and its elevation during flight. Insect Biochem 10:393–397

Goosey MW, Candy DJ (1982) The release and removal of octopamine by tissues of the locust *Schistocerca americana gregaria*. Insect Biochem 12:681–685

Hanstrom B (1953) Neurosecretory pathways in the head of crustaceans, insects and vertebrates. Nature (Lond) 171:72–73

Hanumante MM, Fingerman M (1982) Inhibitory effect of histamine on the release of melanin-dispersing hormone in the fiddler crab, *Uca pugilator*. Biol Bull 162:256–272

Hoyle G (1975) Evidence that insect dorsal unpaired median (DUM) neurones are octopaminergic. J Exp Zool 193:425–431

Hoyle G, Colquhoun W, Williams M (1980) Fine structure of an octopaminergic neuron and its terminals. J Neurobiol 11:103–126

Jones MT, Hillhouse EW, Burden J (1976) Effect of various putative neurotransmitters on the secretion of corticotropin-releasing hormone from the rat hypothalamus in vitro – a model of the neurotransmitters involved. J Endocrinol 69:1–10

Kakucska I, Makara GB (1983) Various putative neurotransmitters affect growth hormone (GH) release in rats with anterolateral hypothalamic deafferentation of the medial basal hypothalamus: evidence for mediation by a GH-releasing factor. Endocrinology 113:318–323

Kleinholz LH (1976) Crustacean neurosecretory hormones and physiological specificity. Am Zool 16:151–166

Klemm N (1983) Monoamine-containing neurons and their projections in the brain (supraoesophageal ganglion) of cockroaches. Cell Tissue Res 229:379–402

Klemm N, Axelsson S (1973) Determination of dopamine, noradrenaline and 5-hydroxytryptamine in the brain of the desert locust, *Schistocerca gregaria* Forsk. (Insecta, Orthoptera). Brain Res 57:289–298

Klemm N, Falck B (1978) Monoamines in the pars intercerebralis-corpus cardiacum complex of locusts. Gen Comp Endocrinol 34:180–192

Kravitz EA, Glusman S, Harris-Warrick RM, Livingstone MS, Schwarz T, Goy MF (1980) Amines and a peptide as neurohormones in lobsters: action on neuromuscular preparations and preliminary behavioural studies. J Exp Biol 89:159–175

Kriger FL (1981) Neuroendocrine regulation of ovulation in an insect, *Rhodnius prolixus* Stal. Ph.D. Thesis, York Univ, Toronto, Canada

Krogh IM, Normann TC (1977) The corpus cardiacum neurosecretory cells of *Schistocerca gregaria*. Electron microscopy of resting and secreting cells. Acta Zool (Stockh) 58:69–78

Krulich L (1979) Central neurotransmitters and the secretion of prolactin, GH, LH and TSH. Annu Rev Neurosci 41:603–615

Krulich L, Giachetti A, Marchlewska-Koj A, Hefco E, Jameson HE (1977) On the role of the central noradrenergic and dopaminergic systems in the regulation of TSH secretion in the rat. Endocrinology 100:496–505

Lafon-Cazal M (1981) Monoamines in the corpora cardiaca of locusts. Adv Physiol Sci 22:255–267

Lafon-Cazal M, Arluison M (1976) Localization of monoamines in the corpora cardiaca and the hypocerebral ganglion of locusts. Cell Tissue Res 172:517–527

Livingstone MS, Schaeffer SF, Kravitz EA (1981) Biochemistry and ultrastructure of serotonergic nerve endings in the lobster: serotonin and octopamine are contained in different nerve endings. J Neurobiol 12:27–54

Masner P, Huot L, Corrivault G-W, Prudhomme JC (1970) Effect of reserpine on the function of the gonads and its neuroendocrine regulation in tenebrionid beetles. J Insect Physiol 16:2327–2344

McCann SM (1980) Control of anterior pituitary hormone release by brain peptides. Neuroendocrinology 31:355–363

McCann SM, Kalra PS, Donoso AO, Bishop W, Schneider HPG, Fawcett CP, Krulich L (1972) The role of monoamines in the control of gonado-tropin and prolactin secretion. In: Brain-endocrine interaction. Median eminence: structure and function. Int Symp Munich 1971. Karger, Basel, pp 224–235

McCann SM, Lumpkin MD, Mizunuma H, Khorram O, Ottlecz A, Samson WK (1984) Peptidergic and dopaminergic control of prolactin release. Trends Neurosci 7:127–131

McNeil TH, Sladek JR (1977) Correlative fluorescence-immunocytochemical localization of monoamines and neurophysin, vasopressin and gonadotropin-releasing hormone in the rat and monkey hypothalamus. Soc Neurosci Abstr 3:351

Meyer JS, McElroy JF, Yehuda R, Miller J (1984) Serotonergic stimulation of pituitary-adrenocortical activity in rats: evidence for multiple sites of action. Life Sci 34:1891–1898

Migliori-Natalizi G, Pansa MC, D'Ajello V, Casaglia O, Bettini S, Frontali N (1970) Physiologically active factors from corpora cardiaca of *Periplaneta americana*. J Insect Physiol 16:1827–1836

Nakai Y, Shioda S, Ochiai H, Kudo J, Hashimoto A (1983) Ultrastructural relationship between monoamine- and TRH-containing axons in the rat median eminence as revealed by combined autoradiography and immunocytochemistry in the same tissue section. Cell Tissue Res 230:1–14

Negro-Vilar A, Ojeda SR, McCann SM (1979) Catecholaminergic modulation of luteinizing hormone-releasing hormone release by median eminence terminals in vitro. Endocrinology 104:1749–1757

Oksche A (1976) The neuroanatomical basis of comparative neuroendocrinology. Gen Comp Endocrinology 29:225–239

Orchard I (1982) Octopamine in insects: neurotransmitter, neurohormone, and neuromodulator. Can J Zool 60:659–669

Orchard I (1983) Neurosecretion: morphology and physiology. In: Downer RGH, Laufer H (eds) Insect endocrinology. Liss, New York, pp 13–38

Orchard I (1984) The role of biogenic amines in the regulation of peptidergic neurosecretory cells. In: Borkovec EB, Kelly TJ (eds) Insect neurochemistry and neurophysiology. Plenum, New York

Orchard I, Lange AB (1983a) Release of identified adipokinetic hormones during flight and following neural stimulation in *Locusta migratoria*. J Insect Physiol 29:425–429

Orchard I, Lange AB (1983b) The hormonal control of haemolymph lipid during flight in *Locusta migratoria*. J Insect Physiol 29:639–642

Orchard I, Loughton BG (1981a) Is octopamine a transmitter mediating hormone release in insects? J Neurobiol 12:143–153

Orchard I, Loughton BG (1981b) The neural control of release of hyperlipaemic hormone from the corpus cardiacum of *Locusta migratoria*. Comp Biochem Physiol 68A:25–30

Orchard I, Loughton BG, Webb RA (1981) Octopamine and short-term hyperlipaemia in the locust. Gen Comp Endocrinol 45:175–180

Orchard I, Carlisle JC, Loughton BG, Gole JWD, Downer RGH (1982) In vitro studies on the effect of octopamine on locust fat body. Gen Comp Endocrinol 98:7–13

Orchard I, Gole JWD, Downer RGH (1983a) Pharmacology of aminergic receptors mediating an elevation in cyclic AMP and release of hormone from locust neurosecretory cells. Brain Res 288:349–353

Orchard I, Ruegg RP, Davey KG (1983b) The role of central aminergic neurons in the action of 20-hydroxyecdysone on neurosecretory cells of *Rhodnius prolixus*. J Insect Physiol 29:387–391

Orchard I, Loughton BG, Gole JWD, Downer RGH (1983c) Synaptic transmission elevates adenosine 3′,5′-monophosphate (cyclic AMP) in locust neurosecretory cells. Brain Res 258:152–155

O'Shea M, Witten J, Schaffer M (1984) Isolation and characterization of two myoactive neuropeptides: further evidence of an invertebrate peptide family. J Neurosci 4:521–529

Rademakers LHPM (1977a) Effects of isolation and transplantation of the corpus cardiacum on hormone release from its glandular cells after flight in *Locusta migratoria*. Cell Tissue Res 184: 213–224

Rademakers LHPM (1977b) Identification of a secretomotor centre in the brain of Locusta migratoria, controlling the secretory activity of the adipokinetic hormone producing cells of the corpus cardiacum. Cell Tissue Res 184:381–395

Rademakers LHPM, Beenakkers AMT (1977) Changes in the secretory activity of the glandular lobe of the corpus cardiacum of *Locusta migratoria* induced by flight. Cell Tissue Res 180:155–171

Rao KR, Brannan AC (1978) Color changes induced by peptide derivatives of lysergic acid in the fiddler crab, *Uca panacea*. Comp Biochem Physiol 59C:97–100

Ruegg RP, Kriger FL, Davey KG, Steel CGH (1981) Ovarian ecdysone elicits release of a myotropic ovulation hormone in *Rhodnius* (Insecta: Hemiptera). Int J Invertebr Reprod 3:357–361

Ruegg RP, Orchard I, Davey KG (1982) 20-Hydroxyecdysone as a modulator of electrical activity in neurosecretory cells of *Rhodnius prolixus*. J Insect Physiol 28:243–248

Scharrer B, Scharrer E (1944) Neurosecretion VI. A comparison between the intercerebralis cardiacum-allata system of insects and the hypothalamo-hypophysial system of the vertebrates. Biol Bull 87:242–251

Schneider HPG, McCann SM (1970) Mono- and indolamines and control of LH secretion. Endocrinology 86:1127–1133

Schooneveld H (1974) Ultrastructure of the neurosecretory system of the Colorado potato beetle, *Leptinotarsa decemlineata* (Say) II. Pathways of axonal secretion, transport and innervation of neurosecretory cells. Cell Tissue Res 154:289–301

Stone JV, Mordue W, Batley KE, Morris HR (1976) Structure of locust adipokinetic hormone, a neurohormone that regulates lipid utilization during flight. Nature (Lond) 263:207–211

Sullivan RE (1979) A proctolin-like peptide in crab pericardial organs. J Exp Zool 210:543–552

Tribollet E, Clarke G, Dreifuss JJ, Lincoln DW (1978) The role of central adrenergic receptors in the reflex release of oxytocin. Brain Res 142:69–84

Warton S (1981) Effect of disulfiram on the ultrastructure of the peptidergic and aminergic cells in the pars intercerebralis of *Galleria mellonella* (Lepidoptera). Cell Tissue Res 215:417–424

Warton S, Dutkowski AB (1977) Ultrastructure of the neurosecretory cells of the pars intercerebralis of *Galleria mellonella* (Lepidoptera) after noradrenaline administration. Gen Comp Endocrinol 33:179–186

Warton S, Dutkowski AB (1978) Ultrastructural analysis of the action of reserpine on the brain neuroendocrine system of the waxmoth, *Galleria mellonella* L., Lepidoptera. Cell Tissue Res 192:143–155

Weiner RI, Ganong WF (1978) Role of brain monoamines and histamine in regulation of anterior pituitary secretion. Physiol Rev 58:905–976

Yagi K, Iwasaki S (1977) Electrophysiology of the neurosecretory cell. Int Rev Cytol 48:141–186

Normal and Abnormal Animal Behaviour: Importance of Catecholamine Release by Nerve Impulses for the Maintenance of Normal Behaviour

S. AHLENIUS and T. ARCHER [1]

1 Introduction

The availability of a wide range of chemical tools that affect particular aspects of brain neurotransmission has greatly improved our possibilities for studying brain-behaviour relationships. Much attention has been focussed upon the particular functions modulated by the catecholamines, dopamine (DA) and noradrenaline (NA). This is understandable, since the physiology of central and peripheral catecholamine pathways has been extensively investigated. Presently, a great number of pharmacological tools interfering with particular aspects of the neurotransmission, from synthesis and uptake to release, receptor interactions, and inactivation are available (for rev see Moore and Bloom 1978, 1979). In this article, certain results that demonstrate the importance of catecholamine release by nerve impulses for the maintenance of normal behaviour will be reviewed. Against this background, the functional importance of DA and NA will be discussed, and finally, some recent experiments from our laboratory on localization of functions within the brain by means of intracerebral application of DA and NA will be described.

All experiments were performed on mice or rats, although where possible reference will be made to data from other species. Spontaneous behavior of the animals was monitored in photocell-equipped activity cages. Various conditioning procedures have been used to study the acquisition and performance of learned behaviours. These will be described in their turn.

2 A Pharmacological Model for Separating Effects due to Nerve-Impulse-Regulated Receptor Activation from Effects due to Pharmacological Activation Independent of the Nerve-Impulse Flow

It has been shown that an extragranular accumulation of catecholamines in the cytosol, as induced e.g. by an inhibitor of monoamine oxidase, inhibits release by nerve impulses (Malmfors 1965; Almgren and Lundborg 1971; see Smith and Winkler 1972). Thus, the neuronal accumulation of catecholamines by L-DOPA administration in animals pretreated with reserpine or tetrabenazine, which both inhibits the granular uptake-storage mechanism of catecholamine neurons (see Carlsson 1965), will not cause any

1 Astra Läkemedel AB, Research and Development Laboratories, Pharmacology,
  151 85 Södertälje, Sweden

Neurobiology
(ed. by R. Gilles and J. Balthazart)
© Springer-Verlag Berlin Heidelberg 1985

release onto pre- or postsynaptic receptors, except by diffusion. In contrast, the administration of L-DOPA to animals pretreated with the inhibitor of catecholamine syntheses, α-methyl-p-tyrosine (α-MT) (see Moore and Dominic 1971), will cause catecholamine refillment of empty granules, and provide the prerequisites for a physiological release (Corrodi et al. 1966; Corrodi and Fuxe 1967; Ahlenius et al. 1973). It is important to note that what has been mentioned above only applies to "low" doses of L-DOPA (see Fig. 1). With increasing dose there will be effects (see below) due to a pharmacologically induced diffusion onto receptors.

A series of experiments will be described wherein the behavioural consequences of these various manipulations have been investigated. The general procedure has been to observe the effects of various doses of L-DOPA in normal animals, and in animals pretreated with α-MT or reserpine as shown in Fig. 1. The "low" dose, species- and parameter-dependent, was defined in biochemical experiments as the dose required to refill α-MT-depleted catecholamine neurons (Ahlenius et al. 1973; Corrodi et al. 1966; Corrodi and Fuxe 1967). A "high" dose of L-DOPA, producing effects due to diffusion as evidenced by behavioural activation in reserpine-treated animals, was usually about ten times higher. This means, in the rat, doses in the range of 10-100 mg kg^{-1} IP of L-DOPA, after inhibition of peripheral aromatic amino acid decarboxylase by means of benserazide or carbidopa.

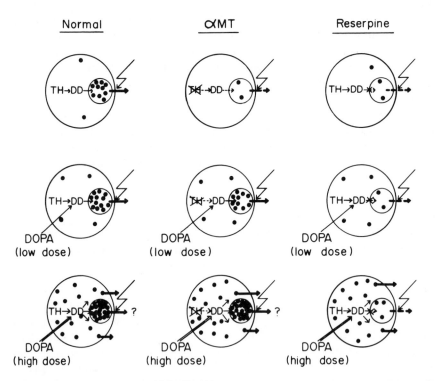

Fig. 1. Availability of catecholamines for release by nerve impulses after L-DOPA administration in *α-MT* or *reserpine* pretreated animals. *TH* tyrosine hydroxylase; *DD* L-DOPA decarboxylase. For details see text. (Courtesy of Nils-Erik Andén)

3 Behavioural Effects due to Pharmacologically Induced Release, or Effects due to Activation of Catecholamine Receptors by Directly Acting Agonists

It is well known that the akinesia and hypomotility induced by reserpine in mice or rats can be antagonized by the administration of L-DOPA (e.g. Carlsson et al. 1957; Smith and Dews 1962) or by apomorphine (e.g. Andén et al. 1973), which directly activates central DA receptors (Andén et al. 1967; Ernst 1967). Furthermore, the suppression of a conditioned avoidance response (CAR), induced by reserpine, can be antagonized by L-DOPA administration (see Seiden et al. 1976). Also, L-DOPA or apomorphine stimulate motor activity in normal animals (e.g. Maj et al. 1972). However, as noted earlier (Vander Wende and Spoerlein 1962) the animals thus treated do not always display the normal range of behaviour.

The effects obtained by L-DOPA after reserpine should be due to a pharmacological release (see Fig. 1), and in order to investigate the quality of behavioural change thus produced, rats or mice were trained to perform a visual successive discrimination or a spatial discrimination in the conventional two-way avoidance shuttle-box (Ahlenius 1974a). Thus, in order to avoid shock the animals had not only to cross to the safe compartment, but also to pass into this compartment via one of two passages, guided by visual or spatial cues. Using this procedure it was shown that, although the CAR performance suppressed by reserpine or tetrabenazine could be restored, this occurred only after high doses of L-DOPA and the animals performed at chance level on the discrimination (Ahlenius 1974b,c). Administration of high doses of L-DOPA or apomorphine to normal animals also appears to produce an abnormal behaviour as characterized in this procedure (Ahlenius and Engel 1976), i.e. loss of discriminative performance.

This abnormal behaviour induced by L-DOPA has been shown to be blocked by the DA receptor blocking agents, pimozide or haloperidol, but not by the NA receptor blocking agent phenoxybenzamine (Ahlenius and Engel 1976). Reserpine, tetrabenazine or α-MT by themselves did not affect discriminative performance (see below).

4 Evidence that Normal Motor Activity and Discriminative Performance is Dependent on Physiological Catecholamine Release

L-DOPA causes a dose-dependent antagonism of locomotor activity suppressed by α-MT (see Fig. 2). There was a significant reversal of the suppression by both low ($<$ 50 mg kg^{-1}) and high doses ($>$ 100 mg kg^{-1}) of L-DOPA (see Ahlenius 1976). The evidence that L-DOPA-induced reversal by low doses may differ qualitatively comes from experiments in the CAR situation where a visual or spatial discrimination is required in order to avoid shock. Using this procedure it was shown that the α-MT-induced suppression of CAR performance in rats or mice was restored by both low and high doses of L-DOPA, however, the discriminative performance remains unaffected at low doses only (Ahlenius 1974b,c). Thus, it appears that a granular uptake and physiological release of DA is required for normal behaviour and, although the animals

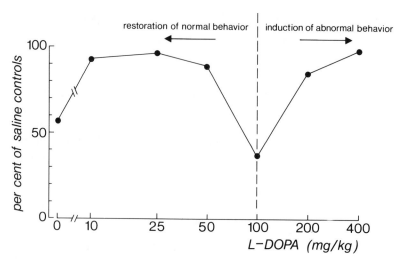

Fig. 2. Effects of L-DOPA on spontaneous locomotor activity in mice pretreated with α-MT. (After Ahlenius et al. 1973; Ahlenius 1976)

are behaviourally restored by high doses, this activation can be characterized as abnormal when appropriately studied. The abnormal behaviour is produced by high doses of L-DOPA, irrespective of pretreatment (cf. Fig. 1).

The inhibitory effects of autoreceptor activation are clearly illustrated in Fig. 2. By increasing the dose of L-DOPA to about 100 mg kg^{-1}, the overflow of catecholamines, primarily DA, formed from L-DOPA, probably begins. This overflow will activate initially autoreceptors on the presynaptic neuron (Carlsson 1975). This activation of autoreceptors will produce sedative effects.

5 Additional Evidence for the Functional Importance of Nerve-Impulse-Regulated Release by use of Different Doses of d-Amphetamine

d-Amphetamine is generally considered to increase the nerve-impulse-dependent release of newly synthesized catecholamines (Obianwu 1969a,b: Löffelholz and Muscholl 1970; von Voigtlander and Moore 1973). With increasing doses, however, there is also a nerve-impulse independent displacement of granularily stored catecholamines (Kehr 1976). Considering these facts, it is interesting to note that at 2 mg kg^{-1} there is an increase in general motility in the rat, and an intact ability to make a visual discrimination. By increasing the dose to 4 mg kg^{-1}, d-amphetamine produces a near identical increase in motility but at this dose discriminative behaviour is apparently lost (Ahlenius et al.

→

Fig. 3. Blockade of rearing and total activity counts induced by a 2 mg kg^{-1} dose of amphetamine, but not that induced by the 1, 4, or 8 mg kg^{-1} doses of amphetamine, following pretreatment with DSP4 (50 mg kg^{-1}, IP) 2 weeks previously. DSP4-treated and control rats were administered amphetamine or saline 60 min after placement in the test boxes wherein the rearing, locomotion and total activity components of behaviour were measured by an automated device

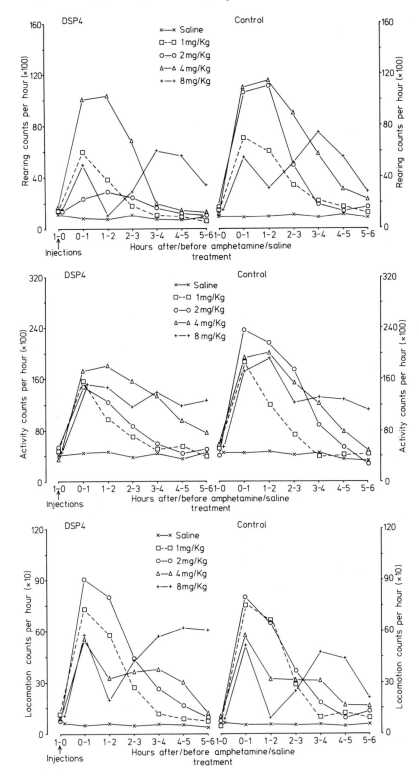

Fig. 3

1975). Similar behavioural effects are obtained when the animals have been trained to perform a temporal discrimination using a DRL schedule of reinforcement (Differential reinforcement of Low Rates of Responding). Using this behavioural situation, it has been shown that low doses of d-amphetamine produce an increase in response rate, with the temporal patterning of responding intact. In analogy with results obtained in the CAR-discrimination procedure described above a high dose of d-amphetamine also increase the response rate, but the temporal discrimination is not possible (Ahlenius 1976; Ahlenius and Engel 1972).

Additional support for a qualitative difference in the effects obtained by low and high doses of d-amphetamine-induced activity was measured in NA-depeleted rats. Thus, the hyperactivity induced by the 2 mg kg^{-1} dose of d-amphetamine only was antagonized by DSP4 pretreatment (see Fig. 3).

6 Attentional Deficits as a Result of Central Noradrenaline Depletion

N-(2-chloroethyl)-N-ethyl-2-bromobenzylamine(DSP4) is a relatively selective depletor of NA in the cortex, hippocampus, cerebellum, and spinal cord of rat and mouse CNS (less than 10% of control values remain after two weeks). 5-hydroxytryptamine and DA are only slightly affected or not at all (Archer et al. 1984; Jaim-Etcheverry and Zieher 1980; Jonsson et al. 1981; Ross 1976). DSP4-treated rats demonstrate considerable and consistent two-way active avoidance acquisition deficits and these impairments are reliably blocked by pretreatment with the selective NA uptake inhibitor, desipramine (Archer 1982; Archer et al. 1982; Ögren et al. 1980). In the typical two-way avoidance task rats are given trials consisting of 10-s tone (1,000 Hz) and 5-s scrambled shock (1.0 mA) presentations with a 40-s intertrial interval. Avoidance responses terminate the tone signal whereas escape responses terminate the signal + shock stimulus compound. Figure 4 demonstrates a typical experiment in which DSP4-treated rats showed a clear and consistent two-way active avoidance acquisition deficit. The two-way avoidance impairment has been reliably produced under a variety of different parameters. DSP4-induced two-way avoidance lesions confirm that of Crow et al. (1977) who inflicted electrolytic lesions in the dorsal pontine tegmental area.

Latent inhibition, the "Lubow effect" (Lubow 1965; Lubow and Moore 1959), may be useful for studying selective attentional processes in conditioning. As a result

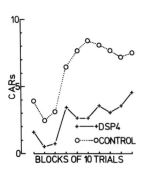

Fig. 4. The effect of DSP4 treatment upon two-way active avoidance acquisition by rats. DSP4-treated and control rats were given a single 100-trial session. The DSP4-treated rats performed significantly fewer Conditioned Avoidance Responses (CAR's) from the fourth block of 10 trials onwards. (Tukey's HSD test)

of latent inhibition, the non-reinforced preexposure of rats to the conditioned stimulus (CS), subsequent conditioning to the CS is retarded. Since much taste-aversion conditioning research has been directed toward the role of contextual cues in taste-aversion learning (cf. Archer et al. 1985), several experiments to study the interaction of taste

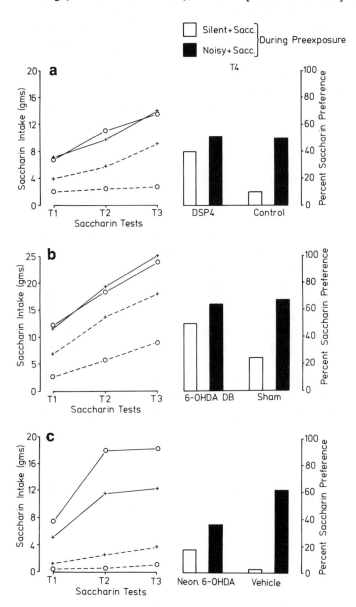

Fig. 5a–c. Effect of noradrenaline depletion upon latent inhibition following preexposure to either the saccharin stimulus (silent + sacc) by itself, or the saccharin plus noisy bottle stimulus compound (noisy + sacc). Noradrenaline was depleted either via *DSP4* (a), or 6-hydroxydopamine into the dorsal bundle, 10 μg side^{-1} bilaterally (b), or intraperitoneal 6-hydroxydopamine neonatally on days 1, 3, 5, 7, and 9 after birth (c). (Mohammed et al., unpublished)

(saccharin) and contextual stimulus preexposure and subsequent taste aversion conditioning in NA-depleted and control rats have been performed (e.g. Archer et al. 1983). When the contextual conditions were arranged so that there was a contextual "mismatch" from the saccharin preexposure to the saccharin-aversion conditioning phase, the NA-depleted rats showed some considerable enhancement of latent inhibition (see Fig. 5). The NA-depleted and control rats, preexposured to either saccharin alone or together with the noisy bottle context demonstrated an equivalent degree of latent inhibition to the compound (saccharin plus context). However, the NA-depleted animals showed much more latent inhibition although saccharin alone was presented, i.e. they failed to attend adequately to the contextual variable. These and other findings seem to confirm an important role of the locus coeruleus NA system in attentional processes (e.g. Mason 1981; McEntee and Mair 1978, 1980).

7 Failure to Initiate Behaviour due to Blockade of Central Dopamine Neurotransmission

There is strong evidence that the suppression of behaviour due to catecholamine depletion or receptor blockade does not interfere with associative brain mechanisms like learning and memory (see Beninger 1983). The administration of α-MT during acquisition of a CAR, in mice, suppressed performance during drug administration, but did not delay final level of performance when tested on saline (Fig. 6 and Ahlenius 1973). Similar results have been obtained in experiments using chlorpromazine or haloperidol (Fibiger et al. 1975; Posluns 1962; Stolerman 1971). The phenomenon of "latent learning" provides a convenient procedure to separate effects on performance from effects on associative brains mechanisms. Briefly, an animal that e.g. has been preexposed to a maze, is more efficient in finding food in the same apparatus some time later, as compared to naive animals not preexposed to the maze. An animal administered haloperidol during preexposure, in a dose sufficient to suppress the exploratory activity, displays

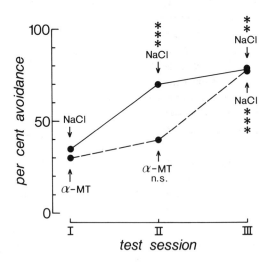

Fig. 6. Effects of α-MT on the acquisition of a conditioned avoidance response in mice. The animals were administered α-MT, 200 mg kg^{-1} SC, or physiological saline, 6 h before each of 3 weekly test sessions (*I–III*), as indicated in the Fig. Shown are the medians based on 10–24 observations. Progress in acquisition in *II* as compared to *I*, and in *III* as compared to *II* test session was statistically evaluated by means of Wilcoxon matched-pairs signed-ranks test. For further details see Ahlenius (1973). n.s. $P > 0.05$; **$P < 0.02$; ***$P < 0.01$

"latent learning" equal to saline treated controls (Ahlenius et al. 1977). The "latent learning" procedure described above has also been used to investigate the quality of behavioural change induced by low doses of apomorphine, preferentially activating dopaminergic autoreceptors (Strömbom 1976). The results show that apomorphine, suppresses exploratory locomotor activity, but when later trained to find food in the maze, the animals perform as well as saline-treated controls (Ahlenius et al. 1977). However, by increasing the dose of apomorphine, central postsynaptic DA receptors will be activated in an uncontrolled, not feed-back regulated, manner. Interestingly, these animals, which do not markedly differ in exploratory activity during preexposure, do not perform better than naive animals when later trained in the maze. Thus, we have further evidence that an uncontrolled activation of central catecholamine receptors disturbs associative brain mechanisms and can produce abnormal behaviour.

Spontaneous locomotor activity and conditioned behaviour are suppressed by catecholamine receptor blockers, with preference for DA receptors, like pimozide, and a selective blocker of central NA receptors, like phenoxybenzamine is ineffective (Ahlenius and Engel 1977; see Beninger 1983). Furthermore, using the model discussed above to refill α-MT-depleted catecholamine stores by administration of low doses of L-DOPA, shows that normal locomotor behaviour can be restored also when an inhibitor of DA-β-hydroxylase, FLA-63, has been added (Ahlenius 1976).

It is obvious that the akinesia produced by haloperidol or α-MT in animal experiments – a failure to initiate motor behavioural acts – is similar to the akinesia seen in Parkinson's disease. Furthermore (1) in both cases the motor disturbances is associated with a deficiency in brain DA neurotransmission and is consequently antagonized by administration of the DA precursor L-DOPA; (2) in either case the akinesia is at least partially antagonized by the administration of anticholinergics (see e.g. Wauquier et al. 1975); (3) the akinesia can also be overcome by strong sensory stimulation as shown in the human (e.g. Schwab and Zeiper 1965) and as further described in animal experiments (Marshall et al. 1976).

8 Some Function Effects of Local Applications of Drugs Interfering with Catecholamine Neurotransmission

Brain DA is primarily localized to the neostriatum and in limbic forebrain areas like the nucleus accumbens and the tuberculum olfactorium. These areas are innervated by a more or less continuous band of cell groups in the mesencephalon: The neostriatum being innervated by cells in the substantia nigra, pars compacta (nigrostriatal pathway), and limbic forebrain areas by cells in the ventral tegmental area, medial to the substantia nigra, but also from a smaller group of DA cells lateral and caudal to the substantia nigra (mesolimbic pathway) (see Beckstead et al. 1979). Based on clinical and laboratory observations it is generally considered that the nigrostriatal pathway is important for extrapyramidal motor functions, whereas the mesolimbic pathway is of importance for functions like motivation and drive (see Mogenson et al. 1980; Denny-Brown and Yanagisawa 1976).

The local application of DA to the neostriatum of the rat produces stereotypies, like sniffing and gnawing, whereas local application to the nucleus accumbens produces forward locomotion (Fog and Pakkenberg 1971; Costall and Naylor 1975; Jackson et al. 1975; Pijnenburg and van Rossum 1973). However, in most of these experiments the animals have been pretreated with reserpine and/or an inhibitor of monoamine oxidase. As discussed above, these pretreatments may interfere with the normal nerve-impulse induced catecholamine release and a normal behaviour is probably not obtained after such pretreatments (Wachtel et al. 1979).

In a recent series of experiments we have investigated the effects of local application of DA and NA to the neostriatum and the nucleus accumbens of normal rats. Guide cannulas were placed stereotaxically on the rat skull under general anesthesia. When the animals had recovered from the operation (48 h), injections were made in awake, unrestrained animals and their behaviour was observed in a 0.5 m^2 arena equipped with photocells to register movements. The most prominent effect of DA, when applied to the nucleus accumbens, is a suppression of the locomotor activity (Fig. 7) (Svensson and Ahlenius 1982, 1983). This inhibition of locomotion is probably due to activation of dopaminergic autoreceptors. This interpretation is supported by results obtained with the putative dopaminergic autoreceptor agonist (−)3-(3-hydroxyphenyl)-N-n-propylpiperidine (3-PPP) (Hjorth et al. 1983). Local application of (−) 3-PPP to the nucleus accumbens has been shown to suppress locomotor activity, and this effect can be antagonized by haloperidol pretreatment (Ahlenius et al. 1984). Furthermore, intra-accumbens application of B-HT 920, which, like (−) 3-PPP has been shown to stimulate

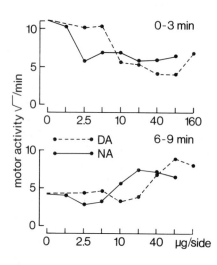

Fig. 7. Effects of local application of *DA* or *l-NA* into the rat nucleus accumbens on locomotor activity. Bilateral injections were made 8 min before the rat was placed in the activity meter (Svensson and Ahlenius 1982)

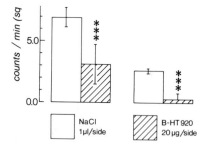

Fig. 8. Effects of local application of *B-HT 920* into the rat nucleus accumbens on locomotor activity. Bilateral injections were made 5 min before the animals were placed in the activity meter. Shown are the means ± S.D. based on the performance of four rats given physiological saline or B-HT 920. Half of the animals received saline first and the remaining 2 animals were given B-HT 920 first (Ahlenius and Hillegaart, unpublished). *** $P < 0.001$ (paired t-test)

dopaminergic autoreceptors (Andén et al. 1982) also suppressed spontaneous loco-motor activity (Fig. 8). By increasing the dose at DA, locally applied to the nucleus ac-cumbens, a stimulation of locomotor activity was obtained in agreement with a number of previous reports (see above). This hyperactivity is probably due to an uncontrolled activation of postsynaptic DA receptors.

In parallel experiments 1-NA was applied to the nucleus accumbens. Surprisingly, the efficacy of 1-NA was not only the same, but it was also about four times as potent as DA. This applies both to the locomotor suppressant and stimulatory effects, as can be seen in Fig. 7. Results obtained after systemic administration of NA antagonists or agonists do not suggest that central NA influences locomotor activity to any greater extent (see above). Unspecific effects do not appear to be likely, however, since d-NA was far less active than 1-NA (Svensson and Ahlenius 1983). An interesting possibility is an action by 1-NA on NA sensitive autoreceptors on the DA neurons. This possibility receives some support from recent electrophysiological experiments, where is has been shown that iontophoretic application of NA onto DA cell bodies inhibits neuronal firing (Wang and White 1984).

In control experiments DA and NA were locally applied to the neostriatum. How-ever, in this area there were no, or only small effects on the locomotor activity. There was a slight increase in the locomotor activity by DA, and suppression by 1-NA. In both cases the doses required to produce these effects were about 10 times higher than those needed to produce an effect in the nucleus accumbens.

9 Clinical Implications

There are two major clinical syndromes strongly associated with brain DA; Parkinson's disease and schizophrenia. The development of Parkinson's disease has been shown to be due to a degeneration of nigrostriatal DA neurons (see Carlsson 1972). The DA pre-cursor L-DOPA has logically become the most important drug therapy. However, there has been much research aimed at finding directly acting DA agonists, like apomorphine, that would be clinically useful. Apomorphine itself possesses antiparkinson properties but is not clinically useful due to unfavorable pharmacokinetic properties, possible tolerance development and side effects (see Cotzias et al. 1976). An important conclu-sion from the present work is that L-DOPA uptake in remaining neurons, and feedback controlled release, is necessary for a complete restoration of normal function and that directly acting DA agonists by themselves will be less effective than L-DOPA as anti-parkinson drugs. Against this background the intrastriatal neuronal graft technique, demonstrated in rats, is particularily interesting, since this would be expected not only to markedly enhance the efficacy of L-DOPA therapy (see Björklund and Stenevi 1984), but also the quality of the response.

The association between DA and schizophrenia is only indirect. However, circum-stantial evidence from the clinic and the laboratory have allowed the formulation of a DA hypothesis of schizophrenia (see Carlsson 1978). E.g. all known antipsychotic drugs do inhibit central DA neurotransmission. Not surprisingly, extrapyramidal motor dis-turbance as in Parkinson's disease is a common side effect. However, these side effects can be overcome by concomitant administration of anticholinergic drugs without loss of clinical response (see Sovner and DiMascio 1978). In animal experiments it has been shown that anticholinergic agents can antagonize the antipsychotic-induced increase in DA turnover in the neostriatum, but not in limbic forebrain dopaminergic areas (Andén 1972), providing support for a functional separation between DA mechanisms of the neostriatum and the limbic forebrain. Thus, according to the DA hypothesis of schizophrenia, the disease is associated with an increase in DA release and receptor activation in the limbic forebrain. It is interesting to note that an overdose of d-amphetamine in the human may produce a behavioural syndrome indistinguishable from acute schizophrenia (see Snyder et al. 1974). By use of a test situation requiring a visual discrimination it is possible to demonstrate abnormal behaviour after high doses of 1-DOPA or d-amphetamine as described above, and the behaviour can be normalized by administration of antipsychotics (Ahlenius and Engel 1976). Thus, the abnormal animal behaviour produced by uncontrolled activation of DA receptors as shown here, possibly in limbic forebrain areas, may be useful in the evaluation of new potential antipsychotic drugs.

References

Ahlenius S (1973) Inhibition of catecholamine synthesis and conditioned avoidance acquisition. Pharmacol Biochem Behav 1:347–350

Ahlenius S (1974a) Reversal by L-DOPA of the suppression of locomotor activity induced by inhibition of tyrosine-hydroxylase and DA-β hydroxylase in mice. Brain Res 69:57–65

Ahlenius S (1974b) Effects of low and high doses of L-DOPA on the tetrabenazine or α-methyltyrosine-induced suppression of the behavior in a successive discrimination task. Psychopharmacologia 39:199–212

Ahlenius S (1974c) Effects of L-DOPA on conditioned avoidance responding after behavioural suppression by α-methyltyrosine or reserpine in mice. Neuropharmacology 13:729–739

Ahlenius S (1976) Neurochemical control of behavior: on the functional significance of drug-induced changes in central catecholamine receptor activation. Diss Abstr Int, vol 37. Univ Microfilms No 76-21,061, pp 1/1446C

Ahlenius S, Engel J (1972) Effects of a dopamine (DA-β-hydroxylase) inhibitor on timing behaviour. Psychopharmacologia 24:243–246

Ahlenius S, Engel J (1976) Normalization by antipsychotic drugs of biochemically induced abnormal behaviour in rats. Psychopharmacology 49:63–68

Ahlenius S, Engel J (1977) Potentiation by α-methyltyrosine of the suppression of food-reinforced lever-pressing behaviour induced by antipsychotic drugs. Acta Pharmacol Toxicol 40:115–125

Ahlenius S, Andén N-E, Engel J (1973) Restoration of locomotor activity in mice by low L-DOPA doses after suppression by α-methyltyrosine but not by reserpine. Brain Res 62:189–199

Ahlenius S, Carlsson A, Engel J (1975) Antagonism by baclophen of the d-amphetamine-induced disruption of a successive discrimination in the rat. J Neural Transm 36:327–333

Ahlenius S, Engel J, Zöller M (1977) Effect of apomorphine and haloperidol on exploratory behaviour and latent learning in mice. Physiol Psychol 5:290–294

Ahlenius S, Svensson L, Hillegaart V, Thorberg O (1984) Antagonism by haloperidol of the suppression of exploratory locomotor activity induced by the local application of (−) 3-(3-hydroxyphenyl)-N-n-propylpiperidine into the nucleus accumbens of the rat. Experientia (Basel) 40:858–859

Almgren O, Lundborg P (1971) Correlation of the recovery of the granular uptake-storage mechanism and the nerve impulse induced release of (3H) noradrenaline after reserpine. J Pharm Pharmacol 23:671–677

Andén N-E (1972) Dopamine turnover in the corpus striatum and the limbic system after treatment with neuroleptic and anti-acetylcholine drugs. J Pharm Pharmacol 24:905–906

Andén N-E, Rubenson A, Fuxe K, Hökfelt T (1967) Evidence for dopamine receptor stimulation by apomorphine. J Pharm Pharmacol 19:627

Andén N-E, Strömbom U, Svensson TH (1973) Dopamine and noradrenaline receptor stimulation: reversal of reserpine-induced suppression of motor activity. Psychopharmacologia 29:289–298

Andén N-E, Golembiowska-Nikitin K, Thornström U (1982) Selective stimulation of dopamine and noradrenaline autoreceptors by B-HT 920 and B-HT 933, respectively. Naunyn-Schmiedeberg's Arch Pharmacol 321:100–104

Archer T (1982) DSP4-(N-2-chloroethyl-N-2-bromobenzylamine), a new noradrenaline neurotoxin, and the stimulus conditions affecting acquisition of two-way active avoidance. J Comp Physiol Psychol 96:476–490

Archer T, Ögren S-O, Johansson G, Ross SB (1982) DSP-4-induced two-way active avoidance impairment in rats: involvement of central and not peripheral noradrenaline depletion. Psychopharmacology 76:303–309

Archer T, Mohammed AK, Järbe TUC (1983) Latent inhibition following systemic OSP4: effects due to presence and absence of contextual cues in taste-aversion learning. Behav Neural Biol 38: 287–306

Archer T, Söderberg U, Johansson G, Ross SB (1984) Role of olfactory bulbectomy and DSP4 treatment in avoidance learning in the rat. Behav Neurosci 98:496–505

Archer T, Sjödén P-O, Nilsson L-G (1985) Contextual control of taste-aversion conditioning and extinction. In: Balsam PD, Tomie A (eds) Context and learning. Erlbaum, Hillsdale, pp 225–271

Beckstead RM, Domesick VB, Nauta WJH (1979) Efferent connections of the substantia nigra and ventral tegmental area in the rat. Brain Res 175:191–217

Beninger RJ (1983) The role of dopamine in locomotor activity and learning. Brain Res Rev 6: 173–196

Björklund A, Stenevi U (1984) Intracerebral neural implants: neuronal replacement and reconstruction of damaged circuitries. Annu Rev Neurosci 7:279–308

Carlsson A (1965) Drugs which block the storage of 5-hydroxytryptamine and related amines. Handb Exp Pharmacol 19:529–592

Carlsson A (1972) Biochemical and pharmacological aspects of parkinsonism. Acta Neurol Scand Suppl 51:11–42

Carlsson A (1975) Receptor-mediated control of dopamine metabolism. In: Usdin E, Bunney WE (eds) Pre- and postsynaptic receptors. Brunner/Mazel, New York

Carlsson A (1978) Antipsychotic drugs, neurotransmitters, and schizophrenia. Am J Psychiatry 135: 164–173

Carlsson A, Lindqvist M, Magnusson T (1957) 3,4-Dihydroxyphenylalanine and 5-hydroxytryptophan as reserpine antagonists. Nature (Lond) 180:1200

Corrodi H, Fuxe K (1967) The effect of catecholamine precursors and monoamine oxidase inhibition on the amine levels of central catecholamine neurons after reserpine treatment or tyrosine hydroxylase inhibition. Life Sci 6:1345–1350

Corrodi H, Fuxe K, Hökfelt T (1966) Refillment of the catecholamine stores with 3,4-dihydroxyphenylalanine after depletion induced by inhibition of tyrosine hydroxylase. Life Sci 5:605–611

Costall B, Naylor RJ (1975) The behavioural effects of dopamine applied intracerebrally to areas of the mesolimbic system. Eur J Pharmacol 32:87–92

Cotzias GC, Papavasiliou PS, Ginos JZ (1976) Therapeutic approaches in Parkinson's disease: possible roles of growth hormone and somatostatin. Res Publ Assoc Res Nerv Ment Dis 55:305–313

Crow TJ, Longden A, Smith A, Wendlandt S (1977) Pontine tegmental lesions, monoamine neurones, and varieties of learning. Behav Biol 20:184–196

Denny-Brown D, Yanagisawa N (1976) The role of the basal ganglia in the initiation of movement. Res Publ Assoc Res Nerv Ment Dis 55:115–148

Ernst AM (1967) Mode of action of apomorphine and dexamphetamine on gnawing compulsion in rats. Psychopharmacologia 10:316–323

Fibiger HC, Zis AP, Phillips AG (1975) Haloperidol-induced disruption of conditioned avoidance responding: attenuation by prior training or by anticholinergic drugs. Eur J Pharmacol 30:309–314

Fog R, Pakkenberg H (1971) Behavioral effects of dopamine and *p*-hydroxyamphetamine injected into corpus striatum of rats. Exp Neurol 31:75–86

Hjorth S, Carlsson A, Clark D, Svensson K, Wikström H, Sanchez D, Lindberg P, Hacksell U, Arvidsson L-E, Johansson A, Nilsson JLG (1983) Central dopamine receptor agonist and antagonist actions of the enantiomers of 3-PPP. Psychopharmacology 81:89–99

Jackson DM, Andén N-E, Dahlström A (1975) A functional effect of dopamine in the nucleus accumbens and in some other dopamine-rich parts of the rat brain. Psychopharmacologia 45: 139–149

Jaim-Etcheverry G, Zieher LM (1980) DSP4-A novel compound with neurotoxic effects on noradrenergic neurons of adult and developing rats. Brain Res 188:513–523

Jonsson G, Hallman H, Ponzio F, Ross SB (1981) DSP4-(N-2-chloroethyl-N-ethyl-2-bromobenzyl-amine) – A useful denervation tool for central and peripheral noradrenaline neurons. Eur J Pharmacol 72:173–188

Kehr W (1976) Wechselwirkung von Dopamin-Rezeptoragonisten und -antagonisten hinsichtlich Dopamin-Synthese und -Metabolismus. Drug Res 26:1086–1088

Löffelholz K, Muscholl E (1970) Der Einfluß von *d*-Amphetamin auf die Noradrenalinabgabe aus dem isolierten Kaninchenherzen. Naunyn-Schmiedeberg's Arch Pharmacol 266:393–394

Lubow RE (1965) Latent inhibition: effect of frequency of nonreinforced preexposure of the CS. J Comp Physiol Psychol 60:454–457

Lubow RE, Moore AV (1959) Latent inhibition: the effect of nonreinforced preexposure of the CS. J Comp Physiol Psychol 52:415–419

Maj J, Grabowska M, Gajda L (1972) Effect of apomorphine on motility in rats. Eur J Pharmacol 17:208–214

Malmfors T (1965) Studies on adrenergic nerves. Acta Physiol Scand 64 Suppl 248:1–93

Marshall JF, Levitan D, Stricker EM (1976) Activation-induced restoration of sensorimotor functions in rats with dopamine-depleting brain lesions. J Comp Physiol Psychol 90:536–546

Mason ST (1981) Noradrenaline in the brain: progress in theories of behavioral function. Prog Neurobiol (NY) 16:263–303

McEntee ST, Mair RL (1978) Memory impairment in Korsakoff's psychosis: a correlation with brain noradrenaline activity. Science (Wash DC) 202:905–907

McEntee ST, Mair RL (1980) Memory enhancement in Korsakoff's psychosis by clonidine: further evidence for a noradrenergic deficit. Ann Neurol 5:466–470

Mogenson GJ, Jones DL, Yim CY (1980) From motivation to action: functional interface between the limbic system and the motor system. Prog Neurobiol (NY) 14:69–97

Moore KE, Dominic JA (1971) Tyrosine hydroxylase inhibitors. Fed Proc 30:859–870

Moore RY, Bloom FE (1978) Central catecholamine neuron systems: anatomy and physiology of the dopamine systems. Annu Rev Neurosci 1:129–169

Moore RY, Bloom FE (1979) Central catecholamine neuron systems: anatomy and physiology of the norepinephrine and epinephrine systems. Annu Rev Neurosci 2:113–168

Obianwu HO (1969a) Possible functional differentiation between the stores from which adrenergic nerve stimulation, tyramine and amphetamine release noradrenaline. Acta Physiol Scand 75: 92–101

Obianwu HO (1969b) Some studies on the mechanism by which *d*-amphetamine antagonized guanethidine induced adrenergic neuron blockade. Acta Physiol Scand 75:102–110

Ögren SO, Archer T, Ross S (1980) Evidence for a role of the locus coerulens noradrenaline system in learning. Neurosci Lett 20:351–356

Pijnenburg AJJ, van Rossum JM (1973) Stimulation of locomotor activity following injection of dopamine into the nucleus accumbens. J Pharm Pharmacol 25:1003–1005

Posluns D (1962) An analysis of chlorpromazine-induced suppression of the avoidance response. Psychopharmacologia 3:361–373

Ross SB (1976) Long-term effects of N-2-chloroethyl-N-ethyl-2-bromozylamine hydrochloride on noradrenergic neurons in the rat brain and heart. Br J Pharmacol 26:458–459

Schwab RS, Zeiper I (1965) Effects of mood, motivation, stress and alertness on the performance in Parkinson's disease. Psychiatr Neurol 150:345–357

Seiden LS, MacPhail RC, Oglesby MW (1976) Catecholamines and drug-behavior interactions. In: Weiss B, Laties VG (eds) Behavioral pharmacology: the current status. Plenum, New York, pp 137–153

Smith AD, Winkler H (1972) Fundamental mechanisms in the release of catecholamines. Handb
Exp Pharmacol 33:538–617
Smith CB, Dews PB (1962) Antagonism of locomotor suppressant effects of reserpine in mice.
Psychopharmacologia 3:55–59
Snyder SH, Banerjee SP, Yamamura HI, Greenberg D (1974) Drugs, neurotransmitters, and schizo-
phrenia. Science (Wash DC) 184:1243–1253
Sovner R, DiMascio A (1978) Extrapyramidal syndromes and other neurological side effects of
psychotropic drugs. In: Lipton MA, DiMascio A, Killam KF (eds) Psychopharmacology: a gener-
ation of progress. Raven, New York, pp 1021–1032
Stolerman IP (1971) Analysis of the acquisition and extinction of food-reinforced behaviour in
rats after the administration of chlorpromazine. Psychopharmacologia 20:266–279
Strömbom U (1976) Catecholamine receptor agonists. Effects on motor activity and rate of tyrosine hydroxylation in mouse brain. Naunyn-Schmiedeberg's Arch Pharmacol 292:167–176
Svensson L, Ahlenius S (1982) Functional importance of nucleus accumbens noradrenaline in the
rat. Acta Pharmacol Toxicol 50:22–24
Svensson L, Ahlenius S (1983) Suppression of exploratory locomotor activity by the local application of dopamine or l-noradrenaline to the nucleus accumbens of the rat. Pharmacol Biochem
Behav 19:693–699
Vander Wende C, Spoerlein MT (1962) Psychotic symptoms induced in mice by the intravenous
administration of solutions of 3,4-dihydroxyphenylalanine (dopa). Arch Int Pharmacodyn Ther
137:145–154
Voigtlander PF von, Moore KE (1973) Involvement of nigro-striatal neurons in the in vivo release
of dopamine by amphetamine, amantadine and tyramine. J Pharmacol Exp Ther 184:542–552
Wachtel H, Ahlenius S, Andén N-E (1979) Effects of locally applied dopamine to the nucleus accumbens on the motor activity of normal rats and following α-methyltyrosine or reserpine.
Psychopharmacology 63:203–206
Wang RY, White FJ (1984) Pharmacological characterization of A10 dopamine autoreceptors:
microiontophoretic studies. Clin Neuropharmacol 7 Suppl 1:72–73
Wauquier A, Niemegeers CJE, Lal H (1975) Differential antagonism by the anticholinergic dexetim-
ide of inhibitory effects of haloperidol and fentanyn on brain self-stimulation. Psychopharmacologia 41:229–235

Symposium V

Photo-Transduction in Invertebrate Visual Cells

Organizers T. YOSHIZAWA and H. LANGER

Phototransduction in Invertebrate Visual Cells. The Present State of Research – Exemplified and Discussed Through the *Limulus* Photoreceptor Cell

H. STIEVE[1]

1 Introduction

Phototransduction in invertebrates differs in at least two conspicuously important aspects from that of vertebrates:

- In invertebrates the visual pigment is converted by light to a thermostable meta-state which is not, or only very slowly, metabolically regenerated.
- The electrical signal of visual excitation in invertebrates is based upon an increase in membrane conductance as opposed to the conductance decrease in the vertebrates, resulting in membrane voltage signals (receptor potentials) of opposite polarity.

These two apparent distinctions may indicate fundamental differences in transduction mechanisms of the two groups of animals. It is most reasonable to assume that vertebrate vision has developed from the invertebrate mechanism. How fundamental the differences are and how much we can learn from the comparative study of invertebrate transduction to understand the transduction mechanism of vertebrates, remains still to be explored.

This lecture is supposed to give an overview on invertebrate vision.

Photoreceptors of invertebrates show a great variety of morphological appearances. The mechanism of phototransduction seems to have less variation, but up to now only little is known how much the mechanism differs between different groups of invertebrates.

Due to limited space, I will concentrate on the transduction mechanism of the *Limulus* ventral nerve photoreceptor while making some remarks and suggestions about possibilities and restrictions for generalization.

2 The Ventral Photoreceptor of Limulus

The ventral photoreceptor of *Limulus* consists of two main parts (Fig. 1), the rhabdomeric lobe which contains the photosensory membrane folded to microvilli and the arhabdomeric lobe (Calman and Chamberlain 1982; Stern et al. 1982). Light absorp-

---

1 Institut für Neurobiologie der Kernforschungsanlage Jülich GmbH, Postfach 1913, 5170 Jülich, FRG

Neurobiology
(ed. by R. Gilles and J. Balthazart)
© Springer-Verlag Berlin Heidelberg 1985

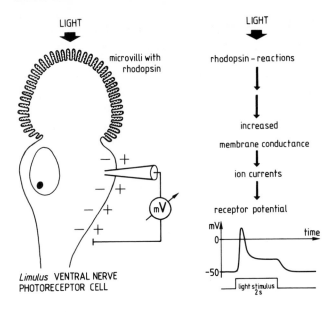

LIGHT

microvilli with rhodopsin

Limulus VENTRAL NERVE PHOTORECEPTOR CELL

LIGHT

rhodopsin – reactions

↓

↓

increased

membrane conductance

↓

ion currents

↓

receptor potential

mV

0

time

-50

light stimulus 2 s

Fig. 1. Functional diagram of the ventral nerve photo-receptor cell of *Limulus*. It has a diameter of 50 to 100 μm. The cell membrane of its distal lobe has glove finger-like protrusions, the microvilli, which contain the visual pigment rhodopsin. Such a cell contains about 10^6 microvilli ca. 1 μm long and 100 nm in diameter; they contain altogether a total of about 10^9 rhodopsin molecules. (Stieve 1984)

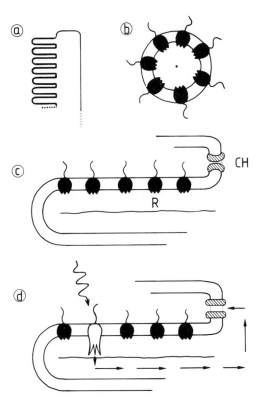

ⓐ

ⓑ

ⓒ

CH

R

ⓓ

Fig. 2a–d. Schematic diagram of the photosensory membrane: **a** Part of a photoreceptor cell with the glove finger-like protrusions of the cell membrane, the microvilli which contain rhodopsin. **b** Cross-section through a microvillus with the rhodopsin molecules. The "tails" of the rhodopsin-molecules are sugar chains which protrude into the extracellular environment. **c** Longitudial section through a microvillus which contains rhodopsin molecules and, presumably at its basis, one or a few ion channels CH. **d** Absorption of a photon causes conformational changes of one rhodopsin molecule. A chain of reactions leads to the transient opening of trans-membrane ion channels which may be far away from the light absorbing rhodopsin molecule. (Stieve 1984)

tion by the visual pigment rhodopsin causes a sequence of rhodopsin reactions followed by enzymatic reactions which lead to a transient increase in membrane conductane for cations. This permits ionic membrane currents which cause a signal in membrane voltage, the receptor potential.

Many rhodopsin molecules are contained in the photosensory membrane as opposed to a probably much smaller number of ion channels which are responsible for the light-induced conductance increase. The successful absorption of a single photon by a rhodopsin molecule suffices to evoke a measurable increase in membrane conductance. The message of the light absorption by a rhodopsin molecule has to be transmitted over relatively large distances in the visual cell (Brown and Coles 1979; Fig. 2). The light induced rhodopsin reactions in *Limulus* lead after less then 5 ms to an active state Rh* which is after a certain life time, converted to a thermostable meta-state. Hamdorf (1979) has proposed a sceme of rhodopsin reactions which has been veryfied more and more in the last years (Fig. 3). The active state of rhodopsin appears to be ended by rhodopsin phosphorylation which can be reverted quickly after rhodopsin has been regenerated due to absorption of another photon by metarhodopsin (Paulsen and Bentrop 1984).

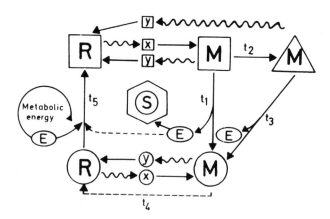

Fig. 3. Hypothetical reaction scheme of visual pigment in the microvillus membrane of invertebrate photoreceptors, according to Hamdorf (1979). The successful absorption of a photon by dark-adapted rhodopsin $\boxed{R}$ transforms the latter to "energy-rich" metarhodopsin $\boxed{M}$, which can activate a site $\textcircled{S}$ of the membrane with the release of energy. In this process $\boxed{M}$ is deactivated to $\textcircled{M}$. Absorption of another photon can transform $\textcircled{M}$ to $\textcircled{R}$, which can be restored to the active form $\boxed{R}$ with the help of metabolic energy. This cycle is dominant under normal, physiological light intensities. Unphysiologically intense illumination increases the transitions R $\leadsto$ M. Since the rate t_1 is limited by the rate at which the membrane can use energy some $\boxed{M}$ molecules go over into a storage state $\triangle\!\!\!\!_M$. This state is transformed in a much slower deactivating reaction ($t_3 \ll t_1$) into $\textcircled{M}$, producing a prolonged depolarizing afterpotential (PDA). The intermediate states of the reactions in the forward and backward directions are indicated by $\boxed{x}$ and $\boxed{y}$. The *dashed arrows* indicate the possibility of energy transfer from $\boxed{M}$ or $\triangle\!\!\!\!_M$ directly to $\textcircled{R}$. The rates t_1 to t_5 of the dark reactions are thermally controlled; t_4 indicates the possibility of a very slow metabolic dark regeneration of the visual pigment. (Hamdorf 1979)

3 Bumps, the Elementary Excitatory Events

If the dark-adapted photoreceptor of *Limulus* is stimulated by light flashes which are so weak that not every flash evokes a light response, one observes the so called bumps, responses of the photoreceptor to the successful absorption of single photons (Yeandle and Fuortes 1964). These bumps can be recorded as membrane voltage signals or as membrane current signals (Fig. 4). Bumps evoked by identical light flashes, i.e. response to absorption of identical photons, exhibit even under constant experimental conditions considerable variations (Fig. 4, left and Fig. 5, DA).

A bump is based on a transiently, considerably increased cation conductance of the photosensory membrane, mainly for sodium ions, which follows photon absorption after a delay. This delay is considerably large compared to the time needed by rhodopsin to reach the activated state (Lisman and Sheline 1976; Ostroy 1977).

The bump current amplitude is about 1–6 nA. We do not know the smallest size of the bumps since we only can detect bumps when they are larger than the noise level of our registration, which means larger than about 20 pA. The time course of the bump has three characteristic sections (Fig. 6; Keiper et al. 1984).

1. The latency phase (ca. 20 ms),
2. the almost linear phase of the bump rise (ca. 30 ms), and
3. the exponential phase of the bump decay (ca. 40 ms).

A large bump of a dark adapted *Limulus* photoreceptor is based upon a cation conductance increase of about 10–20 ns in bump maximum. The plausible assumption, that a bump is based on the superposition of many uncompletely synchronized opened ion channels is supported by the registrations of single channel events (Bacigalupo and Lisman 1983). One can estimate, that in the maximum of a large bump up to 10^3 to 10^4 ion channels, with a single channel conductance of 10–20 ps, are opened simultaneously. Bump generation thus involves a considerable (10^3- to 10^4-fold) amplification.

Bumps have been observed in many photoreceptors but seem to be missing in others like the barnacle *Balanus* and the bee *Apis*. The degree of amplification of the single photon event of the dark adapted photoreceptor may vary from species to species. In *Limulus* (and in locusts) it appears to be very large, in the fly smaller. Possibly the degree of amplification, that is the maximal number of ion channels involved in a bump of a dark adapted photoreceptor cell, is a characteristic value for a specific photoreceptor.

4 Bump Summation

The number of bumps evoked by a light stimulus increases linearly with the energy of the light stimulus, that is to say, with the number of absorbed photons (Yeandle and Fuortes 1964). With stronger light stimuli bumps superimpose and fuse to a fairly smooth signal, the macroscopic receptor current.

Figure 7 shows a test that the macroscopic receptor current mainly consists of fused bumps. A macroscopic receptor current is compared with artificially summated bump

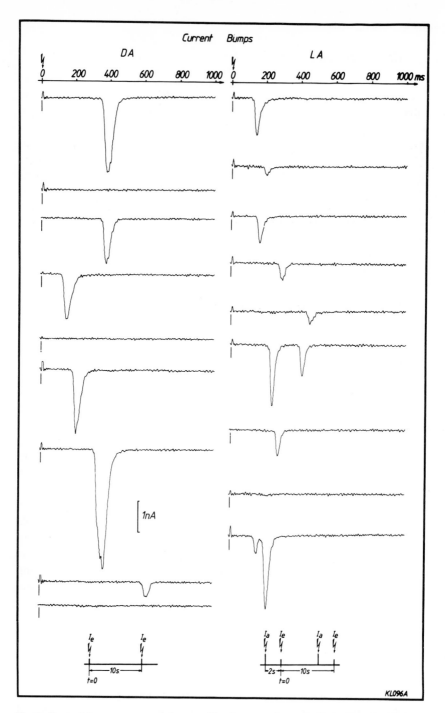

Fig. 4. Current bumps measured from a *Limulus* ventral nerve photoreceptor cell under voltage clamp conditions. *Left column* dark adapted photoreceptor (DA); *right column* photoreceptor weakly light adapted (LA) by a conditioning light flash, 2 s prior to the bump-evoking flash. Bump-evoking flash: E_e ca. 6×10^7 photons cm^{-2}, duration 50 μs, repetition time 10 s; light-adapting flash: E_a ca. 2×10^9 photons cm^{-2}, duration 10 ms both flashes 450 nm, membrane potential constant -40 mV; 15 °C. *Bottom:* stimulus regime.

On the average bumps recorded in the dark adapted state are larger and have a longer latency as compared to bumps which are recorded under weakly light adapted conditions. (Stieve 1984)

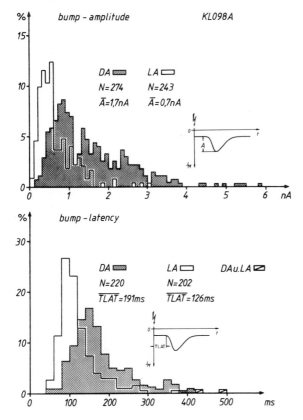

Fig. 5. Frequency distributions of bump amplitudes (*above*) and bump latencies (*below*) of a *Limulus* ventral nerve photoreceptor cell in dark adapted (DA) and weakly light adapted (LA) condition. The stimulus programme is described in Fig. 4. Only latencies of first bumps following the bump evoking flash are plotted; amplitudes plotted from all single bumps. N is the number of the bumps accounted, $\overline{A}$, $\overline{TLAT}$ are the arithmetical averages of the bump amplitudes and bump latency periods. (Stieve 1984)

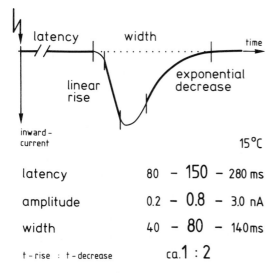

Fig. 6. Time course of a current bump (schematically) with specification of the variation of some shape parameters. (Stieve 1984)

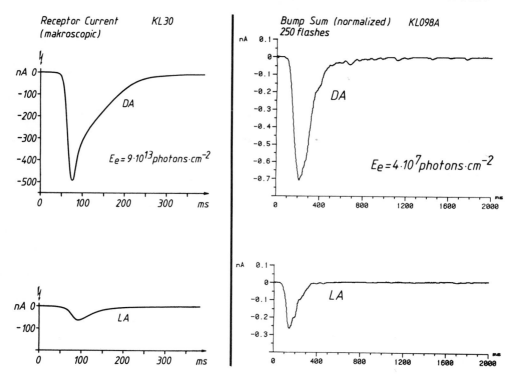

Fig. 7. Comparison of the macroscopic receptor currents (*left*) of a dark-adapted resp. light adapted photoreceptor cell with the artificially summated current bump responses (*right*) of another cell in the dark-resp. light-adapted state. Experimental conditions: *left* receptor current – evoking flash E_e ca. 1.9×10^{14} photons cm^{-2}, duration 10 ms, membrane potential constant –50 mV; record of the light-adapted state: 18 s prior to the receptor current-evoking flash the cell was illuminated for 2 s by a conditioning illumination (intensity ca. 2.3×10^{15} photons cm^{-2} s^{-1}); *right* Bump-evoking flash E_e 8.8×10^7 photons cm^{-2}, flash duration 50 μs, flash repetition time 10 s, membrane potential constant –40 mV; records in light-adapted state: 2 s prior to the bump-evoking flash the cell was illuminated by a 10 ms conditioning flash (8.2×10^9 photons cm^{-2}). Wavelength of stimulating and conditioning light 540 nm; temperature 15 °C. The bump-sum was built by linear summation, millisecond for millisecond, starting from the light stimulus. *Left* and *right* curves show significant differences in their time course which are only partially due to the large difference in the intensities of the response-evoking stimuli and the different degrees of light adaptation. (Stieve 1984)

registrations of another cell. The artificial bump sum shows the characteristic features of a macroscopic receptor current. The similarities between the two signals are obvious, although there are observable significant differences which are only partially due to different experimental conditions (different cells, different light intensities, and different light adaptation).

The amplitude of the macroscopic receptor current raises with increasing stimulus intensity (Fig. 8). In a double logarithmic plot it raises with a steep slope up to a certain intensity, at higher intensities the rise is less steep. The point of transition from the steeper to the less steep slope is in the dark adapted photoreceptor cell according to Brown and Coles (1979) at about 350 rhodopsin photo-isomerizations.

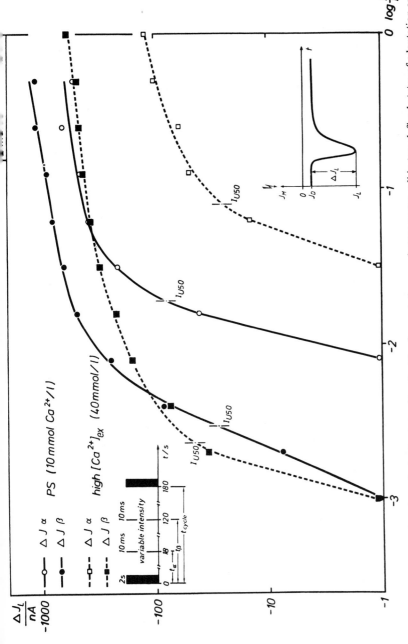

Fig. 8. Amplitude of receptor current as function of stimulus intensity of a *Limulus* ventral nerve photoreceptor cell in two defined states of adaptation and two external Ca^{2+}-concentrations. The *upper left inset* shows the stimulus programme, which was repeated every 3 min (cycle time t_c). A strong constant light adapting illumination (duration 2 s, intensity ca. 1.8×10^{16} photons cm^{-2} s^{-1}; 540 nm) is followed after 18 s (t_α) and 120 s (t_β) by 10 ms test flashes, the intensity of which was varied in order to obtain two stimulus-response curves. I_0 ca. 3.7×10^{16} photons cm^{-2} s^{-1}, 540 nm, 15 °C; membrane potential constant -50 mV. The first test stimulus (α) stimulates the relatively light adapted photoreceptor, the second test flash (β) the fairly dark adapted photoreceptor. The amplitude ΔJ_L of the light induced receptor current (*inset right below*) is plotted versus the test light intensity in a double logarithmic scale. The extent of the shift of the light adapted curve in respect to the dark adapted, depends upon the degree of light adaptation (Stieve and Klomfaß, 1981). The *solid curves* were recorded while the photoreceptor was superfused by saline containing 10 mmol l^{-1} calcium, while the *dashed curves* were recorded when the superfusate contains 40 mmol l^{-1} Ca^{2+}. At each curve I_{U50} is marked, the stimulus intensity which evokes a half saturated amplitude of the membrane voltage response (receptor potential)

5 Adaptation

The photoreceptor cell adjusts its sensitivity according to the mean ambient brightness within a large range. In the foregoing we have considered the visual cell in a state of maximal sensitivity, dark-adapted after a very long stay in the dark. Figure 7, left below, shows that after light adaptation the same light stimulus causes a macroscopic receptor current which is much smaller than that of the dark-adapted cell. In Fig. 8 it can be seen that light adaptation causes the receptor current vs. stimulus intensity curve to shift to the right, to higher stimulus intensities; the amount of shift depends upon the degree of light adaptation. The point of transition from the large steepness to the lower steepness of the curve is also shifted to the right. According to the "adapting bump model" suggested by Adolph (1968) and formulated by Dodge et al. (1968), the macroscopic receptor current of the light-adapted cell is smaller than that of the dark-adapted cell, since the size of the bumps constituting the receptor current is diminished by light adaptation. This was shown by Dodge et al. (1968) and Wong et al. (1982) using noise analysis, and could be shown for directly observed bumps by us (Stieve and Bruns 1980, 1983). Figure 4, right column, shows bumps evoked by identical flashes as in the left (dark-adapted) column, but here the bump-evoking flashes were delivered 2 s after a light-adapting, desensitizing flash had been administered. On the average these bumps of the weakly light-adapted photoreceptors are smaller than those of the dark-adapted one. Figure 5 shows that the frequency distributions of bump amplitudes and bump latencies are narrowed and shifted to smaller values. Artificially summated bump responses under those light-adapted conditions (Fig. 7) result in a light-adapted bump sum which shows characteristic features of light adaptation, diminution of the bump size and shortening of the latency period. This can be compared to the light-adapted response of the macroscopic receptor current which reveals characteristic similarities and differences. The differences are probably again partially due to the different stimulus conditions namely stimulus intensity and degree of adaptation.

There are several, at least four, processes causing desensitization in light adaptation of invertebrate photoreceptors:

1. A feedback mechanism regulating the light sensitivity of the cell by controlling the intracellular concentration of free calcium ions. This was first shown by Lisman and Brown (1972) and Fein and Charlton (1977). Light-adapting illumination causes a transient increase in intracellular free calcium ion concentration which causes a desensitization of the cell (Brown and Blinks 1974; Brown et al. 1977; Maaz and Stieve 1980; Nagy and Stieve 1983). The transient increase in internal calcium ions, monitored by the calcium indicator Arsenazo III, depends upon the membrane voltage (Fig. 9; Ivens and Stieve 1984). The amplitude of the light induced calcium increase becomes smaller, the recovery of the calcium signal, that is the decrease in internal calcium concentration, becomes slower, the more positive the membrane voltage is. This indicates that a substantial part of the calcium increase is due to a calcium influx through the cell membrane, possibly through the light activated ion channels and the existence of a large not electroneutral outward transport of calcium ions.

The calcium dependent feedback loop for sensitivity control can also be demonstrated in the shift of the response versus stimulus intensity curve due to light adaptation in

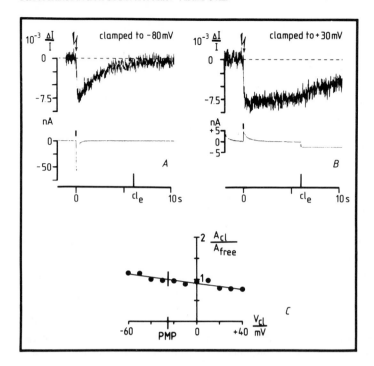

Fig. 9A–C. The change in intracellular concentration of ionized calcium monitored by the calcium indicator Arsenazo III. **A** Arsenazo signal (*upper trace*) and receptor current (*lower trace*) of the *Limulus* ventral nerve photoreceptor cell clamped to −80 mV in response to a 10 ms bright stimulus. **B** Arsenazo signal and receptor current of the cell clamped to +30 mV. In each case two signals are averaged. Clamp is switched off at cl_e; 17 °C. The superfusate contained 10 mmol l^{-1} Ca^{2+}. **C** Normalized amplitude A_{cl}/A_{free} of the Arsenazo signal, relative units, is plotted versus the membrane voltage to which the cell is clamped (V_{cl}). By linear extrapolation of the regression line a hypothetical reversal potential of the Arsenazo signal is calculated to be +250 mV. Normalization is done by dividing the amplitude of the Arsenazo signal of the clamped cell by the average of the amplitudes of the two Arsenazo signals 3 min prior and 3 min after the clamped signal was recorded. PMP is the prestimulus membrane potential. (Ivens and Stieve 1984)

different external calcium concentrations. Whereas the dark-adapted curve is almost uninfluenced by external calcium concentration, the shift due to light adaptation is the greater the higher the external calcium concentration is (Fig. 8; Stieve et al. 1984).

2. There is, however, a not, or at least much less, calcium-dependent mechanism of light adaptation.

Figure 10 shows the recovery of sensitivity during dark adaptation after a light-adapting illumination. It proceeds in two phases. Only the first phase shows a significant dependence upon external calcium concentration. In the second phase the photoreceptor is already relatively dark-adapted. The sensitivity increase during this second phase is not accompanied by a concomitant decrease in intracellular calcium as monitored by Arsenazo (Nagy and Stieve 1983).

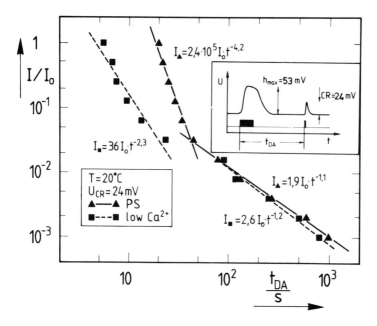

Fig. 10. Time course of sensitivity recovery during dark adaptation of *Limulus* ventral nerve photo-receptor monitored by the intensity of the test stimulus which evokes a criterion amplitude $U_{CR} = 24$ mV of the receptor potential. The stimulus sequency (*inset*) was repeated several times while the delay between light-adapting illumination and test stimulus was varied. In the double logarithmic plot the dark adaptation exhibits two phases, an initial fast one followed by a second slower phase. Only the first phase is markedly influenced by changes in extracellular calcium concentration: On lowering the external calcium concentration from 10 mmol l^{-1} (PS) to 250 μmol l^{-1}, the slope of the first phase is decreased. 1 s light adapting stimulus; I_{LA} about 4.4 × 10^{16} (540 nm) photons cm^{-2} s^{-1}; test stimulus 300 μs; E_0 about 1.4 × 10^{14} (540 nm) photons cm^{-2}; 20 °C. (Claßen-Linke and Stieve 1981)

Furthermore the weak light adaptation used by us to observe single bumps does not show a significant dependence upon external calcium (Stieve and Bruns 1983). The basis of this adaptation mechanism is not yet elucidated.

3. The third mechanism of desensitization in light adaptation can not be demonstrated in *Limulus* properly, due to the fact that in *Limulus* ventral photoreceptor the absorption spectra of rhodopsin and metarhodopsin practically coincide. If (in photoreceptors of other invertebrates) larger amounts of visual pigment are converted from rhodopsin to metarhodopsin, a PDA (prolonged depolarizing afterpotential) is evoked (Hilman et al. 1977; Minke 1979; Hamdorf and Razmjoo 1979) which causes, besides the depolarization, a long-lasting desensitization. This desensitization, as could be shown in mutants by Minke et al. (1975), is not due to depolarization. It may have much in common with light adaptation of the vertebrate photoreceptor (Blumfeld et al. 1984).

4. Desensitization due the migration of screening pigment is not present in the *Limulus* ventral nerve photoreceptor which does not contain screening pigment.

6 A Proposed Bump-Generating Mechanism

This model which is outlined in the following has been developed in cooperation with
J. Schnakenberg and W. Keiper (Keiper et al. 1984). Brown and Coles (1979) have
shown that a light-activated rhodopsin molecule in the dark adapted *Limulus* ventral
photoreceptor causes the opening of sodium channels in regions of the cell membrane
beyond the microvillus in which the photon was absorbed, but not necessarily more
than about 2 μm away.

Rhodopsin photoisomerization causes opening of ion channels in a surface area, the
"bump-speck", which may include about 1,000–2,000 microvilli, respective 1,000 to
2,000 light-activated ion channels. The break in the slope of the intensity dependency
of the receptor current (Fig. 8) is at a stimulus intensity where the stimulating flash
evokes about 400 bumps in the dark-adapted photoreceptor. This intensity corresponds
to a density of absorbed photons in the photosensory membrane where the bump specks
starts to touch each other and overlap.

For the spread of information over the bump speck the hypothesis of diffusing
internal transmitter molecules seems to be a reasonably plausible hypothesis (Fig. 11),

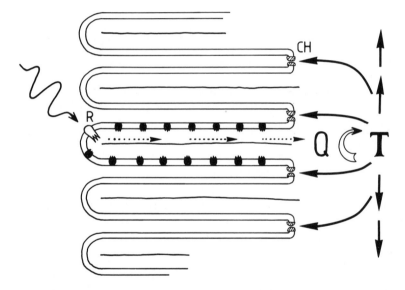

Fig. 11. Schematical diagram of proposed mechanism of bump generation in *Limulus* ventral nerve
photoreceptor. A light-activated rhodopsin molecule R in a microvillus starts the activation of an
enzyme (cascade) which finally leads to the activation of a transmitter source Q. This may be situated at the basis of this microvillus. The transmitter source there-upon produces, activates or releases many transmitter molecules which are built from precursors. The transmitter T diffuses along
the bases of the microvilli and is bound by the ion channels CH which plausibly may be situated
close to the bases of the microvilli. Following transmitter binding the ion channels are transiently
opened. Thus develops a more or less circular "bump-speck" which in the dark adapted photoreceptor cell should have a diameter of about 4 μm. On the average a bump-speck of a light adapted
photoreceptor cell is smaller. The bump amplitude is proportional to the number of simultaneously
opened ion channels and should be thereby more or less proportional to the area of the bump-speck.
(Stieve 1984)

although up to now excitatory transmitter has not been identified in the invertebrate photoreceptor. However, no serious alternative to the diffusing transmitter hypothesis which was first proposed by Cone (1973), has been formulated up to now.

The high amplification results in the opening of 10^3-10^4 ion channels during one bump, which leads to the assumption that at least as many transmitter molecules have to be formed, released or activated in the process of bump generation. This large amplification is most probably brought about by enzymatic reactions. In the vertebrate photoreceptor cell an enzyme cascade could be demonstrated which causes the degradation of cAMP. The high amplification is responsible for the high maximal sensitivity of the *Limulus* ventral photoreceptor, enabling the cell to detect single photons way above the noise level. The great variation in bump size evoked by identical photons under identical experimental conditions indicates that reactions of only a few molecules are determinative for the bump size amplification.

7 Latency

The considerable duration of the bump latency (100-200 ms) depends strongly on temperature (Q_{10} ca. 4; Wong et al. 1980), calcium ion concentration (Stieve and Bruns 1983) and state of adaptation (Stieve et al. 1982). The latency of the macroscopic response depends strongly upon stimulus intensity and density of photon absorption in the photosensory membrane.

The latency is not mainly determined by diffusion; it is longer by a factor of about 100 than the time needed for unhindered diffusion in homogeneous cytoplasma. The long latency is probably caused by time-consuming chemical reactions after the light-induced conversion of rhodopsin to the activated state. We think it is most probable that the process of activation of an enzyme (in the enzyme cascade) is the time-consuming step for the latency. The drastic shortening of the latency of the macroscopic receptor current with increasing stimulus intensity is first of all a statistical phenomenon: The more photons are absorbed from a flash the more bumps with short latencies (which are less probable in the frequency distribution of bump latencies) will occur. That is to say, the more photons, the higher the probability for rare, short latencies. The large fluctuations in the bump latencies indicate that again the reactions of only a few molecules determine the length of the latency; that is to say, the latency is determined by steps in the causal chain of bump generation which do not yet involve major amplification.

Hamdorf and Kirschfeld (1980) have shown that photon absorption in neighbouring microvilli of the fly photoreceptor cell cause a drastical shortening of bump latencies; and even more drastic shortening of the latency occurs when two photons are absorbed by the same microvillus. These phenomena have not yet been clearly demonstrated in the *Limulus* ventral photoreceptor.

It has been shown by Wong et al. (1980), Stieve and Bruns (1983), Keiper et al. (1984), and Goldring and Lisman (1984) that a latency and amplification are determined by distinctly different processes.

8 What is the Molecular Role of Rhodopsin?

After photon absorption rhodopsin most probably does not form an ion channel through the photosensory membrane itself, but rather, as shown for the vertebrate photoreceptor, activates an enzyme. There is however yet not strong evidence that G-protein plays an important act in the phototransduction in *Limulus*, although some remarkable indications for the importance of G-protein exist in the photoreceptor of *Limulus* and other invertebrates (Corson and Fein 1983; Saibil and Michel-Villaz 1984; Brown et al. 1984; Blumfeld et al. 1984; Corson et al. 1983).

Light-activated enzyme reactions should provide the source of production, activation or release of transmitter molecules. Active transmitter molecules should start to occur at the end of the latency period and open sodium channels probably by binding to them. It seems plausible that the linear raising phase of the bump is caused by the diffusion of the transmitter over the "bump speck" opening more and more peripher ion channels (Fig. 11). The longer and the stronger the source produces active transmitter-molecules, the larger becomes the bump.

The bump raise ends when the transmitter production dwindles. There seem to be two possible explanations for the exponential phase of the bump decay: It could be due to the stochastics of the channel closure or an exponential decay of the transmitter concentration, as suggested by Bacigalupo and Lisman (1983). We think the first ex-

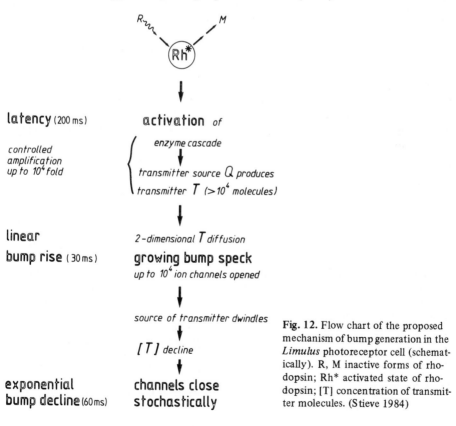

Fig. 12. Flow chart of the proposed mechanism of bump generation in the *Limulus* photoreceptor cell (schematically). R, M inactive forms of rhodopsin; Rh* activated state of rhodopsin; [T] concentration of transmitter molecules. (Stieve 1984)

planation more probable. The scheme in Fig. 12 summarizes our model for bump generation.

In light adaptation the bumps becomes smaller because the amplification is lower and (compare Fig. 8) the bump specks become smaller. The raising phase of the bumps becomes shorter, possibly because the source produces transmitter for a shorter time; the bump decay becomes faster, either because the life time of the channel becomes shorter or because the decrease in transmitter concentration becomes faster.

9 Conclusion

We have described the phenomena of phototransduction and proposed a model for the mechanism of bump generation in the *Limulus* photoreceptor. We think that many phenomena are general for invertebrate photoreceptors. The average size of the dark-adapted bump may vary between different species as well as the relative contribution of the different kinds of processes which cause sensitivity diminution in light adaptation.

References

Adolph A (1968) Thermal and spectral sensitivities of discrete slow potentials in Limulus eye. J Gen Physiol 52:584–599

Bacigalupo J, Lisman JE (1983) Singel-channel currents activated by light in Limulus ventral photo-receptors. Nature (Lond) 304 (5923):268–270

Blumfeld A, Selinger Z, Minke B (1984) Biochemical and electrophysiological evidence of light-activated GTPase in fly photoreceptors. In: Abstr 6th Int Congr Eye Res, vol 4. Alicante, Spain

Brown JE, Blinks JR (1974) Changes in intracellular free calcium concentration during illumination of invertebrate photoreceptors. J Gen Physiol 64:643–665

Brown JE, Brown PK, Pinto LH (1977) Detection of light induced changes of intracellular ionized calcium concentration in Limulus ventral nerve photoreceptors using Arsenazo III. J Physiol (Lond) 267:299–320

Brown JE, Coles JA (1979) Saturation of the response to light in Limulus ventral photoreceptors. J Physiol (Lond) 296:373–392

Brown JE, Kaupp UB, Malbon CC (1984, in press) 3′,5′-cyclic adenosine monophosphate and adenylate cyclase in phototransduction by Limulus ventral photoreceptors. J Physiol (Lond) 2832

Calman BG, Chamberlain SC (1982) Distinct lobes of Limulus ventral photoreceptors II. Structure and ultrastructure. J Gen Physiol 80:839–862

Claßen-Linke I, Stieve H (1981) Time course of dark adaptation in the Limulus ventral nerve photo-receptor – measured as constant response amplitude curve –, and its dependence upon extra-cellular calcium. Biophys Struct Mech 7:336

Cone RA (1973) The internal transmitter model of visual excitation, some quantitative implications. In: Langer H (ed) Biochemistry and physiology of visual pigments. Springer, Berlin Heidelberg New York, pp 275–282

Corson DW, Fein A (1983) Chemical excitation of Limulus photoreceptor I. J Gen Physiol 82:639–657

Corson DW, Fein A, Walthall WW (1983) Chemical excitation of Limulus photoreceptors II. J Gen Physiol 82:659–667

Dodge FA, Knight BW, Toyoda JI (1968) Voltage noise in Limulus visual cells. Science (Wash DC) 160:88–90

Fein A, Charlton JS (1977) A quantitative comparison of the effects of intracellular calcium injection and light adaptation on the photoresponse of Limulus ventral photoreceptor. J Gen Physiol 70:591–600

Goldring MA, Lisman JE (1984, in press) The quantum bump area distribution in voltage-clamped Limulus ventral photoreceptors

Hamdorf K (1979) Comparative physiology and evolution in vision in invertebrates. In: Autrum H (ed) Handbook for sensory physiology, vol 7. Springer, Berlin Heidelberg New York

Hamdorf K, Kirschfeld K (1980) "Prebumps": evidence for double-hits at functional subunits in a rhabdomeric photoreceptor. Z Naturforsch Sect C Biosci 35:173–174

Hamdorf K, Razmjoo S (1979) Photoconvertible pigment states and excitation in calliphora; the induction and properties of the prolonged depolarising after-potential. Biophys Struct Mech 5:137–161

Hillman P, Keen ME, Winterhager J (1977) V. Discussion of selected topics about the transduction mechanism in photoreceptors. Biophys Struct Mech 3:183–189

Ivens I, Stieve H (1984) Influence of the membrane potential due to light adaptation depending on the extracellular calcium ion concentration in Limulus ventral nerve photoreceptor. Z Naturforsch Sect C Biosci 39:662–679

Keiper W, Schnakenberg J, Stieve H (1984) Statistical analysis of quantum bump parameters in Limulus ventral photoreceptor. Z Naturforsch Sect C Biosci 39:781–790

Lisman JE, Brown JE (1972) The effects of intracellular iontophoretic injection of calcium and sodium ions in the light response of Limulus ventral photoreceptors. J Gen Physiol 59:701–719

Lisman JE, Sheline Y (1976) Analysis of the rhodopsin cycle in Limulus ventral photoreceptors using the early receptor potential. J Gen Physiol 68:487–501

Maaz G, Stieve H (1980) The correlation of the receptor with potential the light induced transient increase in intracellular calcium-concentration measured by absorption change of arsenazo III injected into Limulus ventral nerve photoreceptor cell. Biophys Struct Mech 6:191–208

Minke B (1979) Transduction in photoreceptors with bistable pigments: intermediate processes. Biophys Struct Mech 5:163–174

Minke B, Wu C-F, Pak WL (1975) Induction of photoreceptor voltage noise in the dark in Drosophila mutant. Nature (Lond) 258:84–87

Nagy K, Stieve H (1983) Changes in intracellular calcium ion concentration, in the course of dark adaptation measured by arsenazo III in the Limulus photoreceptor. Biophys Struct Mech 9:207–223

Ostroy SE (1977) Rhodopsin and the visual process. Biochim Biophys Acta 463:91–125

Paulsen R, Bentrop J (1984, in press) Reversible phosphorylation of opsin induced by irradiation of blowfly retinae. J Comp Physiol

Saibil H, Michel-Villaz M (1984) Squid rhodopsin and GTP-binding protein cross react with vertebrate photoreceptor enzymes. Proc Natl Acad Sci USA 81:5111–5115

Stern J, Chinn K, Bacigalupo K, Lisman J (1982) Distinct lobes of Limulus ventral photoreceptors I. Functional and anatomical properties of lobes revealed by removal of glial cells. J Gen Physiol 80:825–837

Stieve H (1984) Biophysik des Sehvorgangs. Physikalische Blätter 40(7):205–211

Stieve H, Bruns M (1980) Dependence of bump rate and bump size in Limulus ventral nerve photoreceptor on light adaptation and calcium concentration. Biophys Struct Mech 6:271–285

Stieve H, Klomfaß J (1981) Calcium dependence of light evoked membrane current signal and membrane voltage signal and their changes due to light adaptation in Limulus photoreceptor. Biophys Struct Mech 7(4):345

Stieve H, Bruns M (1983) Bump latency distribution and bump adaptation of Limulus ventral nerve photoreceptor in varied extracellular calcium concentration. Biophys Struct Mech 9:329–339

Stieve H, Klomfaß J (1983) Distribution of bump latency and bump shape parameters in dependence on adaptation on external Ca^{2+}-concentration in Limulus photoreceptor. Abstract Jahrestagung der Dtsch Ges f Biophysik, 10.10.–12.10.1983, Neuherberg

Stieve H, Bruns M, Klomfaß J (1982) The distribution of bump parameters under various stimulus conditions of the ventral nerve photoreceptor of Limulus. Abstr Eye Res Congr Einhoven 03.10.−08.10.1982

Stieve H, Bruns M, Gaube H (1984) The sensitivity shift due to light adaptation depending on the extracellular calcium ion concentration in Limulus ventral nerve photoreceptor. Z Naturforsch Sect C Biosci 39:662−679

Wong F, Knight BW, Dodge FA (1980) Dispersion of latencies in photoreceptors of Limulus and the adapting bump model. J Gen Physiol 76(5):517−537

Wong F, Knight BW, Dodge FA (1982) Adapting bump model for ventral photoreceptors of Limulus. J Gen Physiol 79:1089−1113

Yeandle S, Fuortes MGF (1964) Probability of occurrence of discrete potential waves in the eye of Limulus. J Gen Physiol 47:443−463

Hypersensitivity in the Anterior Median Eye
of a Jumping Spider

H. TATEDA[1] and S. YAMASHITA[2]

1 Introduction

It has been shown that Ca^{2+} plays important roles in controlling sensitivity of invertebrate photoreceptors. Lisman and Brown (1972) showed that during intracellular iontophoretic injection of Ca^{2+} into *Limulus* ventral photoreceptors, there was a progressive
diminution of the light response. They postulated that light stimulation leads to an
increase in intracellular Ca^{2+} which in turn reduces responsiveness to light stimulation.
Direct measurement of intracellular Ca^{2+} concentration in *Limulus* ventral photoreceptors and *Balanus* photoreceptors indicates that illumination does induce an increase
in the intracellular Ca^{2+} concentration (Brown and Blinks 1974). Hanani and Hillman
(1976) showed that the barnacle photoreceptor sensitivity either decreased or increased
after exposure to illumination, and both phenomena were influenced by external Ca^{2+}
concentration. In a study on the retina of the honey bee drone, Bader et al. (1976)
showed that an increase in intracellular Ca^{2+} concentration played a central role in
light adaptation.

In this chapter, we will show that photoreceptor cells of the anterior median eye of
the jumping spider *Menemerus* are more sensitive for a brief period following illumination than they are during complete dark adaptation, and the hypersensitivity is greatly
affected by the concentration of Ca^{2+}.

2 Materials and Methods

Jumping spiders, *Menemerus confusus*, were used in this study. A small portion of the
dorsal cuticle of the cephalothorax was removed with a sharp razor blade, exposing
the retinal portion of the anterior median eye. Electroretinograms (ERG's) were recorded by means of glass pipette microelectrodes (10-30 MΩ) filled with 2.5 M KCl,
or suction electrodes (0.1-0.2 mm tip diameter) filled with physiological saline. Intracellular potentials were recorded by means of glass pipette microelectrodes (50-100 MΩ)
filled with 2.5 M KCl. For recording ERG's from the intact eye, a glass pipette micro-
electrode (30-50 MΩ) filled with physiological saline was inserted through a small hole

1 Department of Biology, Faculty of Science, Kyushu University, Fukuoka 812, Japan
2 Biological Laboratory, Kyushu Institute of Design, Fukuoka 815, Japan

Neurobiology
(ed. by R. Gilles and J. Balthazart)
© Springer-Verlag Berlin Heidelberg 1985

in the cuticle covering the anterior median eye. Two 6–8 V tungsten lamps (lamp I, II) placed side by side were used for white light stimulation. Lamp I was used as the control light and the test light, and lamp II was used as the conditioning light. Initially, the control light, serving also as the test light, was presented. This was followed by the conditioning light and after various time intervals by a test light (Fig. 2A). The control light was used on the completely dark-adapted eye. In some cases, the conditioning light was used also for background illumination. The composition of the normal physiological saline was as follows: NaCl, 217 mM; KCl, 5 mM; $CaCl_2$, 4 mM; $MgCl_2$, 1.1 mM; $NaHCO_3$, 3 mM (Rathmayer 1965). Low-Na^+ saline containing 112 mM, 46 mM and 3 mM-Na^+ were made by replacing NaCl with equimolar choline chloride, and K^+-free saline by replacing KCl with choline chloride. Low-Ca^{2+} saline (0.1 mM-Ca^{2+}) was made by replacing $CaCl_2$ with equivalent NaCl, and high-Ca^{2+} saline (10 mM Ca^{2+}) by replacing NaCl with $CaCl_2$. Mg^{2+}-free saline was made by replacing $MgCl_2$ with equivalent NaCl. After a change in the perfusing solution, a period of 3–10 min was usually required to establish the steady-state effects of the new solution upon the eye's light response. Reported results were obtained repeatedly under these steady-state conditions.

3 Results

3.1 Hypersensitivity

Responses to repetitive flashes of 250 ms were recorded intracellularly from the dark-adapted photoreceptor cells of the anterior median eye (Fig. 1A). The amplitude of the response to the first flash is about 1 mV. The responses to the following flashes are progressively larger, with a maximum amplitude of about 2 mV. There is a small continuous depolarization during repetitive stimulation. It is probably not due to injury since a similar phenomenon occurs in the ERG of the intact eye (Fig. 1B). In most fresh preparations, the maximum increase was observed when the stimulus interval was 3–5 s.

The increase in response following repetitive stimulation suggests that photoreceptor cells may become more sensitive to ensuing stimuli. This was investigated by ERG

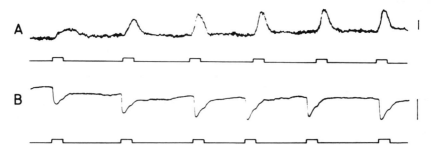

Fig. 1A,B. Receptor potentials to repetitive light flashes. **A** Increased responsiveness of a single photoreceptors. **B** Increase in the ERG of the intact eye, for which saline was not used. All stimuli were 250 ms duration and 1–1.5 s apart. Calibrations: 1 mV. (Yamashita and Tateda 1976b)

intensity-response curves to white light stimuli obtained from completely dark-adapted eyes and from eyes 5 s after a constant conditioning stimulus of 1-s duration (Fig. 2B). The intensity-response curves obtained before and after conditioning stimuli were almost parallel; any one of them could be superimposed on the other by a shift along the abscissa. This result shows that the sensitivity of the photoreceptors after illumination is indeed greater than they are during complete dark adaptation. We call this phenomenon "hypersensitivity".

Changes in the sensitivity after the conditioning stimulus were studied. The relative sensitivity was defined as the reciprocal of the relative intensity required to elicit a response amplitude 50% that of the saturated response, and the sensitivity of the completely dark-adapted eye was taken as 1.0. An intensity-response relation was obtained for the completely dark-adapted eye. ERG's to constant test lights at various light intervals were obtained before and after a constant conditioning light stimulus of 1 s duration. Assuming that the intensity-response curves at any time are all parallel to that of the completely dark-adapted eye, one can then obtain a measurement of the change in sensitivity. In Fig. 2C, the relative sensitivity is plotted against the time after the end of the conditioning stimulus. The sensitivity is very low just after the conditioning stimulus, but increases rapidly beyond the dark-adapted level and then recovers gradually. The increase lasts for about 60 s after illumination. In fresh preparations, the maximum relative sensitivity was about 1.5–1.8, and occurred 3–5 s after illumination.

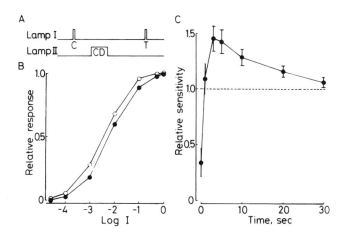

Fig. 2A–C. A Schematic drawing of the control stimulus (C) given by lamp I, conditioning stimulus (CD) given by lamp II and test stimulus (T) given by lamp I. **B** ERG intensity-response relations obtained during the dark (*closed circles*) and 5 s after (*open circles*) the cessation of a 1 s duration CD. The CD was the same throughout. The saturated value of the intensity-response curve for the dark-adapted eye is set at 1.0. The relative response to each light stimulus obtained from one experiment is plotted against the relative intensity. **C** Changes of sensitivity following a CD of 1 s duration. Relative sensitivity obtained from six experiments is plotted against time after the end of CD. *Vertical bars* indicate the size of the standard deviations. (Yamashita and Tateda 1982)

3.2 Loss of Hypersensitivity

The magnitude of the hypersensitivity appeared to decline with time following the removal of a small portion of the dorsal cuticle of the cephalothorax in physiological saline (Fig. 3). Two hours after the operation, hypersensitivity was clearly observed (maximum relative sensitivity = 1.5). Seven hours after the operation, there was a marked depression of hypersensitivity (maximum relative sensitivity = 1.1). At that time, however, the intensity-response curve for the dark-adapted eye was almost identical to that of the fresh preparation. Twenty hours after the operation, no hypersensitivity was observed. When the pedicel was transected and the abdomen was removed from the intact animal, loss of hypersensitivity occurred within a few minutes. Since the respiratory organs of the spiders are located in the abdomen, these observations suggest that respiration may be necessary for maintenance of hypersensitivity.

Since the jumping spiders *Menemerus* were too small (0.6–0.8 cm body length) to examine the effect of respiration on hypersensitivity, further experiments were done on orb weaving spiders *Argiope* of about 2.5 cm in body length. The anterior median eye of the orb weaving spider has three types of receptor cells, UV, blue, and green cells, and the green cells show a hypersensitivity (Yamashita and Tateda 1978). The pedicel of *Argiope* was constricted repeatedly by means of a V-shaped wire (Fig. 4A). Figure 4B shows the effect of pedicel constriction on the ERG response to a test light. The test light was presented to the eye 10 s after the conditioning stimulus. In unconstricted animals, the amplitude of the response to the control light is about 1.3 mV and that to the test light is about 1.6 mV. The response apparently increases after illumination. Five minutes after pedicel constriction, the amplitude of the response to the control light is about 1.1 mV and that to the test light is also about 1.1 mV. The increase in response following illumination apparently disappears. Five minutes after the release of the pedicel both the response to the control and test light recovered to the level observed in the normal preparation. Also, the response to the test light is apparently greater than to the control light. The effect of pedicel constriction was observed repeatedly. These results shows that respiration is necessary for maintenance of hypersensitivity.

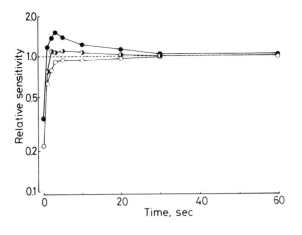

Fig. 3. Post-operative loss of hypersensitivity. Changes of sensitivity during dark adaptation were recorded 2 h (*closed circles*), 7 h (*half-closed circles*), and 20 h (*open circles*) following operation. Relative sensitivities are plotted against the time after the cessation of a 1 s CD. (Yamashita and Tateda 1976b)

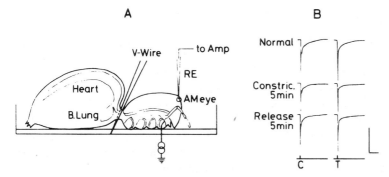

Fig. 4A, B. Effect of pedicel constriction on hypersensitivity. **A** Diagrammtic representation of the method of pedicel constriction and the recording method from the intact animal. B. Lung, book lung; V-wire, V-shaped wire for pedicel constriction; RE, recording electrode. **B** ERG's recorded from the anterior median eye before and after a CD. Traces at the *left* are ERG's of the dark-adapted eye following C (Fig. 2A). Traces at the *right* are ERG's of the same eye following T presented 10 s after the CD. Time after pedicel constriction and the time after release of the constriction are shown to the *left* of the figure. Calibrations: 1 mV, 0.5 s. (Yamashita and Tateda 1978)

3.3 Process of Hypersensitivity

The shape of the ERG during long term illumination of the normal eye of *Menemerus* was compared with that from the same eye following loss of hypersensitivity (Fig. 5). The ERG consists of a rapid initial phase followed by a slow phase. For the normal eye, the amplitude of the slow phase of the ERG increases a few seconds after the onset of illumination and continues to increase gradually (Fig. 5A). Hypersensitivity of this same eye was almost lost about 7 h after the removal of the cuticle. At that time, the increase of the slow phase as observed in the normal eye was also lost (Fig. 5B). Fifteen hours after the operation, the ERG itself became small (Fig. 5C). These results suggest that the light adaptation processes are different for the normal eye and the non-hypersensitive eye. The course of the light adaptation process was also studied together with the dark adaptation process (Fig. 6). In the normal eye, the sensitivity decreases rapidly, but then increases shortly after the onset of illumination. This increase is maintained throughout the course of the light adaptation. About 7 h after the operation, hyper-

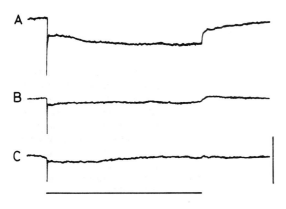

Fig. 5A–C. ERG's of the normal and non-hypersensitive eye elicited by illumination of 60-s duration. **A** Normal eye. **B** Seven hours after surgery. **C** About 15 h after surgery. Calibrations: 1 mV, 60 s. (Yamashita and Tateda 1976b)

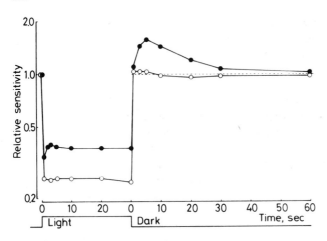

Fig. 6. Light and dark adaptation of the normal (*closed circles*) and non-hypersensitive eye (*open circles*). Relative sensitivity is plotted against time after the beginning and after the end of the 30-s CD. (Yamashita and Tateda 1976b)

sensitivity was markedly depressed. At that time the decrease of the sensitivity during light adaptation was greater than that in the normal eye, and the small increase following the onset of illumination was also lost. These data suggest that the process underlying hypersensitivity is initiated at the onset of illumination.

We assume that there are two antagonistic processes in the photoreceptors of the anterior median eye (Fig. 7). One process decreases the sensitivity during illumination (process I), the other process increases the sensitivity (process II). The hypothetical time course of these processes is shown in Fig. 7. We assume that a saturation of process II occurs more slowly than that of process I. If process I and II summate, the light and the dark adaptation process may follow a third time course (process III). The actual time course for light and/or dark adaptation in the normal eye (closed circles in Figs. 2, 3, 6) may correspond to the time course for process III.

Process I is similar to the light and dark adaptation process of the ordinary photoreceptors. Therefore, it may be related to the photochemical cycle or to the electrical properties of the membrane. On the other hand, process II may be related to the ionic concentration of the saline, since calcium ions are important in controlling the sensitivity of photoreceptors in other arthropods (Lisman and Brown 1972, 1975; Brown and Lisman 1972, 1975; Brown and Blinks 1974; Fein and Lisman 1975; Bader et al. 1976;

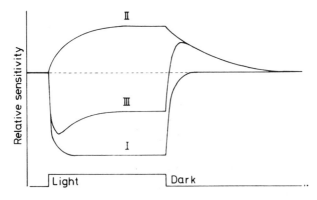

Fig. 7. Hypothetical time courses of process *I, II,* and *III*. Process *I*, the decrease of sensitivity during illumination. Process *II*, the increase of sensitivity during illumination. Process *III*, the summation sensitivity of the two processes. The light and dark adaptation process may have the same time course as process *III*. (Yamashita and Tateda 1976b)

Hanani and Hillman 1976; Fein and Charlton 1977; Brown et al. 1977; Lisman and Strong 1979). In the following sections, the effects of the four major cations on hypersensitivity will be reported.

3.4 Effects of Cations on Hypersensitivity

3.4.1 Sodium and Potassium Ions

ERG light responses before and 5 s, 10 s, and 30 s after a constant conditioning stimulus were obtained in normal and in low-Na^+ saline (Fig. 8). In normal saline (220 mM-Na^+) and in 112 mM-Na^+ saline, the amplitude of the responses increased after the conditioning stimulus. In 46 mM-Na^+ saline, the response showed little increase after the conditioning stimulus, and in 3 mM-Na^+ saline, it markedly decreased.

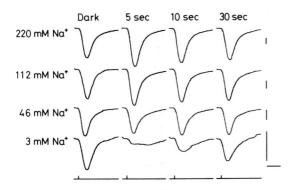

Fig. 8. Effects of decreased sodium concentration of the external saline on ERG light responses before and after a CD of 1 s duration. C (Fig. 2A) was presented to the dark-adapted eye and T was presented, 5, 10, and 30 s after the end of CD. Calibrations: 150 μV, 0.1 s. (Yamashita and Tateda 1982)

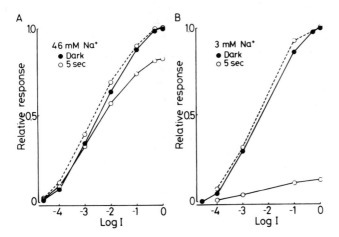

Fig. 9A,B. Effects of reducing Na^+ from the perfusate on ERG intensity-response relations. The curves for the dark-adapted eye (*closed circles*) and for the eye 5 s after the end of a CD of 1 s duration (*open circles*) were obtained in 46 mM-Na^+ saline (A) and in 3 mM-Na^+ saline (B). In both A and B, *solid lines* were drawn relative to the saturated value for the dark-adapted eye. *Dashed curves* were normalized to the saturated value after the end of CD. (Yamashita and Tateda 1982)

In 46 mM and in 3 mM-Na⁺ saline, the intensity-response function for the dark-adapted eye and that for the eye 5 s after the cessation of the conditioning stimulus show that the saturated values markedly decreased after illumination compared with those before illumination (Fig. 9). Note that sensitivities increased after the conditioning stimulus at both reduced Na⁺ levels. The relative sensitivity 5 s after conditioning was 1.51 in 46 mM-Na⁺ saline and 1.31 in 3 mM-Na⁺ saline. These values were approximately the same as those in normal saline (cf. Fig. 2).

In 112 mM-Na⁺ saline both the intensity-response curve during the dark and the change in sensitivity after illumination were almost identical with those in normal saline (Fig. 10). Therefore, it is unlikely that Na⁺ plays a significant role in the hypersensitiv-

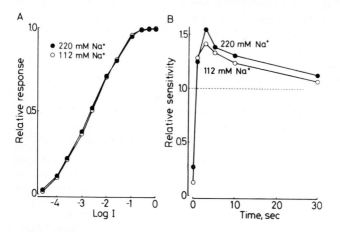

Fig. 10A,B. Effects of reducing Na⁺ from the perfusate on **A** normalized ERG intensity-response curves for the dark-adapted eye and **B** changes in sensitivity after a CD of 1-s duration obtained in normal saline containing 220 mM-Na⁺ (*closed circles*) and in 112 mM-Na⁺ saline (*open circles*). (Yamashita and Tateda 1982)

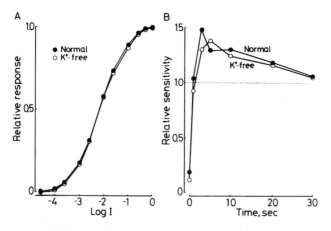

Fig. 11A,B. Effects of reducing K⁺ from the perfusate on **A** normalized ERG intensity-response curves for the dark-adapted eye and **B** changes in sensitivity after a CD obtained in normal saline (*closed circles*) and in K⁺-free saline (*open circles*). (Yamashita and Tateda 1982)

ity. The role of Na^+ in regulating the saturated value of the ERG after the conditioning illumination was not investigated.

In K^+-free saline, the dark-adapted intensity-response curve and the change in sensitivity after illumination were about the same as with those in normal saline (Fig. 11). Therefore, it is unlikely too that K^+ plays a significant role in the hypersensitivity.

3.4.2 Calcium Ions

In contrast, Ca^{2+} had marked effects on the hypersensitivity. Figure 12 shows the effects of changes in external Ca^{2+} concentration on ERG light responses to control light (C) presented to the completely dark-adapted eye, and test light (T) presented 5 s after the onset of a conditioning stimulus (T_1) and 5 s after the cessation of the conditioning stimulus (T_2). The amplitudes of the responses to C, T_1, and T_2 are given in Table 1.

Changes in external Ca^{2+} concentration had a small effect on light responses during the completely dark-adapted state, but a large effect during and after illumination. The intensity-response curves show that the sensitivity of the dark-adapted eye was somewhat greater in low-Ca^{2+} saline, and somewhat lower in high-Ca^{2+} saline (Fig. 13A). Hypersensitivity after illumination markedly increased to a maximum of about 2.0 in low-Ca^{2+} saline and markedly decreased to about 1.1 in high-Ca^{2+} saline (Fig. 13B). Maximum sensitivity was about 1.5 in normal saline. These results show that external Ca^{2+} plays an important role in determining the sensitivity of the eye especially during and after illumination.

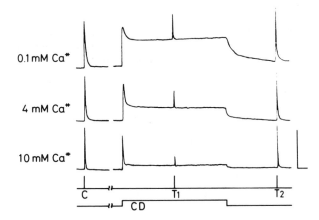

0.1 mM Ca*

4 mM Ca*

10 mM Ca*

C   T₁   T₂

CD

Fig. 12. Effects of changes in external Ca^{2+} concentration on ERG light responses obtained in 4 mM-Ca^{2+} (normal), 0.1 mM-Ca^{2+}, and 10 mM-Ca^{2+} saline. C was given to the completely dark-adapted eye. T_1 was presented 5 s after the onset of a CD, and T_2 5 s after the cessation of the CD. Calibrations: 1 mV, 1 s. (Yamashita and Tateda 1982)

Table 1. Effects of Ca^{2+} on ERG amplitude (mV)

Perfusate/stimulus	C	T_1	T_2
0.1 mM-Ca^{2+} saline	1.24	0.68	1.48
4 mM-Ca^{2+} saline	1.20	0.44	1.33
10 mM-Ca^{2+} saline	1.11	0.23	1.13

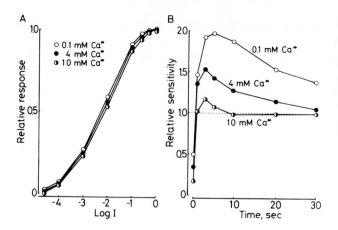

Fig. 13A,B. Effects of Ca^{2+} concentration on A normalized ERG intensity-response curves for the dark-adapted eye and B changes in sensitivities after a CD obtained in 4 mM-Ca^{2+} (normal), 0.1 mM-Ca^{2+}, and 10 mM-Ca^{2+} saline. (Yamashita and Tateda 1982)

3.4.3 Magnesium Ions

Intensity-response relations during the dark (Fig. 14A) and the changes in sensitivities after illumination (Fig. 14B) obtained with normal and Mg^{2+}-free saline show that Mg^{2+} had no effect in the dark-adapted eye. Mg^{2+}, however, had a marked effect on hypersensitivity. In normal saline, maximum sensitivity after illumination was about 1.4 but in Mg^{2+}-free saline, it was only about 1.05. These results show that Mg^{2+} is necessary for maintenance of hypersensitivity in the *Menemerus* eye.

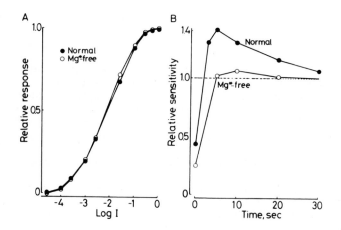

Fig. 14A,B. Effects of reducing Mg^{2+} from the perfusate on A normalized ERG intensity-response curves for the dark-adapted eye and B changes in sensitivities after a CD obtained in normal saline (*closed circles*) and in Mg^{2+}-free saline (*open circles*). (Yamashita and Tateda 1982)

4 Discussion

As susggested in the present report, there are two antagonistic processes in the photoreceptors. One process decreases the sensitivity during illumination (process I) and the other increases the sensitivity (process II). Respiration was necessary to maintain hypersensitivity. This suggests that process II may be related to an active mechanism. Brown and Lisman (1972) showed the existence of an electrogenic sodium pump in the ventral photoreceptors of *Limulus*. They concluded that an electrogenic sodium pump generates the hyperpolarization following illumination. In the photoreceptors of the anterior median eye of the jumping spider, however, after-hyperpolarization did not occur (Yamashita and Tateda 1976a). Moreover, if there is an electrogenic sodium pump, it must be activated by external potassium ions, since hyperpolarization is abolished by removal of external potassium ions (Brown and Lisman 1972). In the jumping spider, however, hypersensitivity occurred even in potassium-free saline. Therefore, hypersensitivity cannot be explained by a sodium pump.

On the other hand, Ca^{2+} plays important role in controlling sensitivity of invertebrate photoreceptors (see Introduction). As shown in the present report, sensitivity of the spider antero-median eye was also greatly affected by Ca^{2+}. When the external Ca^{2+} concentration is low, the sensitivity of the dark-adapted eye increases a little and hypersensitivity after illumination markedly increases. The hypersensitivity phenomenon in spider eye may be explained by the following hypothesis. A light-dependent Ca^{2+}-pump which may be related to process II is present in the photoreceptors. Efflux of Ca^{2+} from the photoreceptors mediated by the light-dependent Ca^{2+}-pump is greater than influx of Ca^{2+} during illumination. The resulting decrease of intracellular Ca^{2+} concentration may continue for a short period after the cessation of illumination. As a result, the sensitivity of the photoreceptors after illumination may increase for a short period. When the external Ca^{2+} concentration is high, or Mg^{2+} concentration is low, influx of Ca^{2+} may be greater and/or the Ca^{2+}-pump may be less activated than in normal saline.

References

Bader CR, Baumann F, Bertrand D (1976) Role of intracellular calcium and sodium in light adaptation in the retina of the honey bee drone (*Apis mellifera* L.). J Gen Physiol 67:475–491

Brown JE, Blinks JR (1974) Changes in intracellular free calcium concentration during illumination of invertebrate photoreceptors: detection with aequorin. J Gen Physiol 64:643–665

Brown JE, Brown PK, Pinto LH (1977) Detection of light-induced changes of intracellular ionized calcium concentration in *Limulus* ventral photoreceptors using arsenazo III. J Physiol (Lond) 267:299–320

Brown JE, Lisman JE (1972) An electrogenic sodium pump in *Limulus* ventral photoreceptor cells. J Gen Physiol 59:720–733

Brown JE, Lisman JE (1975) Intracellular Ca modulates sensitivity and time scale in *Limulus* ventral photoreceptors. Nature (Lond) 258:252–253

Fein A, Charlton JS (1977) A quantitative comparison of the effects of intracellular calcium injection and light adaptation on the photoresponse of *Limulus* ventral photoreceptors. J Gen Physiol 70:591–600

Fein A, Lisman J (1975) Localized desensitization of *Limulus* photoreceptors produced by light or intracellular calcium ion injection. Sciences (NY) 187:1094–1096

Hanani M, Hillman P (1976) Adaptation and facilitation in the barnacle photoreceptor. J Gen Physiol 67:235–249

Lisman JE, Brown JE (1972) The effects of intracellular iontophoretic injection of calcium and sodium ions on the light response of *Limulus* ventral photoreceptors. J Gen Physiol 59:701–719

Lisman JE, Brown JE (1975) Effects of intracellular injection of calcium buffers on light adaptation in *Limulus* ventral photoreceptors. J Gen Physiol 66:489–506

Lisman JE, Strong JA (1979) The initiation of excitation and light adaptation in *Limulus* ventral photoreceptors. J Gen Physiol 73:219–243

Rathmayer W (1965) Neuromuscular transmission in a spider and the effect of calcium. Comp Biochem Physiol 14:673–687

Yamashita S, Tateda H (1976a) Spectral sensitivities of jumping spider eyes. J Comp Physiol 105: 29–41

Yamashita S, Tateda H (1976b) Hypersensitivity in the anterior median eye of a jumping spider. J Exp Biol 65:507–516

Yamashita S, Tateda H (1978) Spectral sensitivities of the anterior median eyes of the orb web spiders, *Argiope bruennichii* and *A. amoena*. J Exp Biol 74:47–57

Yamashita S, Tateda H (1982) Importance of calcium and magnesium ions for postexcitatory hypersensitivity in the jumping spider (*Menemerus*) eye. J Exp Biol 97:187–195

Sensitizing Pigments and Their Significance for Vision

K. KIRSCHFELD[1]

1 Introduction

The primary process induced by absorption of a quantum of light in a visual pigment molecule is the isomerization of the chromophore retinaldehyde from the all-cis to the all-trans form (Wald 1968). I will show here that besides this direct interaction between light and visual pigment another process can take place: the light quantum can be absorbed by an accessory pigment which then transfers energy to the normal, Schiff-base linked chromophore of the visual pigment, which then will be isomerized. The photostable, accessory pigment therefore is acting as a sensitizing pigment. We have investigated the process of sensitization in some detail in the most common type of receptor of the fly (type R1-6); we show, however, that sensitization of visual pigments is realized in other types of receptors of the fly and in many other insect species as well.

2 Fly Photoreceptors Type R1-6

In the compound eye of the fly six of the eight receptor cells called R1-6 have a receptor potential action spectrum with two maxima: one close to 500 nm, the other, usually still higher one, in the near ultraviolet, close to 350 nm (Burkhardt 1962; Horridge and Mimura 1975). Dual peak sensitivity of this type cannot be explained on the basis of extinction spectra of known visual pigments. These pigments have only a small peak (β-peak) at shorter wavelengths, in the order of 25% of the maximum. For long time this dual peak spectral sensitivity was a matter of debate. Suggested explanations have included: two different pigments in one and the same photoreceptor (Horridge and Mimura 1975; Rosner 1975), waveguide effects that can selectively enhance short wave-lenght extinction of light (Snyder and Pask 1973) or electrical coupling of receptors with different spectral sensitivities. More recently it has been suggested, that the high UV sensitivity might be due to an unusually enhanced β-peak of the visual pigment (Paulsen and Schwemer 1979).

With electrophysiological techniques it can be excluded that there is substantial coupling between photoreceptors with different spectral sensitivities and, as I have discussed already earlier (Kirschfeld 1979), older experiments in which the spectral sensitiv-

1 Max-Planck-Institut für Biologische Kybernetik, Spemannstr. 38, 7400 Tübingen, FRG

Neurobiology
(ed. by R. Gilles and J. Balthazart)
© Springer-Verlag Berlin Heidelberg 1985

ity of white eyed mutants was measured by means of the ERG exclude the waveguide concept as a possible explanation. The following experiments show also that the two pigment as well as the enhanced β-peak hypotheses cannot explain the high UV-sensitivity in the photoreceptors of the fly.

3 Microspectrophotometry

A direct method of investigating visual pigments is by means of microspectrophotometry. In Musca photoreceptors R1-6, a difference spectrum can be measured which has a minimum at 470 nm, an isosbestic point at 510 nm and a maximum at 570 nm (Fig. 1). This difference spectrum is similar to that measured in *Calliphora* (Hamdorf et al. 1973; Stavenga et al. 1973) and corresponds to a visual pigment with maximal absorption at 490 nm and a metapigment with an absorption maximum at 580 nm.

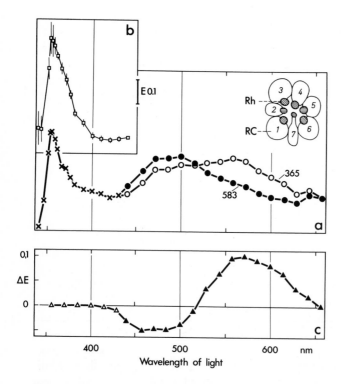

Fig. 1. a Extinction spectrum of rhabdomeres type R1-6 of *Musca* as measured in a microspectrophotometer. At regular intervals during the measurement the preparation was illuminated with either strong orange (λ = 583 nm) light, in order to shift most of the pigment into the xanthopsin state, or with ultraviolet (λ = 365 nm) light, in order to shift some xanthopsin into metaxanthopsin. *Inset* Cross-section through ommatidium indicating receptor cells *RC* and rhabdomeres *Rh*. b Mean extinction spectrum in the ultraviolet of 6 ommatidia. c Difference spectrum of a. (After Kirschfeld et al. 1977)

It is possible to show: (1) that UV-light creates the same metapigment as blue light; (2) that there is, nevertheless, no significant decrease of extinction in the UV, and (3) that instead a conspicuous decrease in extinction in the blue can be observed. These observations together with the fact that in the absolute extinction spectrum there is stable high extinction in the UV (Fig. 1) led to the concept that there could be an energy transfer from a photostable, UV-absorbing pigment onto the blue-absorbing visual pigment. This sensitizing pigment hypothesis can be formulated as follows:

$$X \ \ + h\nu \ \rightarrow X^*$$
$$X^* + P \ \ \rightarrow P^* + X$$
$$P^* \ \ \ \ \ \ \rightarrow M$$

X is the sensitizing pigment, X^* its activated state, P, P^* are the visual pigment and its activated state, respectively, and M is the visual pigment in the metastate (Kirschfeld et al. 1977). In the meantime we have collected a variety of experimental evidence that unanimously supports the sensitizing pigment hypothesis.

4 Further Evidence for a Sensitizing Function

Flies reared on a vit. A-deprived diet lose absolute sensitivity, which indicates that vit. A or a derivative might be essential for their visual pigment (Goldsmith et al. 1964; Stark et al. 1976). Unexpectedly, however, the loss in sensitivity in the UV is much stronger than in the visible. This is not to be expected if the sensitivity in the UV and visible is due to a single pigment. The sensitizing pigment concept, however, allows an easy explanation of this finding: the sensitizing pigment in conditions of vitamin A deprivation is no longer present or at least not capable of transfering energy.

The photoreceptors R1-6 exhibit polarization sensitivity (PS), however, only in the visible and not in the UV (Hardie 1978; Guo 1981). Presumably the dipoles, responsible for UV sensitivity, are aligned in a different way compared to the normal chromophores of the visual pigment. If we measure the polarization sensitivity in the UV in receptors of vit. A-deprived flies we expect again polarization sensitivity, since now the β-band absorption should be responsible for the remaining UV sensitivity. That this is actually the case is illustrated in Fig. 2. We can conclude from these results that the visual pigment in fly rhabdomeres is quite normal with respect to the height of the β-band absorption, and hence that an unusual β-band is not the explanation for the high UV sensitivity (Vogt and Kirschfeld 1983a).

A prediction from the sensitizing pigment concept is that energy transfer from the sensitizing pigment is to be expected not only onto the visual pigment but also onto the metapigment. This follows at least if we assume that the energy transfer occurs according to Förster's (1951) theory: the fluorescence spectrum of the sensitizing pigment should overlap not only with the visual pigment but also with the metapigment absorption spectrum because both are close together on the wavelength scale (Minke and Kirschfeld 1979). This prediction has been confirmed by determining the photosensitivity spectrum of the metapigment which also has a high UV maximum.

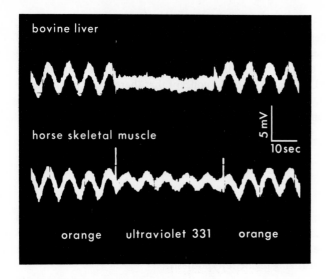

Fig. 2. Response of receptor cells of type R1-6 to light delivered through a continuously rotating polarization filter. First orange light was applied and then the colour was switched to UV light, adjusted in intensity to evoke approx. the same mean response. Then again orange light was applied. While there is no modulation during UV in the fly raised on bovine liver (*upper trace*), a response to the angle of the e-vector of the light is obvious in the carotenoid deprived fly, raised on horse skeletal muscle. (Vogt and Kirschfeld 1983a)

The quantum efficiency of energy transfer to the visual pigment was estimated by electrophysiological methods (Vogt and Kirschfeld 1982). The remarkable high value of $\geqslant 0.8$ infers a distance of less than 25 Å between the sensitizing pigment and the normal chromophore, a distance considerably smaller than the diameter of the visual pigment (Vogt and Kirschfeld 1983a, see Fig. 6a).

A different kind of support for the sensitizing pigment concept comes from experiments that have been performed in order to evaluate the chemical identity of the sensitizing pigment as described below.

5 A New Chromophore in Fly Photoreceptors

In order to identify the sensitizing pigment Vogt (1983) prepared extracts of retinae from compound eyes of flies. In these extracts he was unable to find any retinal but, instead, a more polar aldehyde. Several lines of evidence discussed in the original paper led to the conclusion, that his molecule must be the chromophoric group of the visual pigment. This means, however, that the visual pigment in flies cannot be a rhodopsin which should have retinal as chromophore. Because the precursors of this new chromophore are most likely hydroxy-xanthophylls, Vogt proposed the name "Xanthopsin" for the visual pigment. More detailed biochemical analysis has shown that the chromophore is 3-hydroxyretinal (Fig. 3; Vogt and Kirschfeld 1984).

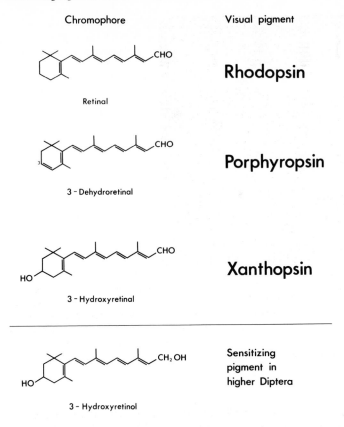

Fig. 3. Chemical structure of visual and sensitizing pigments

6 The Sensitizing Pigment in Fly Photoreceptors: 3-Hydroxyretinol

In order to recognize the sensitizing pigment spectrophotometrically a finding by Gemperlein et al. (1980) was important. These authors developed a special method (Fourier spectroscopy) that allows spectral sensitivity to be rapidly measured with high spectral resolution. They found that the UV peak in *Calliphora* exhibits a vibrational fine structure with peaks at 332, 350, and 369 nm. We improved our microspectrophotometer for better spectral resolution and were able to measure the same vibrational fine structure in the UV of extinction spectra in individual rhabdomeres of receptors R1-6. If flies are reared on a vit. A-deprived diet, however, extinction in the UV can no longer be detected (Fig. 4): the substance that exhibits the UV-extinction must be the sensitizing pigment and, in the diet-flies, the substance obviously is no longer present in the rhabdomeres (Kirschfeld et al. 1983). Parallel to this observation thin layer chromatography analysis has shown that there is, besides the 3-hydroxyaldehyde which represents the normal chromophore of the visual pigment, a still more polar compound exhibiting strong fluorescence. This compound is also considerably reduced in flies grown on a vit. A deprived diet and therefore fulfills one of the prerequisites of the sensitizing pig-

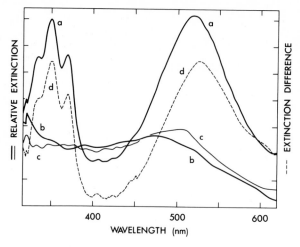

Fig. 4. Extinction spectra of receptors type R1-6 from *Musca*; *a* fly grown on normal diet; *b, c* two spectra from two different flies, grown on a carotenoid deprived medium; *d* difference between *a* and *c*. (Kirschfeld et al. 1983)

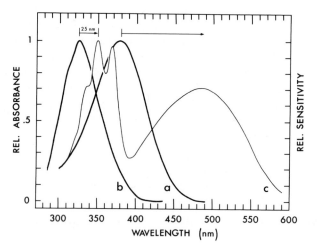

Fig. 5. Absorbance spectra of the fly chromophore aldehyde (*a*) and alcohol (*b*). The *thin line* (*c*) represents the spectral sensitivity of the most common fly photoreceptor (R1-6). (Vogt and Kirschfeld 1984)

ment. This compound was shown to be 3-hydroxy retinol (Fig. 3; Vogt and Kirschfeld 1984).

At first sight, however, it seemed unlikely, that this alcohol could represent the sensitizing pigment because the peak absorbance of 3-hydroxyretinol is at 325 nm and has no vibrational fine structure (Fig. 5). This discrepancy may be explained, however, by analogy with retinol: if, in retinol, the ionon ring is fixed relative to the side chain at the C6-C7 bond and approximately coplanar, then a shift of the extinction maximum of some 25 nm and a fine structure become obvious (Ong and Chytil 1978). Such a fixation and coplanarity can be achieved either by a retro structure (C6 = C7 double bond) or by binding of retinol to a protein. For reasons discussed in detail in the original paper, we suggest a structure of the visual pigment complex as drawn in Fig. 6a (Vogt and Kirschfeld 1984).

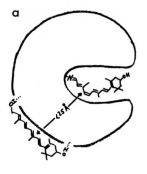 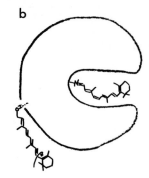

Fig. 6a,b. Suggested composition of the visual pigment complex within the photoreceptors in higher diptera (a according to Vogt and Kirschfeld 1984) and in *Simuliids* (b according to Kirschfeld and Vogt, in prep.)

7 Other Photoreceptors in the Fly with a Sensitizing Pigment

The most common type of photoreceptor in the fly's eye is the type called R1-6. These receptors, though anatomically distinct, all have the same spectral sensitivity, and as we have seen, a sensitizing pigment. Besides the 6 receptors R1-6, there are two more receptors in each ommatidium, called R7 and R8. These receptors are not a homogeneous population: in the dorsal marginal eye region they are anatomically distinct from normal R7 and R8, and even in the regular ommatidia, in which they look structurally rather similar, they are functionally different. Finally, the ocellar receptors have to be taken into account. As can be seen from Table 1, most of these receptors (11 out of 15)

Table 1. Musca photoreceptors

Receptor type	Anatomical location	UV sensitizing pigment	Visual pigment λ_{max} (nm)	Remarks	
R1-6	Regular and marginal ommatidia	+	490	a	specialized for high absolute sensitivity
R7y	In 2/3 of the regular ommatidia statistically distributed	+	430	b	
R7p	In 1/3 of the regular ommatidia	–	335	c	
R7r	"Love spot" of males	+	490	d	
R8y	As R7y	+	515	e	
R8p	As R7p	–	460	f	
R8r	"Love spot" of males	+	490	g	
R7marg	Dorsal marginal eye region	–	335 ⎫		specialized for high polarization sensitivity
R8marg	As R7m	–	335 ⎭	h	
Ocelli receptors	Ocelli	+	430	i	

References: (a) Kirschfeld et al. 1977, 1983; (b) Hardie et al. 1979; Hardie and Kirschfeld 1983; (c) Hardie and Kirschfeld 1983; (d) Franceschini et al. 1981; Hardie et al. 1981; (e), (f) as (c); (g) Hardie et al. 1981; (h) Hardie 1984; (i) Kirschfeld and Vogt, in prep

have a UV-sensitizing pigment as characterized from the vibrational fine structure in the UV. In the case of R7y it was shown also with MSP, that the isomerisable pigment has $\lambda_{max} \approx 430\,nm$ (Kirschfeld, Hardie and Vogt, in prep.).

8 Evolutionary Aspects

The existence of an up to now unknown visual pigment in flies leads to the question where else in the animal kingdom can this pigment be found. It turns out that, in insects, groups such as Caelifera, Heteroptera, Coleoptera, and Hymenoptera have retinal, whereas groups as Lepidoptera and Diptera have 3-hydroxyretinal (Vogt 1984a). This result is in favour of the view that the new chromophore has a monophyletic origin, and has been "invented" only once, some 300 million years ago, during the Carboniferous. Because of its monophyletic origin the chromophore can be used as an indicator for phylogenetical relationships. For instance the presence of retinal or 3-hydroxyretinal, respectively, favours the view that Neuropteroidea and Mecopteroidea together are a monophyletic group. This is against the view favoured today (Fig. 7), but corresponds to older family trees (see e.g. Ross 1965).

The next obvious question concerns the problem of which insect groups have a sensitizing pigment. In order to get an easy check we developed an experimental setup similar to that of Gemperlein et al. (1980) that allows a fast registration of spectral sensitivity with high spectral resolution (Kirschfeld and Vogt, in prep.). The outcome of the comparative study (Vogt and Kirschfeld, in prep) is: (1) the insect groups with rhodopsin never have UV-sensitivity with the vibrational fine structure. (2) In the groups with *xanthopsin* there are two different cases: either there is UV-sensitivity with vibrational fine structure, indicative of a sensitizing function, or any UV-vibrational fine structure is lacking. Actually, the higher diptera such as Bibioniformia, Empidiformia, Acalyptratae, and Calyptratae have a vibrational fine structure, whereas the more primitive diptera such as Tipuloidea and the Lepidoptera do not (examples in Fig. 8).

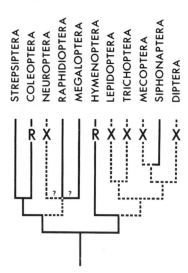

Fig. 7. Family tree of holometabolic insects according to Kristensen (1975). The letters R and X indicate in which orders rhodopsin or xanthopsin was found, respectively. (After Vogt 1984b)

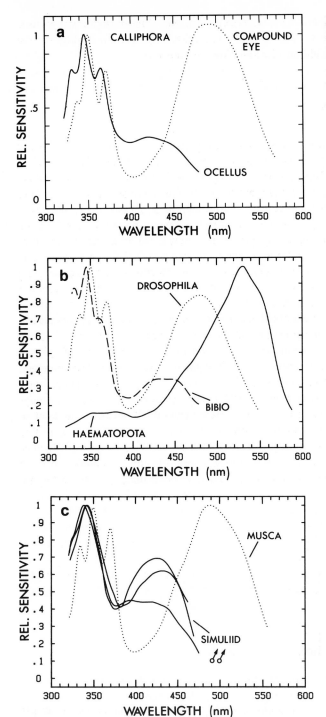

Fig. 8a–c. a Spectral sensitivity of the compound eye of *Calliphora* and of the ocellus. Data from white-eyed mutant. (Kirschfeld and Vogt, in prep.) **b** Spectral sensitivity of *Drosophila* compound eye (white-eyed mutant), of the dorsal eye of Bibio male and of the tabanid Haematopota compound eye. (Vogt and Kirschfeld, in prep.) **c** Spectral sensitivity of *Musca* compound eye (white-eyed mutant) and of the dorsal eye of three different *Simuliid* males. (Kirschfeld and Vogt, in prep.)

They lack a sensitizing pigment. This result indicates that in order to exhibit a vibrational fine structure, the sensitizing pigment seems to need the second OH-group at the iononring: only then there is a fixation of the C6-C7 double bond, as indicated in Fig. 6a (Vogt and Kirschfeld, in prep.). A further conclusion from this study is that it took some 80 million years after the occurence of xanthopsin until the sensitizing pigment was "invented".

9 Is 3-Hydroxyretinol the Only Sensitizing Pigment?

In most cases one of the characteristic properties of spectral sensitivity in photoreceptors with a sensitizing pigment is high sensitivity in the UV combined with a second peak, or at least a shoulder, at longer wavelengths. During the measurements we found one group of flies — *Simuliids* — which also have this general property. However, the UV sensitivity in *Simuliids* is unusual: (1) It does not show the vibrational fine structure but only one maximum and (2) this maximum is shifted significantly to shorter wavelengths, i.e. at 340 instead at 350 nm (Fig. 8c). Several observations are indicative of a UV-sensitizing pigment combined with a visual pigment of $\lambda_{max} \approx 430$ nm: there is a considerable variability between the heights of the two peaks (as if the diet of the individuals had been different) and, furthermore, it is not possible to modify the relative heights of both peaks by means of selective chromatic adaptation.

We analyzed the visual pigment in the rhabdomeres by means of microspectrophotometry and found, indeed, an isomerisable visual pigment with $\lambda_{max} \approx 430$ nm which fits with the position of the peak of sensitivity in the visible, the metapigment has a $\lambda_{max} \approx 510$ nm (Kirschfeld and Vogt, in prep.). The situation insofar is quite similar to that in receptors R1-6. However, why is there no vibrational fine structure as in all other sensitizing pigments analyzed up to now?

A possible explanation comes from the biochemical analysis of heads of *Simuliid* flies. Here we found – the only exception in diptera up to now – retinal instead of 3-hydroxyretinal (Vogt and Kirschfeld, in prep.). If our explanation of the UV-vibrational fine structure is correct, namely that it depends upon the fixation of the C6-C7 double bond due to two hydrogen bonds (Fig. 6a), then we do not expect such a vibrational fine structure in the *Simuliids*, because the second hydrogen bond, responsible for the fixation of the C6-C7 bond in the other flies is lacking (Fig. 6b). If retinol is the sensitizing pigment then the spectral sensitivity in the UV should be similar to the absorption spectrum of retinol in solution, which it actually is. These data suggest that not only can 3-hydroxyretinol act as a sensitizing pigment, but that there is still at least one other molecule, which is most likely retinol.

10 Functional Consequences of Sensitization

Highly evolved photoreceptors should absorb light with a high probability. This can be important for an animal for several reasons: in order to allow vision at low ambient intensities where only a few quanta are available, or, when the animal has to detect small optical signals (small modulation of intensity) in a short time. The detection of such signals can be a problem even in bright light because the light quantum noise must be smaller than the signal. The only way to achieve a low quantum noise is to absorb many quanta per unit time. Normally the absorption probability in photoreceptors is limited by membrane density, visual pigment concentration and length of the absorbing photoreceptor organelle. One of the functional consequences of sensitizing pigments is that this limitation may be overcome: The advantage of a sensitizing pigment is that the sensitizing molecules need not to be large since they do not directly mediate transduction and hence can be incorporated into the photoreceptor membranes in addition to the visual pigment without demanding much space.

Another functional consequence of sensitizing pigments is that in principle they may extend the spectral range over which the receptor is sensitive. That is, besides the gain in number of collected quanta, also patterns can be seen (e.g. structures visible in the ultraviolet spectral range only), that otherwise would be undetectable.

Finally, sensitizing pigments can be a means to overcome the problem of photooxidation in photoreceptors. Light is capable of destroying cells or their components by photooxidation, and it is especially light of short wavelengths that is dangerous. The dipteran photoreceptors called R7y illustrate one possibility of how this problem can be overcome: In these cells there is a UV-sensitizing pigment that sensitizes a 430 nm xanthopsin (Hardie and Kirschfeld 1983; Table 1). This blue absorbing visual pigment itself is protected from direct access of light by means of a C_{40}-carotenoid that acts as a blue absorbing light filter (Kirschfeld et al. 1978). The C_{40}-carotenoid has been identified as zeaxanthin (Vogt and Kirschfeld 1983b). By this means a UV-sensitive photoreceptor is created, in which parts of the energy of the UV-quanta is dissipated as heat during the energy transfer to the normal chromophore. The C_{40}-carotenoid in addition most likely acts as a "quencher" for dangerous activated states of molecules. The complex setup leads to a receptor that is extremely resistant against short wavelength irradiation (Kirschfeld 1982; Zhu and Kirschfeld 1984).

It is surprising that sensitization of visual pigment which is so common amongst insects has not yet been described in vertebrates. When it became clear that the sensitizing pigment in fly photoreceptors type R1-6 is 4-hydroxyretinol we thought that the reason might be that vertebrates do not have 3-hydroxyretinol and 3-hydroxyretinal, which could have been a prerequisite for sensitization. Since the *Simuliids* also lack these chromophores but nevertheless have a sensitizing pigment, it appears, in principle, that animals with rhodopsin or porphyropsins could also use sensitization as an improvement of their photoreceptors.

Acknowledgement. I thank Dr. R. Hardie and Dr. K. Vogt for discussion and reading the manuscript.

References

Burkhardt D (1962) Spectral sensitivity and other response characteristics of single visual cells in the arthropod eye. Symp Soc Exp Biol 16:86–109

Förster T (1951) Fluoreszenz organischer Verbindungen. Vandenhoeck und Ruprecht, Göttingen

Franceschini N, Kirschfeld K, Minke B (1981) Fluorescence of photoreceptor cells observed in vivo. Science (Wash DC) 213:1264–1267

Gemperlein R, Paul R, Lindauer E, Steiner A (1980) UV fine structure of the spectral sensitivity of flies visual cells. Naturwissenschaften 67:565–566

Goldsmith TH, Barker RJ, Cohen CF (1964) Sensitivity of visual receptors of carotenoid-depleted flies: a vitamin A deficiency in an invertebrate. Science (Wash DC) 146:65–67

Guo AK (1981) Elektrophysiologische Untersuchungen zur Spektral- und Polarisations-Empfindlichkeit der Sehzellen von *Calliphora erythrocephala* III. Scientia Sinica XXIV:272–286

Hamdorf K, Paulsen R, Schwemer J (1973) Photoregeneration and sensitivity control of photoreceptors of invertebrates. In: Langer H (ed) Biochemistry and physiology of visual pigments. Springer, Berlin Heidelberg New York, pp 155–166

Hardie RC (1978) Peripheral visual function in the fly. Ph.D. Thesis, ANU Canberra

Hardie RC (1984) Properties of photoreceptors R7 and R8 in dorsal marginal ommatidia in the compound eyes of *Musca* and *Calliphora*. J Comp Physiol A Sens Neural Behav Physiol 154: 157–165

Hardie RC, Kirschfeld K (1983) Ultraviolet sensitivity of fly photoreceptors R7 and R8: evidence for a sensitising function. Biophys Struct Mech 9:171–180

Hardie RC, Franceschini N, McIntyre PD (1979) Electrophysiological analysis of fly retina II. Spectral and polarisation sensitivity in R7 and R8. J Comp Physiol 133:23–39

Hardie RC, Franceschini N, Ribi W, Kirschfeld K (1981) Distribution and properties of sex-specific photoreceptors in the fly *Musca domestica*. J Comp Physiol 145:139–152

Horridge GA, Mimura K (1975) Fly photoreceptors I. Physical separation of two visual pigments in *Calliphora* retinula cells 1–6. Proc R Soc Lond B Biol Sci 190:211–224

Kirschfeld K (1979) The function of photostable pigments in fly photoreceptors. Biophys Struct Mech 5:117–128

Kirschfeld K (1982) Carotenoid pigments: their possible role in protecting against photooxidation in eyes and photoreceptor cells. Proc R Soc Lond B Biol Sci 216:71–85

Kirschfeld K, Franceschini N, Minke B (1977) Evidence for a sensitising pigment in fly photoreceptors. Nature (Lond) 269:386–390

Kirschfeld K, Feiler R, Franceschini N (1978) A photostable pigment within the rhabdomere of fly photoreceptors no 7. J Comp Physiol 125:275–284

Kirschfeld K, Feiler R, Hardie R, Vogt K, Franceschini N (1983) The sensitizing pigment in fly photoreceptors. Properties and candidates. Biophys Struct Mech 10:81–92

Kristensen N (1975) The phylogeny of hexapod "orders". A critical review of recent accounts. Z Zool Syst Evolutionsforsch 13:1–44

Minke B, Kirschfeld K (1979) The contribution of a sensitizing pigment to the photosensitivity spectra of fly rhodopsin and metarhodopsin. J Gen Physiol 73:517–540

Ong DE, Chytil F (1978) Cellular retinol-binding protein from rat liver. J Biol Chem 253:828–832

Paulsen R, Schwemer J (1979) Vitamin a deficiency reduces the concentration of visual pigment protein within blowfly photoreceptor membranes. Biochim Biophys Acta 557:385–390

Rosner G (1975) Adaptation und Photoregeneration im Fliegenauge. J Comp Physiol 102:269–295

Ross HH (1965) A textbook of entomology, 3rd edn. Wiley, New York

Snyder AW, Pask C (1973) Spectral sensitivity of dipteran retinula cells. J Comp Physiol 84:59–76

Stark WS, Ivanyshyn AM, Hu KG (1976) Spectral sensitivities and photopigments in adaptation of fly visual receptors. Naturwissenschaften 63:513–518

Stavenga DG, Zantema A, Kuiper JW (1973) Rhodopsin processes and the function of the pupil mechanism in flies. In: Langer H (ed) Biochemistry and physiology of visual pigments. Springer, Berlin Heidelberg New York, pp 175–180

Vogt K (1983) Is the fly visual pigment a rhodopsin? Z Naturforsch Sect C Bio Sci 38:329–333

Vogt K (1984a) The chromophore of the visual pigment in some insect orders. Z Naturforsch Sect C Bio Sci 39:196–197

Vogt K (1984b) Zur Verteilung von Rhodopsin und Xanthopsin bei Insekten. Verh Dtsch Zool Ges 1984. Fischer, Stuttgart, p 258

Vogt K, Kirschfeld K (1982) Die Quantenausbeute der Energieübertragung von Photorezeptoren von Fliegen. Verh Dtsch Zool Ges 1982. Fischer, Stuttgart, p 337

Vogt K, Kirschfeld K (1983a) Sensitizing pigment in the fly. Biophys Struct Mech 9:319–328

Vogt K, Kirschfeld K (1983b) C_{40}-carotinoide in Fliegenaugen. Verh Dtsch Zool Ges 1983. Fischer, Stuttgart, p 330

Vogt K, Kirschfeld K (1984) Chemical identity of the chromophores of fly visual pigment. Naturwissenschaften 71:211–213

Wald G (1968) The molecular basis of visual excitation. Nature (Lond) 219:800–807

Zhu H, Kirschfeld K (1984) Protection against photodestruction in fly photoreceptors by carotenoid pigments. J Comp Physiol A Sens Neural Behav Physiol 154:153–156

Visual, Mitochondrial, and Pupillary Pigments of Fly Photoreceptor Cells

D.G. STAVENGA[1]

1 Introduction

Photoreceptor cells, the biological transducers of light into an electrical signal, are extremely sophisticated amplifiers. They are constructed from a large variety of substances some of which absorb substantially at the (so-called) visible wavelengths. Of these pigments, the most important one is by definition the visual pigment. We will argue in this paper that the pigments of the mitochondrial respiratory chain and the screening pigments rank virtually equally high. We shall illustrate this claim on the case of fly photoreceptor cells.

Treating the various pigments of fly photoreceptors in concert has a simple technical reason. Pigments can be favourably studied in vivo by optical methods. The photoreceptor pigments and their functional interrelationship can hence be investigated in intact eyes of living animals.

2 Fly Visual Pigment: Xanthopsin

2.1 Fluorescence of Metaxanthopsin M

The chromophore of the visual pigments of flies has recently shown not to be common retinal but 3-hydroxyretinal (Vogt 1983; Vogt and Kirschfeld 1984; see Kirschfeld 1985, this Vol.).

The 3-hydroxyretinal-based pigments have been christened xanthopsins. The thermostable photoproducts, previously called metarhodopsins, are now called metaxanthopsins.

Note: the tortuous evolution of visual pigment nomenclature (Lythgoe 1979) has now reached the point where three chromophore types, i.e. retinal, 3-dehydroretinal, and 3-hydroxyretinal define three classes of visual pigment: rhodopsins, porphyropsins, and xanthopsins, respectively. Rhodopsins have been found throughout the animal kingdom, porphyropsins in Agnatha, fishes, amphibia, reptiles (Lythgoe 1979, p. 49, 87), and crayfish (Suzuki et al. 1984), and xanthopsins in several insects (Vogt 1984).

---

1 Department of Biophysics, Rijksuniversiteit Groningen, Westersingel 34, Groningen, The Netherlands

Neurobiology
(ed. by R. Gilles and J. Balthazart)
© Springer-Verlag Berlin Heidelberg 1985

Fly xanthopsin X, absorbs in the blue-green and its metaxanthopsin M absorbs in the orange. The latter visual pigment state exhibits a distinct fluorescence, which can be studied in vivo (Stavenga 1983; Franceschini 1983; Stavenga et al. 1984). Measurements of both transmission and fluorescence of the eye of a living housefly *Musca domestica*, mutant white, are presented in Fig. 1. All visual molecules exist initially in the xanthopsin state. Illumination with blue light (477 nm) induces conversion of part of the molecules into the metaxanthopsin state. In the photosteady state, which is established after a few seconds of illumination with 5.7×10^{15} quanta cm^{-2} s^{-1} (Leitz objective NPL 10,0.20) the transmission in the orange, at 572 nm, is low, and the emission in the far-red (> 665 nm) is high, both being due to the created large amount of metaxanthopsin molecules. Reconversion of these molecules by red light (613 nm) to their native xanthopsin state results in a rise in transmission (i.e. in a drop in absorbance) and in a drop in fluorescence. We note that the initial value of the blue-induced emis-

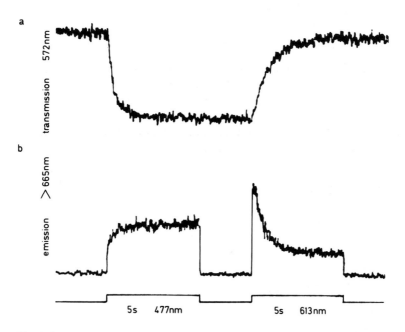

Fig. 1a,b. Transmission and fluorescence measurements performed on the eye of the housefly *Musca domestica* mutant white. Antidromic transmission was measured at 572 nm, where absorption by xanthopsin is low and by metaxanthopsin is high. Creation of metaxanthopsin by orthodromic blue (477 nm) light results in a decrease in transmission (a *left*). The orthodromic beam is sufficiently intense to establish a photosteady-state within a few seconds. The high metaxanthopsin fraction is maintained after termination of the 5-s lasting orthodromic illumination. The metaxanthopsin fraction is lowered by red (613 nm) orthodromic light (a *right*). The transmission changes were only about 20% because a major part of the transmission signal is due to stray light. Emission changes (measured above 665 nm) occurring during photoconversion are shown in **b**. An increase in emission accompanies metaxanthopsin creation and a decrease in emission occurs when metaxanthopsin is photoreconverted back to xanthopsin. (Metaxanthopsin emission is seen superimposed upon a background emission from non-visual pigments in the eye tissue.) The intensities were 5.7×10^{15} quanta cm^{-2} s^{-1} (477 nm) and 5.2×10^{15} quanta cm^{-2} s^{-1} (613 nm). (Stavenga et al. 1984)

sion and the final value of the red-induced emission are due to non-visual pigments which abundantly exist in the fly eye.

2.2 Fluorescence Quantum Efficiency

The fluorescence signals of Fig. 1 were obtained by applying rather intense light; the fluorescence of visual pigments is weak. We have not yet attempted to estimate the fluorescence efficiency of fly metaxanthopsin, but we expect that it will be similar to that of the fluorescence efficiency of crayfish metharhodopsin being $(1.6 \pm 0.4) \times 10^{-3}$ (Cronin and Goldsmith 1981). As we were unable to discriminate a fluorescence signal which could be assigned to the native state of the fly's visual pigment we may expect that its fluorescence quantum efficiency is comparable to that of squid and bovine rhodopsin being $(1.3 \pm 0.7) \times 10^{-5}$ and $(1.9 \pm 0.7) \times 10^{-5}$ respectively (Doukas et al. 1983; for further references see Cronin and Goldsmith 1981).

2.3 Fluorescence as a Visual Pigment Monitor

The fluorescence of fly metaxanthopsin can be utilized to monitor the content and composition of the visual pigment in eyes of intact living animals. This is exemplified in Fig. 2 showing photoconversions induced by red light (613 nm), measured from a white eyed mutant (chalky) blowfly *Calliphora erythrocephala*.

Previous to Fig. 2 violet light (Balzers K40) had been applied during various periods: 10, 20, 40, 60, and 120 s, respectively. Because always at the onset of the violet expo-

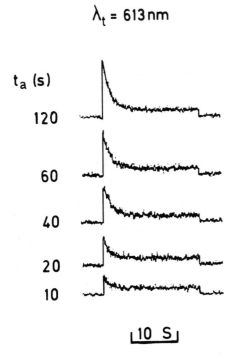

$$\lambda_t = 613 \, nm$$

t_a (s)

120

60

40

20

10

$\lfloor$ 10 S $\rfloor$

Fig. 2. Emission above 665 nm measured during reconversion of metaxanthopsin into xanthopsin induced by 613 nm light after preadaptation for 10, 20, 40, 60, and 120 s to violet light (Balzers K40). Through the Leitz objective NPL10, numerical aperture = 0.20, the 613 nm light produced a quantum flux of 3.0×10^{15} quanta cm^{-2} s^{-1}; the violet light contained 1.7×10^{14} quanta cm^{-2} s^{-1} (*Calliphora* chalky)

sures all molecules were in the xanthopsin state the illuminations caused an increase in metaxanthopsin content. This was evident from the increased far-red fluorescence induced by the subsequent red test light: the initial fluorescence signal increased with the duration of the previous violet light.

The initial value of the red-induced fluorescence was plotted as a function of the total violet quantum flux previously delivered (Fig. 3). Measurements performed at two temperatures (21 and 4 °C, respectively) are shown. Four intensity levels of violet light were applied separated from each other by approx. 1 log unit. With increased intensity the illumination time was proportionally shortened. The data of Fig. 3 show that photopigment conversion is a function of $I \times t$ (I = intensity of illumination, t = time); this is expected from a photochromic pigment (see Hochstein et al. 1978; Hamdorf 1979; Stavenga and Schwemer 1984). The rate of conversion then is $(K_X + K_M) It$. The sum of the photosensitivites of the two visual pigment states $K_X + K_M$, does not appear to depend appreciably on temperature. When the photosteady state of a photochromic substance is established (in Fig. 3, after delivering $\geqslant 3 \times 10^{16}$ quanta cm^{-2}) prolongation of the illumination, or, alternatively, its intensification does not change the distribution of pigment molecules between the two states. In the case of fly visual pigment, however, very bright light populates another visual pigment state, previously called metharhodopsin M', and now metaxanthopsin M'.

2.4 Fluorescence of Metaxanthopsin M'

Prolonged illumination with very bright light yields fluorescence signals deviating from those presented above.

The experiment shown in Fig. 4, performed also on a blowfly mutant chalky, started with all visual pigment molecules in the xanthopsin state. The far-red emission induced by broad-band blue light (390–490 nm) and red light (606 nm) was measured. A flash intense blue light (a) created rapidly a photosteady state with a high content of meta-xanthopsin, as revealed by the ensuing red flash (b). Prolonged intense blue light (c) induces the conversion of the visual pigment molecules to the metaxanthopsin M' state. M' is highly fluorescent (d) and, relative to M, quite stable, as only after a prolonged illumination period with the red light (e) it was reconverted.

Emission spectra with the visual pigment in predominantly the metarhodopsin states M and M', respectively, were obtained from a housefly mutant white (Fig. 5). The excitation light was broad-band blue (390–490 nm). In the "fresh" eye (curve 1) the fluorescence of M in the red ($\geqslant 600$ nm) is noticeable, together with an emission in the green originating from non-visual pigments in the eye tissue. After bright blue light (curve 2) a dominant red emission, due to the created M', emerges. The emission spectrum after prolonged red illumination (curve 3) shows the depopulation of the M' state.

In order to obtain the pure emission spectra of M and M' the background signal and the instrumental properties have to be accounted for. The M'-emission spectrum, thus arrived at, shows an emission peak at 660 nm (see Stavenga et al. 1984). The emission spectrum of M is virtually identical to that of M' except for the much lower efficiency (Kruizinga and Stavenga, in prep.).

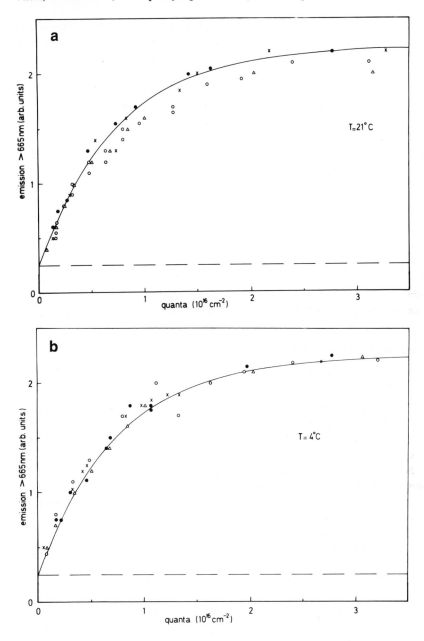

Fig. 3a,b. Initial value of emission induced by 613 nm (as in Fig. 2) plotted as a function of the preceding illumination. Violet light (K40) was applied during various illumination times t at four intensities I: $\triangle$ I = 1.7 × 10^{14} , o I = 1.6 × 10^{15} , x I = 1.7 × 10^{16} , ● I = 1.5 × 10^{17} quanta cm^{-2} s^{-1}. a Temperature 21 °C. b Temperature 4 °C. The same exponential function has been drawn in the two figures (*Calliphora* chalky)

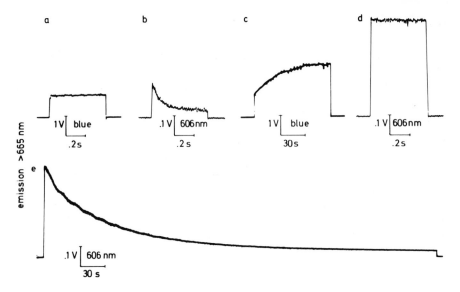

Fig. 4a–e. Demonstration of the conversion of the visual pigment population into the metaxanthopsin M′ state. The fly's eye (*Calliphora* chalky) was preadapted with 606 nm light. A short bright broad-band blue (390–490 nm) flash (**a**) establishes a high metaxanthopsin content, as shown by the subsequent 606 nm flash (**b**). However, a long (1.5 min) intense blue exposure (**c**) puts virtually all visual molecules in the M′ state, as is shown by the subsequent 606 nm flash (**d**), which induces no transient, but only a high plateau. Only prolonged red light (**e**) can reconvert M′ back into the native xanthopsin state

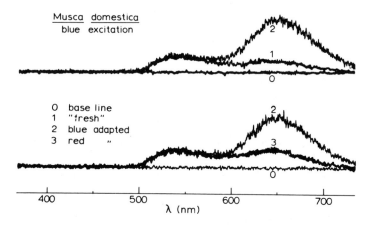

Fig. 5. Experimental emission spectra under blue excitation (390–490 nm). Curve 1 is "fresh", no M′ present, although a substantial amount M is already created. Prolonged blue light shows a much-enhanced emission in the red due to M′ formation (curve 2). Subsequent red adaptation reduces the M′ concentration, i.e. reduces the emission in the red (curve 3); housefly *Musca* white, dorsal frontal area of a male eye. (Stavenga et al. 1984)

3 Mitochondrial Pigments

Applying blue excitation light and measuring the induced emission in the green (from the eyes of white-eyed mutants) we failed to see any indication for fluorescence from xanthopsin. However, we observed a transient increase in green fluorescence when the excitation light was delivered to the eye after a few seconds of darkness. After longer dark times a biphasic process occurred which could be repeated at will, at least for several hours (Stavenga and Tinbergen 1983). We argued that the fluorescence changes originated from redox changes in the pigments of the respiratory chain, and we indeed found that hypoxia substantially lowered the green fluorescence. We supposed that this phenomenon was due to the reduction of flavoproteins, which are known to fluoresce highly when oxidized, and much less when being in the reduced state. We therefore measured the transmission of the retina in the normal (air) situation and under hypoxia, respectively. The spectrum of Fig. 6 presents the change in transmittivity (Rushton

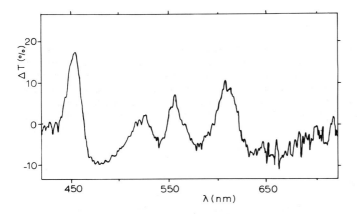

Fig. 6. Difference in transmittivity between the normal and the hypoxia state (white-eyed blowfly mutant chalky *Calliphora erythrocephala*)

1972) of the eye occurring upon hypoxia. The peaks at 605 and 555 nm are characteristic for cytochromes a, a3, and c, c1, respectively. The trough at 480 nm can be assigned to flavoproteins (Chance and Williams 1956; Lehninger 1970; Piantadosi and Jobsis-Vandervliet 1984).

The transmission measurements substantiated the hypothesis that the fluorescence changes occurring upon hypoxia (Fig. 7) are due to reduction of the flavoproteins of the mitochondrial respiratory chain (Stavenga and Tinbergen 1983). The light-induced changes, interpreted as a transient increase in oxidation of the mitochondria, accord with findings by Hamdorf and Schwemer (1975) and Tsacopoulos et al. (1983), namely that illumination induces an increase in oxygen consumption by the photoreceptors of blowfly and bee, respectively.

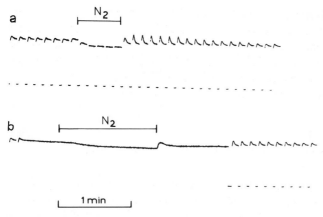

Fig. 7a,b. The influence of hypoxia on blue-induced green fluorescence from the eye of a blowfly mutant chalky. Flashes of 5-s duration were given with 30-s dark time interval (during which the recorder stopped). Hypoxia lowers the fluorescence and blocks the light-induced dynamics. After hypoxia fluorescence increases and the dynamics recovers (a). Essentially the same effects occur during continuous light (b). (Stavenga and Tinbergen 1983)

4 Pupillary Pigment

The screening pigments, which inhabit the pigment cells in wild type flies, are absent in white-eyed mutants. Moreover, in the mutants the pigment granules in the visual sense cells are lacking. In the wild type the pigment granules are able to migrate inside the photoreceptor soma presumably due to a cytoskeletal system as in crayfish photoreceptors (e.g. Frixione 1983). Illumination drives the pigment granules towards the rhabdomere, the structure containing the visual pigments, thus bleeding light from the rhabdomere. In the dark the pigment granules retirate. This so-called pupillary process

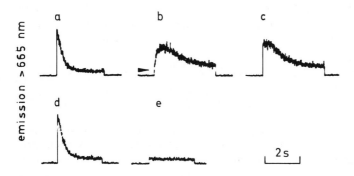

Fig. 8a–e. Emission above 665 nm induced by red (613 nm; a, d, e) and blue (488 nm; b, c) light; wild type blowfly. The (constant intensity) illumination activates the pupil, which subsequently relaxes during the 1-min dark interval time, given between the illuminations. Photoconversions occur transiently in a, b, and d. The influence of the pupil is distinctly noticeable with blue illumination; it is negligible with red illumination, since the pupil absorbs highly in the blue and little in the red. (Stavenga 1983)

can be followed in reflected and transmitted light (Kirschfeld and Franceschini 1969; Stavenga 1979) but also in fluorescence (Franceschini 1977; Stavenga 1983). Figure 8 demonstrates the absorbing action of the pupillary granules on metaxanthopsin fluorescence. Because the pupil absorbs predominantly in the blue (Vogt et al. 1982) it selectively reduces the light flux in the rhabdomeres as well as the conversion of xanthopsin to metaxanthopsin (Stavenga et al. 1973; Stavenga 1980).

5 Functional Interrelationships of Photoreceptor Pigments

The three classes of pigments treated above serve quite different functions. Firstly, the function of the visual pigments is to absorb light, so that the chain of phototransduction processes is triggered, thus resulting in a change in the potential across the photoreceptor cell membrane (Hamdorf 1979).

Secondly, the pigments of the mitochondrial respiratory chain are constituents of the machinery which supplies the metabolic energy for numerous cell functions, as there are the Na^+/K^+-ion pump, the renewal of cell organelles, and the control systems which act on ion channels in the membrane and on other components of the phototransduction chain (Tsacopoulos et al. 1983; Paulsen and Bentrop 1984).

Thirdly, the function of the pupillary pigment is to control the light flux incident on the visual pigment, thus extending the visual range of the photoreceptor cell (Blakeslee et al. 1984). Although the functions of the three pigment classes are quite distinct they are still intimately related. For instance, the action spectra measured electrophysiologically are virtually identical to those of light-induced mitochondrial (Tinbergen and Stavenga, in preparation) and pupillary activities (Bernard and Stavenga 1979); we recall that the spectral sensitivity of a photoreceptor is essentially determined by the spectral absorption properties of the visual pigment.

The mechanism underlying the light-induced increase in mitochondrial activity is unknown, as yet. As discussed by Tsacopoulos et al. (1983), an important agent may be the cytosolic Ca^{2+} concentration, which is known to stimulate mitochondrial respiration. Furthermore, Ca^{2+} is involved in the pupillary pigment control system (Kirschfeld and Vogt 1981; Howard 1984). In this respect it is interesting that the intensity ranges for mitochondrial and for pupillary activation (blowfly mutant chalky and wild-type, respectively) virtually coincide (Tinbergen and Stavenga, in preparation).

Since illumination of invertebrate photoreceptors induces a transient increase in cytosolic Ca^{2+} both mitochondrial and pupillary systems may have a same input.

Acknowledgements. J. Tinbergen and B. Kruizinga are acknowledged for their constant encouragement and collaboration. The Dutch Organization for the Advancement of Pure Research (Z.W.O.) provided financial support through the Foundation for Biophysics (Stichting voor Biofysica). fysica).

References

Bernard GD, Stavenga DG (1979) Spectral sensitivities of retinular cells measured in intact living flies by an optical method. J Comp Physiol 134:95–107

Blakeslee B, Howard J, Laughlin S (1984) The role of the fly pupil mechanism in regulating the signal – to – noise ratio of light-adapted photoreceptors. Neurosci Lett 15:20

Chance B, Williams GR (1956) The respiratory chain and oxidative phosphorylation. Adv Relat Areas Mol Biol 17:65–134

Cronin TW, Goldsmith TH (1981) Fluorescence of crayfish metarhodopsin studied in single rhabdoms. Biophys J 35:653–664

Doukas AG, Junnarkar MR, Chandra D, Buchert J, Alfano RR, Callender RH, Honig B (1983) Quantum yield measurements of rhodopsin: theoretical implications. Photochem Photobiol 37: S109

Franceschini N (1977) In vivo fluorescence of the rhabdomeres in an insect eye. Proc Int Union Physiol Sci XIII. 26th Int Congr Physiol Sci, Paris, p 237

Franceschini N (1983) In vivo microspectrofluorimetry of visual pigments. In: Cosens DJ, Vince-Price D (eds) The biology of photoreception. Soc Exp Biol Symp, vol 36, p 53

Franceschini N, Kirschfeld K, Minke B (1981) Fluorescence of photoreceptor cells observed in vivo. Science (Wash DC) 213:1264–1267

Frixione E (1983) Firm structural associations between migratory pigment granules and microtubules in crayfish retinula cells. J Cell Biol 96:1258–1265

Hamdorf K (1979) The physiology of invertebrate visual pigments. In: Autrum H (ed) Handbook of sensory physiology, vol 7/6A. Springer, Berlin Heidelberg New York, p 145

Hamdorf K, Schwemer J (1975) Photoregeneration and the adaptation process in insect photoreceptors. In: Snyder AW, Menzel R (eds) Photoreceptor optics. Springer, Berlin Heidelberg New York, p 263

Hochstein S, Minke B, Hillman P, Knight BW (1978) The kinetics of visual pigments I. Mathematical analysis. Biol Cybern 30:23–32

Howard J (1984) Calcium enables photoreceptor pigment migration in a mutant fly. J Exp Biol 113:471–476

Kirschfeld K, Franceschini N (1969) Ein Mechanismus zur Steuerung des Lichtflusses in den Rhabdomeren des Komplexauges von Musca. Kybernetik 6:13–22

Kirschfeld K, Vogt K (1981) Calcium ions and pigment migration in fly photoreceptors. Naturwissenschaften 67:516–518

Lehninger AL (1970) Biochemistry. Worth, New York

Lythgoe JN (1979) The ecology of vision. Clarendon, Oxford

Paulsen R, Bentrop J (1984) Reversible phosphorylation of opsin induced by irradiation of blowfly retinae. J Comp Physiol 155:39–46

Piantadosi CA, Jobsis-Vandervliet FF (1984) Spectrophotometry of cerebral cytochrome a, a3 in bloodless rats. Brain Res 305:89–94

Rushton WAH (1972) Visual pigments in man. In: Dartnall HJA (ed) Handbook of sensory physiology, vol 7/1. Springer, Berlin Heidelberg New York, p 364

Stavenga DG (1979) Pseudopupils of compound eyes. In: Autrum H (ed) Handbook of sensory physiology, vol 7/6A. Springer, Berlin Heidelberg New York, p 357

Stavenga DG (1980) Short wavelength light in invertebrate visual sense cells – Pigments, potentials and problems. In: Senger H (ed) The blue light syndrome. Springer, Berlin Heidelberg New York, p 5

Stavenga DG (1983) Fluorescence of blowfly metarhodopsin. Biophys Struct Mech 9:309–317

Stavenga DG, Schwemer J (1984) Visual pigments of invertebrates. In: Ali MA (ed) Photoreception and vision in invertebrates. Plenum, New York, p 11

Stavenga DG, Tinbergen J (1983) Light dependence of oxidative metabolism in fly compound eyes studied in vivo by microspectrofluorometry. Naturwissenschaften 70:618–620

Stavenga DG, Zantema A, Kuiper JW (1973) Rhodopsin processes and the function of the pupil mechanism in flies. In: Langer H (ed) Biochemistry and physiology of visual pigments. Springer, Berlin Heidelberg New York, p 175

Stavenga DG, Frenceschini N, Kirschfeld K (1984) Fluorescence of housefly visual pigment. Photochem Photobiol 40:653−659

Suzuki T, Makino-Tasaka M, Eguchi E (1984) 3-dehydroretinal (vitamin A2 aldehyde) in crayfish eye. Vision Res 24:783−788

Tsacopoulos M, Orkand RK, Coles JA, Levy S, Poitry S (1983) Oxygen uptake occurs faster than sodium pumping in bee retina after a light flash. Nature (Lond) 301:604−606

Vogt K (1983) Is the fly visual pigment a rhodopsin? Z Naturforsch Sect C Bio Sci 38:329−333

Vogt K (1984) The chromophore of the visual pigment in some insect orders. Z Naturforsch Sect C Biosci 39:196−197

Vogt K, Kirschfeld K (1984) Chemical identity of the chromophores of fly visual pigment. Naturwissenschaften 71:211−213

Vogt K, Kirschfeld K, Stavenga DG (1982) Spectral effects of the pupil in fly photoreceptors. J Comp Physiol 146:145−152

Two-Dimensional Gel Analysis of Polypeptides in Drosophila Compound Eyes

H. MATSUMOTO and W. L. PAK [1]

1 Introduction

Several years ago, we undertook an analysis of *Drosophila* eye proteins in the hope of identifying eye-specific proteins that might be involved in molecular mechanisms of visual excitation. We chose *Drosophila melanogaster* as an experimental organism because of its well-known genetics and the availability of a large number of mutants defective in visual function (Pak 1975; Pak 1979; Hall 1982). The approach we took was to apply two-dimensional polyacrylamide gel electrophoresis (2-D gel) to the analysis of proteins in the compound eye of both wild-type and mutant flies. Fujita and Hotta (Fujita and Hotta 1979; Hotta 1979) first applied this technique to *Drosophila* eyes and showed that three polypeptides observed in 2-D gel originate from the compound eye. In addition to these three, we found at least three other polypeptides that are specific to the photoreceptor layer (Matsumoto et al. 1982). Moreover, the three polypeptides we identified (designated as 80 K, 49 K, and 39 K) were found to alter their isoelectric points in response to a light stimulus in vivo (Matsumoto et al. 1982).

Subsequently, we found evidence that reversible, light-induced phosphorylation of these polypeptides is responsible for changes in their isoelectric points (Matsumoto and Pak 1984). On the basis of kinetic studies and mutant studies, we further suggested that these polypeptides and their light-dependent phosphorylation are likely to be involved in the molecular mechanisms of the visual process (Matsumoto and Pak 1984; Matsumoto et al. 1983). The purpose of this paper is to summarize our evidence that supports the above hypothesis.

2 Materials and Methods

2.1 Drosophila Melanogaster Stocks

Wild-type flies of the Oregon R strain and two allelic mutants of the *norpA* (no receptor potential A) gene, *P24* and *P47*, were used. The *norpA* mutants were isolated in chemical mutagenesis (Hotta and Benzer 1969; Pak et al. 1969; Heisenberg 1971), and the gene has been localized to 6.5 ± 0.7 on the X chromosome by recombination mapping (Pak 1975) and to 4B5-6 by cytogenetic mapping (Banga et al., in prep.) The *norpA* muta-

---

1 Department of Biological Sciences, Purdue University, West Lafayette, Indiana 47907, USA

Neurobiology
(ed. by R. Gilles and J. Balthazart)
© Springer-Verlag Berlin Heidelberg 1985

tion causes reduction in amplitude, or even complete elimination, of the photoreceptor cell types, R1-6, R7, and R8. The severity of expression of the *norpA* mutant
phenotype depends on the particular mutant allele carried by the flies. For example,
norpA^{P24}, one of the strongest alleles, completely eliminates the photoreceptor potential. As a result of the *norpA*^{P24} flies are blind and show no phototactic behaviour.
However, no obvious defect in the light-microscopic anatomy of the compound eye
structure has been found at least in the young *norpA* mutant flies. In contrast, a weak
allele, *norpA*^{P47}, allows the photoreceptor potential to be generated, though reduced
in amplitude and slow in time course.

2.2 Preparation of Drosophila Compound Eyes

The flies were raised on normal cornmeal-agar medium under 12 h dark/12 h light cycle
at 25 °C. About 80 flies were frozen in a test tube (2 cm $\times$ 20 cm) at liquid nitrogen
temperature and dismembered by vigorous vortexing. The photoreceptor layer preparation was obtained by a method similar to that of Fujita and Hotta (1979). About
10 ml of chilled acetone was added to the test tube and routinely left overnight at
– 20 °C to dehydrate the flies. Acetone was evaporated on a Buchner funnel before dissecting the dehydrated heads with a tungsten needle under a stereo-microscope. The
dissection gave compound eyes free from lamina. If necessary, the cornea was also
removed from the preparation.

The acetone treatment dehydrated the flies completely. It is highly unlikely that
any biochemical reactions could take place under these conditions. We have never observed any inconsistent results which could be attributed to residual biochemical reactions that might take place even under these extreme conditions.

2.3 Light- or Dark-Adaptation of Flies

The flies were dark-adapted either for 24 h or 12 h prior to each experiment. Flies
dark-adapted for longer than 12 h gave two-dimensional gel profiles indistinguishable
from those obtained from flies dark adapted for 12 h. The dark-adapted flies were
separated into two groups, one of which was frozen in the dark and treated with acetone. The other group was light-adapted under normal room light (160 μW cm^{-2}) for
5 min and then frozen in the light. Longer adaptation under these conditions did not
give gel profiles that are any different from those obtained after 5-min light adaptation.

Illumination of the flies at lower intensities was accomplished by introducing adapting light through a light guide inserted into the lid of a light-tight Dewer containing
approximately 70 dark-adapted flies in a test tube. The intensity of light was controlled
using neutral density filters. The light intensity at logI = 0 was 8,800 μW cm^{-2}. Electroretinograms (ERG) were measured as reported elsewhere (Lo and Pak 1981). The
stimulus intensities used in ERG measurements were adjusted to be approximately
the same as those of the illumintion in the Dewer.

2.4 Labelling of Phosphorproteins in vivo and in vitro

The labelling of the flies in vivo was achieved as described previously (Matsumoto and
Pak 1984). The protein phosphorylation in vitro was carried out by incubating the

homogenate of 20 compound eyes with ^{32}P-ATP. The standard reaction mixture contained the following ingredients in a 35 μl volume: 12 mM phosphate buffer, pH 7.5; 0.1 mM ATP; 5 mM MgSO$_4$; 1 μCi [α-^{32}P]ATP or [γ-^{23}P]ATP (3,000 Ci/mmol); and the homogenate from 20 eyes. After incubating for 10 min at 25 °C, the reaction mixture was centrifuged at 3,000 rpm for 10 min, and the pellet was subjected to electrophoresis.

2.5 Two- and One-Dimensional Gel Electrophoreses

For a 2-D gel analysis, one hundred, or in some cases 140, compound eyes were homogenized in 60 μl 8 M urea/2% Triton X-100/2% Bio-Lyte 3/10 (Bio-Rad). The supernatant (ca. 55 μl) was recovered after centrifugation at 3,000 rpm for 5 min, and subjected to 2-D gel electrophoresis as described by O'Farrell (1975) with a modification of Miyazaki et al. (1978). The procedures for the first dimension, isoelectric focusing (IEF), and the following second dimension, sodium dodecylsulfate-10% polyacrylamide gel electrophoresis (SDS-PAGE) according to Laemmli (1970), have been described elsewhere (Matsumoto et al. 1982; Matsumoto and Pak 1984). For one-dimensional gel, the procedures for the second dimension of the 2-D gels were adopted. The gels were fixed in 25% *iso*-propanol/10% acetic acid and stained in 0.05% Coomassie Brilliant Blue R-250/25% *iso*-propanol/10% acetic acid. After destaining, the gels were dried on filter papers and photographed. For autoradiography, Kodak XAR-5 films were exposed to the dried gels at −80 °C. A DuPont Lightning Plus screen was used to enhanced the signals.

3 Results

In Fig. 1 are shown acetone treated, dehydrated *Drosophila* heads at various stages of dissection. Figures 1E, P, and C show, respectively, a dissected compound eye, photoreceptor layer, and cornea. Shown also in the figure is the remainder of the head from which these parts were removed. It may be seen that the pigmented surface which forms the boundary between the photoreceptor and the laminar layers (see Fig. 8) are still attached to the residual part of the head (Fig. 1, insets 2, 3), insuring that the lamina did not come off with the dissected compound eye or photoreceptor layer preparations.

Under optimal conditions, the compound eye preparation run on a polyacrylamide slab gel of 14 cm × 28 cm × 1.5 mm and stained with Coomassie blue yielded more than 400 polypeptide spots in the range of ca. pI 4 to 9 and mol. wt. 14 K to 200 K daltons (data not shown), consistent with the earlier observations of Fujita and Hotta (1979). Among them more than 30 polypeptides appeared as major spots. These major spots were readily identifiable even in smaller gels (14 cm × 15 cm × 0.75 mm) used in most of the experiments.

To determine tissue specificity of each polypeptide, we compared the 2-D gel patterns of the compound eye preparation with those of the rest of the head. Figures 2a and 2b show the gel profiles of the compound eye and "eyeless" head preparations, respectively, obtained from the dissection of 70 dark-adapted, wild-type flies. Except

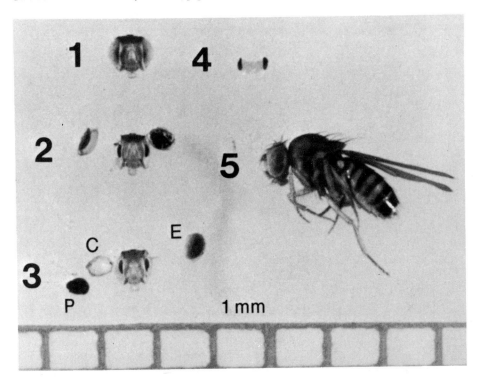

Fig. 1. Microdissection of *Drosophila melanogaster* head shown in sequence. *1* whole head; *2* the compound eyes are removed; *3* the cornea is removed from the compound eye; *4* brain and the optic lobe; *5* whole fly. *P* photoreceptor layer preparation; *C* cornea; *E* compound eye

for the differences to be noted below, the patterns of the major spots are similar in these two gels. Thus, the major spots indicated by the downward pointing arrows in Fig. 2b are found in gels obtained from both the compound eye and head preparations. The polypeptides indicated by arrows in Fig. 2a (a, b, c, d, e, f, g, h, i, 80 K, 49 K, and 39 K), on the other hand, appeared in gels of the compound eye preparation, but not in those of the rest of the head (Fig. 2b). Therefore, these polypeptides are specific for the compound eye within the detection limit of the Coomassie blue staining. Of these compound eye specific polypeptides, those labelled e, f, g, and h were found to originate from the cornea from electrophoretic examination of the isolated cornea (Fig. 2c). These analyses, thus, identified the polypeptides that are specific to the layer of tissues containing primarily the photoreceptors and the associated pigment cells. We will refer to these polypeptides as being photoreceptor layer- or retina-specific.

If any of the retina-specific polypeptides are involved in visual processes, it seemed likely that they are altered by illumination. We reasoned that at least some of these alterations might be detectable in 2-D gel analysis. We, therefore, examined the possibility that illumination might modify the 2-D gel profile of the major retina-specific polypeptides. Wild-type flies were dark-adapted for 24 h and then separated into two groups. One group was frozen in the dark, and the other group was exposed to normal room light ($160 \mu W \, cm^{-2}$) for 5 min and then frozen.

H. Matsumoto and W. L. Pak

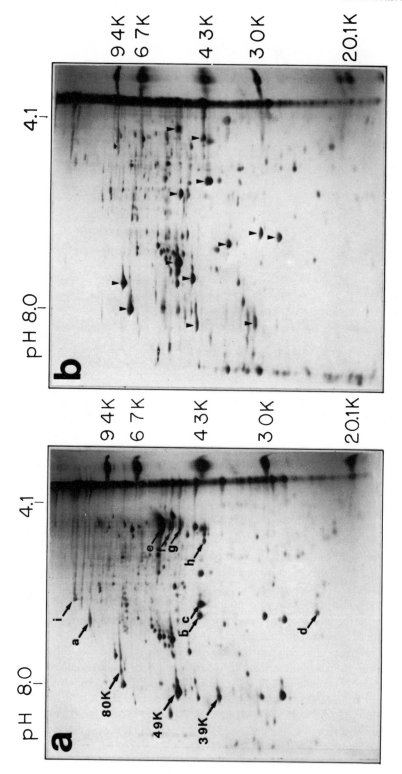

Fig. 2a,b

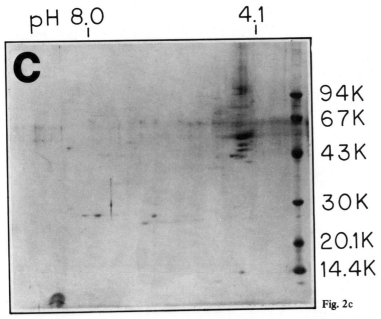

Fig. 2c

Fig. 2a–c. Two-dimensional gel profiles of *Drosophila melanogaster* head tissue samples. a compound eyes (cornea and photoreceptor layer). b heads from which the eyes have been removed. c cornea. In Fig. a *arrows a, b, c, d, e, f, g, h, i, 80 K, 49 K,* and *39 K* are all compound eye-specific poly-peptide spots. In Fig. b *arrow-heads* pointing downwards indicate typical major polypeptide spots found in gel profiles of both the head and the compound eye samples. The mol. wt. markers on the *right edge* of each gel are: phosphorylase b (*94 K*), bovine serum albumin (*68 K*), ovalbumin (*43 K*), carbonic anhydrase (*30 K*), soybean trypsin inhibitor (*20.1 K*), and α-lactalbumin (*14.4 K*), respectively

Illustrated in Figs. 3a and b are the gels obtained from the dark-adapted and illuminated flies, respectively. Figures 3c and d display computer generated contour profiles of Figs. 3a and b, respectively. (These figures do not show the entire gel but only that portion containing the three classes of polypeptides to be discussed.) The results show that illumination induces pI shifts in three classes of retina-specific polypeptides toward the acidic direction. These polypeptides were designated as 80 K, 49 K, and 39 K according to their approximate mol. wt. calibrated by internal mol. wt. markers (Matsumoto et al. 1982). Each polypeptide consisted of two or more pI states. These states are designated by letters A through F in Figs. 3c and d. In each case, the dark-adapted state is designated by the letter A (80 A, 49 A, and 39 A), while the light-adapted states are designated by letters B through F. Note the considerable pI heterogeneity displayed by the 80 K polypeptide, particularly following illumination.

To test the idea that the light-induced pI shifts of these polypeptides are due to phosphorylation, wild-type flies fed with ^{32}P-labelled phosphate were analyzed on 2-D gels. The labelled flies were separated into two groups, one of which was dark-adapted and the other light-adapted, and the 2-D gel analysis was carried out on each sample. The results obtained in such experiments are illustrated in Fig. 4. Figures 4a and b are

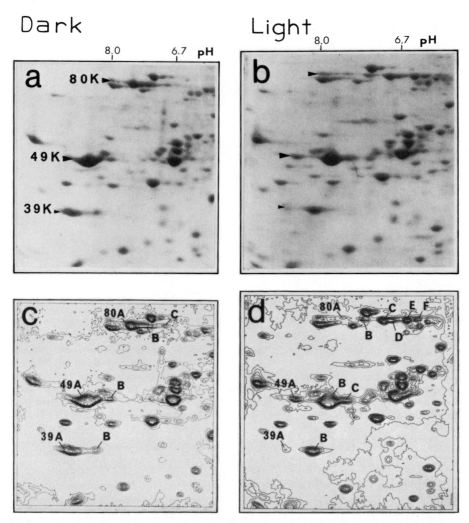

Fig. 3a–d. Light-induced pI changes of the *80 K, 49 K,* and *39 K* polypeptides. **a** compound eye sample dissected from dark-adapted flies. **b** light-adapted for 5 min in room light (160 μW cm^{-2}). **c** and **d** contour map profiles corresponding to **a** and **b**, respectively. The *horizontal arrows* in **a** and **b** indicate: large, *49 K*; medium, *80 K*; small, *39 K* polypeptide. The various pI states of each polypeptide are labelled by letters *A* through *F* in Figs. **3c** and **3d**. In each case, the dark-adapted state is designated by the letter *A*

the Coomassie blue-stained gels of the dark- and light-adapted samples, respectively. The corresponding autoradiograms are shown in Figs. 4c and d, respectively. The results showed that the ^{32}P-radioactivity was incorporated into the light-adapted states of the 80 K, 49 K, and 39 K polypeptides, but not into their dark-adapted states, indicating that, indeed, light-induced phosphorylation of these polypeptides is responsible for the light-induced pI shifts.

Figure 5 demonstrates the effect of the *norpA* mutation on the light-induced pI shifts of the 80 K, 49 K, and 39 K polypeptide. We examined two *norpA* alleles, *P24*

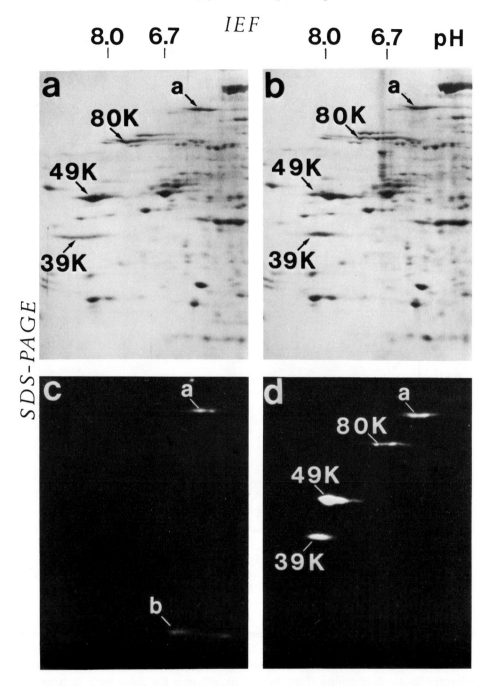

Fig. 4a–d. In vivo incorporation of [^{32}P]phosphate into the light-adapted states of *80 K, 49 K,* and *39 K* polypeptides. **a** and **b** Coomassie blue-stained gels from the dark- and light-adapted flies fed with [^{32}P]phosphate, respectively. **c** and **d** Autoradiograms corresponding to **a** and **b**, respectively. (Matsumoto and Pak 1984, copyright 1984 by the AAAS)

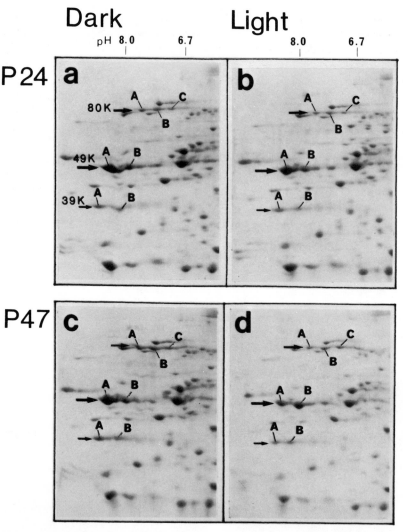

Fig. 5a–d. The effect of the *norpA* mutation on the light-induced pI shifts of the 80 K, 49 K, and 39 K polypeptides in vivo. **a** and **b** dark- and light-adapted *norpA*[P24], respectively. **c** and **d** dark- and light-adapted *norpA*[P47], respectively. The *horizontal arrows* indicate: large, *49 K* polypeptide; medium, *80 K*; small, *39 K*. Letters *A, B, C* have the same meaning as in Fig. 3

and *P47*, a strong and a weak allele, respectively. The *norpA*[P24] flies exhibited no detectable changes in these polypeptides following illumination (Figs. 5a and b). The weaker allelic mutant, *norpA*[P47], on the other hand, did show shifts in the pI of these polypeptides on illumination (Figs. 5c and d), although the shifts were incomplete compared to those seen in wild-type flies (Fig. 3a and b).

Phosphorylation of the 80 K, 49 K, and 39 K polypeptides were examined in vitro to address the following two questions: (1) whether the polypeptides accept phosphoryl groups only from the γ-position of ATP, as they should in phosphorylation reactions, or indiscriminately from any position and (2) whether the phosphorylation of these polypeptides are blocked in *norpA* mutants in vitro as well as in vivo. For this purpose, eye homogenates of dark-adapted wild-type or *norpA* flies were incubated with $[\alpha\text{-}^{32}\text{P}]$-ATP or $[\gamma\text{-}^{32}\text{P}]$ATP in room light and examined on one-dimensional SDS gels, as described in Methods. One-dimensional gels were used because of their relative simplicity. We found that the three polypeptides could be unequivocally identified in autoradiograms of 1-D gels when they were labelled with ^{32}P (Fig. 6, lanes 6 and 8). In Fig. 6, lanes 5 and 6 are the autoradiograms of 1-D (lanes 1 and 2) gels obtained from *norpA* eye homogenates incubated with $[\alpha\text{-}^{32}\text{P}]$ATP and $[\gamma\text{-}^{32}\text{P}]$ATP, respectively. The autoradiograms obtained in the corresponding experiments with wild-type eye homogenates are shown in lanes 7 and 8. Lanes 1 through 4 are the Coomassie blue-stained gels from which the autoradiograms were taken. These results indicate that the 80 K, 49 K, and 39 K polypeptides of the *norpA* flies as well as those of wild-type flies were phosphorylated in vitro when $[\gamma\text{-}^{32}\text{P}]$ATP was used as a phosphoryl group donor (Fig. 6, lanes 6

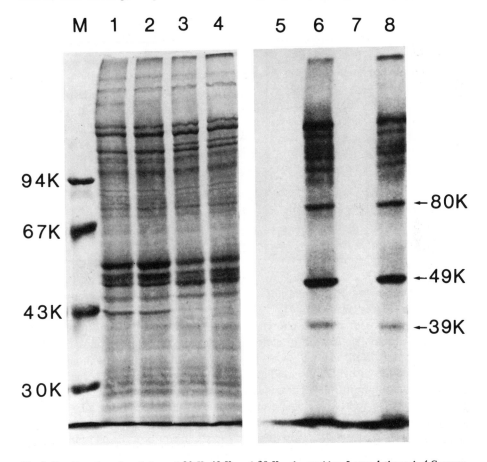

Fig. 6. In vitro phosphorylation of *80 K, 49 K,* and *39 K* polypeptides. Lanes *1* through *4* Coomassie blue-stained gels; lanes *5* through *8* corresponding autoradiograms; *1* and *5 norpA*[P24] incubated with $[\alpha\text{-}^{32}\text{P}]$ATP; *2* and *6 norpA*[P24] incubated with $[\gamma\text{-}^{32}\text{P}]$ATP; *3* and *7* wild type incubated with $[\alpha\text{-}^{32}\text{P}]$ATP; *4* and *8* wild type incubated with $[\gamma\text{-}^{32}\text{P}]$ATP; *M* mol. wt. markers

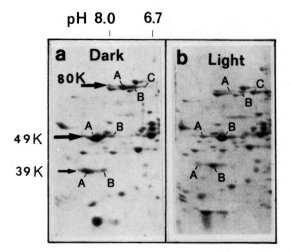

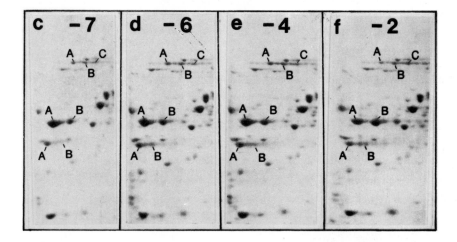

Fig. 7a–f. Phosphorylation of the 49 K polypeptide observed as a function of light intensity. **a** and **b** Dark- and light-adapted controls, respectively. **c, d, e,** and **f** The flies exposed to illuminations of increasing intensities. The intensities are indicated at the top of each panel in log units. Log I = 0 corresponds to 8,800 μW cm^{-2}. The pI states of individual spots are indicated by letters as in Fig. 3

and 8). However, [α-^{32}P]ATP did not donate the labelled phosphoryl group to these polypeptides (Fig. 6, lanes 5 and 7).

The dependence of the phosphorylation of these polypeptides on light intensity was examined to obtain some information about the sensitivity of the phosphorylation reactions to light. Dark-adapted wild-type flies were illuminated for two minutes with various intensities of light, frozen in liquid nitrogen, and prepared for 2-D gel analysis. The results are shown in Fig. 7. These indicate (1) that the phosphorylation of the 49 K polypeptide began to be detectable even at very low light intensities (log I = –7 or –6) and (2) that the amount of 49 K phosphorylation gradually increased with light intensities approximately logarithmically (log I = –7 to 0). In contrast, the phosphorylations of the other two polypeptides, 80 K and 39 K, required much higher light intensities (log I = –2 to 0).

4 Discussion

A horizontal section through the compound eye and the brain of *D. melanogaster* observed at the optical level, prepared by K. Isono of our laboratory, is shown in Fig. 8, together with a corresponding schematic diagram. There are three anatomically distinct classes of photoreceptors in the *Drosophila* compound eye: R1-6, R7, and R8 photoreceptors. The axons of the majority class of photoreceptors synapse with the second-order neurons in the lamina (La in Fig. 8), whereas R7 and R8 photoreceptor axons from synapses in the medula (Me) (Trujillo-Cenóz and Melamed 1966; Braitenberg 1967).

Microdissection of dehydrated heads (see Fig. 1) cleaved the eye tissues primarily at the basement membrane, which forms the boundary between the compound eye (CE in Fig. 8) and the lamina (La), thus leaving the lamina still attached to the medulla (insets 2 and 3 in Fig. 1). However, the dissection sometimes caused the cleavage at the first optic chiasm between the lamina (La) and the medulla (Me) rendering the compound eye preparation contaminated with the lamina. Even in such cases, the lamina which was attached to the compound eye could be removed by further dissection. Since the cornea could also be removed from the compound eye (inset 3, Fig. 1), we found it possible to collect a pure preparation consisting only of isolated laminas, corneas, or tissues in the photoreceptor layer.

Comparison of the compound eye, "eyeless head," and cornea preparations showed that, among the "major" polypeptides seen on a 2-D gel, those labelled, a, b, c, d, i, 80 K, 49 K, and 39 K in Fig. 2a are specific for the photoreceptor layer. The specificity of these polypeptides for a particular class of specialized tissues makes it highly unlikely

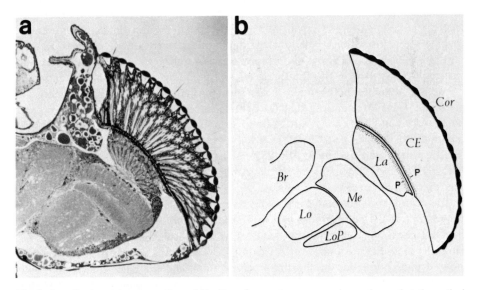

Fig. 8a,b. a Horizontal cross section of the *D. melanogaster* compound eye observed at the optical level. **b** Corresponding schematic diagram. Wild-type fly of the Oregon R strain was used. *CE* compound eye; *Cor* cornea; *La* lamina; *Me* medulla; *Lo* lobula; *LoP* lobula plate; *Br* brain; *P* pigment granules

that they are involved in such general housekeeping functions as respiration or metabolism. Rather, they are likely to have some specialized functions for the photoreceptor. Moreover, since our compound eye and photoreceptor layer preparations do not contain photoreceptor synapses, as discussed above (see also Fig. 1 and Results), it is likely that the specialized photoreceptor functions performed by these polypeptides do not include those directly related to synaptic transmission.

Fujita and Hotta (1979) first described compound eye specific polypeptides of *Drosophila* observed on a 2-D gel. Some of the compound eye specific polypeptides we found in the present work seem to correspond to those reported by Fujita and Hotta previously. Thus, our polypeptides labelled b, e, and i in Fig. 2a seem to correspond to their "ocular", "nebular", and "eyebrow", respectively (Hotta 1979). To the best our knowledge, the rest of the compound eye specific polypeptides labelled by arrows in Fig. 2a were identified for the first time in this work.

Each of the three polypeptides that undergo light-induced pI changes consists of two or more pI states that are identified by capital letters A through F in Figs. 3b and c. The probability of occupancy of these states seems to depend on the state of adaptation. Thus, in dark-adapted flies, these polypeptides are mainly in the A state, with a residual amount in the B state (Fig. 3a and c). In light-adapted flies, on the other hand, the 80 K polypeptide occupies mainly the C, D, E, and F states, the 49 K polypeptide occupies the B and C states, and the 39 K polypeptide the B state, with a small residual amount in the A state in each case (Fig. 3b and d). Occupancy of the 80 B state appears to be transient in that the amount of the 80 K polypeptide in this state first increases with light adaptation and then decreases again upon complete light adaptation.

The time course of the pI shifts determined in vivo varies considerably among these polypeptides, with the 49 K polypeptide having the fastest and the 39 K the slowest time courses (Matsumoto et al. 1982). Even the slowest pI shift, however, takes place within minutes (Matsumoto et al. 1982). These relatively fast time courses seem to exclude the contribution of de novo syntheses of proteins to these changes. Rather, posttranslational modifications of the proteins appear to be responsible for the observed changes. Consistent with this interpretation, we found light-induced incorporation of ^{32}P activity into these polypeptides in vivo when the flies are fed with labelled inorganic phosphate (Fig. 4), indicating that the light-dependent pI changes are due to protein phosphorylation. This view is strongly supported by the observation that $[\gamma\text{-}^{32}P]ATP$, but not $[\alpha\text{-}^{32}P]ATP$, donates its radioactivity to these three polypeptides in vitro (Fig. 6, lanes 7 and 8). The $[\alpha\text{-}^{32}P]ATP$ result unequivocally excludes the possibility that any non-specific binding or any covalent binding involving the α-position of ATP contributes to the pI shift.

The *norpA* mutation has been found to reduce or block the light-induced phosphorylation of the polypeptides in vivo. In the two *norpA* alleles examined, the biochemical phenotype qualitatively correlates with the electrophysiological phenotype. Thus, the allele that has a severe effect on the ERG also has a severe effect on the light-induced phosphorylation of the three polypeptides, and the allele that is mild with respect to the ERG phenotype is also mild with respect to the phosphorylation phenotype. This tendency holds true even in other *norpA* alleles examined (data not shown). The finding suggests a common causal relationship between the biochemical and electrophysiological defects.

In sharp contrast to the results in vivo, the 80 K, 49 K, and 39 K polypeptides of the $norpA^{P24}$ flies can be phosphorylated in vitro just as well as those of wild type (Fig. 6, lane 6). The result indicates that endogeneous protein kinases that can utilize these polypeptides as substrates are present even in the most severely affected mutants of $norpA$. Thus it is highly unlikely that the $norpA$ mutation directly affects protein kinases. As for the substrates, i.e. the 80 K, 49 K, and 39 K polypeptides themselves, we have observed neither any noticeable reduction in their amount nor changes in their pIs or mol. wt. in any of the $norpA$ mutants examined by means of 2-D gels. These observations suggest that the substrates are probably normal in these mutants. Thus, the block in the protein phosphorylation observed in vivo in $norpA$ mutants (Matsumoto et al. 1982) probably is due to an abnormality in the regulation mechanism of protein kinases. In many cases, protein kinases are known to exhibit rather wide substrate specificity in vitro (Weller 1979). The regulation of their substrate specificity and catalytic action in vivo may be achieved through compartmentalization of the enzyme and the substrate. Conceivably, the $norpA$ mutation might express its phenotype through abnormality in such compartmentalization and/or in light-induced changes in this compartmentalization.

One of the striking findings of this work is the extraordinary sensitivity of the 49 K phosphorylation to illumination. The threshold for the activation of the 49 K phosphorylation was found to be −6 or −7 log units in the units defined in Fig. 7. In a separate experiment, the ERG threshold was found to be approximately −6 log units. Thus, the 49 K phosphorylation begins to be activated at light intensities that barely evoke the ERG responses. Such an extreme sensitivity to light suggests that the 49 K phosphorylation reaction involves an enormous amplification process, as would be the case if it were involved in the later stages of the visual excitation process.

We have shown in this report (1) that the 80 K, 49 K, and 30 K polypeptides undergo reversible, light-induced phosphorylation, (2) that these polypeptides are localized specifically to the photoreceptor cell layer, (3) that the time courses of the light-dependent phosphorylation of these polypeptides are rather fast (Matsumoto and Pak 1984; Matsumoto et al. 1983), and (4) that the $norpA$ mutation blocks these light-dependent changes in vivo (Matsumoto et al. 1982). These findings strongly suggest that the 80 K, 49 K, and 39 K polypeptides and their light-dependent phosphorylations are likely to play an important role in photoreceptor function. Because of its very rapid time courses ($<$ 400–600 ms) and its extreme sensitivity to light, we further suggest that the 49 K polypeptide and its phosphorylation reaction are likely to be involved in photoreceptor potential generation and/or modulation.

Acknowledgements. This work was supported by grants BNS 80-15599 and BNS 83-11203 from the National Science Foundation and grant EY 00033 from the National Eye Institute of NIH. Dr. Joseph E. O'Tousa was involved in the early stage of the experiments. We thank Dr. Kunio Isono for histology and many fruitful discussions and Lydia L. Randall for reading the manuscript.

References

Banga SS, Bloomquist BT, Brodberg RK, Pye QN, Larrivee DC, Mason JM, Boyd JB, Pak WL. Cytogenetic characterization of the 4BC region on the X chromosome of *Drosophila melanogaster* (in preparation)

Braitenberg V (1967) Patterns of projection in the visual system of the fly. I. Retina-lamina projections. Exp Brain Res 3:271–298

Fujita S, Hotta Y (1979) Two-dimensional electrophoretic analysis of tissue specific proteins of *Drosophila melanogaster*. Protein, Nucl Acid Enzyme 24:1336–1343 (in Japanese)

Hall JC (1982) Genetics of the nervous system in *Drosophila*. Q Rev Biophys 15:223–479

Heisenberg M (1971) Isolation of mutants lacking the optmotor response. Dros Inf Serv 46:68

Hotta Y (1979) A biochemical analysis of visual mutations in *Drosophila melanogaster*. changes in major eye proteins. In: Ebert, Okada (eds) Mechanism of cell change. Wiley, New York, pp 169–182

Hotta Y, Benzer S (1969) Abnormal electroretinograms in visual mutants of *Drosophila*. Nature (Lond) 222:354–356

Laemmli LK (1970) Cleavage of structural proteins during the assembly of the head of bacteriophage T4. Nature (Lond) 227:680–685

Lo M-V, Pak WL (1981) Light-induced pigment granule migration in the retinular cells of *Drosophila melanogaster*. J Gen Physiol 77:155–175

Matsumoto H, O'Tousa JE, Pak WL (1982) Light-induced modification of *Drosophila* retinal polypeptides in vivo. Science (Wash DC) 217:839–841

Matsumoto H, Isono K, Pak WL (1983) Light-induced phosphorylation of *Drosophila* retinal proteins. Invest Ophthalmol Visual Sci Suppl 24:115

Matsumoto H, Pak WL (1984) Light-induced phosphorylation of retina-specific polypeptides of *Drosophila* in vivo. Science (Wash DC) 223:184–186

Miyazaki K, Hagiwara H, Yokota M, Kakuno T, Horio T (1978) Two-dimensional gel electrophoresis. In: Ui, Horio (eds) Isoelectric focusing and isotachophoresis. (in Japanese) Kyoritsu Shuppan, Tokyo, pp 183–196

O'Farrell PM (1975) High resolution two-dimensional electrophoresis of proteins. J Biol Chem 250:4007–4021

Pak WL, Grossfield J, White NV (1969) Nonphototactic mutants in a study of vision of *Drosophila*. Nature (Lond) 222:351–354

Pak WL (1975) Mutants affecting the vision of *Drosophila melanogaster*. In: King RC (ed) Handbook of genetics, vol 3. Plenum, New York, pp 703–733

Pak WL (1979) Study of photoreceptor function using *Drosophila* mutants. In: Breakefield XO (ed) Neurogenetics: genetic approaches to the nervous system. Elsevier, North Holland

Trujillo-Cenóz O, Melamed J (1966) Compound eye of dipterans: anatomical basis for integration-an electron microscope study. J Ultrastruct Res 16:395–398

Weller M (1979) Protein phosphorylation. Pion, London

Subject Index